Pathology of Bone and Joint Disorders

Pathology of Bone and Joint Disorders

with Clinical and Radiographic Correlation

Edward F. McCarthy, MD

Associate Professor of Pathology
and Orthopedic Surgery
The Johns Hopkins School of Medicine
Baltimore, Maryland

Frank J. Frassica, MD

Associate Professor of Orthopedic Surgery
and Oncology
The Johns Hopkins School of Medicine
Baltimore, Maryland

W.B. SAUNDERS COMPANY
A Division of Harcourt Brace & Company
Philadelphia   London   Toronto   Montreal   Sydney   Tokyo

W.B. SAUNDERS COMPANY
A Division of Harcourt Brace & Company

The Curtis Center
Independence Square West
Philadelphia, Pennsylvania 19106

Library of Congress Cataloging-in-Publication Data

McCarthy, Edward F.
  Pathology of bone and joint disorders with clinical and radiographic correlation / Edward F. McCarthy, Frank J. Frassica.—1st ed.
      p.   cm.
  ISBN 0-7216-6336-2
  1. Bones—Diseases.   2. Joints—Diseases.   I. Frassica, Frank J.
    II. Title.   [DNLM: 1. Bone Diseases—pathology.   2. Joint Diseases—pathology.   WE 225 M748p 1998]
  RC930.4.M43   1998
  616.7′ ′107—dc21
  DNLM/DLC   97-27845

PATHOLOGY OF BONE AND JOINT DISORDERS WITH
CLINICAL AND RADIOGRAPHIC CORRELATION   ISBN 0-7216-6336-2

Copyright © 1998 by W.B. Saunders Company.

All rights reserved. No part of this publication may be reproduced or transmitted in any form or by any means, electronic or mechanical, including photocopy, recording, or any information storage and retrieval system, without permission in writing from the publisher.

Printed in the United States of America.

Last digit is the print number: 9   8   7   6   5   4   3   2   1

To our parents
Ed and Muriel McCarthy
and
Peter and Mary Ann Frassica

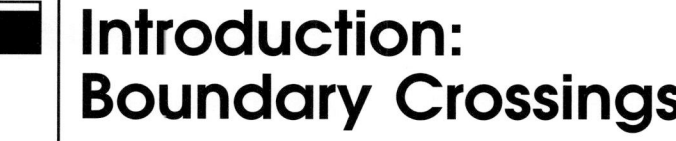

Introduction: Boundary Crossings

This book is an introduction to orthopedic pathology cowritten by a bone pathologist and an orthopedic surgeon. It is based on our day-to-day collaboration at The Johns Hopkins Hospital. Not only do we work together in clinical medicine, but we also teach together, and in composing this book, we draw from both our daily practice and our in-service course in bone pathology. We instruct residents in pathology and orthopedic surgery, and it is for these students that this book is primarily intended. In addition, however, we believe it provides practicing physicians with a useful survey of bone and joint disease. Although we keep our discussions at an introductory level, we supply appropriate references for those readers who want to inquire further. In our view, the information in this volume represents the minimum that residents in pathology and orthopedic surgery should know by the completion of their training.

Our underlying assumption throughout is that bone and joint diseases are best viewed from multiple angles. Diagnosing skeletal disorders requires the close interaction of pathologists, orthopedists, and radiologists. Therefore, we emphasize the correlation of pathologic features with clinical history and radiographic images. We believe that this multidisciplinary approach should inform students' learning from the beginning. That is, when pathologists begin to learn about bone diseases, they should at the same time learn to read radiographs. The radiographs represent the gross pathology of bone and joint disease, and they provide the context for interpreting the histologic features. Conversely, orthopedists and radiologists must learn to look at pathology slides. Seeing tissues under the microscope will help them better understand what a disease is doing to the patient.

In sum, working with bones requires physicians to cross boundaries between specialties. When pathologists cross into the realm of images and learn to converse with radiologists, they return to their own discipline with a better understanding of it. And when orthopedists speak with pathologists, they see their patients in new light. These boundary crossings may be likened to the enriched comprehension of English that results from studying French. This multidisciplinary approach is what we practice and teach, and it is what we encourage in this book.

We organize this volume into 18 chapters, and they are best read in order, from first to last. We begin in Chapter 1 with an overview of skeletal diseases and the principles of their diagnosis. In Chapter 2, we leave this general picture to begin building the foundational vocabulary needed to study bone disorders. That is, we summarize the anatomy and physiology of normal bone, subjects required to understand abnormal bone. In subsequent chapters we explore each of the major bone disease categories that we outline in Chapter 1: genetic, metabolic, traumatic, infectious, circulatory, and neoplastic. In addition to bone disease, we also discuss joint diseases and the pathology of failed total joint arthroplasty. We provide historical background in most of these chapters, detailing archeological evidence of skeletal disorders and honoring individuals whose work has led to our current knowledge. This is to remind us that, in the words of Sir Isaac Newton, "We stand on the shoulders of giants." It also helps us remember that humans have suffered from these diseases for thousands of years.

EDWARD F. MCCARTHY
FRANK J. FRASSICA

Acknowledgments

Many people have supported us during the writing of this book. Lucille McCarthy read the entire manuscript and helped us make it "reader friendly." She also supplied encouragement when the authors' spirits were low. Kelli Earnest kept track of all of the illustrations and helped with proofreading.

Pamela Godwin photographed all of the radiographs, and Norman Barker took almost all of the photomicrographs. We owe them thanks for their skill and patience. Stacy Lund and Carmela Clifford creatively translated our ideas into visually instructive art.

Special thanks go to Ursula Jacob, who, with tireless devotion, typed many versions of the manuscript and managed the more than 1200 references. Without her competence and good humor, this book could not have been written.

Contents

Color Insert follows page 98

CHAPTER 1
Diagnosing Bone Disease 1
- The Spectrum of Skeletal Disease 1
- The Multidisciplinary Approach to Diagnosis 7

CHAPTER 2
Anatomy and Physiology of Bone 25
- Anatomy of Bone 25
- Development of Bone 37
- Physiology of Bone 42

CHAPTER 3
Genetic Diseases of Bones and Joints 51
- Mendelian Inheritance 51
- Genetic Diseases Indirectly Affecting the Skeleton 52
- Genetic Diseases Directly Affecting the Skeleton—The Skeletal Dysplasias 58
- Focal Developmental Disorders 70
- Role of the Pathologist in the Skeletal Dysplasias 71

CHAPTER 4
Metabolic Bone Diseases 75
- Specific Endocrine Disorders 75
- Renal Osteodystrophy 83
- Osteoporosis 88
- Evaluating Patients Whose Bones Fracture Easily 95
- Localized Osteoporosis 96

CHAPTER 5
The Pathophysiology of Fractures 105
- Fracture Mechanics 105
- Classification of Fractures 108
- Fracture Healing 108
- The Histology of Fracture Healing 109
- Delayed Union and Nonunion 112
- Special Types of Fractures 112
- Pathologic Fractures 117

CHAPTER 6
Skeletal Manifestations of Systemic Disease 119
- Reticuloendothelial Diseases 119
- Hematologic Disorders 125
- Hypertrophic Osteoarthropathy 131

CHAPTER 7
Osteonecrosis 135
- Osteonecrosis Due to Intravascular Occlusion 135
- The Osteochondroses 145
- Radiation Osteodysplasia 148

CHAPTER 8
Infections of Bones and Joints 153
- History 153
- Hematogenous Bacterial Osteomyelitis 154
- Subacute Osteomyelitis 155
- Secondary Osteomyelitis 155
- Chronic Osteomyelitis 156
- The Pathology of Osteomyelitis 156
- Vertebral Osteomyelitis 158
- Osteomyelitis in Patients at Risk 159
- Treatment of Osteomyelitis 160
- Septic Arthritis 161
- Tuberculosis and Fungal Infection of Bone 162
- Syphilitic Bone Infection 162
- Chronic Multifocal Osteomyelitis 163

CHAPTER 9
Paget's Disease 165
- History 165
- Epidemiology 165
- Clinical Factors 166
- Etiology 166
- Histopathology 166
- Radiologic Features 167
- Laboratory Studies 158
- Complications 169
- Differential Diagnosis 171
- Treatment 172

CHAPTER 10
Metastatic Carcinoma in Bone 175
Incidence 175
Clinical Settings 175
Pathophysiology 176
Clinical Features 177
Radiographic Features 178
Pathologic Features of Metastatic Bone Tumors 180
Treatment of Metastatic Carcinoma in Bone 180

CHAPTER 11
Plasma Cell Dyscrasia 185
Monoclonal Gammopathy of Undetermined Significance 185
The Pathology of Plasma Cell Dyscrasias 185
Multiple Myeloma 186
Solitary Myeloma of Bone 190
Osteosclerotic Myeloma 190
Amyloidoma of Bone 190
Treatment of Plasma Cell Neoplasms 191

CHAPTER 12
Primary Bone Tumors 195
History 196
General Principles of Primary Bone Tumors 197
Osseous Lesions 198
Cartilage Lesions 220
Fibrous Lesions 244
Giant Cell Tumor of Bone 252
Lymphoma of Bone 256
Hodgkin's Disease of Bone 257
Ewing Sarcoma/Peripheral Neuroectodermal Tumor 258
Osteofibrous Dysplasia 261
Adamantinoma 263
Vascular Neoplasms 264
Chordoma 268
Sarcomas Arising in Irradiated Bone (Postradiation Sarcomas) 269

CHAPTER 13
Bone Cysts 277
Unicameral Bone Cyst 277
Aneurysmal Bone Cyst 279
Subchondral Cysts 284
Intraosseous Lipoma 286
Epidermal Inclusion Cyst 289

CHAPTER 14
Tumor-Like Lesions 291
Tumoral Calcinosis 291
Tumoral Calcium Pyrophosphate Deposition Disease 293
Calcifying Pseudotumor of the Neural Axis 294
Heterotopic Bone 294
Heterotopic Bone in the Hands and Feet 299
Infantile Cortical Hyperostosis 302
Giant Cell Reparative Granuloma 303
Hemophilic Pseudotumor 305

CHAPTER 15
Diseases of Synovial Membrane 307
Synovial Chondromatosis 307
Pigmented Villonodular Synovitis 310
Synovial Hemangioma 312
Synovial Lipomatosis 313

CHAPTER 16
Diseases of Joints 317
History 317
The Normal Joint 319
Osteoarthritis 324
Special Forms of Osteoarthritis 332
Inflammatory Arthritis 336
Rheumatoid Arthritis 337
Juvenile Rheumatoid Arthritis 342
Ankylosing Spondylitis 343
Reactive Arthritis 344
Psoriatic Arthritis 346
Arthritis of Systemic Lupus Erythematosus 346
Gout 346
Calcium Pyrophosphate Deposition Disease 348

CHAPTER 17
The Pathology of Failed Total Joint Arthroplasty 353
History 354
Features of Asymptomatic Well-Functioning Prostheses 355
Aseptic Loosening 356
The Biological Response to Total Joint Prostheses 359
Granulomatous Pseudotumors 359
Septic Loosening 360
Malignant Neoplasms Arising in Association with Total Joint Prostheses 362
The Role of the Pathologist in Total Joint Failure 362

CHAPTER 18
Management of Orthopedic Pathology Specimens from the Operating Room to Microscope 365
The Conference 365
The Biopsy 365
Handling Orthopedic Specimens 366
Processing Bone Specimens 370

Index 373

NOTICE

Pathology of bone and joint disorders is an ever-changing field. Standard safety precautions must be followed, but as new research and clinical experience broaden our knowledge, changes in treatment and drug therapy become necessary or appropriate. Readers are advised to check the product information currently provided by the manufacturer of each drug to be administered to verify the recommended dose, the method and duration of administration, and contraindications. It is the responsibility of the treating physician relying on experience and knowledge of the patient to determine dosages and the best treatment for the patient. Neither the Publisher nor the editor assumes any responsibility for any injury and/or damage to persons or property.

THE PUBLISHER

CHAPTER 1 — Diagnosing Bone Disease

THE SPECTRUM OF SKELETAL DISEASE

Looking at bones in a museum or a gross anatomy teaching box may leave the impression that they are inert, rocklike substances. However, this is not true. Bones are alive and dynamic just like other tissues. They atrophy if they are not used; they become infected; they die if deprived of blood; they develop neoplasms; they respond to systemic changes; and they heal themselves.

Considering these dynamic reactions, bone diseases should be conceptualized like diseases of other body systems. Therefore, an initial approach to diagnosing a skeletal disorder is to place the lesion in one of seven major disease categories. These categories, which are common to all diseases, are congenital, metabolic, traumatic, circulatory, neoplastic, infectious, and changes due to systemic disease (Table 1–1). In some cases, choosing the correct category is the first step toward making the correct diagnosis. In other cases, the disease category is known only after the correct diagnosis has been made. Because understanding these categories is essential to diagnosing bone disease, we begin with a brief summary. Detailed discussions of these categories are presented in subsequent chapters.

Table 1–1 ■ **THE SEVEN MAJOR BONE DISEASE CATEGORIES**

Category	Examples
Congenital	Achondroplasia, osteogenesis imperfecta
Metabolic	Rickets, osteoporosis
Traumatic	Fracture, avulsion injuries, myositis ossificans
Circulatory	Osteonecrosis
Neoplastic	Metastatic carcinoma, osteosarcoma
Infectious	Osteomyelitis
Bone changes in systemic disease	Hypertrophic pulmonary osteoarthropathy

Congenital Diseases

The first category of bone disease, disease due to gene mutations, usually manifests in childhood. These congenital diseases affect the skeleton either directly or indirectly. A direct effect on the skeleton is caused by mutations in any of the huge number of genes that control the growth and development of bone or cartilage. These disorders are called the *skeletal dysplasias,* and at least 140 have been defined.[1] In addition to gene mutations that affect the skeleton directly, mutations in genes that regulate other tissues, such as the reticuloendothelial system, affect bones indirectly. All told, gene mutations that directly or indirectly affect the skeleton result in at least 500 diseases. Despite this large number of disease entities, congenital bone diseases are uncommon in general clinical practice.

Skeletal Dysplasias (Gene Mutations Directly Affecting the Skeleton)

The skeletal dysplasias manifest in three principal ways: short stature, abnormally shaped bones, and skeletal fragility. For the diagnostician, an important feature of these manifestations is their symmetry in the skeleton. An asymmetric disorder is unlikely to be a skeletal dysplasia.

Recognizing the abnormal size and shape of bones (and whether the changes are symmetric) is best done with plain radiographs. In fact, the nomenclature of the skeletal dysplasias, although always in a continuous state of flux, is based almost exclusively on radiographic features—which bones and bone segments are involved. Therefore, radiologists usually diagnose and classify skeletal dysplasias. Moreover, because most of these diseases are rare and the manifestations so numerous, a difficult diagnosis requires a radiologist with a special expertise in congenital bone diseases.

Whereas the skeletal dysplasias can be distinguished by plain radiographic features, their pathologic features are nonspecific. All of these diseases appear very similar under the microscope. For example, a pathologist cannot distinguish, at least with routine light microscopy, an abnormal growth plate of a patient with achondroplasia from one with pseudoachondroplasia. Moreover, in some cases, the bone or cartilage from a patient with skeletal dysplasia is histologically normal. Therefore, the diagnosis of skeletal dysplasias is not the province of the pathologist. The pathologist, however, must be familiar with these diseases to ensure that tissue is available for special studies, including electron microscopy, tissue culture, or genetic investigations.

Although skeletal dysplasias are currently classified by radiologic features, future classification systems may be based on genetic information. Advances in molecular genetics have led to the identification of many of the mutations that cause these diseases. Every year, at least one skeletal dysplasia is elucidated by identifying its causative mutation. The first genetic bone disease to be so characterized was osteogenesis imperfecta. This disease, the most common of all the skeletal dysplasias, results in brittle bones. In 1975, a mutation in one of the two genes encoding type 1 collagen was discovered to be its cause.[2] More recently, it was discovered that achondroplasia, another common skeletal dysplasia, is caused by a mutation in the gene encoding the receptor for fibroblast growth factor.[3] Identifying causative gene mutations not only results in clarifying specific diseases, it also increases the understanding of normal skeletal growth and development.

Skeletal dysplasias exhibit a wide range of clinical severity. Severe dysplasias are evident at birth or even in utero. Some of these, such as thanatophoric dysplasia, are incompatible with life. Infants die at birth from respiratory failure due to chest cage deformity. Less severe dysplasias, such as pseudoachondroplasia, become manifest in childhood. Even milder dysplasias, such as the mild variant of multiple epiphyseal dysplasia, become evident only in early adulthood with the onset of early osteoarthritis. Finally, a skeletal dysplasia, such as osteopoikilosis, may be asymptomatic throughout a patient's life.

Clinical severity also differs among patients with the same dysplasia. Recent molecular genetic discoveries suggest that in some dysplasias, the varying degrees of severity are due to different point mutations in the same gene. For example, over 150 different mutations in the two genes encoding type 1 collagen have been discovered.[4] These different mutations account for the wide range of clinical presentations of osteogenesis imperfecta.

Since the skeletal dysplasias usually affect only bones and cartilage, patients have normal intelligence and a near normal life span. Most patients with these disorders lead productive lives. However, their abnormally shaped bones often lead to physical disability; some are severely disabled. Many require orthopedic surgery to correct deformities, stabilize frequent fractures, or treat early osteoarthritis. In addition to orthopedic problems, patients with skeletal dysplasias must contend with the emotional burden of their deformities. They usually help each other with these problems. For example, Little People of America is a mutual support group with almost 10,000 members.

Gene Mutations Indirectly Affecting the Skeleton

In addition to the skeletal dysplasias, genetic diseases targeting other tissues can secondarily affect the skeleton. For example, neurofibromatosis 1, the most common single-gene disorder of humans, primarily causes neural tumors and café au lait spots. It can also affect bones in a variety of ways. Patients may develop scoliosis, pseudarthrosis, and bone erosions. Other genetic diseases, such as those involving the reticuloendothelial system, also affect the skeleton. In Gaucher disease, for example, abnormal cells accumulate in the bone marrow and cause osseous lesions.

Metabolic Bone Disease

Whereas congenital bone disease results from gene mutations, metabolic bone disease results from alterations in the chemical environment of the body. This chemical environment consists of hormones, vitamins, minerals, and other systemic factors—all interacting in complicated ways with physical activity. Disturbances in this environment adversely affect the two components of bone, calcium and the organic matrix, causing osteopenia, a generalized decrease in skeletal mass. Thus, the characteristic feature of metabolic bone disease is weak bones. When osteopenia is severe enough to result in clinical symptoms, such as fractures or bone pain, it is called osteoporosis. Therefore, when patients present with fractures associated with little or no trauma, physicians should be alert to the likelihood of metabolic bone disease.

Osteopenia Associated with Endocrine Disorders

Metabolic bone diseases may be grouped into three categories: problems due to endocrine disorders, osteopenia associated with aging, and disuse osteoporosis. First, of the many endocrine disorders that adversely affect the skeleton, the most damaging are those that disturb calcium homeostasis. Calcium homeostasis is critical for two reasons. First, calcium participates in many of the body's physiologic reactions, and therefore its serum level must be precisely regulated. Second, calcium must be available to mineralize bone.

Calcium homeostasis depends on several factors. First calcium intake must be adequate. Second, vitamin D, which gets calcium into the system, must also be present. Third, parathyroid function must be normal because parathyroid hormone regulates the serum calcium level. Finally, the interaction of these factors requires healthy kidneys. Because of the complexity of calcium homeostasis, disorders of any aspect of this system lead to metabolic bone disease. These disorders include rickets and osteomalacia, hyperparathyroidism, and renal disease. Generally, these endocrine disorders are characterized by specific histopathologic changes and can be diagnosed by looking at bone biopsies.

Osteopenia Associated with Aging

Osteopenia associated with aging is the second major category of metabolic bone disease. Unlike the osteopenia of endocrine disease in which calcium homeostasis is abnormal, in this category, calcium homeostasis appears normal. The osteopenia of aging is due to a reduction in the organic matrix. Also, unlike disorders of calcium homeostasis, no specific histopathologic features characterize osteopenia of aging. The bone is normal; there is just too little of it.

Osteopenia of aging is caused by imbalanced bone remodeling. From birth to death, the human skeleton is remodeling; old bone is gradually removed by osteoclasts, and new bone is added by osteoblasts, a process known as bone turnover. Theoretically, the remodeling process is necessary to remove bits of damaged bone. In the normal adult skeleton, the remodeling process is balanced: The amount of bone replaced equals the amount removed. However, in osteopenia of aging, the amount of bone replaced is less than the amount removed, an imbalance known as uncoupling. After multiple remodeling cycles over many years, the accumulated effect of uncoupling results in osteopenia.

Two overlapping syndromes of age-related osteopenia have been described: senile osteoporosis and postmenopausal osteoporosis.[5] Senile osteoporosis is a natural result of aging. After a person reaches peak skeletal mass, usually in the mid-20s, bone mass begins to decline gradually. This age-related bone loss occurs in both men and women of all ethnic groups and cultures. In this syndrome, the bone turnover rate is normal, but uncoupling, probably due to decreased osteoblast longevity, gradually reduces bone mass.

Postmenopausal osteoporosis, by contrast, is a syndrome of rapid bone loss. Beginning at the menopause and lasting only a few years, some women suffer a rapid bone loss that is engrafted on the normal age-related bone loss. These women are acutely sensitive to estrogen withdrawal. As a result, their bone turnover rate increases. This increased turnover rate leads to a rapid bone loss because of age-related remodeling imbalance.

These two syndromes of age-related bone loss are very common. In fact, osteoporosis is one of the most important public health problems in developed countries. Thirty percent of postmenopausal women have clinical osteoporosis.[6] Men also suffer from this disease. These women and men have suffered, or are at risk to suffer, vertebral fractures, hip fractures, and distal radius fractures. Osteoporosis accounts for 300,000 hip fractures in the United States each year. The annual cost to treat these fractures exceeds seven billion dollars.[7]

Although orthopedic surgeons treat the fractures that complicate osteoporosis, endocrinologists usually diagnose and treat the metabolic bone disease itself. Because up to 30% of bone may be lost before plain radiographic changes are evident, early osteoporosis is often difficult to diagnose.[8] Therefore, the most important diagnostic tool used by endocrinologists is the dual x-ray absorptiometry (DEXA) scan. This diagnostic modality compares a person's bone mass with that of a control group. In addition, a wide variety of laboratory tests are also available to diagnose metabolic bone disease. These include measurements of serum hormones, vitamin D levels, and indices of bone turnover. Although prevention is crucial in managing osteoporosis, a wide variety of drugs are available to prevent further bone loss and, with lesser success, to restore bone that has been lost.

Disuse Osteoporosis

The final major category of metabolic bone disease includes the osteoporotic syndromes that result from disuse. Bones need to be stressed and strained to stay healthy. Although the relationship between bone use and maintenance of bone mass is not fully understood, electrical activity in bone probably plays a vital role. Bone is minimally deformed each time it is stressed, and the deformation results in the generation of piezoelectricity and electric streaming potentials. These tiny electric currents somehow maintain balanced bone turnover. Failure to generate these currents results in increased osteoclastic resorption. For example, prolonged bed rest or long-term weightlessness results in significant generalized osteoporosis. Syndromes of focal osteoporosis also occur. For example, prolonged non–weight bearing of one leg results in bone loss in that leg.

Traumatic Bone Disease

The third category of bone disease includes those disorders caused by trauma. These disorders are discussed in detail in Chapter 5. Healthy bones can withstand stress and strain well beyond that required in daily use. However, once forces exceed this safety range, bones break. Fractures are by far the most common bone disease; however, bones have a remarkable healing ability. In fact, bone is one of the few tissues in which the healing process is so complete and the original structure so well restored that evidence of injury is obliterated. Whereas other tissues, such as liver, brain, and kidney, heal with a fibrous scar, bone heals with bone. Moreover, the bone's architecture is restored by a process of remodeling after the healing tissue, known as fracture callus, completely ossifies. Stress and strain stimulate osteoclasts and osteoblasts to sculpt the bone back to its original shape. Depending on the bone involved, a fracture takes a few weeks to a few months for the bone ends to unite, but it takes a few years for bone to remodel to its original shape.

The impetus for healing is so strong that even fractures through abnormal bone heal normally. This even includes severely osteoporotic bone. Furthermore, fracture healing is seldom adversely affected by diseases of other organ systems. Only diabetes and cigarette smoking are associated with poor fracture callus formation.

However, complications occasionally occur at fracture sites. For example, a fracture may disrupt the blood supply to a portion of bone, resulting in focal osteonecrosis. The dead bone cannot heal to the viable bone. A second complication is a nonunion. This complication, which occurs most commonly in tibial fractures, is a failure of the fracture callus to ossify. A fibrous, rather than a bony, bridge occurs between the fractured bone ends. As a result, motion occurs at the fracture site, a condition known as a pseudarthrosis. Why does the fracture callus fail to ossify? One cause is extensive stripping of the osteogenic periosteum, a problem that occurs in particularly violent injuries or from vigorous surgical manipulation. Nonunion also results if a portion of muscle or fibrous tissue becomes trapped in the fracture site. Nonunions can be successfully treated. Surgery is required to start the fracture over again by removing the fibrous bridge. Often, internal stabilization and bone grafting are required.

Although abnormal bones heal like normal ones, they break more easily. Whereas significant trauma is required to break normal bone, abnormal bone fractures with little trauma. Fractures through bones with either focal or generalized diseases are known as pathologic fractures. For example, an aggressive lytic bone tumor greatly weakens a bone, and pathologic fractures occur. Although both primary and metastatic bone tumors cause pathologic fractures, this complication is more common in metastatic carcinoma to bone. In fact, treating or preventing pathologic fractures is one of the most important aspects of managing patients with terminal cancer. In addition to focal bone lesions, generalized bone disease also predisposes to fractures. Thus, fractures through severely osteoporotic bones are pathologic fractures. In these patients, the pathologic fracture is often the presenting symptom of the generalized disease.

Although fractures are the most common and easily recognized form of traumatic bone disease, two special types of bone injury present diagnostic problems: stress fractures and avulsion injuries. A stress fracture is the reaction of bone to repetitive trauma. Although none of the individual traumas are sufficient to produce injury, the cumulative effect eventually weakens the bone. The repetitive stress stimulates a zone of increased bone remodeling, and a discrete line of rarefaction—the stress fracture—occurs. Typically, a patient who develops a stress fracture has taken up a new activity, such as jogging, and particular activities are associated with stress fractures in specific bones. For example, military recruits, unaccustomed to long marches, develop metatarsal stress fractures. Because stress fractures are painful and cause subtle radiographic changes, they are occasionally mistaken for neoplasms or other bone diseases. Awareness of the varied presentations of stress fractures is the key to their diagnosis.

Avulsion injuries, another manifestation of trauma, may also be mistaken for neoplasms. These injuries, most common in children, result from repetitive muscular activity that pulls off a portion of periosteum from the bone surface. Occasionally, a portion of underlying bone is also avulsed, and it is the resulting periosteal bone reaction and adjacent intraosseous or soft tissue edema that mimics a neoplasm. This problem most frequently occurs on the medial femoral condyle. However, avulsion injuries can occur anywhere a tendon is attached to bone.

Circulatory Diseases

The fourth category of bone disease that we summarize here includes disorders resulting from disturbances in blood circulation. We discuss these in detail in Chapter 7. Bone is a richly vascular tissue; it receives 10 to 20% of the cardiac output. The blood supply to bone comes from many sources: large nutrient arteries that penetrate the diaphysis, smaller arteries that enter the epiphysis and metaphysis, and many small arterioles that penetrate the cortex from the periosteum. Focal bone death, the most common circulatory disease, results from disruption of blood flow of any of these vessels. Histologic changes that follow bone death are known as osteonecrosis.

Bone dies when blood flow is disrupted. This happens in one of three clinical settings: fracture, infection, or intravascular occlusion. The first setting, fracture, causes bone death by rupture or compression of an artery. Such injuries occur if the fracture is severely displaced or if an associated joint dislocation has occurred. For example, osteonecrosis of the femoral head may occur after a displaced femoral neck fracture. Other bones particularly susceptible to fracture-related osteonecrosis are the talus and the carpal navicular.

The second setting in which bone death may occur is infection. Spreading inflammatory tissue isolates a segment of bone by surrounding it with a purulent exudate and isolating it from its blood supply. The dead bone fragment, known as a sequestrum, harbors causative microorganisms and protects them against the body's defenses and antibiotics. The sequestra must be removed to allow the infection to heal.

The third setting of osteonecrosis is a variety of clinical conditions that predispose to intravascular occlusion. Vascular occlusion is followed by infarction of the bone supplied by that vessel. However, unlike other organs, such as the brain or the heart, in which infarction is caused by atherosclerosis, bone infarction is usually caused by intravascular coagulation. This process occurs most frequently at either end of the femur and results in distinct clinical syndromes. The most common syndrome is osteonecrosis of the femoral head. From 10,000 to 20,000 new cases of osteonecrosis of the femoral head occur in the United States each year.[9] Usually, men between the ages of 20 and 40 years are affected. The clinical symptoms of this disease are due to the nearness of the osteonecrotic segment to the articular surface. Dead bone is brittle, and weight bearing causes microfractures through the brittle trabeculae. As a result, the articular surface eventually collapses and secondary osteoarthritis develops in the joint. Affected patients usually have at least one of multiple risk factors. Risk factors include alcohol abuse, steroid therapy, and hypercoagulable blood.

Bone Infection

Infection in bone is the next category of bone disease. Bone, like any other tissue, can become infected, a condition known as osteomyelitis. In fact, organisms grow readily in bone. However, osteomyelitis is difficult to diagnose. Although most patients with osteomyelitis present with systemic signs of infection, the clinical and radiographic patterns vary considerably. Because of these various presentations, osteomyelitis is known as the "great imitator." It must always be considered as a diagnostic possibility in any medullary bone lesion, particularly in children.

Osteomyelitis occurs by two mechanisms—direct inoculation of organisms into bone and the hematogenous spread of organisms to bone from an infection elsewhere in the body. Infection from direct inoculation, known as secondary osteomyelitis, occurs most commonly after an open fracture. Before antibiotics, bone infection almost always complicated an open fracture. Today, only 5% of open fractures become infected.

Hematogenous osteomyelitis, known as primary osteomyelitis, is usually a pediatric disease.[10] Children present acutely with symptoms of infection: fever, pain, and leukocytosis. Radiographs reveal bone destruction and a periosteal reaction, usually in the metaphysis of a long bone. The cause of these bone changes is the proliferation of granulation tissue with varying amounts of an acute purulent exudate. *Staphylococcus aureus* is the usual causative organism. Adults may on occasion develop acute osteomyelitis. In adults, the spine is the most common site. Usually, they have had prior genitourinary tract manipulation or they are immunocompromised.

Acute osteomyelitis must be diagnosed and treated decisively. Otherwise, organisms gain a foothold, in part facilitated by the bone's reactive response, which tends to protect the organisms. Incomplete eradication of acute osteomyelitis, a problem that occurs in 5% of cases, leads to chronic osteomyelitis. Unfortunately, chronic osteomyelitis is extremely difficult, and sometimes impossible, to cure. Chronic osteomyelitis is characterized by the long-term interaction, usually for decades, of the bone and the infecting organism. Periodic flare-ups occur, and radiographs show ill-defined areas of radiolucency mixed with areas of increased density. The radiodense areas are the bone's reactions to the infection. In addition, radiodense sequestra (dead bone fragments) appear in the lucent areas. Extensive surgical débridement and antibiotic therapy are required to treat chronic osteomyelitis.

Although most bone infections are caused by bacteria, any type of microorganism can cause osteomyelitis. For example, fungal and mycobacterial organisms can infect bone, particularly in immunocompromised patients. In addition, viruses and parasites, such as the echinococcal worm, cause unusual presentations. Therefore, the orthopedist must culture a suspected osteomyelitic lesion for all organisms.

Neoplastic Bone Disease

Bone neoplasms are generally divided into two major categories—those that arise in bones, known as primary bone tumors, and those that have metastasized to bone from neoplasms elsewhere. Primary bone tumors may be benign or malignant. Metastatic bone tumors are always malignant, and they indicate an advanced stage of cancer.

Metastatic lesions in bone are extremely common because of the high incidence of cancer in developed countries (it is the second leading cause of death) and the natural history of the disease. Most people dying of cancer have bone metastases. Therefore, any patient with a bone lesion who is older than 40 years should be presumed to have metastatic cancer until proven otherwise. Although any malignant tumor can spread to bone, carcinomas of the lung, breast, and prostate account for 80% of bone metastases.

Unlike the distinctive radiographic features of most other bone lesions, metastatic carcinoma in bone has a wide range of radiographic patterns. This variability occasionally makes diagnosis difficult. Lesions may be radiodense (blastic metastases) or radiolucent (lytic metastases). Lesions may be well defined or poorly defined, and they may be centered in the medullary canal or on the bone surface. Despite their variable radiographic presentations, however, metastatic carcinomas occur in predictable locations. They usually develop in the axial skeleton and are most common in the spine. Other sites frequently involved are the pelvis, proximal femurs, and proximal humeri. Metastatic carcinoma is rare in the distal extremities. Although metastatic carcinoma may present in one site, most patients develop multiple lesions.

Two clinical settings characterize metastatic carcinoma to bone. First, some patients with a bone lesion have no history of a primary carcinoma. In these patients, the diagnosis of metastasis requires a search for the primary site. Unfortunately, the site of the primary cannot always be discerned from the histopathologic features of the metastasis. Therefore, finding the primary is a clinical and radiographic problem. Sometimes it is never found.

The second and more common presentation of bone metastases occurs in patients with a known primary. In these patients, the diagnosis of metastasis establishes the advanced stage of the disease. Orthopedists must direct their attention to the prevention or treatment of pathologic fractures, a common complication of metastatic lesions in bone. These procedures are moderately successful in relieving pain and restoring function for the remainder of the patient's life, usually not more than 2 years.

After metastatic carcinoma in bone, multiple myeloma is the most common bone neoplasm. Approximately 13,800 new cases develop per year in the United States. Multiple myeloma is a neoplastic proliferation of plasma cells that almost always presents with bone lesions. Although plasma cells are not native to the bone marrow, multiple myeloma is considered a primary bone neoplasm because most of the neoplastic cells are in the bone marrow. However, other organs are also affected.

Multiple myeloma affects older adults; usually patients are older than 50. Unlike many other neoplastic proliferations, multiple myeloma has a very insidious onset. In the early stages, bone lesions, almost always multiple, are difficult to see with plain radiographs. In fact, diffuse osteopenia may be the only radiographic feature. As the disease progresses, punched-out osseous lesions begin to appear. Patients develop pain and, occasionally, pathologic fractures.

In almost all cases of multiple myeloma (98%), the neoplastic plasma cells retain their function—they synthesize and secrete immunoglobulins. However, because the neoplastic plasma cells originate from a single cell, the immunoglobulins are monoclonal. These monoclonal immunoglobulins can be recognized in a serum protein electrophoresis. In addition to monoclonal serum immunoglobulins, monoclonal light chains are excreted in the urine. Recognition of these serum and urine protein abnormalities aids in the diagnosis of multiple myeloma. Therefore, serum proteins should be studied in any elderly patient with an undiagnosed lytic bone lesion.

Although multiple myeloma is usually a disseminated bone disease, a solitary lesion is present in 5 to 10% of cases. This manifestation of myeloma, known as solitary myeloma, occurs in slightly younger patients. In addition, serum protein abnormalities are less common (50 to 75% of cases). About half the patients with solitary plasmacytoma eventually develop disseminated disease.

Unlike metastatic bone tumors, which originate in organs other than bone, primary tumors begin in bone. Several important features characterize primary bone tumors. First, primary bone tumors exhibit a wide spectrum of tissue differentiation. There are about 20 different types, and many types have well-defined variants. Generally, these lesions are grouped according to the major pattern of tissue differentiation. Thus, there are cartilage lesions, fibrous lesions, and bone-forming lesions, with benign and malignant versions of each. In addition to these major categories of differentiation, some tumors, such as giant cell tumor and Ewing sarcoma, are of uncertain differentiation. These lesions are regarded as specific entities.

The second important characteristic of primary bone tumors is the age of affected patients. Unlike metastatic tumors or myeloma, which are diseases of older people, primary bone tumors most often occur in adolescents and young adults. The probable cause of this age predilection is the susceptibility of growing or modeling bone to neoplastic transformation. Those bone areas that are most active are most vulnerable. Thus, the distal femur and proximal tibia are the most common locations for primary bone tumors.

The third characteristic of primary bone tumors is that they each have specific radiographic presentations. In general, each type of lesion favors a certain zone of a bone, and each type has very distinctive radiographic features. In many instances, the diagnosis can be made by radiographic features alone. In addition, some of the specific variants of lesions are defined solely by radiographic features. Therefore, when a biopsy is required, awareness of the radiographic features is critical to making the correct diagnosis. Thus, primary bone tumors may be regarded as radiographic-pathologic entities.

The final general characteristic of primary bone tumors is their wide variety of clinical behavior. Some lesions are benign and grow slowly. In fact, some tumors are not neoplasms at all. For example, enchondromas and osteochondromas are developmental lesions (hamartomas) that cease growing after full skeletal maturation. Other bone tumors are difficult to classify as benign or malignant. For example, giant cell tumor is very aggressive locally but only rarely metastasizes. If it does, the metastases are slow growing and are therefore regarded as "benign metastasis." Finally, some primary bone tumors, such as Ewing sarcoma, are highly malignant. Patients with these neoplasms, despite recent therapeutic advances, have a poor prognosis.

Bone Changes in Systemic Disease

The final category of bone disorders includes various skeletal manifestations of systemic disease. Although bone changes in these diseases are usually diffuse and symmetric, focal lesions occasionally occur. Bone change in systemic disease manifests in two manners. In some cases, bone changes are the initial presentation of an underlying systemic disease. In other cases, the systemic disease is long standing and the bone changes are noted incidentally.

The most common systemic conditions that affect bone are diseases of the kidney and the hematologic or reticuloendothelial system. Chronic renal failure is always complicated by widespread bone changes. These changes, known as renal osteodystrophy, are particularly exaggerated in patients on renal dialysis. The changes of renal osteodystrophy may become so severe that the nephrologist must pay constant attention to minimizing this disease when caring for patients with renal failure. Bone changes in renal disease are caused by the impairment of the kidney's ability to regulate calcium and phosphorus metabolism. Therefore, renal osteodystrophy may be regarded as a metabolic bone disease.

Hematologic disorders also produce bone changes, but they are usually diagnosed incidentally during long-term patient care. These changes are usually due to expansion of the marrow. For example, leukemic infiltration of the marrow causes widespread lytic lesions. Similarly, anemias characterized by marrow hyperplasia, such as iron deficiency anemia and thalassemia, also expand the bone marrow space and produce widespread symmetric lytic changes. Some hematologic disorders, however, such as myeloproliferative disease and systemic mastocytosis, produce bone sclerosis.

Unlike the diffuse, symmetric bone changes of hematologic disorders, proliferative disorders of the reticuloendothelial system tend to produce multifocal and asymmetric lesions. Bone lesions occur in these disorders because cells of the reticuloendothelium system, mainly macrophages and histiocytes, reside in the bone marrow. Proliferative disorders of histiocytes include sarcoidosis, Langerhans' histiocytosis, and sinus histiocytosis with massive lymphadenopathy. In contrast to the anemias, bone changes in reticuloendothelial disease are often the presenting problem.

Diseases of other organ systems also involve bone. For

example, neuropathic arthropathy occurs in many patients with neurologic disorders, particularly those with diabetic neuropathy. Chronic pulmonary disease also affects bones. Patients with long-standing lung disease develop extensive deposits of periosteal new bone, a condition called pulmonary hypertrophic osteoarthropathy. In this disorder, chronic hypoxia results in subperiosteal vascular proliferation and new bone formation. Clubbing of the fingers, also a feature of chronic lung disease, is probably caused by the same mechanism.

THE MULTIDISCIPLINARY APPROACH TO DIAGNOSIS

The diagnosis and management of bone disease depends on the close teamwork of the clinician, the radiologist, and the pathologist. This team must consider a bone lesion's clinical presentation, radiographic image, and histomorphology to determine the lesion's behavior and plan effective treatment. Before making a specific diagnosis, the team must answer the following questions about the lesion's behavior: "What is it doing to the patient?" Specifically, "Is the lesion growing?" If so, "How fast?" By answering these questions, a more important one can be asked: "What is the lesion going to do to the patient in the future"? Pondering these questions before making a specific diagnosis allows the team to get a feel for the lesion. After sensing the lesion's behavior, a specific diagnosis is more likely to be correct.

Three principal sources of information are crucial to the process of judging a lesion's behavior: its clinical presentation, laboratory studies, and the practice of radiographic-histologic correlation. In addition, ancillary radiographic and histologic techniques permit more specific diagnoses.

The Clinical Presentation

The clinical presentation of a bone lesion offers numerous clues to its behavior and helps place it in one of the disease categories we have just summarized. Important considerations are age of the patient, location of the lesion, pain, swelling and deformity, the presence of other disease, and systemic symptoms.

Age and Location

Although any lesion can occur at just about any age, most bone lesions are more prevalent in certain age groups. For example, eosinophilic granuloma usually occurs in children and should always be included in the differential diagnosis of lytic lesions in this age group. By contrast, a lytic lesion in an older adult is a metastatic carcinoma or plasmacytoma until proven otherwise.

Location is also a diagnostic clue. Many lesions, particularly neoplasms, occur almost exclusively in certain zones of a bone. For example, nonossifying fibroma occurs only in the metaphysis of long bones. Therefore, this diagnosis should never be rendered for a benign fibrous lesion in other locations, such as the skull or spine. Another lesion, giant cell tumor, almost always involves the epiphysis. Therefore, giant cell–containing lesions in other locations are unlikely to be giant cell tumors. Lesions also favor particular bones. For example, unicameral bone cysts occur most frequently in the proximal humerus, and osteoblastomas favor the spine. Thus, knowing the sites of predilection of the various bone diseases is crucial to accurate diagnosis.

When multiple lesions are present, their distribution is extremely important. Symmetrically distributed lesions, such as the sclerotic foci of osteopoikilosis, usually indicate a systemic or congenital disease, whereas asymmetrically distributed lesions, such as the sclerotic foci of metastatic prostatic carcinoma, often indicate a neoplasm.

Pain

Pain usually indicates that a lesion is growing. Conversely, nongrowing lesions are almost always painless. The pain from growing lesions results from the stimulation of small, unmyelinated nerves in haversian canals or from expansion of the periosteum. Bone pain is a dull aching pain, similar to a toothache, and is characteristically worse at night. The duration of bone pain is a clue to how long a lesion has been growing.

Although growing bone lesions are painful, the clinician must decide if the patient's pain is being caused by the lesion or by something else. Often, a painful joint calls attention to a nearby, unrelated bone lesion. For example, a magnetic resonance imaging (MRI) examination to study degenerative changes in the knee or shoulder occasionally reveals a nearby cartilage lesion. Usually, the lesion is a nongrowing enchondroma that, in the absence of joint pain, would go unnoticed. Two features help distinguish joint pain from bone pain. First, unlike bone pain, joint pain eases at night or with immobilization of the joint. Second, joint pain disappears with an intraarticular injection of an analgesic. If pain persists after these procedures, it is most likely caused by the bone lesion.

On rare occasions, nongrowing lesions are painful, particularly when they occur in weight-bearing bones. In these situations, pain is almost always caused by stress fractures through the lesion. For example, enchondromas and healing nonossifying fibromas, although nongrowing, weaken the bone. As a result, increased activity causes painful intralesional stress fractures and simulates a growing process. In these situations, an MRI often contributes to overdiagnosis. This is because a soft tissue signal increase due to hemorrhage or edema from the stress fracture may be mistaken for neoplastic tissue. In this setting, the clue to the presence of a stress fracture is the disappearance of pain with non–weight bearing. An orthopedist who is aware of this complication of nongrowing lesions is less likely to do unnecessary surgery.

Swelling and Deformity

Swelling and deformity are also clues to the nature of a bone lesion. Swelling is usually caused by the expansion of a surface lesion, such as a parosteal osteosarcoma or an osteochondroma. The duration and rate of swelling usually reflect the speed of the lesion's growth. However, bursae often form over surface lesions, particularly osteochondromas. Inflammation in these bursae increases their size, a change that may be interpreted as rapid growth of the underlying lesion. Therefore, the orthopedist should compare the amount of clinical swelling with the radiographs to avoid misinterpretation.

Deformity produced by bone lesions is best evaluated by radiographs. However, certain skeletal alterations may be appreciated clinically. One alteration is limb length discrepancy. In children, lesions near the epiphyseal plate may either stimulate or retard bone growth. The amount of discrepancy often indicates the duration of the lesion.

Other Diseases and Systemic Signs

Another question in the evaluation of a bone lesion is whether it is a manifestation of disease in another organ system. Because the skeleton is sensitive to many systemic factors, a careful history must be taken. Renal, endocrine, hematologic, and pulmonary disease all may influence the skeleton. The presence of disease in any one of these systems may immediately explain the bone lesion.

Systemic signs are also an important clue to the behavior of a bone lesion. The most important systemic signs are those caused by infection. The presence or history of fever suggests that a bone lesion may be osteomyelitis. High fevers are caused by acute osteomyelitis; low-grade or intermittent fevers characterize chronic osteomyelitis. Also, a history of a remote febrile illness may be a clue to subacute osteomyelitis. In the presence of fever, a leukocytosis or an elevated erythrocyte sedimentation rate increases the suspicion of bone infection.

Although fever usually indicates osteomyelitis, other bone lesions, on rare occasions, also cause fever. For example, rapidly growing neoplasms, such as Ewing sarcoma, may produce fever and leukocytosis, because rapid growth results in extensive tumor necrosis and the release of pyrogens into the circulation. Therefore, because Ewing sarcoma and acute osteomyelitis also have overlapping radiographic features, these two lesions may be difficult to distinguish clinically and radiographically. Sometimes even a biopsy does not solve this diagnostic dilemma. A tissue sample from a necrotic portion of a Ewing sarcoma may be histologically mistaken for infection. Awareness of the potential hazards in distinguishing Ewing sarcoma and acute osteomyelitis is important in making the correct diagnosis.

Laboratory Studies

In addition to evaluating the white blood cell count and erythrocyte sedimentation to rule out infection, other laboratory studies are important in the diagnosis of a bone disease. For example, a complete blood count is necessary to evaluate the health of the bone marrow. Diffuse infiltrative disorders and the osteosclerotic bone dysplasias may present with anemia. Another important laboratory study is the serum protein electrophoresis. This study, necessary for the diagnosis of myeloma, should be performed in any older adult with an undiagnosed lytic bone lesion.

Indices of Bone Turnover

An important group of laboratory tests, ordered mainly by endocrinologists, are the indices of bone turnover.[11] These tests are useful to confirm the diagnosis of a high-turnover bone disease. These diseases may focally involve the skeleton, such as Paget's disease, or they may be diffuse, such as primary hyperparathyroidism or renal osteodystrophy. The indices of bone turnover are measurements of products that reach the serum or urine as a result of osteoblastic and osteoclastic activity. These products are increased in high-turnover bone diseases. Markers of osteoblastic activity are serum alkaline phosphatase and serum osteocalcin. Osteoblasts secrete alkaline phosphatase simultaneous with the secretion of osteoid. Although its exact function is unknown, alkaline phosphatase probably either initiates or facilitates mineralization. The other marker of osteoblastic activity, osteocalcin, is a noncollagenous component of osteoid, but, like alkaline phosphatase, its function in osteoid is unknown. Because 10 to 25% of the synthesized osteocalcin escapes into the circulation, the serum levels reflect the amount of osteoid synthesized.[12]

Markers of osteoclastic activity include tartrate-resistant acid phosphatase, urinary hydroxyproline, and urinary pyridinoline cross-links. Acid phosphatase is secreted by osteoclasts during bone resorption. Although various other tissues, including prostate and spleen, demonstrate acid phosphatase activity, only osteoclast acid phosphatase is tartrate resistant. Therefore, elevated serum levels indicate increased bone resorption.[13] Urinary hydroxyproline and urinary pyridinoline cross-links, the other markers of bone resorption, are breakdown products of collagen. Hydroxylation of proline occurs after collagen synthesis and is necessary for helix formation of the collagen molecules. Hydroxyproline is almost exclusively limited to collagen, and when bone collagen is degraded by osteoclasts during resorption, it is excreted in the urine. Increased urinary levels, therefore, indicate increased collagen breakdown, an indication of increased resorption.[14] In addition to the hydroxylation of proline, another post-translational collagen modification is the covalent cross-linking between lysines or hydroxylysines. These cross-links resist degradation during collagen breakdown. After breakdown, the collagen fragments, held together by these cross-links, form a molecule known as pyridinoline, which is excreted in the urine. Like hydroxyproline, increased urinary levels indicate increased bone resorption.[15]

Radiologic-Histologic Correlation

The plain radiograph represents the gross pathology of bone and joint disease and provides essential clues to the

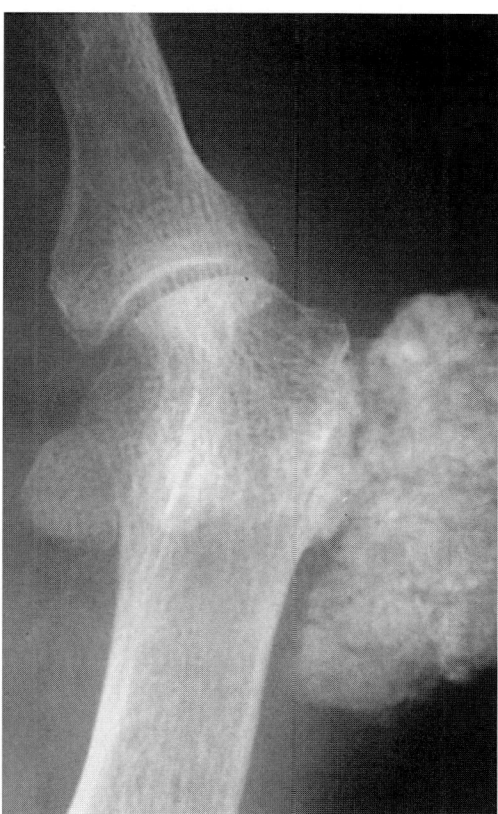

Figure 1-1 ■ First metatarsophalangeal joint of the foot, showing the amorphous calcification of tumoral calcinosis.

behavior of a lesion. In fact, some bone diseases can be diagnosed with certainty with plain radiographs alone. When a biopsy is necessary, the plain radiographs teach the pathologist how to interpret the slides. Therefore, it is not enough to simply look up the radiology report on the hospital computer. Pathologists must examine the radiographs themselves. Also, the clinician and radiologist should come to the pathology department to look at the slides with the pathologist. This sort of communication across disciplinary boundaries results in more accurate diagnosis and better treatment.

Studying the plain radiographs is the most effective way to learn what a bone lesion is doing to the patient. They reveal how long a lesion has been present and, in many cases, what type of tissue it is made of. The best way to study a plain radiograph is through histopathologic lenses.[16-18] That is, the radiologist must imagine what the lesion looks like under the microscope. This approach is most effective when considering the two major categories of radiographic patterns: patterns of radiodensity and patterns of radiolysis.

Patterns of Radiodensity

Radiodensity is produced by calcium. Therefore, increased radiodensity in a bone or new radiodensity on the bone surface is caused by a lesion with extra or new calcium. The histologic manner of the calcium deposition is discernible by plain radiographs, and the radiologist can therefore diagnose what type of tissue is present. Calcium is deposited in three manners: as amorphous calcium, as calcified cartilage, or as bone. Determining which manner of calcification is present is the first step in diagnosing a radiodense lesion.

Amorphous calcification, especially on the bone surface, causes round or oval radiodensities that may be likened to a mass of squashed wet cotton balls (Fig. 1-1). Generally, each oval is uniformly radiodense. The histologic correlate of this pattern of calcification is amorphous calcified debris in soft tissue, often with an extensive histiocytic and foreign body giant cell reaction (Fig. 1-2). The calcium is either amorphous calcium phosphate or plates and laminated spherules (psammoma bodies) of calcium hydroxyapatite. The calcifications are deeply basophilic and are not birefringent in polarized light. In the soft tissues adjacent to the bone, this pattern of calcification characterizes a disease called tumoral calcinosis. Intraosseous amorphous calcification also occurs, particularly in bone infarcts. In this setting, calcified fat necrosis causes ill-defined densities resembling smoke rings (Fig. 1-3). Histologically, this type of calcification occurs in necrotic fat (Fig. 1-4).

Hyaline cartilage calcification is the second major pattern of radiodensity. Cartilage is a radiolucent substance. Therefore, some intramedullary cartilage lesions are entirely radiolytic. However, as cartilage matures, calcifications appear. Typically, hyaline cartilage calcification appears as fine stip-

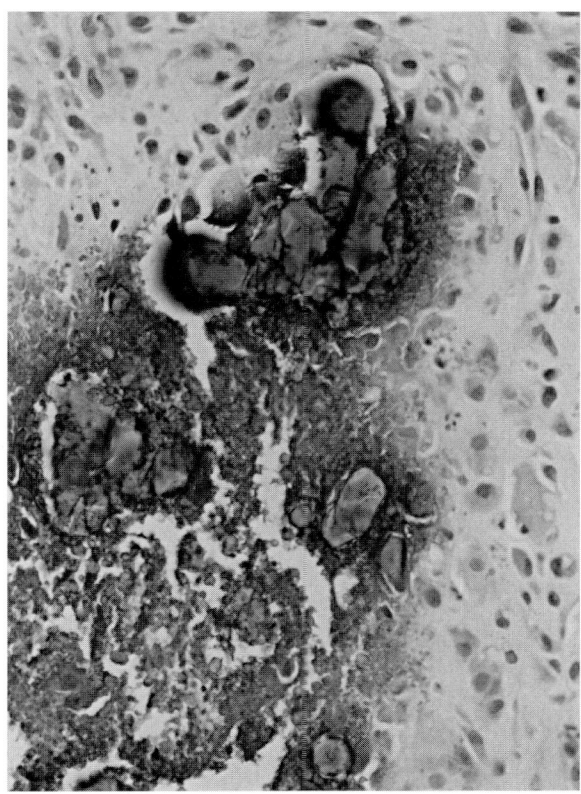

Figure 1-2 ■ Histology of amorphous calcification. Amorphous basophilic powder, as well as plates of calcium hydroxyapatite crystals, can be seen.

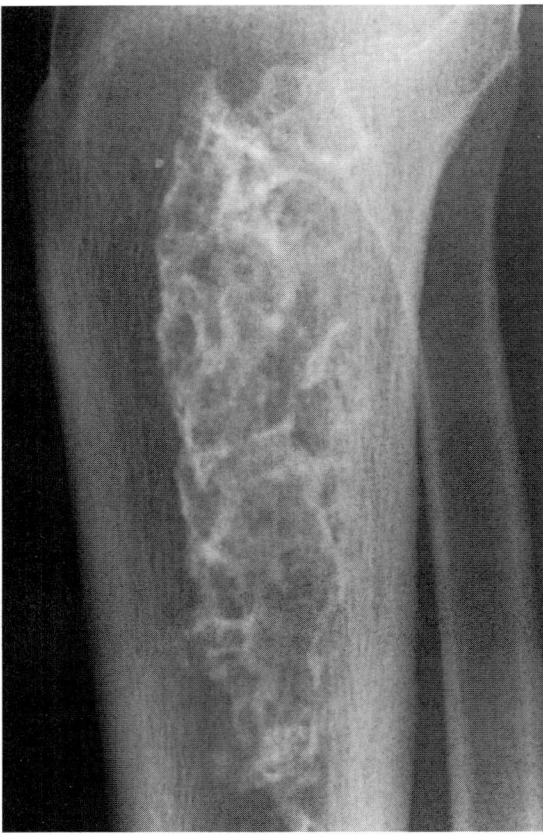

Figure 1-3 ■ Bone infarct of proximal tibia. Calcification of the necrotic marrow has occurred, forming a smoke-ring pattern.

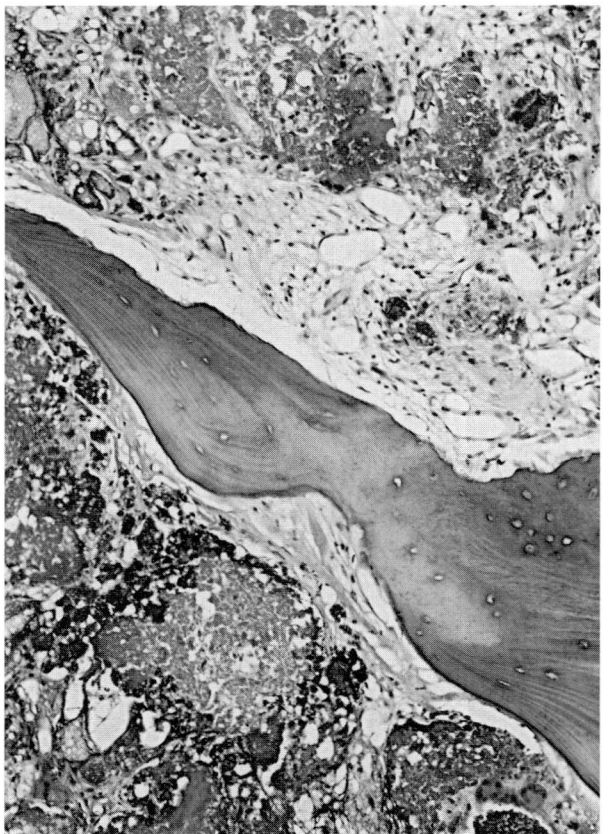

Figure 1-4 ■ Bone infarct showing amorphous calcification of necrotic fat.

ples and small rings, a result of the growth characteristics of cartilage (Fig. 1–5). The clonal proliferation of chondrocytes results in discrete cartilage lobules that undergo a series of programmed changes (Fig. 1–6). First, the center of each lobule calcifies, and a group of these focally calcified lobules produces radiographic stippling. Then, the periphery of each lobule undergoes endochondral ossification (Fig. 1–7). As a result, rimming of each lobule with bone causes ring-shaped densities on plain radiographs. This pattern of calcification—rings and stipples—occurs in both surface and intramedullary hyaline cartilage lesions.

The third pattern of radiodensity is due to *bone formation.* Radiographically, bone formation is characterized by trabecular lines, most evident in surface or soft tissue osseous lesions (Fig. 1–8). Trabeculae of woven or lamellar bone are present histologically (Fig. 1–9). Although less distinct than surface lesions, extra bone is also recognizable in intramedullary bone–forming lesions. Extra intramedullary bone usually manifests by thickening of existing native trabeculae or the addition of new trabeculae between existing trabeculae (Fig. 1–10). The radiographic pattern of bone density may also be correlated with histologic features. New woven or lamellar bone is present either in the marrow space or deposited on native trabeculae (Fig. 1–11).

Although new bone deposition is readily diagnosed radiographically and histologically, the type of new bone—reactive or neoplastic—must also be distinguished. Neoplastic bone deposition is patternless (Fig. 1–12),

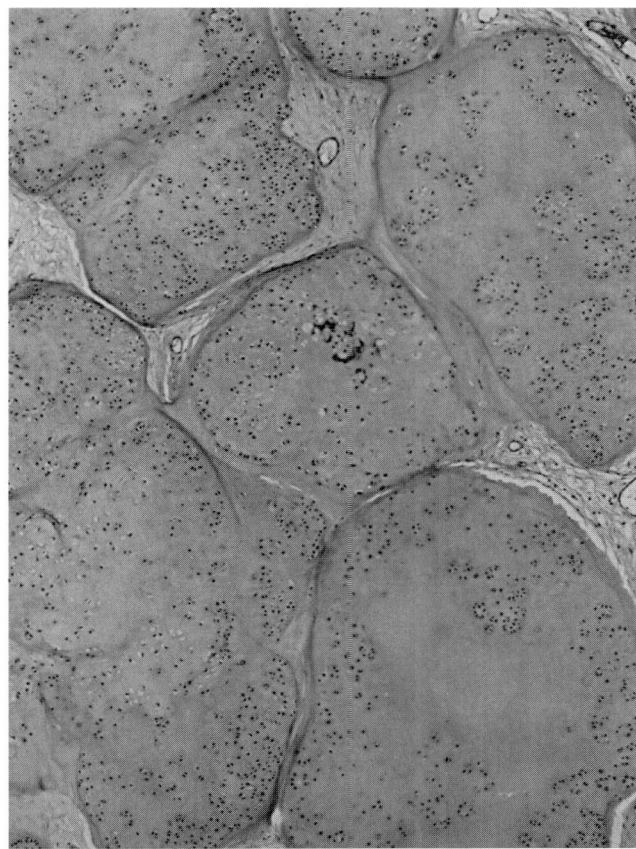

Figure 1-6 ■ Lobular growth pattern of cartilage.

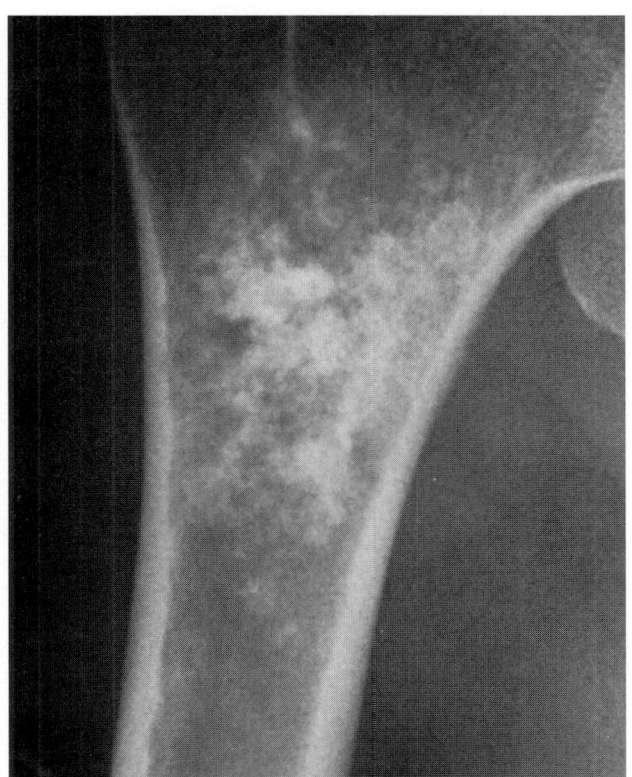

Figure 1-5 ■ Ring-shaped radiodensities of an enchondroma in the proximal humerus.

whereas reactive bone is *zonal.* The zonal pattern of reactive bone can be appreciated both radiographically and histologically. Radiographically, zonation of reactive bone results in a gradient of radiodensity. For example, a radiodense area that gently and evenly blends with the normal bone is likely to be reactive (Fig. 1–13). Another example of reactive bone is a uniform sclerotic rim around a lytic area. In the soft tissue, zonal reactive bone may result in a dense outer shell surrounding a less radiodense central area. Histologically, the zonal pattern of reactive bone is characterized by a gradient of bone maturation and an organized pattern of trabecular arrangement. The trabeculae in a particular zone show similar degrees of maturation. For example, immature woven bone present in one zone gradually changes to mature lamellar bone in another zone (Fig. 1–14). Another histologic pattern of reactive bone is appositional bone formation. Existing trabeculae are thickened by layers of new bone. Appositional reactive bone frequently accompanies marrow infiltrative processes, such as infection or neoplasia.

Patterns of Radiolysis

The growth rate of an intramedullary bone lesion can usually be determined by its pattern of radiolysis. Three radiographic patterns correspond to three growth rates: nongrowing (or healing), slowly growing, and rapidly growing.

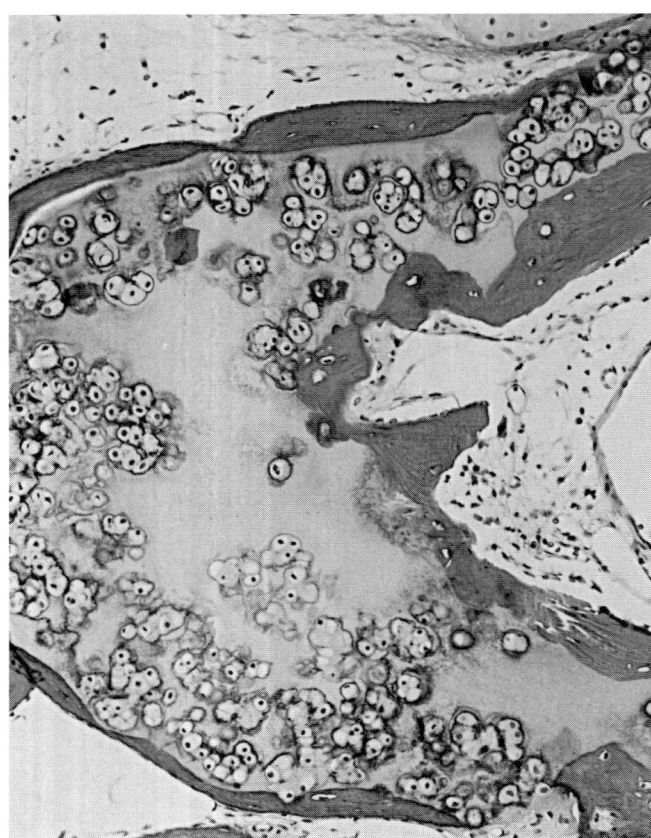

Figure 1-7 ▪ Lobule of cartilage rimmed by endochondral bone. This pattern correlates with the rings seen on plain radiographs.

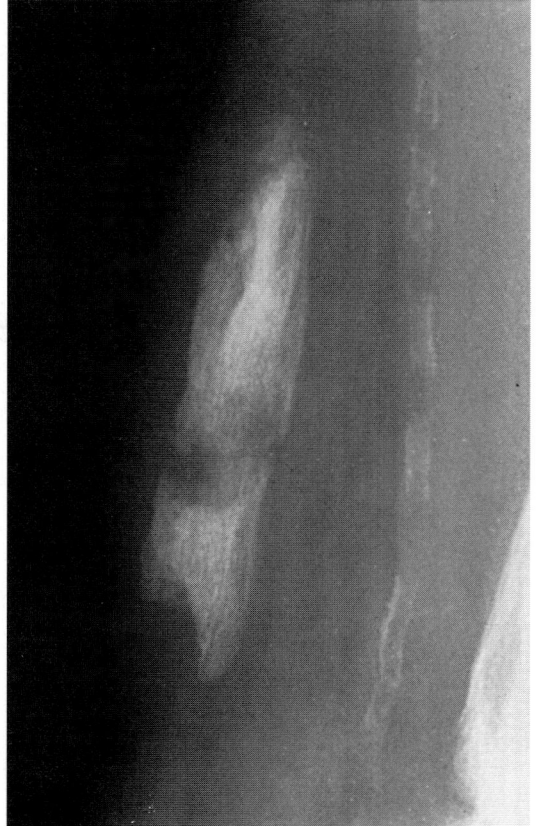

Figure 1-8 ▪ Heterotopic bone in the Achilles tendon. Distinct trabecular lines are present.

Figure 1-9 ▪ Heterotopic bone in soft tissue. Trabeculae of woven bone are present.

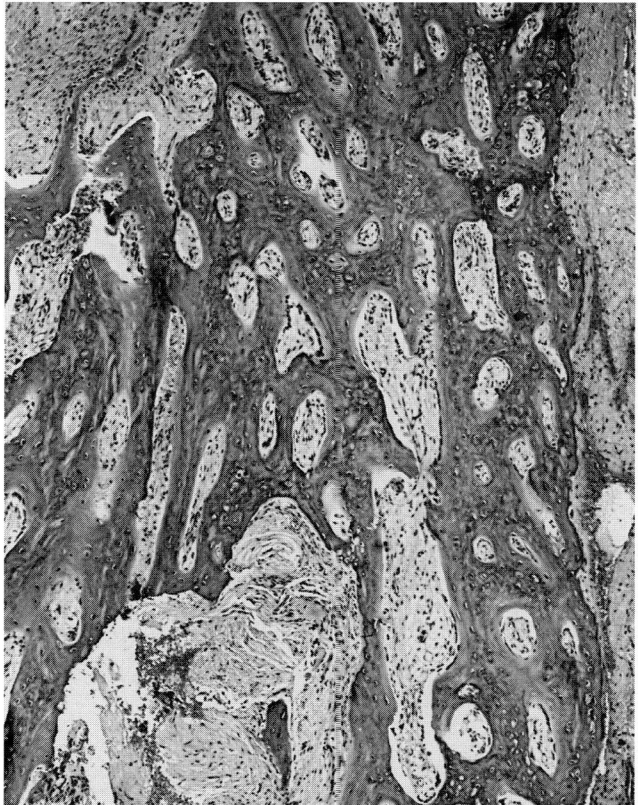

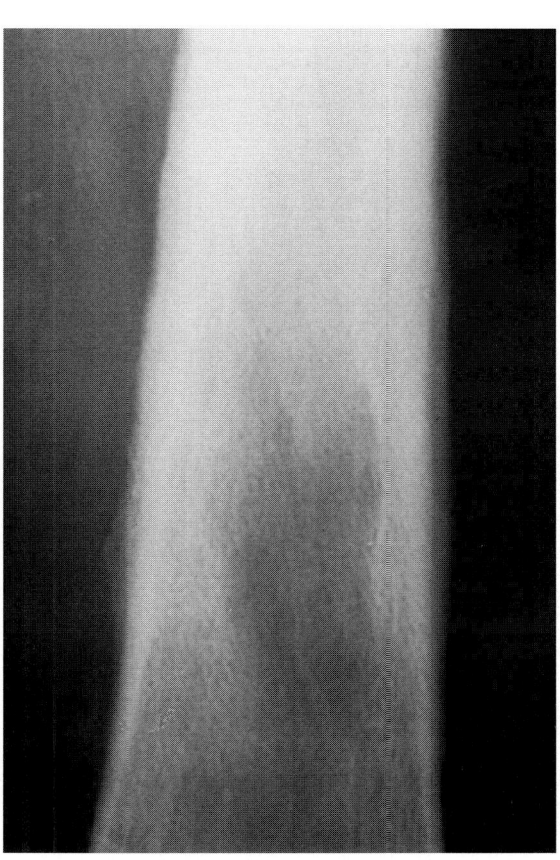

Figure 1-10 ▪ Chronic osteomyelitis of the distal femur. The radiodensity is due to successive layers of appositional bone on native trabeculae. Cortical thickening is also present.

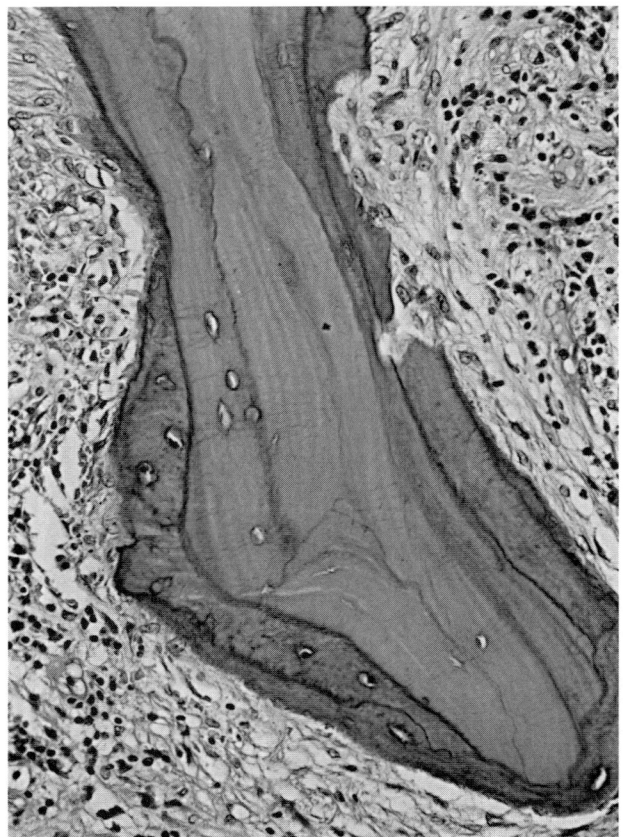

Figure 1-11 ■ Chronic osteomyelitis. The native trabeculae are encased by appositional new bone.

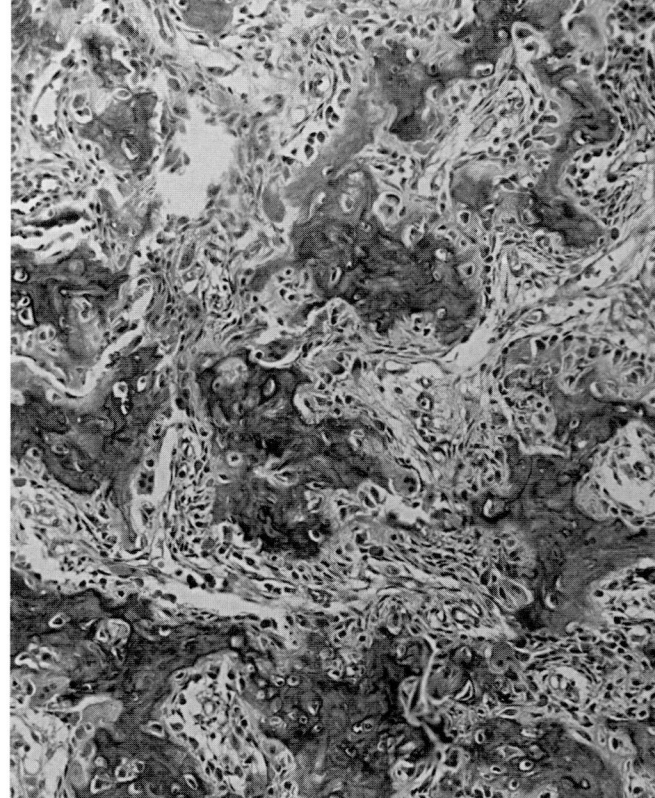

Figure 1-12 ■ Osteoblastoma. A patternless deposition of new bone can be seen. (From Frassica, F. J., Waltrip, R. L., Sponseller, P. D., Ma, L. D., and McCarthy, E. F.: Clinicopathologic features and treatment of osteoid osteoma and osteoblastoma in children and adolescents. *Orthop Clin North Am* 27:559–587, 1996.)

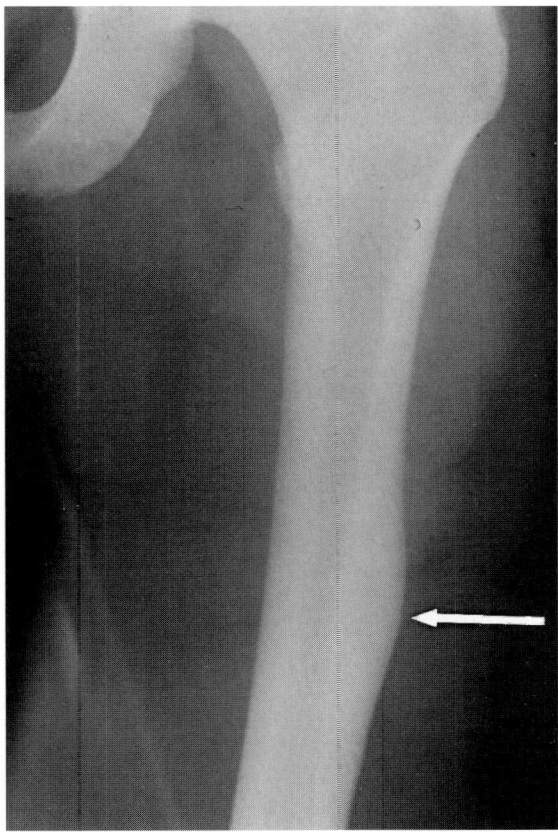

Figure 1-13 ■ Osteoid osteoma of femur. Reactive bone around the nidus (invisible) forms a symmetric fusiform swelling.

growing lesions. These include infections and malignant neoplasms. The radiolucency produced by these lesions is poorly defined, and there is no clear demarcation between the lesion and the native bone. Also, varying amounts of native trabeculae are present within the lytic areas, resulting in the so-called *permeative* radiologic pattern (Fig. 1-19). Occasionally, extensive native trabeculae persist and bone lysis is almost inapparent on plain radiographs. Persistence of native trabeculae in the lesion indicates that the marrow is being infiltrated so rapidly that the bone has not had time to be resorbed. Generally, the more rapidly growing a lesion, the more difficult it is to see on plain radiographs.

The permeative growth pattern of rapidly growing lesions is also evident histologically. Lesional tissue is present in the marrow space, but the native trabeculae, identifiable as mature lamellar bone, are intact (Fig. 1-20). Some trabeculae are completely encased by lesional tissue, and sometimes, because of an interrupted blood supply, they are necrotic. This permeative pattern is virtually diagnostic of malignancy in bone- and cartilage-producing neoplasms. In contrast to the cortical expansion, which characterizes some slowly growing lesions, rapidly growing lesions often cause cortical destruction. If this happens, lesional tissue is present in the periosteum or in the soft tissues

Enneking and colleagues[19] have called these same three lesion patterns inactive, active, and aggressive.

Nongrowing lesions are well circumscribed and have a *sclerotic rim*. The sclerotic rim, which may be a thin line or broad zone of radiodensity, is the bone's attempt to wall off or heal the lytic area (Fig. 1-15). It always means that the lesion is not growing or is growing slowly enough to allow the bone to react. Histologically, varying amounts of reactive bone are present at the periphery of the lesion (Fig. 1-16). Some nonossifying fibromas are examples of nongrowing lesions.

Like nongrowing lesions, slowly growing lesions are well circumscribed. However, slowly growing lesions lack a sclerotic rim. Despite this, the demarcation between the lytic lesion and the native bone is generally quite crisp in the majority of the periphery (Fig. 1-17). Histologically, the tissue of a growing lesion is distinct from the native bone and marrow (Fig. 1-18). The edges of the lesion are clearly demarcated, and little or no native bone is entrapped in the process. Unless a pathologic fracture has occurred, reactive bone is minimal. Some giant cell tumors of bone are examples of slowly growing lesions. In addition to their lack of a sclerotic rim, many slowly growing lesions are characterized by an expanded cortex.

The final pattern of radiolysis is produced by rapidly

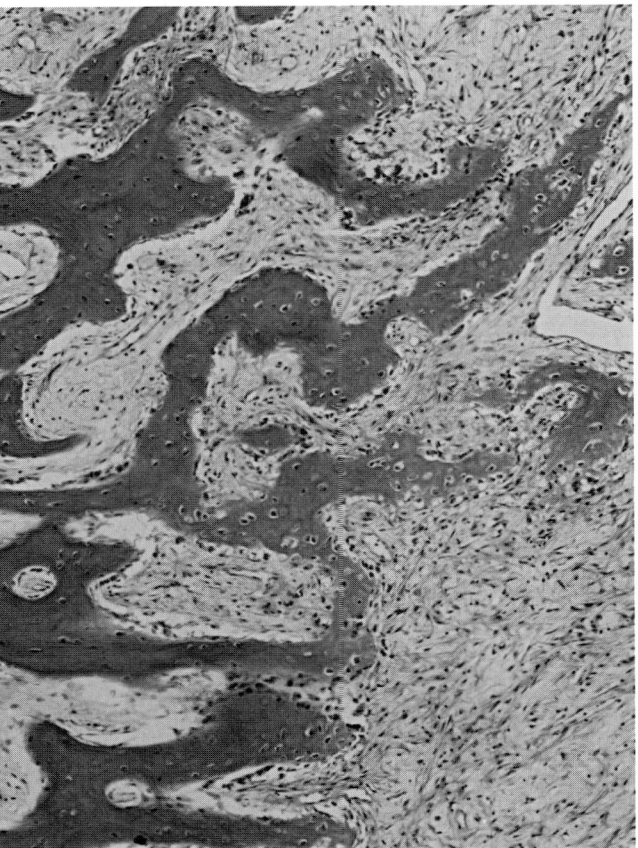

Figure 1-14 ■ Zonal pattern of reactive bone. The trabeculae have a purposeful pattern, and newly formed osteoid blends with more mature new bone.

16 DIAGNOSING BONE DISEASE

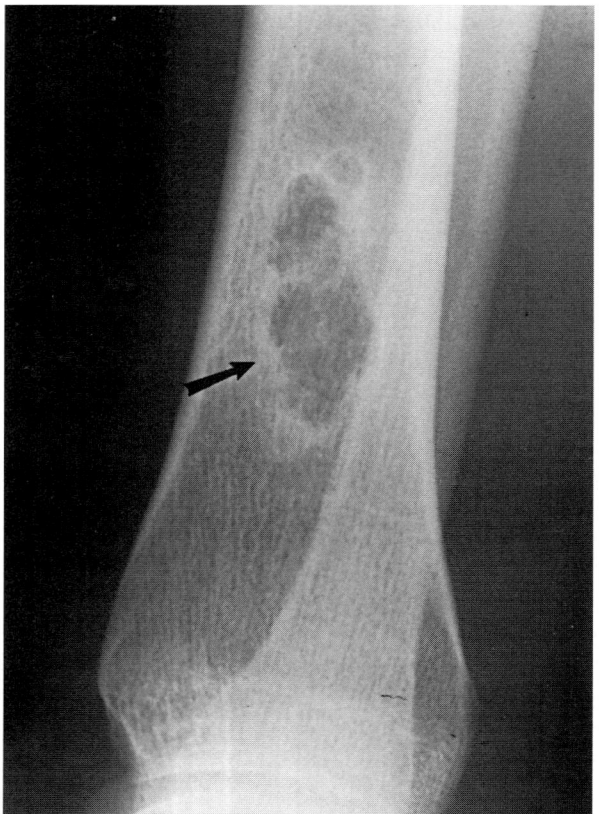

Figure 1-15 ■ Nonossifying fibroma of distal tibia. This nongrowing lesion is encased by a rim of sclerotic bone *(arrow)*.

Ancillary Radiographic Techniques

In addition to plain radiographs, many ancillary radiographic modalities are available to study bone lesions. Four of these modalities are particularly useful in answering specific questions: the radionuclide bone scan, bone densitometry, computerized axial tomography (CT) scan, and MRI. However, these ancillary studies, particularly CT scans and MRIs, should only be interpreted in view of plain radiographic features. Failure to correlate special imaging modalities with plain radiographs, a growing trend in radiology practice, often results in incomplete or, worse, inaccurate diagnoses. Several factors have contributed to this trend. First, many university radiology departments emphasize specialization in imaging modalities rather than organ systems. As a result, an MRI of a bone lesion may be interpreted by an MRI specialist with little interest in skeletal disease. Second, plain radiographs may not be available to radiologists in satellite MRI suites, facilities common in private practice radiology. Third, gatekeepers in the managed care system sometimes order MRIs indiscriminately, and plain radiographs are never obtained.

The problem of inefficient or inaccurate use of ancillary imaging modalities must be solved by the clinician. First, he or she should remember that the diagnosis of a bone lesion can usually be made solely with the plain radiograph. Second, before ordering an ancillary study, the clinician must specify a question that that modality can answer. Without formulating specific questions, most of these studies are wasted.

The Radionuclide Bone Scan

The bone scan, also known as bone scintigraphy, was one of the first ancillary modalities to be used in clinical practice. The bone scan is the most sensitive way to determine if an active lesion is present and to ascertain the presence of multiple lesions (Fig. 1–21).[20] Although the bone scan is nonspecific, its very high sensitivity accurately establishes the presence of lesions even before plain radiographic changes occur. In fact, a bone scan may show changes as early as 1 or 2 days after a bone disease begins. Therefore, in every category of bone disease, scintigraphy identifies skeletal abnormalities that are not yet evident radiographically. Also, in the hands of a skilled nuclear medicine physician, bone scans provide information about the growth rate of specific lesions.

A bone scan is performed by the injection of a radioactive pharmaceutical agent, today almost always technetium 99m phosphate. Within minutes, this radioisotope tracer begins to accumulate in areas of bone disease, and scanning the entire body at specific time intervals with a gamma scintillation

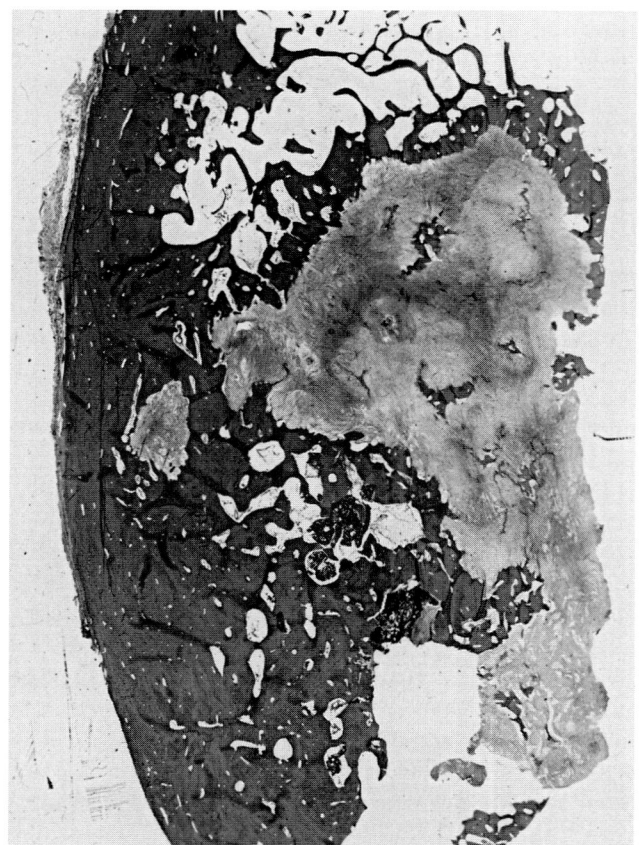

Figure 1-16 ■ Nonossifying fibroma. The lesion is encased by a wall of reactive bone. Cortical thickening, due to endosteal bone deposition, is also present.

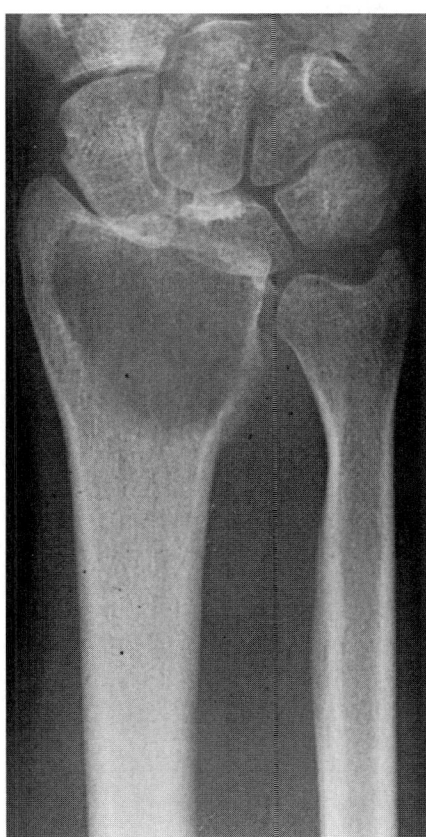

Figure 1-17 ■ Giant cell tumor of distal radius. This slow-growing lesion is well circumscribed but lacks a sclerotic rim.

late tracer. Although plain radiographs suggest that lytic lesions have no osteoblastic activity, tracer accumulation indicates that osteoblasts are active microscopically. Another group of lesions that intensely accumulate tracer are those characterized by high bone turnover. These diseases include Paget's disease and the focal osteoporotic syndromes.

Any tracer not taken up by a bone lesion is rapidly excreted in the urine. Because the radioactive half-life of ^{99m}Tc is 6 hours, the radioactivity in the bone lesions rapidly diminishes.

Computerized Tomography

Computerized tomography is an imaging modality introduced in 1972 by Godfrey Hounsfield, who received the 1979 Nobel prize in medicine for developing this technique. CT creates images of cross-sectional slices of the body. With this modality, the radiologist can study portions of the skeleton, such as the skull, spine, and pelvis, that are difficult to visualize with plain radiographs.

With CT, the patient receives x-rays, but the images are not collected on radiographic film. Instead, sensitive sodium iodide scintillation crystals detect the amount of residual radiation energy after the beam has passed through the patient. The difference between the intensity of the original camera locates these areas. There are three phases of a bone scan based on images made at different time intervals after tracer administration. In the first phase, images are recorded immediately after injection of the radioactive tracer. Tracer accumulation at this time, known as the flow phase, documents mature blood vessels. The flow phase is similar to an angiogram; hemangiomas show marked accumulation. In the second phase, images are made a few minutes after tracer injection. In this portion of the study, known as the blood pool phase, tracer has accumulated at tissue sites with prominent neovascularity. Newly formed, leaky blood vessels allow tracer to pass into the soft tissue of the lesion. Characteristically, granulation tissue and very vascular neoplasms accumulate tracer in this phase of a radionuclide image.

In the final stage of bone scintigraphy, the delayed phase, the body is scanned 2 to 3 hours after radioisotope injection. By this time, tracer has accumulated in bone. The ^{99m}Tc adsorbs onto the surface of newly formed apatite crystals, such that wherever mineralization is occurring, tracer accumulates. Thus, tracer uptake, occurring in zones of newly formed bone, is a marker for osteoblast activity, and accumulations occur in any lesion characterized by neoplastic or reactive bone formation. Tracer accumulation is particularly intense in osteoblastic neoplasms, such as osteosarcoma, and lesions with extensive reactive bone deposition, such as chronic osteomyelitis. However, even lytic lesions accumu-

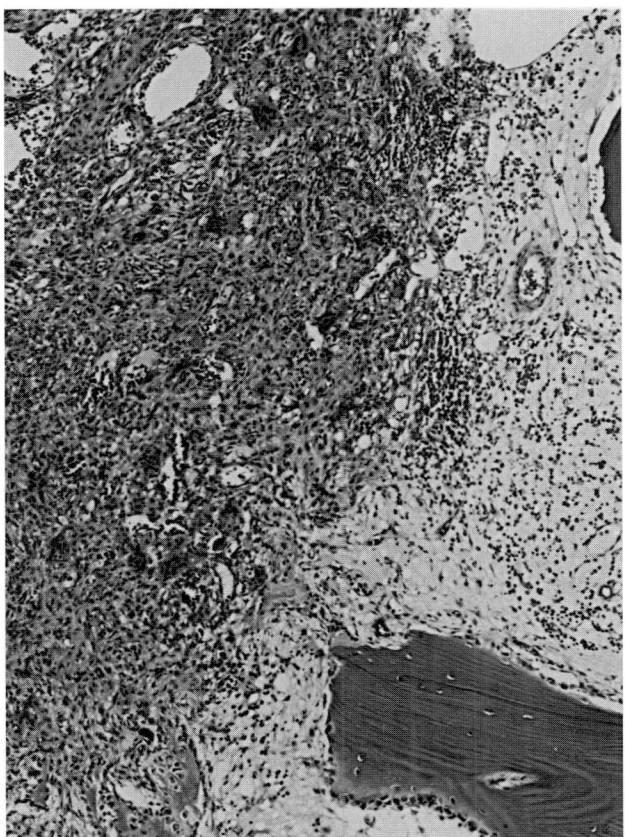

Figure 1-18 ■ Giant cell tumor showing a sharp demarcation of the neoplasm from the native marrow and bone. A margin of reactive bone is not present.

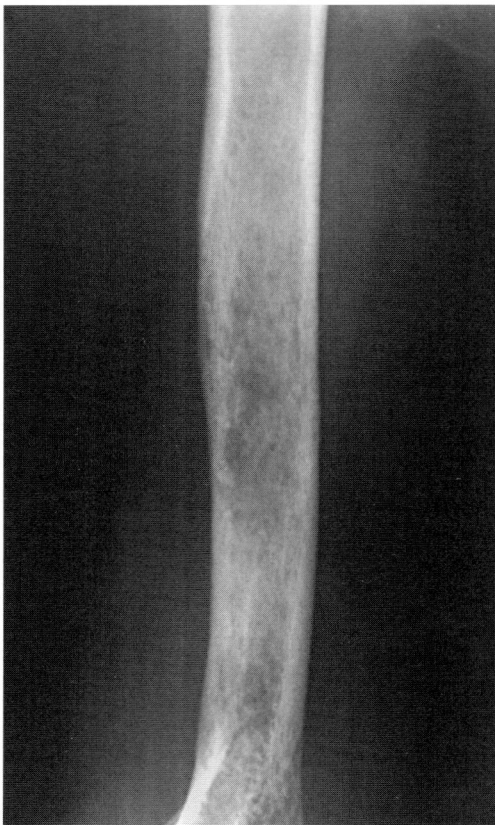

Figure 1-19 ■ Ewing sarcoma of humerus. There is an extensive permeative growth pattern.

record can be obtained. The highest-density substance can be made to appear white, and air, the lowest, black. Intermediate values appear as approximately 16 shades of gray.

Details in tissues of a particular density can be enhanced by altering the gray scale. Thus, "windows" are created by collapsing all the shades of the gray scale into a particular attenuation range. However, using this technique, detail is lost in other attenuation ranges. For example, in bone windows, fine differences in bone structure can be enhanced, but soft tissue detail is obscured.

With plain radiographic correlation, the CT scan is the procedure of choice for imaging the axial skeleton.[21] This modality precisely locates lesions and defines the extent of intraosseous and extraosseous lesional tissue (Fig. 1–22). In addition to its usefulness in the axial skeleton, CT is useful in the long bones. Images clearly define a surface lesion's margins and its relationship to the cortex. Also, the amount of cortical destruction can be quantified.

In addition to imaging thin body slices, newer CT software allows three-dimensional reconstruction of the slices. This three-dimensional image can be rotated on the computer screen and studied from any direction. Hard copies of the computer images can be generated for future reference (Fig. 1–23).

beam and that sensed by the detectors, known as the attenuation value, can be calculated. Different substances have different attenuation values. Bone, for example, has the highest attenuation value, and air has the lowest.

Using these principles, an image of a body slice can be produced in the following way. The patient is placed in a gantry that is circumferentially lined with a multitude of detectors. Then, a precisely collimated x-ray beam, 0.5 to 1.5 cm wide, fans out from an x-ray source located inside the gantry and passes through the patient. However, unlike conventional plain radiographs, the beam is not stationary. With a CT scan, the x-ray source rotates around the patient and sends the beam through the body from various directions. At the same time, the patient is gradually moved through the rotating beam, so that a spiral of radiation passes through the selected body part. As a result, several hundred thousand bits of data, obtained from the circumferentially located detectors, are fed into a computer.

Construction of an image of the selected body slice is done with the computer. To examine a bone lesion, 20 or more slices are created. The readings from each detector are processed and stored on a disc or magnetic tape. They can be displayed as a digital display of numbers or as an analog display. In an analog display, each attenuation value corresponds to a shade of gray, so that a permanent photographic

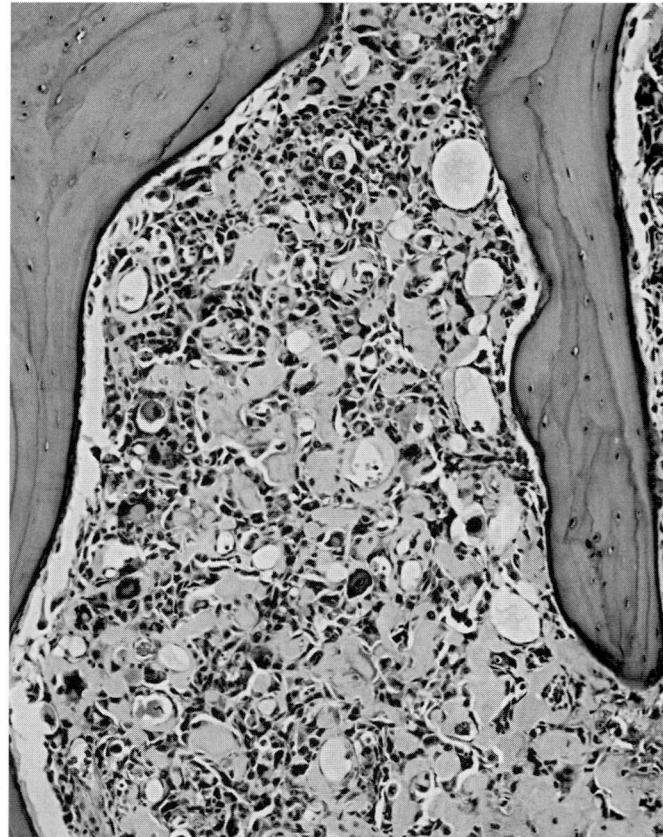

Figure 1-20 ■ Osteosarcoma showing infiltration of marrow spaces with preservation of native bone. This pattern of infiltration correlates with a permeative growth pattern on plain radiographs.

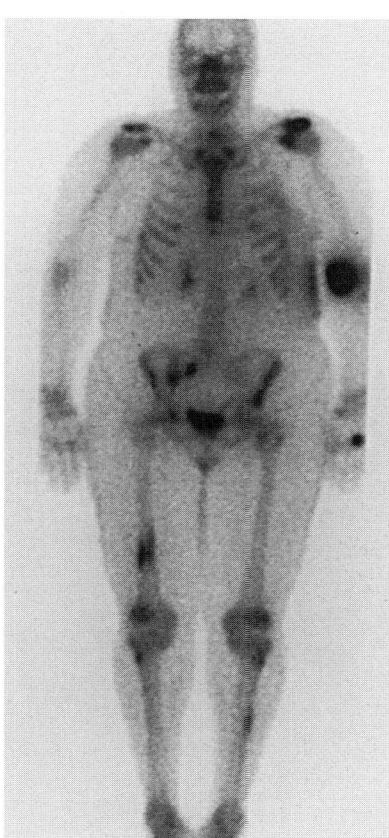

Figure 1-21 ■ Radionuclide bone scan Tracer accumulation is present in several locations including the femur and in the contralateral tibia. Tracer accumulation in the elbow is caused by extravasation of injected tracer.

Magnetic Resonance Imaging

Magnetic resonance imaging, which produces images without the use of ionizing radiation, was introduced into clinical practice in the early 1980s. This powerful imaging modality is most useful in differentiating the textures of various soft tissues. Therefore, it identifies abnormalities in the bone marrow space and in the soft tissues adjacent to bone.[22] MRI has limited value in delineating osseous abnormalities.

This imaging modality depends on the body's own natural magnetism, particularly that present in the protons of the hydrogen nuclei. Because protons naturally spin, their positive charge, which spins with them, generates a tiny magnetic field. When the body is placed inside the field of an external magnet, the protons, due to their own magnetic field, align themselves with the axis of the external magnet. Thus, the first step in an MRI examination is to place the patient (or an extremity) in a large magnet.

The next step is giving the patient pulses of radiofrequency energy. Each pulse is absorbed by the aligned hydrogen nuclei (protons), causing them to realign in a different axis. When the pulse is stopped, the nuclei "relax" back into the state of alignment induced by the external magnet. In so doing, the protons give up energy that takes the form of a radiofrequency that can be captured by a radioreceiver and translated into a computer image.

The MRI works because different body tissues hold on to their protons with varying degrees of intensity. Thus, the hydrogen nuclei in these varying tissues relax at different rates, and this variation in relaxing time and the number of protons present is the basis for image construction. For example, bone holds very tightly to its protons, and the protons return very quickly to their original alignment. Therefore, bone has a short relaxation time and produces no signal in an MRI examination. By contrast, the protons in water are very loose. They absorb much energy with a radiofrequency pulse and take a long time to relax to their original state. Water, therefore, has a slow relaxation time and, with the correct sequence of pulses, emits a heavy signal.

Variations in tissue contrast can be enhanced by varying the manner in which the electromagnetic pulses are given. Three of these variations are known as spin echo, gradient echo, and inversion-recovery. By varying the manner of radiofrequency pulses, the various parameters of proton relaxation are enhanced in different ways.

The images of particular body slices depend on another magnetic system superimposed on the static magnet. The second magnet is a gradient and has different strengths in different locations. Protons in different parts of the body feel the pull of the magnets differently. One way of creating a body slice image is to precisely tune the radiofrequency pulse to resonate with a particular zone of magnetic intensity.

Images are created by the energy produced when the protons relax. Three different parameters of relaxation can be measured. These are known as T_1, T_2, and proton density (Fig. 1–24). The T_1- and T_2-weighted images are most useful. In T_1-weighted images, fat is bright, and water (edema) is dark. This sequence is useful for anatomic detail. Pathologic processes are best visualized with T_2-weighted images. In this sequence, both water and fat are bright; however, because edema usually accompanies neoplasms and infections, these processes are brightly enhanced on T_2-weighted images. Therefore, when correlated with plain radiographs, the MRI accurately assesses the extent of disease. For example, the presence of marrow or soft tissue involvement by a malignant neoplasm, inapparent on plain radiographs, (Fig. 1–25) may be seen on MRI (Fig. 1–26). Thus, the extent of disease can be evaluated and surgical resections planned. The MRI is also extremely useful in the diagnosis of intraarticular disease.

Tissue contrast may be further enhanced by the prescan administration of gadolinium. This paramagnetic agent creates a local magnetic field in tissues and enhances the relaxation of protons. This technique is particularly effective in T_1-weighted images in which the fat signal has been suppressed. Because the gadolinium concentrates in richly vascular areas, viable and necrotic tissue may be differentiated.

Dual Energy X-Ray Absorptiometry

Dual energy x-ray absorptiometry is a sensitive tool for measuring bone mass and is extremely valuable in evaluating

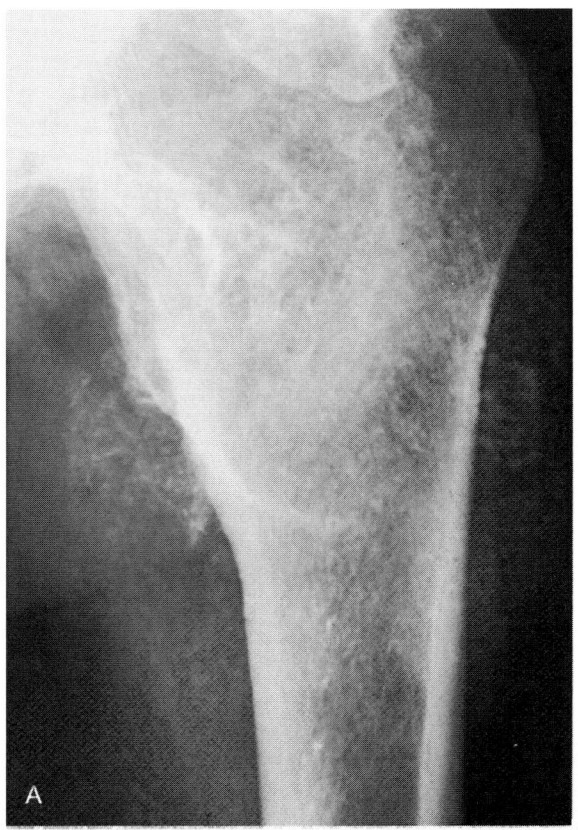
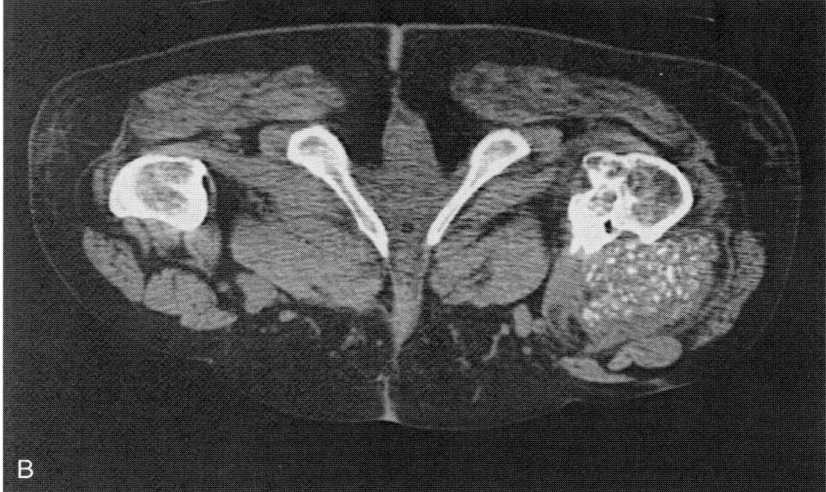

Figure 1-22 ▪ **A,** Synovial chondromatosis associated with an osteochondroma. The relationship of these two processes is not apparent on plain radiographs. **B,** CT scan of proximal femur. The stippled cartilage nodules are well circumscribed and adjacent to the prominence of the osteochondroma.

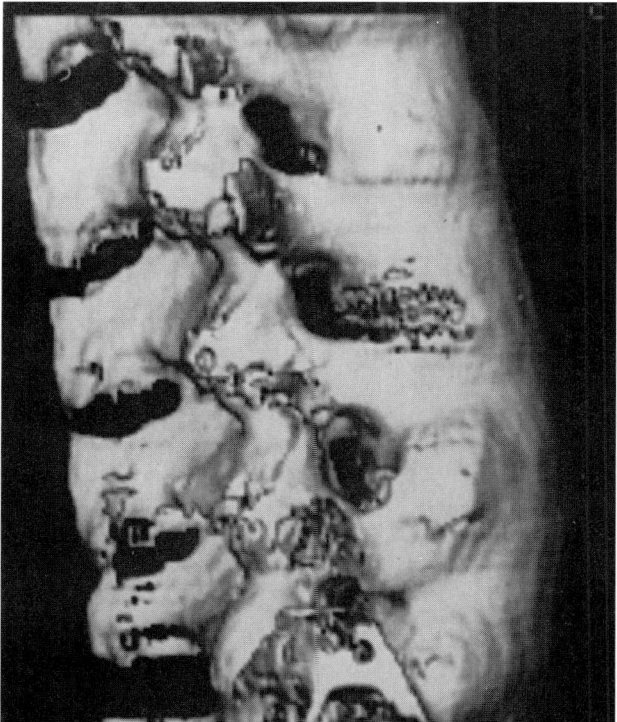

Figure 1-23 ■ Three-dimensional reconstruction of a CT image. This reconstruction demonstrates ankylosing spondylitis of the cervical spine. The vertebral bodies are fused into a continuous mass.

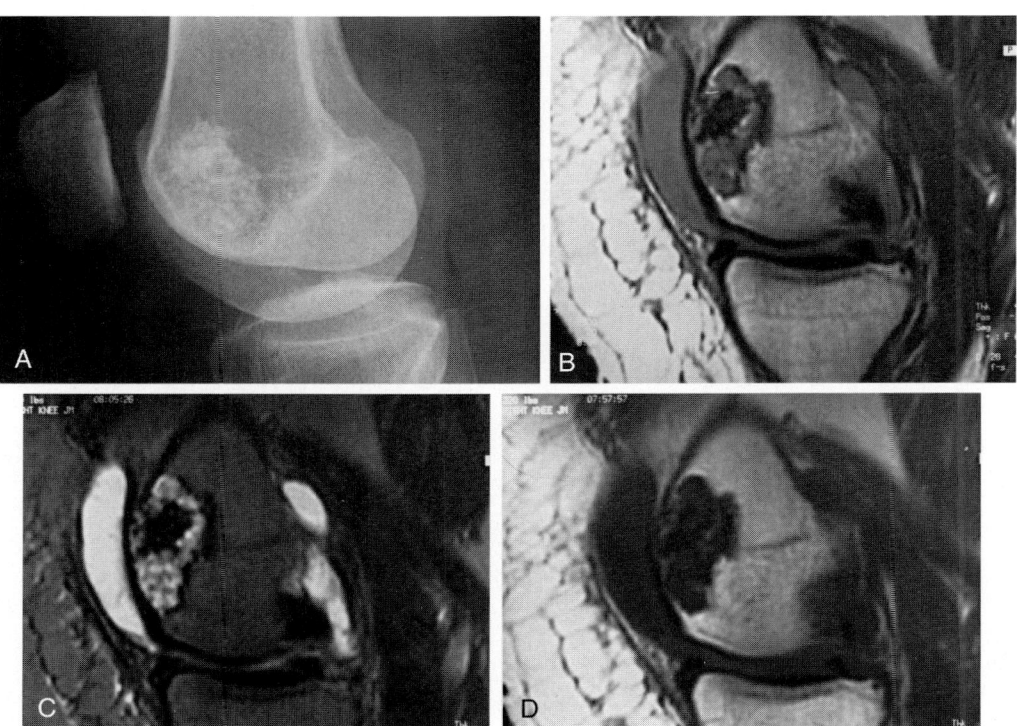

Figure 1-24 ■ Enchondroma of the distal femur. **A,** Plain radiograph showing a well-circumscribed group of stippled radiodensities. **B,** Proton density weighted MRI. **C,** T_2-weighted MRI showing increased signal from the cartilage lesion. This image also shows fluid present in the bursa anterior to the knee. **D,** T_1-weighted MRI. In this sequence the fat shows increased signal.

22 DIAGNOSING BONE DISEASE

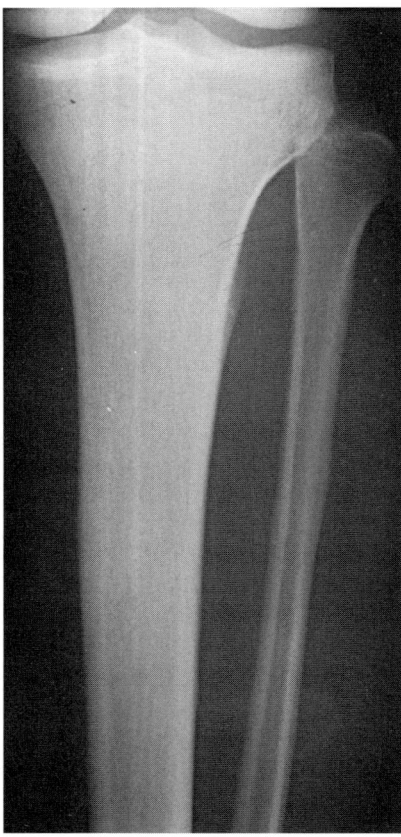

Figure 1-25 ■ Malignant lymphoma of the tibia. The process is not apparent on plain radiographs.

osteoporosis.[23] This is because bone mass must be decreased by at least 30% before osteopenia is visible on plain radiographs. By contrast, DEXA is far more sensitive.

With this modality, specified sites of the skeleton are scanned with a very fine x-ray beam in a procedure that takes about 10 minutes per site. A detector with an attached computer translates the degree of beam attenuation into a series of numbers. Although an image is also generated, it is only used to map variations in the generated numbers. These numbers reflect bone mass (measured as grams per unit area) at precise points in the skeleton. The scan is interpreted by comparing the generated numbers with those from a reference population. Abnormality is expressed as the amount of standard deviation from normal. The most common bones scanned are the femoral neck, the spine, and the distal radius.[24] This imaging procedure, also known as *densitometry,* is used primarily by endocrinologists who care for patients with metabolic bone disease. Some physicians believe that all women with osteoporosis risk factors should have densitometry studies around the time of the menopause. In patients with established osteoporosis, it is the most effective way to monitor the effects of treatment.

Ancillary Histologic Techniques

Just as ancillary radiographic studies greatly contribute to the diagnosis of bone lesions, special histologic techniques also aid in making specific diagnoses. Two important special histologic techniques are immunohistochemistry and histomorphometry of undecalcified bone.

Immunohistochemistry

Since their advent in the early 1970s, immunohistochemical stains have revolutionized the practice of diagnostic pathology. Immunohistochemistry identifies proteins specific to various types of tissue differentiation by using immunologic techniques.[25] Antibodies to specific proteins are artificially prepared and placed on a histologic preparation of the lesional tissue. The antibodies react with the specific antigens and can then be localized with a chromogen. Fortunately, this reaction is not disturbed by decalcification.[26] Immunohistochemical stains are most useful in identifying the differentiation of cells. For example, stains with antibodies to keratin identify the epithelial cells of metastatic carcinoma. Also, stains with antibodies to lymphoid antigens identify lymphoma cells. Many other lesions can be specifically diagnosed. Ewing sarcoma, for example, contains a gene product called C99. This protein can be identified with an O13 stain. Also, the Langerhans' cells of eosinophilic granuloma are positive with an S-100 stain. Using this stain, eosinophilic granuloma can be distinguished from chronic osteomyelitis.

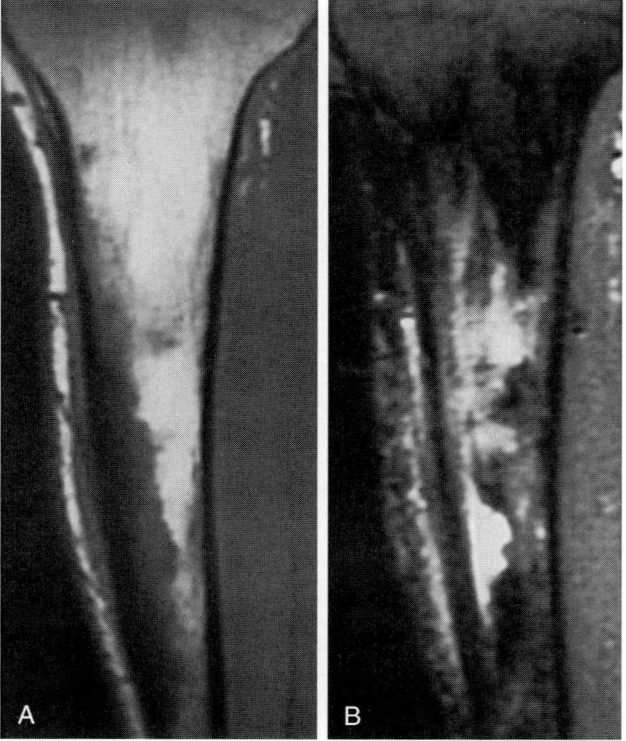

Figure 1-26 ■ **A,** T_1-weighted MRI of lesion present in Figure 1–25. An area of decreased signal corresponds to displacement of fat by neoplasm. **B,** T_2-weighted inversion-recovery sequence of the lymphoma. The irregular bright signal corresponds to the neoplasm.

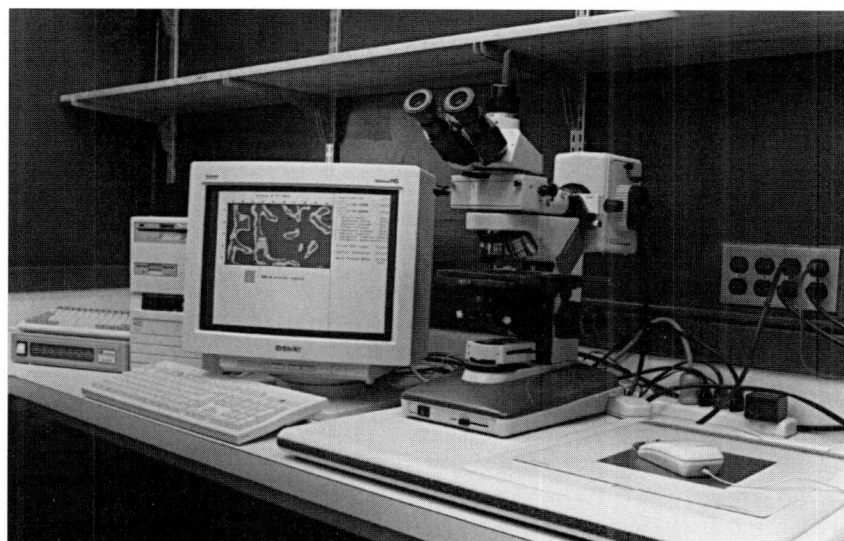

Figure 1-27 ■ System for the histomorphic analysis of undecalcified bone biopsies. The system consists of a digitizing board, microscope, camera, and computer.

Histomorphometry of Undecalcified Bone

The histomorphometry of undecalcified bone sections is another special histologic technique. Once the province of bone biologists for studying normal bone metabolism, it is now a useful diagnostic tool. With this procedure, specific metabolic bone diseases can be diagnosed and studied and their response to treatment evaluated.

Using undecalcified bone, a computer-assisted analysis of at least 50 microscopic fields generates precise data about four major parameters of bone metabolism (Fig. 1–27). First, the amount of bone, measured as cortical thickness and trabecular volume, is quantified. Second, the rate of bone turnover can be calculated from the amount of osteoblastic and osteoclastic activity. Third, the functional capacity of osteoblasts can be evaluated by measuring their bone formation rate. Fourth, the efficiency of mineralization, as measured by the mineralization lag time, can be calculated. When studying a biopsy from a particular patient, data in each of these parameters are compared to data from normal, age-matched control groups.

Two special techniques of bone histomorphometry enable the various indices of bone metabolism to be calculated—the use of undecalcified bone and tetracycline labeling. Most diagnostic bone pathology is performed with decalcified sections. However, decalcification obliterates the distinction between unmineralized osteoid and bone. However, by analyzing undecalcified sections, the amount of unmineralized osteoid provides information about the efficiency of mineralization.

Undecalcified bone sections also permit the use of tetracycline to study bone metabolism.[27] This antibiotic has two properties useful to bone histomorphometry. First, it fluoresces in ultraviolet light, and second, it adsorbs onto newly formed calcium hydroxyapatite crystals. Thus, for as long as tetracycline is in a patient's serum, bone formed during that period will be labeled with a fluorescent line. If two tetracycline labels are given about 7 days apart, the distance between the two fluorescent lines in the bone biopsy represents the amount of bone formed during that 7-day interval.[28]

Careful planning is required for the histomorphometric study of an undecalcified bone biopsy specimen. First, the tetracycline labels must be correlated with the scheduled

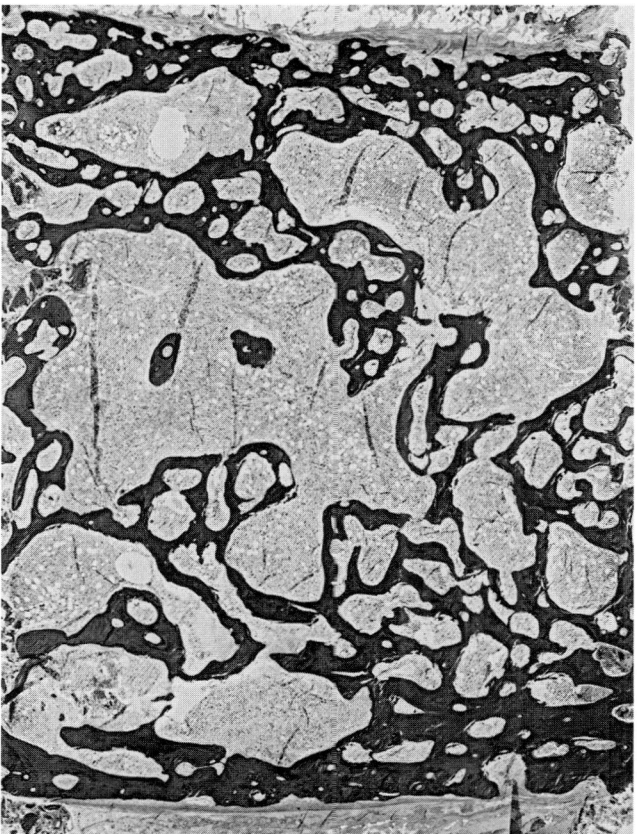

Figure 1-28 ■ Macrosection of a transiliac undecalcified bone biopsy specimen. This biopsy specimen, stained with a trichrome stain, shows renal osteodystrophy.

date of the biopsy. A transiliac core biopsy provides adequate cancellous bone, and most published normal data are based on bone from this region. In addition, the transiliac core biopsy, an outpatient procedure, lasts only a few hours and has few complications.[29]

After the biopsy, the specimen is prepared in special ways. First, for undecalcified sectioning, the specimen is embedded in methyl methacrylate, a process that takes about 2 weeks. After embedding is complete, sections are prepared with a special motorized microtome and stained in a variety of ways. A trichrome stain best differentiates bone from osteoid (Fig. 1–28).

Bone histomorphometry has several important clinical applications.[30] First, although the diagnosis of osteomalacia can be strongly suspected from laboratory studies (elevated serum parathyroid hormone levels with a normal serum calcium), bone histomorphometry establishes this diagnosis unequivocally. Second, the degree and pattern of renal osteodystrophy can be assessed. For example, staining for aluminum, only possible with undecalcified bone, assists in the diagnosis of aluminum bone disease, a complication of renal dialysis. Also, the degree of secondary hyperparathyroidism can be calculated. A third application of histomorphometry is distinguishing high-turnover from low-turnover osteoporotic syndromes. This distinction is useful in planning drug therapy and monitoring the results. In addition to these three important applications, bone histomorphometry is an adjunct to the diagnosis of unexplained osteopenia and fractures in young adults and adolescents.

Before turning to a detailed discussion of the specific disease categories, we briefly discuss the anatomy and physiology of bone.

REFERENCES

1. Beighton, P., Giedion, Z. A., Gorlin, R., Hall, J., Horton, B., Kozlowski, K., Lachman, R., Langer, L. O., Maroteaux, P., Poznanski, A., Rimoin, D. L., Sillence, D., and Spranger, J.: International classification of osteochondrodysplasias. *Am J Med Genet* 44:223–229, 1992.
2. Penttinen, R. P., Lichtenstein, J. R., Martin, G. R., and McKusick, V. A.: Abnormal collagen metabolism in cultured cells in osteogenesis imperfecta. *Proc Natl Acad Sci U S A* 72:586–589, 1975.
3. Shiang, R., Thompson, L. M., Zhu, Y.-Z., Church, D. M., Fielder, T. J., Bocian, M., Winokur, S. T., and Wasmuth, J. J.: Mutations in the transmembrane domain of FGFR3 cause the most common genetic form of dwarfism, achondroplasia. *Cell* 78:335–342, 1994.
4. Cole, W. G.: Osteogenesis imperfecta as a consequence of naturally occurring and induced mutations of type 1 collagen. Heersche JKJ (Ed.): *Bone Mineral Research* Amsterdam, Elsevier Science, 1994, pp. 67–204.
5. Riggs, B. L., and Melton, L. J.: Involutional osteoporosis. *N Engl J Med* 314:1676–1686, 1986.
6. Melton, L. J.: How many women have osteoporosis now. *J Bone Miner Res* 10:175–177, 1995.
7. Ray, N. F., Chan, J. K., Thamer, M., and Melton, L. J., III: Medical expenditures for the treatment of osteoporotic fractures in the United States in 1995: Report from the National Osteoporosis Foundation. *J Bone Miner Res* 12:24–34, 1997.
8. Einhorn, T. A.: Osteoporosis and metabolic bone disease. *Adv Orthop Surg* 8:175–184, 1984.
9. Mont, M. A., and Hungerford, D. S.: Current concepts review: Nontraumatic avascular necrosis of the femoral head. *J Bone Joint Surg* 77A:459–474, 1995.
10. Lew, D. P., and Waldvogel, F. A.: Osteomyelitis. *N Engl J Med* 336:999–1007, 1997.
11. Delmas, P. D.: Biochemical marks of bone turnover in osteoporosis. Riggs, L. B., Melton, L. J., III (Eds.): *Osteoporosis: Etiology, Diagnosis, and Management.* New York, Raven Press, 1988, pp. 297–316.
12. Slovik, D. M., Gundberg, C. M., Neer, R. M., and Lian, J. B.: Clinical evaluation of bone turnover by serum osteocalcin measurements in a hospital setting. *J Clin Endocrinol Metab* 59:228–230, 1984.
13. Halleen, J., Hentunen, T. A., Hellman, J., and Vaananen, H. K.: Tartrate-resistant acid phosphatase from human bone: Purification and development of an immunoassay. *J Bone Miner Res* 11:1444–1452, 1996.
14. Hodgkinson, A., and Thompson, T.: Measurement of the fasting urinary hydroxyproline: Creatinine ratio in normal adults and its variations with age and sex. *J Clin Pathol* 35:807–811, 1982.
15. Schlemmer, A., Hassager, C., Jensen, S. B., and Christiansen, C.: Marked diurnal variation in urinary excretion of pyridinium cross-links in premenopausal women. *J Clin Endocrinol Metab* 74:476–480, 1992.
16. Madewell, J. E., Ragsdale, B. D., and Sweet, D. E.: Radiologic and pathologic analysis of solitary bone lesions. Part I: Internal margins. *Radiol Clin North Am* 19:715–748, 1981.
17. Ragsdale, B. D., Madewell, J. E., and Sweet, D. E.: Radiologic and pathologic analysis of solitary bone lesions. Part II: Periosteal reactions. *Radiol Clin North Am* 19:749–783, 1981.
18. Sweet, D. E., Madewell, J. E., and Ragsdale, B. D.: Radiologic and pathologic analysis of solitary bone lesions. Part III: Matrix pattern. *Radiol Clin North Am* 19:785–814, 1981.
19. Enneking, W. F., Spanier, S. S., and Goodman, M. A.: A system for the surgical staging of musculoskeletal sarcoma. *Clin Orthop* 153:106–120, 1980.
20. Holder, L. E.: Clinical radionuclide bone imaging. *Radiology* 176:607–614, 1990.
21. Genant, H. K., Wilson, J. S., Bovill, E. G., Brunelle, F. O., Murray, W. R., and Rodrigo, J. J.: Computed tomography of the musculoskeletal system. *J Bone Joint Surg* 62A:1088–1101, 1980.
22. Moon, K. L., Jr., Genant, H. K., Helms, C. A., Chafetz, N. I., Crooks, L. E., and Kaufman, L.: Musculoskeletal applications of nuclear magnetic resonance. *Radiology* 147:161–171, 1983.
23. Pocock, N. A., Sambrook, P. N., Nguyen, T., Kelly, P., Freund, J., and Eisman, J. A.: Assessment of spinal and femoral bone density by dual x-ray absorptiometry: Comparison of lunar and hologic instruments. *J Bone Miner Res* 7:1081–1084, 1992.
24. Trevisan, C., Gandolini, G. G., Sibilla, P., et al.: Bone mass measurement by DXA: Influence of analysis procedures and interunit variation. *J Bone Miner Res* 7:1373–1382, 1992.
25. Kindblom, L. G.: Histochemistry applied to pathologic diagnosis of soft tissue and bone tumors. Spicer S. S. (Ed.): *Histochemistry in Pathologic Diagnosis.* New York, Marcel Dekker, 1986, pp. 729–754.
26. Mukai, K., Yoshimura, S., and Anzai, M. T.: Effects of decalcification on immunoperoxidase staining. *Am J Surg Pathol* 10:413–419, 1986.
27. Fallon, M., and Teitelbaum, S. L.: The interpretation of fluorescent tetracycline markers in the diagnosis of metabolic bone diseases. *Hum Pathol* 13:416–417, 1982.
28. Frost, H. M.: Tetracycline-based histological analysis of bone remodeling. *Calcif Tissue Res* 3:211–237, 1969.
29. Hodgson, S. F., Johnson, K. A., Muhs, J. M., Lufkin, E. G., and McCarthy, J. T.: Outpatient percutaneous biopsy of the iliac crest: Methods, morbidity, and patient acceptance. *Mayo Clin Proc* 61:28–33, 1986.
30. Bullough, P. G., Bansal, M., and DiCarlo, E. F.: The tissue diagnosis of metabolic bone disease. Role of histomorphometry. *Orthop Clin North Am* 21:65–79, 1990.

CHAPTER 2
Anatomy and Physiology of Bone

ANATOMY OF BONE

The Functions of Bone

Bones serve three crucial functions for the human body: (1) offering structural support, (2) housing the bone marrow, and (3) serving as a reservoir for calcium and phosphate ions. The first function, structural support, is made possible by the hardness of bone, a durability due to the impregnation of an organic matrix with calcium hydroxyapatite crystals. This mineral is abundant, accounting for about 77% of the dry weight of bone. The remainder is organic material. This blend of inorganic crystals in an organic matrix enables bone to withstand both tension and compression forces. The crystals withstand high compressive forces, and the organic matrix resists high tension forces, an arrangement similar to steel-reinforced concrete.

The second function of bone is to protect the bone marrow. This protection is afforded by cavities, known as marrow spaces, inside the bones. Bone marrow is a mixture of fat and hematopoietic cells. In children, the hematopoietic cells occupy most of the bone marrow space. However, in adults, the hematopoietic marrow contracts toward the axial skeleton and is mainly found in the spine. As contraction occurs, the marrow spaces in the distal skeleton become occupied entirely by fat.

The final function of bone is to provide a source of calcium ions. Depending on body size, bones contain 1 to 2 kg of calcium, accounting for 99% of the body's total calcium. Maintaining serum calcium in a very precise range is critical for many of the body's physiologic reactions. Because calcium intake may vary according to diet or hormonal status, release of calcium ions from bone provides a homeostatic buffer.

Macroscopic Organization of Bone

Bone is organized macroscopically in two ways: compact bone and cancellous bone. Most of the bone in the body, about 70%, is *compact bone*. This kind of bone is very dense and has few visible spaces. The dense outer shell of a bone, known as the *cortex,* is made up of compact bone. The cortex provides most of the structural strength of the skeletal frame.

The second macroscopic pattern of bone is *cancellous bone,* also known as spongy bone. Cancellous bone is found inside the cortices and forms an interconnecting network of plates or bars called *trabeculae* (Fig. 2–1). The trabeculae

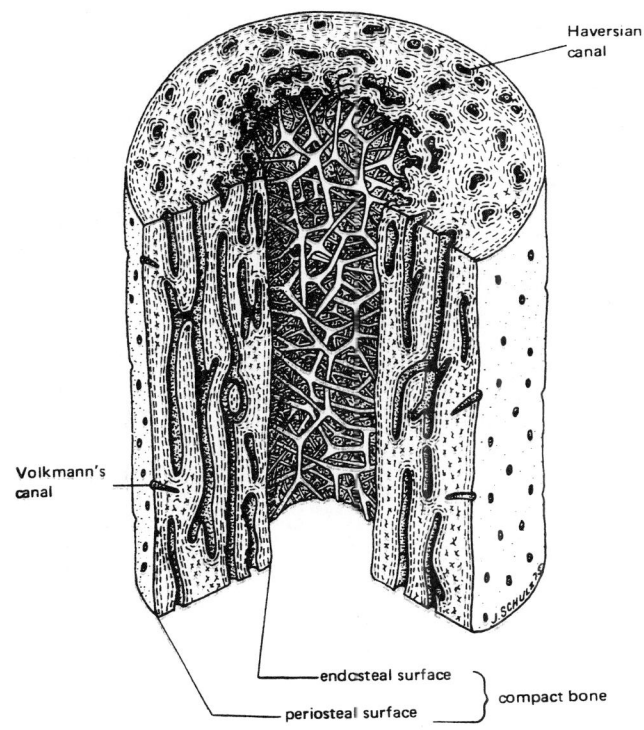

Figure 2-1 ■ A long bone diaphysis. A shell of dense compact bone, the cortex, encases thin spicules of trabecular bone. (From Han, S., and Holmestedt, J. O. V.: *Human Microscopic Anatomy.* New York, McGraw-Hill Book Company, 1981. Reproduced with permission of the McGraw-Hill Companies.)

are continuous with the inner surface of the cortex, and the spaces between them are filled with hematopoietic or fatty bone marrow. Radiologically, trabeculae are thin radiodense lines (Fig. 2–2). Generally, the extensive connectedness of the trabeculae (Fig. 2–3) is not readily apparent with routine histologic preparations (Fig. 2–4).

Cancellous bone has two important features. First, the organization of the trabeculae is purposeful. The plates and bars are oriented along lines of stress and strain inside the bone. Therefore, cancellous bone assists the cortex in structural support. Second, although cancellous bone is not as abundant as compact bone, it is much more metabolically active. The surface area of the body's cancellous bone is hundreds of times greater than the surface area of compact bone. Therefore, most remodeling and calcium exchange occurs in cancellous bone.

The proportion of compact and spongy bone varies in different portions of any particular bone (Fig. 2–5). This variation is most obvious in long bones. The midportion of a long bone, called the *diaphysis*, is a cylindrical rod composed mainly of compact bone. The area between the cortices, called the *medullary canal*, contains marrow and a few spicules of cancellous bone. The end of a long bone is called the *epiphysis*. This segment consists of abundant cancellous bone and a thin shell of cortical bone. Because the epiphysis

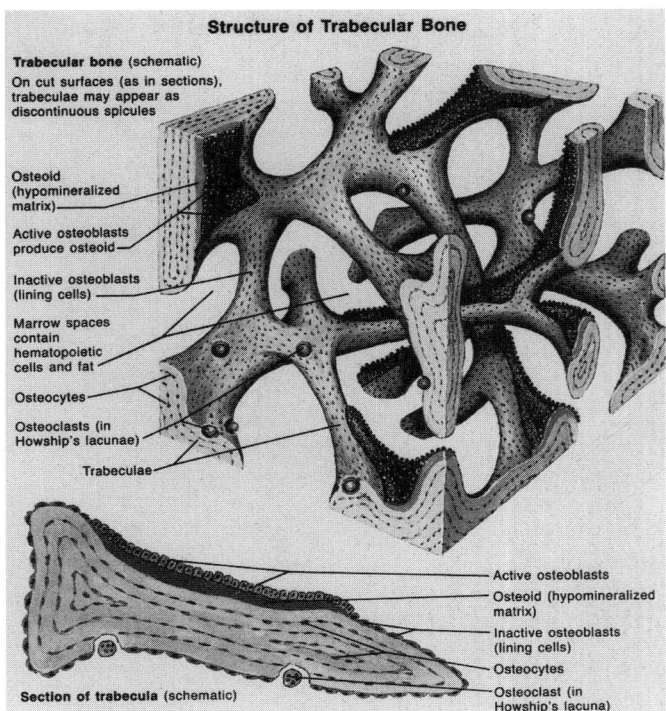

Figure 2-3 ■ The structure of trabecular bone. The trabeculae are interconnected, and some are lined by seams of osteoid synthesized by active osteoblasts. (Copyright 1987 Novartis. Modified with permission from The Ciba Collection of Medical Illustrations, Vol. 8, Part I, Sctn. III, illustrated by Frank H. Netter, MD. All rights reserved.)

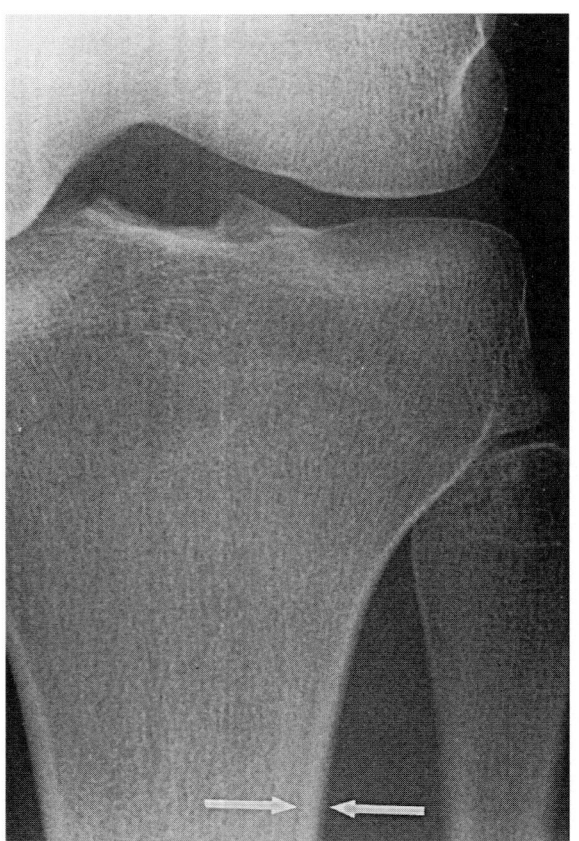

Figure 2-2 ■ Radiograph of proximal tibia. Most of the metaphysis and epiphysis is composed of thin lines of cancellous bone. Dense cortical bone *(arrows)* encases the distal metaphysis and the diaphysis.

often articulates with another bone, it is usually covered by *articular cartilage*. Between the epiphysis and the diaphysis is the *metaphysis*. This segment also contains abundant cancellous bone, which is surrounded by cortex. The metaphysis is the zone where a bone narrows from the wide epiphysis to the narrower diaphysis. In growing children, the epiphysis is separated from the metaphysis by the cartilaginous *epiphyseal plate*, also called the *physis*.

Bones have numerous associated supporting tissues. First, a thin membrane of fibrous tissue, called the *periosteum*, tightly encases the outside surface of most bones. A similar but thinner membrane, called the *endosteum*, lines the inside of the cortex. These membranes have osteogenic potential and are important in repair reactions. The second important supporting tissue is the extensive network of blood vessels that bring oxygen and nutrients. Bones are richly vascular, receiving 10 to 20% of the cardiac output. Blood vessels enter bones in several locations. Usually, several blood vessels enter both the epiphyseal and the metaphyseal segments. In addition, a large nutrient artery enters the diaphysis. Branches of the nutrient arteries anastomose with branches of the epiphyseal and metaphyseal blood vessels. Also, some of the branches of these vessels are open ended, allowing blood to percolate through the marrow spaces. In addition to larger blood vessels, many small blood vessels penetrate the cortex from the periosteum (Fig. 2–6).

ANATOMY AND PHYSIOLOGY OF BONE   27

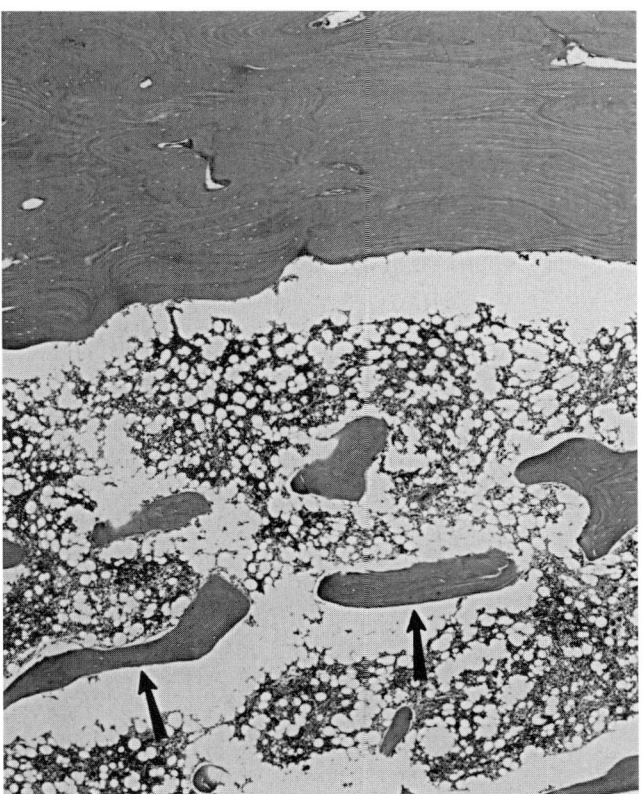

Figure 2-4 ■ Photomicrograph showing dense compact bone adjacent to disconnected spicules of cancellous bone *(arrows)*. Surrounding the cancellous bone is hematopoietic marrow.

Microscopic Organization of Bone

At a microscopic level, bone has two components: cells and an extracellular matrix consisting mainly of collagen. The number of cells is small compared with the great volume of extracellular matrix. A feature of this extracellular matrix not present in any other normal adult tissue is mineral. As a result, microscopic study of bone requires special procedures. Usually the mineral must be removed so that thin sections can be cut for histologic analysis.

The collagen of the extracellular matrix of mature bone is arranged in layers, known as *lamellae,* which are 3 to 7 μm thick (Fig. 2–7). Within each lamella, the collagen fibers are oriented perpendicular to those in the neighboring lamella, an arrangement highlighted by polarized microscopy. Evenly distributed throughout the matrix are small holes, known as *lacunae,* which contain the most abundant cell type of bone, the *osteocyte.* Radiating from each lacuna are tiny channels called *canaliculi.* These canaliculi, almost invisible on routine hematoxylin and eosin (H & E) sections, contain the long cytoplasmic processes of the osteocytes, which interconnect with processes from neighboring osteocytes.

Compact bone is made up of subunits called *osteons* or *haversian systems* (Fig. 2–8). Osteons are microscopic bone cylinders that average 50 μm in diameter and 1 cm in length, and their long axis is oriented parallel to the long axis of the bone (Fig. 2–9). An osteon consists of a central canal, called a *haversian canal,* which contains one or two capillaries and, occasionally, a nerve fiber. Around each canal are 8 to 15 concentric bone lamellae, and osteocytes in their lacunae are scattered throughout. The architecture of an osteon, with a central canal surrounded by concentric lamellae of bone, permits each osteocyte to be no further than 0.1 to 0.2 mm away from a blood vessel. Cancellous bone, like compact bone, is also lamellar and contains numerous cement lines. However, in contrast to compact bone, complete osteons are not usually present due to the thinness of the trabeculae.

In addition to the longitudinally oriented blood vessels in haversian canals, cortical bone contains another system of blood vessels. These blood vessels, present in channels called *Volkmann's canals,* run perpendicular to the osteons and connect the haversian canals with the marrow cavity or the periosteum.

The bone packets between the osteons, known as interstitial systems, connect the osteons like a mosaic. The interstitial systems and osteons are outlined by thin basophilic lines, known either as *cement lines* or *remodeling lines* (Fig. 2–10). These lines are evidence of prior remodeling cycles and indicate that the bone is mature.

The bulk of compact bone is composed of osteons and interstitial systems. However, the outermost and innermost portions of the cortex consist of bone lamellae arranged

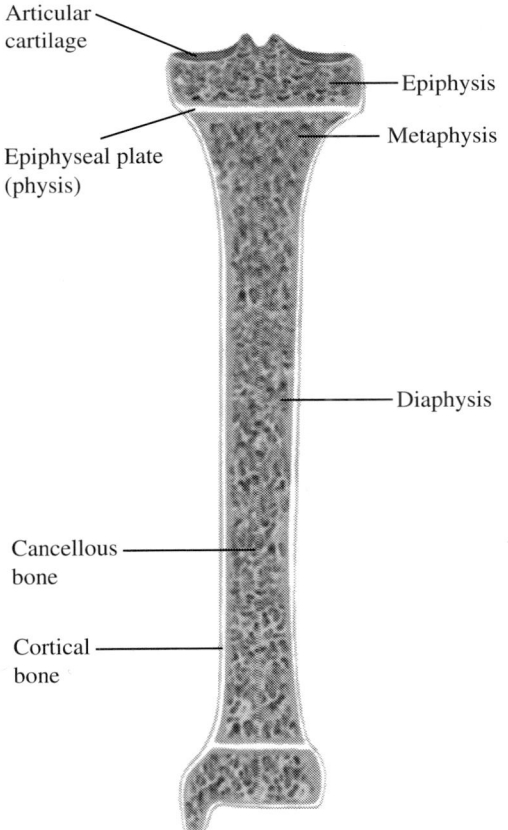

Figure 2-5 ■ The zones of a long bone.

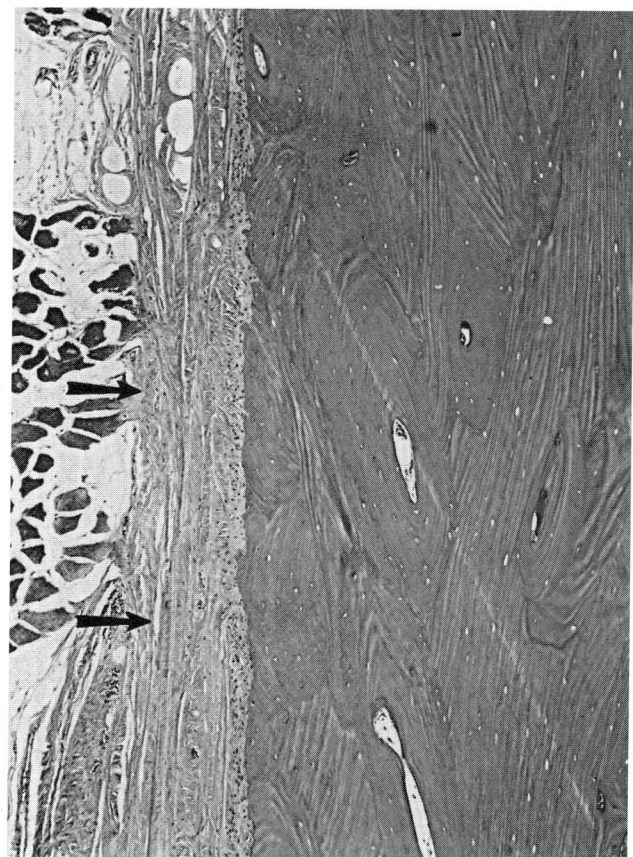

Figure 2-6 ■ Photomicrograph of dense cortical bone. A fibrous tissue membrane, the periosteum, is adjacent to one surface *(arrows)*.

Figure 2-7 ■ Photomicrograph of dense compact bone. Many parallel lamellae are present.

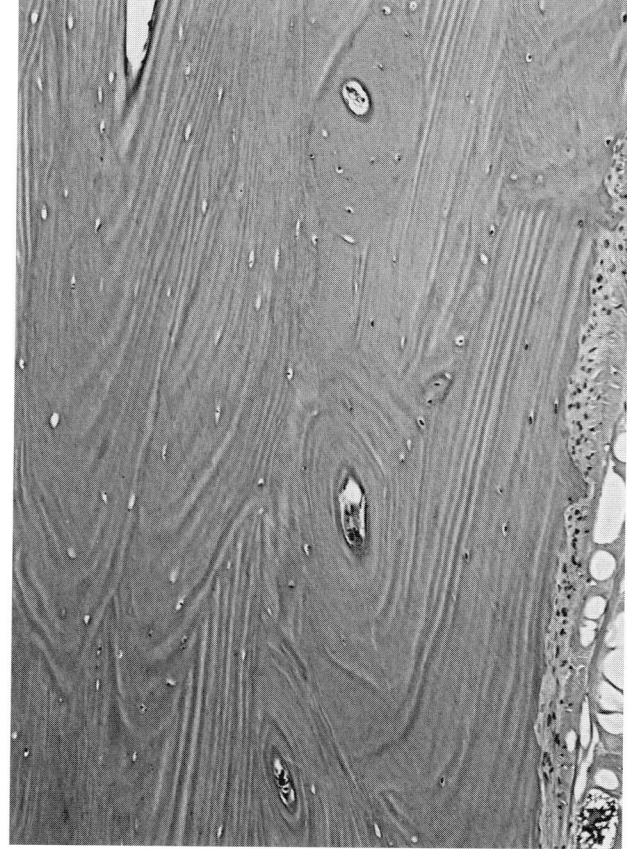

ANATOMY AND PHYSIOLOGY OF BONE

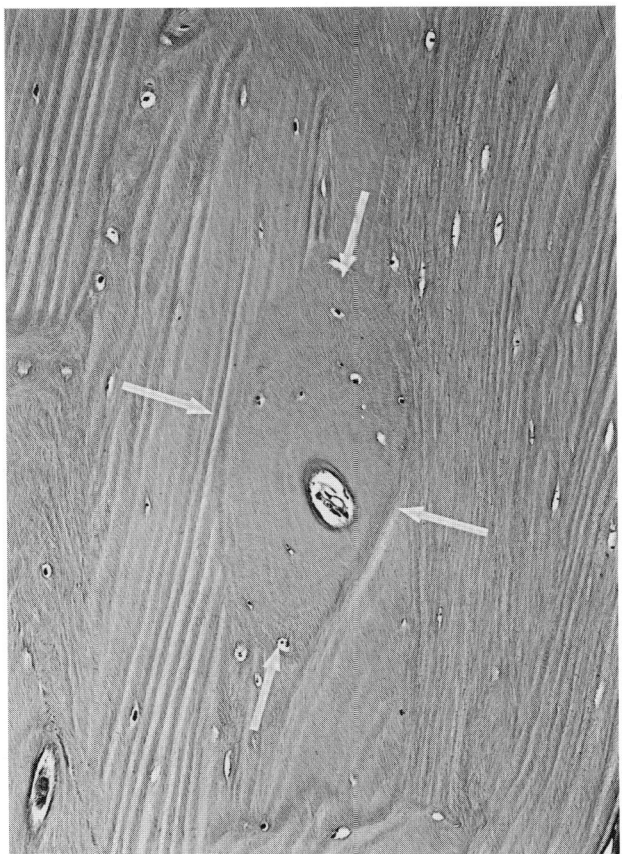

Figure 2-8 ▪ Photomicrograph of dense compact bone showing an osteon *(outlined by arrows)*. In the center of the osteon is a haversian canal. Many lacunae, containing osteocytes, are present in the compact bone.

circumferentially around the bone shaft. These are known as the outer and inner circumferential lamellae.

The Cells of Bone

Osteoblasts

Osteoblasts are the cells that synthesize the organic bone matrix. They are most easily recognized when they are in a row depositing a seam of matrix, known as *osteoid* (Fig. 2–11). Osteoblasts are cuboidal or low columnar cells connected to each other by short cytoplasmic processes. Each osteoblast is polarized so that the nucleus, with a single prominent nucleolus, is at the end of the cell farthest from the bone surface. Osteoblasts have a prominent endoplasmic reticulum and Golgi apparatus, features characteristic of protein-secreting cells. The Golgi apparatus is usually visible with routine H & E stains as an amphophilic area between the nucleus and the bone. This area resembles the paranuclear hof of a plasma cell. Mature osteoblasts are not capable of mitotic division. At the molecular level, a distinguishing feature of osteoblasts (and their precursors) is the presence of receptors for 1,25 $(OH)_2$ vitamin D and parathyroid hormone.

In addition to bone matrix, osteoblasts synthesize the enzyme *alkaline phosphatase*. This enzyme can be demonstrated in the cytoplasm of osteoblasts by special histochemical stains. The alkaline phosphatase synthesized by osteoblasts is similar to the alkaline phosphatase produced by the liver and kidney. Although needed locally for the mineralization process, some osteoblast alkaline phosphatase escapes into the serum. Therefore, increased serum levels, indicating increased osteoblastic activity, suggest certain disease processes. For example, serum alkaline phosphatase is elevated in such disorders as Paget's disease and bone-forming neoplasms.

Origin of Osteoblasts. Osteoblasts are the final stage of differentiation of a pluripotential stem cell in the bone marrow. The same stem cell also differentiates into marrow stromal elements such as fibroblasts, chondroblasts, and adipocytes. The signal for the stem cell to differentiate into an osteoblast is carried by local growth factors such as transforming growth factor β (TGF-β) and bone morphogenic protein (BMP).

Preosteoblasts are an intermediate stage of differentiation between the stem cell and the mature osteoblast. This stage of differentiation lasts 2 or 3 days. Preosteoblasts, although not easily distinguishable from other stromal precursor cells, have pale-staining oval or elongated nuclei and have faintly acidophilic cytoplasm. The presence of intracellular alkaline phosphatase helps identify these cells as osteoblast precursors. Like fully differentiated osteoblasts, preosteoblasts also have receptors for 1,25 $(OH)_2$ vitamin D and parathormone. Unlike mature osteoblasts, however, preosteoblasts are capable of mitotic division.

Osteocytes

Osteocytes, the most abundant cell type of bone, originate from osteoblasts. The life span of a row of osteoblasts averages about 6 months. During active bone formation, 10 to 15% of the osteoblasts are entombed in the newly formed bone matrix. Once entombed, the cells are known as osteocytes. When bone formation is complete, the remaining osteoblasts, those not entrapped in bone, flatten out and line the bone surface. These cells, although technically inactive osteoblasts, are called *lining cells*. Although they no longer secrete osteoid, they remain sensitive to parathyroid hormone and vitamin D.

Osteocytes are rounded cells with an oval nucleus and scanty cytoplasm. They are surrounded by bone and reside in lacunae, which are approximately 15 μm in diameter. A feature of osteocytes, best seen with the electron microscope, is the presence of long cytoplasmic processes that radiate from the cell body. The processes pass through the canaliculi in the mineralized bone and connect with the processes of other osteocytes by gap junctions. They also connect with processes of the lining cells. Thus, osteocytes and lining cells form a vast network of cell-to-cell connections known as the *osteocytic membrane system* (Fig. 2–12).

The osteocytic membrane system has two important functions. First, the system regulates calcium ion flow in and out

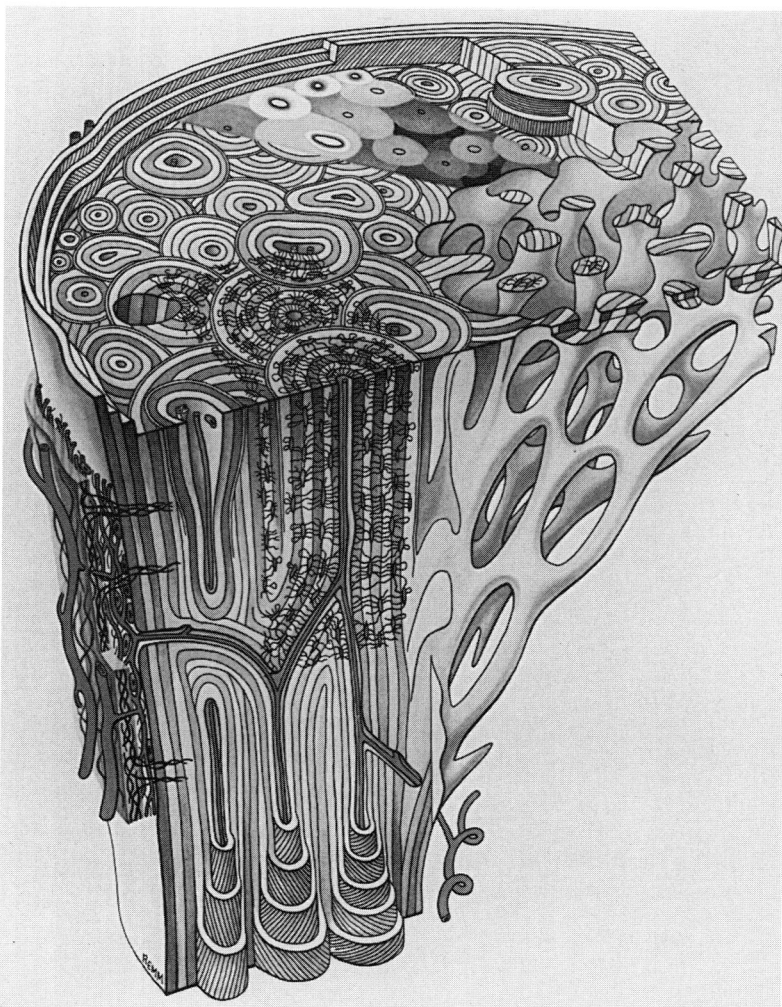

Figure 2-9 ■ Compact and cancellous bone. The osteons with their haversian canals are oriented parallel to the long axis of the bone. Volkmann's canals, containing blood vessels, penetrate the osteons perpendicular to the long axis of the bone. The cancellous bone is continuous with the inner surface of the cortex. (From *Gray's Anatomy,* 35th ed. London, Churchill Livingstone, 1980).

of the mineralized matrix, a function due to the osteocyte's sensitivity to parathyroid hormone. Binding with this hormone causes osteocytes to pump calcium from the mineral into the extracellular fluid by a process known as *osteocytic osteolysis.* As a result, serum calcium rises almost immediately in response to parathyroid hormone before osteoclasts can be recruited to digest bone.

The second function of the osteocytic membrane system is the transmission of electrical signals in bone. Stress and strain during daily activities cause bone deformation, and deformation of mineralized organic matrix produces small piezoelectric currents and streaming potentials. This electrical activity is important in maintaining balanced bone remodeling and increasing remodeling in areas subject to maximal stress and strain.

Osteoclasts

Osteoclasts are cells that resorb bone by enzymatic degradation. They are multinucleated giant cells 20 to 100 μm in diameter and are usually found on the bone surface in resorption craters known as *Howship's lacunae* or in deep resorption cavities called *cutting cones* (Fig. 2–13). Osteoclasts are rarely seen in routine histologic preparations of normal bone. However, their number increases in diseases characterized by increased bone turnover.

The cytoplasmic features of osteoclasts, which enable them to resorb bone are best seen with the electron microscope. The first feature is the ruffled border, a specialized area of the cytoplasmic membrane adjacent to the bone surface. The ruffled border consists of numerous fine, finger-like cytoplasmic projections that form an immense surface area to carry out resorption. Beneath the ruffled border is a clear zone devoid of organelles but rich in actin filaments. This zone enables the osteoclast to tightly affix to bone and seal off the ruffled border to form a microenvironment for bone digestion.

Another feature of osteoclasts is their cytoplasmic lysosomes. These lysosomes contain proteases as well as *tartrate-resistant acid phosphatase,* an enzyme specific to os-

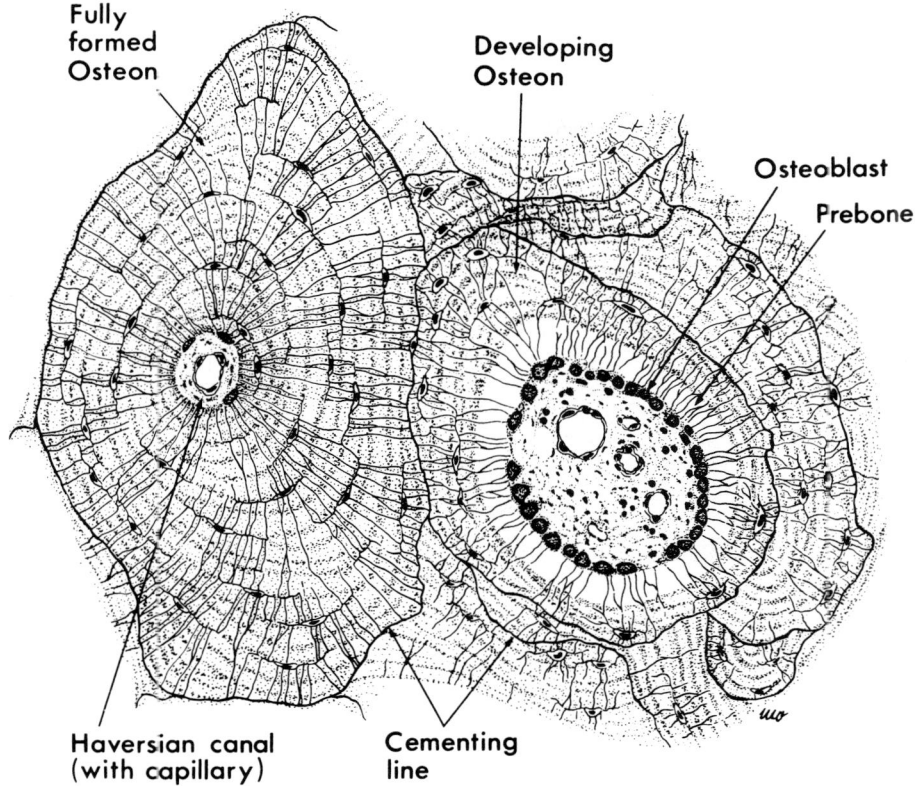

Figure 2-10 ▪ Osteons. The osteons are outlined by cementing lines. (From Cormack, D.: *Ham's Histology,* 9th ed. Philadelphia, Lippincott, 1987.)

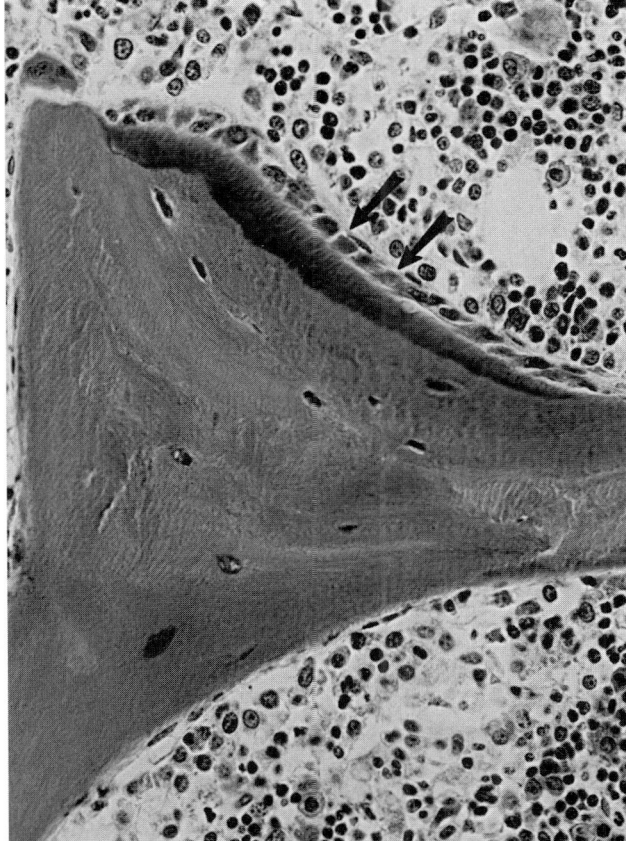

Figure 2-11 ▪ Photomicrograph of cancellous bone. One surface of the bone is lined with an osteoid seam, which is being synthesized by a row of osteoblasts *(arrows).*

32 ANATOMY AND PHYSIOLOGY OF BONE

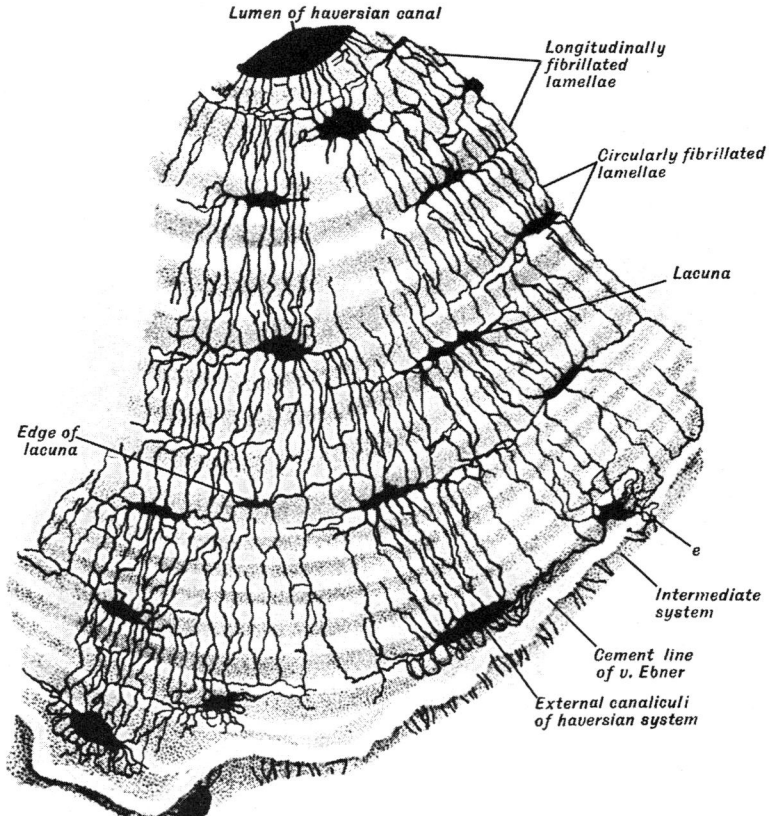

Figure 2-12 ■ A portion of an osteon. The lacunae are interconnected by many long canaliculi. (From Bloom, W., and Fawcett, D. W.: *A Textbook of Histology,* 12th ed. New York, Chapman & Hall, 1994.)

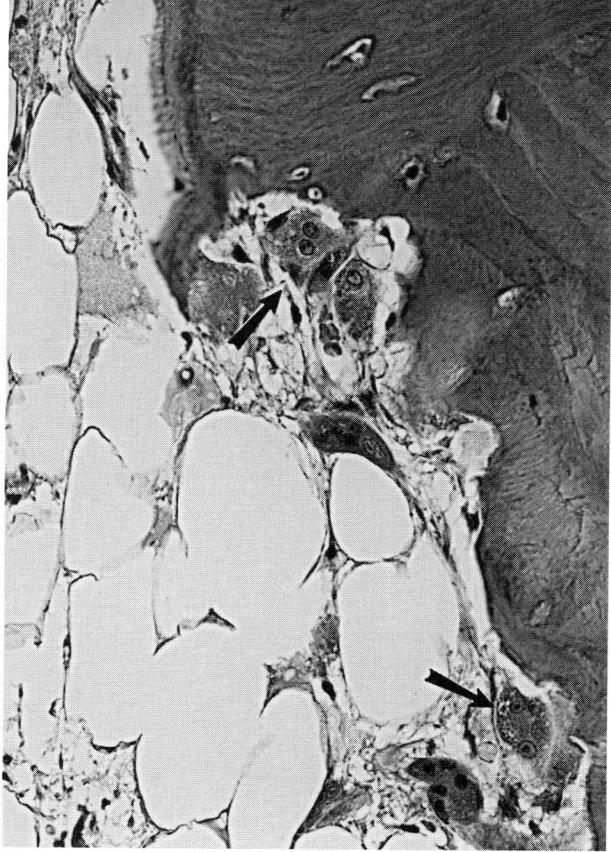

Figure 2-13 ■ Photomicrograph of cancellous bone being eroded by osteoclasts. The osteoclasts are multinucleated cells present in Howship's lacunae *(arrows).*

teoclasts. Osteoclasts and their precursors are strongly positive with histochemical stains for tartrate-resistant acid phosphatase, a reaction that helps the pathologist identify them in tissue sections. The role of tartrate-resistant acid phosphatase in bone resorption is not clear. It is the lysosomal proteases in the lysosomes that resorb the bone matrix.

Bone resorption takes place in several steps. Osteoclasts must be directly adjacent to mineralized matrix for resorption to begin. Therefore, the layer of lining cells must contract and a thin layer of nonmineralized protein on the bone surface must be digested. Contraction of the lining cells is a result of either systemic factors, such as parathyroid hormone, or local factors. The lining cells then secrete a protease to digest the unmineralized layer of matrix.

Once exposed to a mineralized surface, osteoclasts attach themselves and secrete protons that acidify the microenvironment between the projections of the ruffled border and the bone surface. The acid environment dissolves the mineral from the matrix; then proteases released from the lysosomes digest the matrix proteins. In the late stages of resorption, osteoclasts undergo fission to form multiple mononuclear bone–resorbing cells that finalize the resorption process.

Origin of Osteoclasts. Mature multinucleated osteoclasts form by fusion of mononuclear osteoclast precursors. The osteoclast precursors, like preosteoblasts, originate from bone marrow stem cells. However, osteoclasts are the end product of a completely different cell lineage. Osteoclasts are derived from precursors that also differentiate into monocytes, macrophages, and other peripheral blood leukocytes. In fact, the osteoclast precursors that fuse to form osteoclasts express monocyte or macrophage markers, such as CD45 (the leukocyte common antigen), CD13, CD15, and CD54. Vitamin D is required for the fusion of preosteoclasts.

Increased numbers of osteoclasts are found in patients with high levels of parathyroid hormone. However, osteoclasts or their committed precursors do not have receptors for this hormone. Therefore, the stimulus for osteoclasts to resorb bone is mediated by osteoblasts. Osteoblasts do have parathyroid hormone receptors, and they transfer a signal to local osteoclast precursors. In addition to parathyroid hormone, other compounds such as interleukins, prostaglandins, and vitamin D also stimulate osteoclast formation, but osteoblasts are necessary intermediaries for the action of all of these compounds as well.

Although lacking receptors for parathyroid hormone, osteoclasts do have receptors for calcitonin. This hormone inhibits osteoclast function by causing their retraction from the bone surface. However, this effect is short lived. Osteoclasts continuously exposed to calcitonin escape from the hormonal effects due to downregulation of the calcitonin receptors.

The Organic Matrix of Bone—Osteoid

Collagen

The organic matrix of bone, synthesized by osteoblasts, is called *osteoid*. This substance is 90% collagen; the remaining 10% is a mixture of noncollagenous proteins and proteoglycans. Collagens are fibrillar proteins composed of three polypeptide chains, called alpha chains, which are arranged in a *triple helix*. All collagens have a repeating triplet of amino acids, with the order glycine-X-Y. In most collagens, the X is often proline and the Y is often hydroxyproline. The repetitive sequence of a glycine at every third amino acid and frequent prolines and hydroxyprolines is necessary for the molecule to form the triple helix.

At least 15 types of collagen are present in varying amounts in different tissues. The collagen of osteoid is almost exclusively type I collagen, the most abundant collagen in the body. Type I collagen is also present in skin, tendons, and ligaments. However, in these nonosseous locations, type I collagen has slightly different post-translational modifications.

Type I collagen has two identical $alpha_1$ chains and another structurally different $alpha_2$ chain. Two genes, therefore, are necessary to synthesize type I collagen, and one of these genes must synthesize twice as much protein as the other.

Many steps, both intracellular and extracellular, are involved in the synthesis of type I collagen (Fig. 2–14). The first step is the synthesis of the alpha amino acid chains, known as protocollagen. Then, after synthesis, a variety of intracellular post-translational modifications, almost 100 in all, occur in each chain. The principal modification is the hydroxylation of proline and lysine to hydroxyproline and hydroxylysine. The two $alpha_1$ chains and the single $alpha_2$ chain are then able to form the triple helix. At this point, the compound, known as procollagen, is excreted from the cell.

Modifications continue in the extracellular space. First, the procollagen molecule is cleaved at both the N terminal and C terminal ends, removing as much as one third of the protein. The remaining portion, the collagen molecule, is then able to self-aggregate into multiple long, parallel lines forming a *collagen fibril*. Within each fibril, the collagen molecules are staggered one quarter of their length relative to the adjacent collagen molecule. In addition, gaps are present between each molecule, forming "hole zones" in the fibril. The quarter stagger arrangement and the hole zones create the 64-nm periodicity seen when collagen fibrils are viewed with the electron microscope.

After the aggregation of collagen molecules into a collagen fibril, the final stage of synthesis occurs. Aldehyde cross-links form between adjacent collagen molecules. These cross-links, occurring between lysine and hydroxylysine amino acids, stabilize the collagen fibril.

Breakdown of Collagen. When bone collagen is broken down by osteoclasts, various portions of the collagen molecules are released into the serum and excreted in the urine. Measurement of these breakdown products is a useful clinical tool to quantify the rate of bone resorption. One such breakdown product is *hydroxyproline*. The intracellular hydroxylation of proline is unique to bone collagen. Once released from the collagen molecule during bone resorption, hydroxyproline cannot be reused. Therefore, the presence of

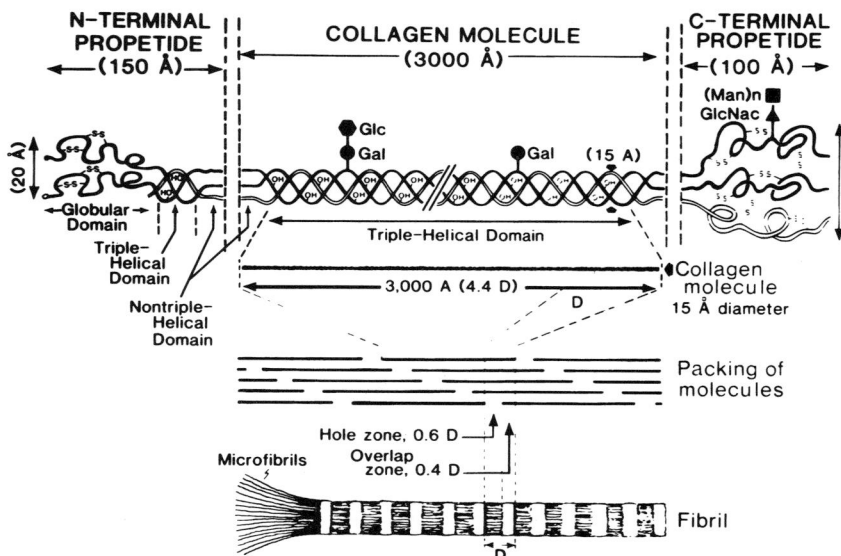

Figure 2-14 ■ The collagen molecule and its orientation in collagen fibrils. The quarter staggered arrangement of the collagen molecules creates holes in the collagen fibrils. (From Riggs, L. B., Melton, L. J. (Eds.): *Osteoporosis. Etiology, Diagnosis, and Management.* Philadelphia, Lippincott, 1988.)

increased levels of urinary hydroxyproline indicate increased osteoclastic bone resorption. Another product of collagen digestion that can be measured in the urine is collagen cross-links. The aldehyde cross-links between the lysine and hydroxylysine molecules are resistant to breakdown. Therefore, when the collagen molecule is digested, the lysines, with their interconnecting aldehyde bonds, form a compound unique to bone known as *pyridinoline.* Increased urinary levels of pyridinoline indicate increased bone resorption. For example, in Paget's disease and hyperparathyroidism, both conditions of increased bone resorption, urinary pyridinoline cross-links are elevated.

Noncollagenous Proteins

Ten percent of the organic matrix of bone consists of numerous noncollagenous proteins (Table 2–1). Although most of these proteins have been well characterized biochemically, their exact function in the organic matrix is not fully understood. Some are probably regulators of bone turnover. Others are undoubtedly important in the mineralization process and may be either initiators of mineralization or regulators of crystal growth. Most noncollagenous proteins are degraded within about a year after bone is mineralized.

Osteocalcin is one of the best characterized noncollagenous proteins. This single-chain protein is also known as bone Gla-protein because of vitamin K–dependent, post-translational carboxylation of glutamic acid residues. Osteocalcin is synthesized by osteoblasts and secreted as a component of osteoid. Vitamin D causes increased synthesis of this protein. The role of osteocalcin is obscure. However, because osteocalcin is known to be chemotactic for osteoclasts, it may help initiate bone turnover. After synthesis, some osteocalcin escapes into the serum, where it can be measured by radioimmunoassay. Therefore, serum osteocalcin levels reflect the level of bone formation. For example, levels are increased in diseases characterized by high bone turnover, such as high-turnover osteoporosis or renal osteodystrophy. Osteocalcin is unique to bone and composes about 15% of the noncollagenous proteins.

Osteonectin, another well-characterized protein, also comprises about 15% of the noncollagenous bone proteins. Osteonectin is a phosphorylated glycoprotein that strongly binds to both collagen and apatite crystals. This binding property suggests that it functions as an initiator or moderator of mineralization. Osteonectin is not unique to bone—it is present in greatly reduced concentrations in other tissues, such as kidney, salivary gland, and platelets. Osteonectin may be identified in tissues by immunohistochemical techniques. Some investigators have suggested that its presence in neoplastic cells indicates osteoblastic differentiation. Although osteoid-producing neoplasms do contain osteonectin, its presence in cartilage neoplasms and other bone tumors limits its diagnostic usefulness.

The bone matrix sialoproteins are also present in osteoid. These include *osteopontin* and *bone sialoprotein.* A particular amino acid sequence in these proteins allows them to bind to cell surfaces and facilitate attachment of the osteoblasts to the bone.

Proteoglycans, extremely abundant in cartilage matrix, are also present in bone matrix. Two bone proteoglycans are biglycan and decorin. The function of these proteoglycans is

Table 2-1 ■ **NONCOLLAGENOUS PROTEINS OF BONE**

Octeocalcin
Osteonectin
Osteopontin
Bone sialoprotein
Proteoglycans (biglycan, decorin)
Growth factors
Serum proteins (albumin, immunoglobulin)

unknown. However, regulation of collagen fibril growth is one proposed role.

Another group of noncollagenous matrix proteins are *growth factors*. Many types are present in bone. Growth factors are small proteins that serve as signaling agents between cells. These include insulin-like growth factor (IGF), TGF-β, platelet derived growth factor, fibroblast growth factor, and various BMPs. Some of these growth factors are secreted by osteoblasts. In addition, some originate from the serum and find their way into the osteoid from nearby blood vessels or bone marrow cells. Although growth factors compose less than 1% of the noncollagenous matrix proteins, they play critical roles. For example, one proposed role of TGF-β is the recruitment of osteoblasts in the remodeling process. Growth factors are also necessary to repair bone after fractures.

A final group of proteins, comprising about 25% of the total of noncollagenous bone proteins, originate in the serum. These include albumin and immunoglobulin G. The function, if any, of these serum proteins is not known.

Mineralization of Osteoid

During bone remodeling, osteoblasts deposit a layer of osteoid about 10 μm thick on preexisting bone. This layer is known as an osteoid seam. Approximately 20 days later, the osteoid begins to mineralize. During this interval, known as the mineralization lag time, changes in osteoid cause the ionic calcium and phosphate in the extracellular fluid to precipitate. The exact nature of these osteoid changes is unknown. In fact, the entire process of mineralization is poorly understood. However, two mechanisms of mineralization have been proposed. In the first proposed mechanism, mineralization is initiated by *matrix vesicles*. In the second, a protein unique to osteoid causes mineral to precipitate. In both mechanisms, alkaline phosphatase plays a crucial role. The calcium/phosphate product in the extracellular fluid is normally high enough to allow crystals to form anywhere in the body. However, mineralization is prohibited by various inhibitors, particularly pyrophosphate. Alkaline phosphatase, secreted by the osteoblasts, hydrolyzes pyrophosphate and allows the calcium and phosphate ions to precipitate in the osteoid.

Matrix vesicles are important initiators of mineralization in epiphyseal plate cartilage and woven bone. Matrix vesicles begin as buds of cytoplasmic membrane on the surface of chondrocytes and osteoblasts. The buds are squeezed off and become free in the extracellular matrix. As seen with electron micrographs, matrix vesicles are extracellular membrane-bound structures, 1 to 2 μm in diameter. Mineralization begins inside these structures because they contain high concentrations of alkaline phosphase. Once formed, crystals penetrate the matrix vesicle membrane and propagate in the extracellular space.

Matrix vesicles play a less important role in the mineralization of lamellar bone. In lamellar bone, mineralization begins within the collagen fibril. Electron micrographs demonstrate that mineralization begins in the "hole zones" left open by the quarter stagger arrangement of the collagen molecules. Mineral appears in each hole zone independently, precipitated most probably by a calcium-binding phosphoprotein. Eventually, the entire collagen fibril becomes encrusted by mineral. Although matrix vesicles are present in the noncollagenous matrix of lamellar bone, mineralization of the collagen fibrils proceeds independently.

The mineralization of osteoid is an evolving process, both quantitatively and qualitatively. First, it takes about a year for newly formed bone to become fully mineralized. After the first crystals appear, mineralization proceeds rapidly for several days until the bone contains 75% of its total mineral. Then, mineral is gradually added over the next year. As a result, older bone contains more mineral than newly formed bone.

The quality of the mineral also changes. Most of the mineral in bone is crystalline calcium hydroxyapatite ($Ca_{10}[PO_4]_6[OH]_2$). Mature apatite crystals are long, flat plates measuring $400 \times 100 \times 20$ angstroms. However, the initial apatite crystals are very poorly formed. In addition, the early mineral contains other calcium compounds, such as amorphous calcium salts and calcium brushite ($Ca\,H\,PO_4\,H_2O$). With time, much of the amorphous calcium is gradually incorporated into apatite crystals. However, some amorphous calcium remains and is the probable source of exchangeable calcium needed for rapid adjustments in the extracellular fluid.

Although the initial apatite crystals are poorly formed, with time they become more crystalline. In addition, other changes occur. For example, the calcium-to-phosphorus ratio increases in the crystal, and water is lost. Thus, older apatite crystals are harder, but they are also more brittle.

Apatite crystals contain other compounds besides calcium and phosphorus. For example, the crystals may adsorb sodium, magnesium, potassium, citrate, and carbonate ions. In addition, various cations or anions may substitute in the crystal. Fluoride, for example, may replace OH and render the crystal harder and less soluble. Also, calcium may be replaced by heavy metals such as strontium, plutonium, lead, uranium, or gold.

A useful property of the apatite crystal is its ability to chelate the antibiotic tetracycline. Any tetracycline present in the extracellular fluid at the time of mineralization chelates with the crystals and becomes trapped by the osteoid. Because tetracycline fluoresces under ultraviolet light, the amount of tetracycline attached to bone can be quantified by fluorescent microscopy, and the rate of mineralization can be calculated. This property is useful in the study of metabolic bone disease.

Bone Remodeling

Bone remodeling is a process by which bone is removed in tiny increments and then replaced by new bone. It is a normal process that occurs throughout life. Just as other tissues, such as intestinal mucosa and skin, are gradually removed and replaced, the skeleton is also continuously replacing itself at an average rate of about 18% per year.

Theoretically, therefore, the entire skeleton is replaced every 5 years. However, bone remodeling rates vary in different parts of the skeleton. For example, remodeling is much more active in the iliac crest than in the distal femur. Rates also vary according to the types of bone, cancellous bone being much more active. Cancellous bone replaces itself at a rate of 25% per year, whereas only 2% of cortical bone is replaced per year.

Therefore, in any area of bone, only 5 to 15% of the bone surfaces are remodeling. Because it occurs focally, the remodeling process of nondiseased bones is not obvious on routine H & E preparations.

Bone remodeling has three important functions. First, remodeling removes injured bone. Aging bone becomes weaker, probably a result of less water content and changes in the collagen. The resulting brittleness leads to microcracks in both the cortical and cancellous bone. Fortunately, the remodeling process removes these damaged areas and adds new bone. Because microcracks occur even with normal skeletal stress, cessation of the remodeling process, which removes the damaged areas, would theoretically lead to skeletal failure in an estimated 2 years.

A second function of remodeling is the reinforcement of bone in areas subject to increased stress. Remodeling is more active in these areas so that the older, more brittle bone is replaced more rapidly. Therefore, microcracks are less likely to occur.

A final function of bone remodeling is its participation in calcium homeostasis. The temporary release of calcium during remodeling may be necessary when the homeostatic system of calcium balance is stressed, particularly during a hypocalcemic challenge. About 500 mg of calcium is immediately available as a result of the remodeling process. However, the calcium released in the initial stages of remodeling is always replaced in the final stages. Therefore, remodeling probably plays very little role in long-term calcium balance.

Bone remodeling is carried out by the bone cells (Fig. 2–15). First, a team of osteoclasts resorb a cavity of bone, and then a team of osteoblasts fill the cavity with new bone. Many teams, known as bone remodeling units (BMUs), work closely together.

A remodeling cycle may be divided into four stages: activation, resorption, reversal, and formation. During the *activation* phase, osteoclasts are recruited to the resorption site. First, the lining cells of the bone surface must shrink, and the thin layer of unmineralized osteoid on the bone surface must be removed to allow the osteoclasts access to the mineralized surface. Then, a signal causes bone marrow macrophages to migrate to the bone surface where they fuse to become osteoclasts.

The exact nature of the activation signal is not known. However, two theories have been proposed. One theory suggests that the signal is a protein, such as osteocalcin,

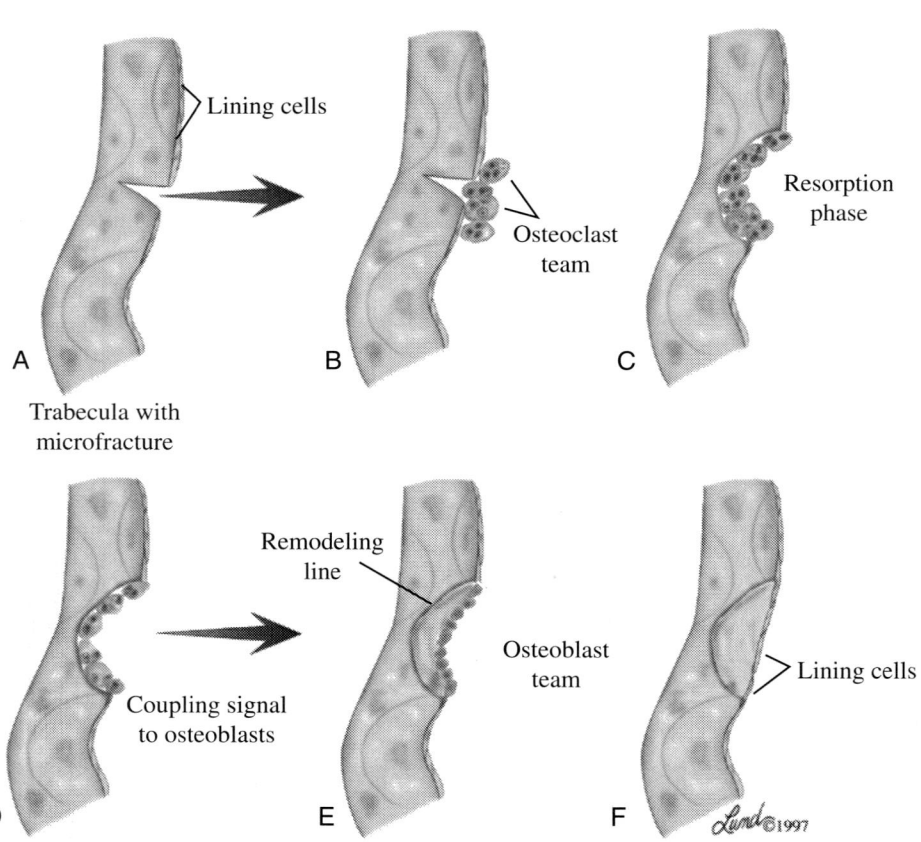

Figure 2-15 ■ Bone remodeling. **A,** A microfracture in a trabecula signals for a team of osteoclasts. **B,** An osteoclast team appears after the lining cells have retracted. **C,** Osteoclasts begin the resorption phase and remove the portion of bone containing the microfracture. **D,** After the osteoclasts have done their work, a coupling signal to osteoblasts is made. **E,** Osteoblasts fill up the resorption cavity with new bone. The interface of the resorption cavity and new bone results in a cement line. **F,** The osteoblasts have completed their work, and the surface is again lined by lining cells.

which is released from the matrix, possibly after a microcrack. This protein then causes macrophage migration. Another theory suggests that electric streaming potentials, known to occur when bone deforms, initiate resorption. The streaming potentials, transmitted by the osteocytic membrane system, cause lining cells to summon the osteoclasts. According to this theory, the stress and strain on bone control the remodeling process.

After activation, the *resorption phase* begins. A group of osteoclasts begins to remove bone and forms a resorption cavity. A resorption cavity in cancellous bone is about 50 μm deep. In cortical bone, the cavity, known as a cutting cone, may be 2.5 mm deep. In the final stages of resorption, osteoclasts undergo fission to form mononuclear osteoclastic cells, which complete the bone removal. The entire resorption phase lasts about 1 month.

To conclude the resorption phase, the mononuclear osteoclasts secrete a collagen-poor and proteoglycan-rich substance that "glues" the new bone into the newly formed cavity. This substance, easily recognized as a blue line, is known as a remodeling line. The number of remodeling lines in a given area of bone reflects the amount of prior bone remodeling. In fact, because remodeling continues throughout life, the number of lines suggests the age of a person. By counting remodeling lines in an unknown bone specimen, forensic osteologists and anthropologists are able to estimate the age of the person at death.

The next phase of remodeling is the *reversal phase*. During this phase, which lasts 7 to 14 days, signals are sent to osteoblasts, attracting them to the resorption cavity. The signaling of osteoblasts is called *coupling*. However, the signal responsible for coupling, like the signal that activates resorption, has not been definitely identified. Likely candidates are growth factors released from bone matrix during resorption. These growth factors include IGF and TGF-β.

After the coupling signal reaches the osteoblasts, the final phase of remodeling, the *formation* phase, begins. A team of osteoblasts line the inside of the resorption cavity and fill it in with new bone. In cancellous bone, the cavity is filled completely. However, in cortical bone, the central region is left unossified. This unossified region becomes the haversian canal of a newly formed osteon. The formation period lasts about 5 months. Thus, the entire remodeling cycle takes a little over 6 months.

In a healthy adult, the remodeling process does not alter the mass of the skeleton. The amount of bone formed equals the amount resorbed. However, as discussed in Chapter 4, certain metabolic bone diseases are characterized by a disturbance in this balance. A slight imbalance in favor of resorption ultimately, over many remodeling cycles, decreases the bone mass and leads to skeletal fragility.

DEVELOPMENT OF BONE

Ossification

The organic matrix of bone, known as osteoid, is synthesized by osteoblasts. The osteoblasts, which derive from differentiation of primitive mesenchymal cells, deposit bone in two ways. In the first way, osteoid is secreted directly in loose fibrous connective tissue, a process known as *intramembranous ossification*. In the second way, osteoid is deposited on scaffolds of cartilage, a process known as *endochondral ossification*. Both manners of bone deposition are necessary for the growth and development of the skeleton. In addition, both intramembranous and endochondral ossification are active in reparative reactions of bone, particularly fracture healing.

Intramembranous Ossification

The flat bones of the skull, part of the mandible, and part of the clavicle form by intramembranous ossification. In addition, thickening of the cortex of bone is due to intramembranous ossification beneath the periosteum. Therefore, intramembranous bone formation is a mechanism for increasing the diameter of bone.

Intramembranous ossification begins in loose, vascular connective tissue. First, thin strands of eosinophilic osteoid appear. Soon thereafter, spindle-shaped connective tissue cells become plump and line the surface of the osteoid strands (Fig. 2–16). These cells, now committed osteoblasts, continue to secrete osteoid to widen the strands (Fig. 2–17). Mineralization of the osteoid occurs shortly after deposition, and the newly formed tissue is now primitive bone. The osteoid strands, known as trabeculae, form a branching and anastomosing network, and the spaces between them are

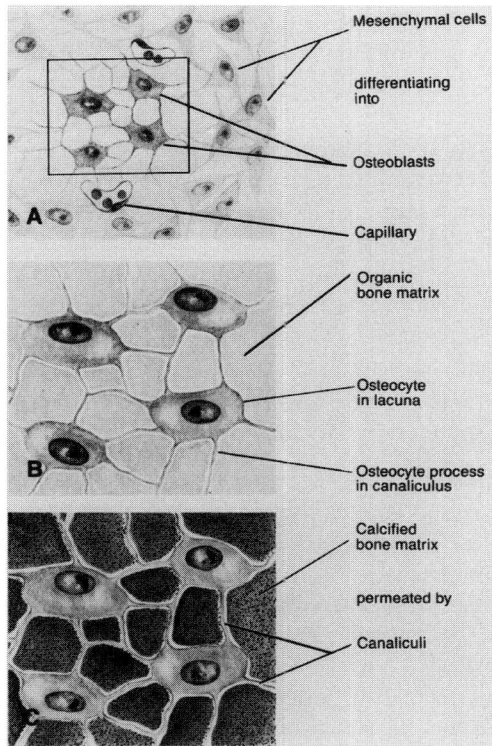

Figure 2–16 ■ Membranous bone formation. (From Cormack, D.: *Ham's Histology*, 9th ed. Philadelphia, Lippincott, 1987.)

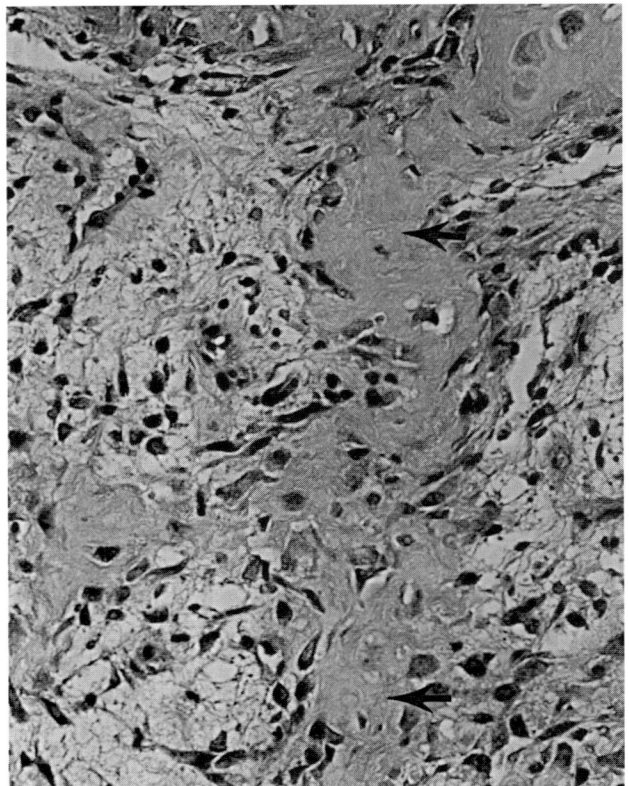

Figure 2-17 ■ Photomicrograph of early membranous bone formation. Pale, organic matrix (osteoid) appears in a background of loose fibrous connective tissue.

filled with vascular connective tissue (Fig. 2–18). As more osteoid is synthesized, the trabeculae become longer and thicker. As a result, many osteoblasts become entombed in the newly secreted osteoid and become osteocytes. Unlike the regular layering of collagen in mature lamellar bone, the collagen fibers in primitive intramembranous bone are haphazardly arranged. The term *woven bone* is used to describe these primitive trabeculae.

Gradually, the woven bone trabeculae thicken, thereby reducing the amount of intertrabecular connective tissue. Thus, primitive compact bone is formed. Gradually, osteoclastic resorption and orderly new bone formation transform woven bone into lamellar bone.

Endochondral Ossification

Endochondral bone formation is a process whereby osteoid is deposited on preexisting cartilage. Most of the skeleton is formed by this process. For example, the bone that forms in the primary and secondary centers of ossification is endochondral bone. Also, continuous endochondral ossification at the epiphyseal plate is responsible for longitudinal bone growth.

Endochondral bone forms after a series of programmed changes in the preexisting cartilage. First, chondrocytes in a distinct zone become hypertrophied. Also, their cytoplasm becomes vacuolated by the accumulation of glycogen, a process that thins the intervening matrix. Then, the cartilage matrix becomes calcified by matrix vesicles originating from the cytoplasmic membranes. This is followed by death of the chondrocytes, which leaves empty spaces between the septae of calcified cartilage, and these spaces are then invaded by blood vessels and adjacent perivascular tissue (Fig. 2–19). This perivascular tissue contains mesenchymal cells that differentiate into osteoblasts. Next, the newly formed osteoblasts secrete a rapidly mineralizing osteoid on the septae of calcified cartilage. Continued osteoid secretion eventually encases the bars of calcified cartilage with new bone. This complex of newly formed bone with a core of calcified cartilage is called *primary spongiosa* (Fig. 2–20). The primary spongiosa is eventually remodeled and replaced by mature lamellar bone.

Centers of Ossification

With the exception of bones in the skull, mandible, and clavicle, the entire skeleton is formed by replacement of cartilage models (Fig. 2–21). Each bone has a cartilage model, although the models of some of the larger flat bones, such as the ilium and scapula, have several parts that later fuse. Ossification begins at genetically predetermined sites in each model. These sites, known as *primary centers of ossification*, become ossified at different points in fetal development, depending on the bone. For example, the primary

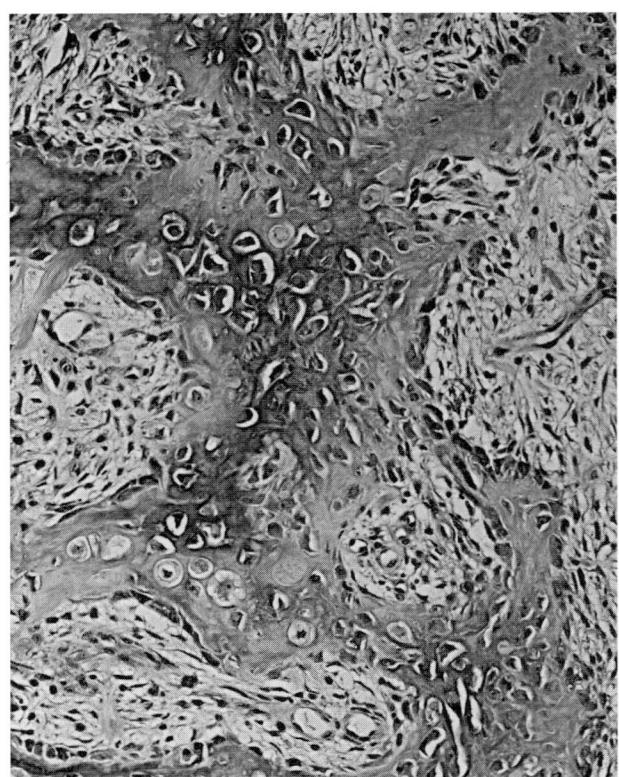

Figure 2-18 ■ Photomicrograph of mineralized membranous bone. The osteoid has entombed numerous osteocytes.

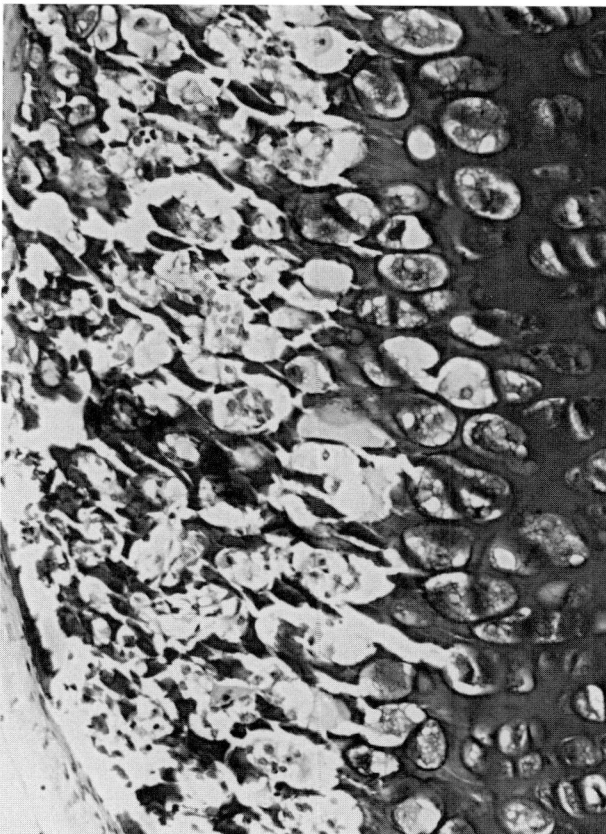

Figure 2-19 ■ Photomicrograph of cartilage with endochondral ossification. The chondrocytes are hypertrophied and undergoing programmed cell death (apoptosis). The cartilage matrix is being calcified.

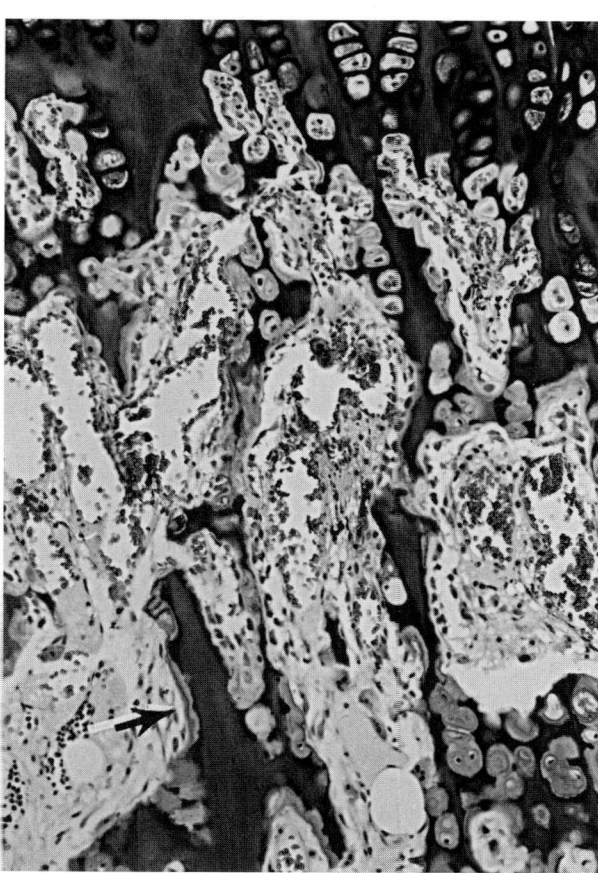

Figure 2-20 ■ Photomicrograph of primary spongiosa. Bars of calcified cartilage are encased by endochondral bone *(arrow)*.

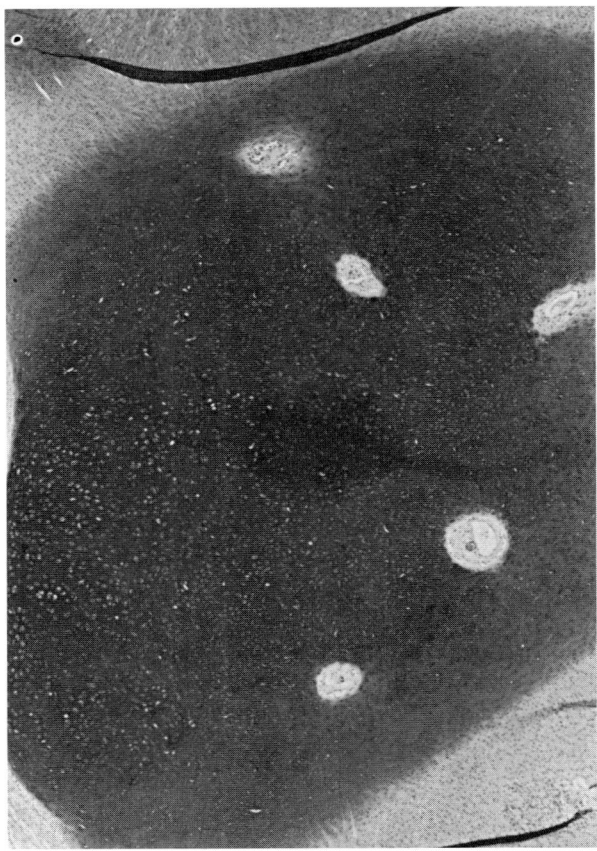

Figure 2-21 ■ Photomicrograph of the cartilage anlage of a vertebral body.

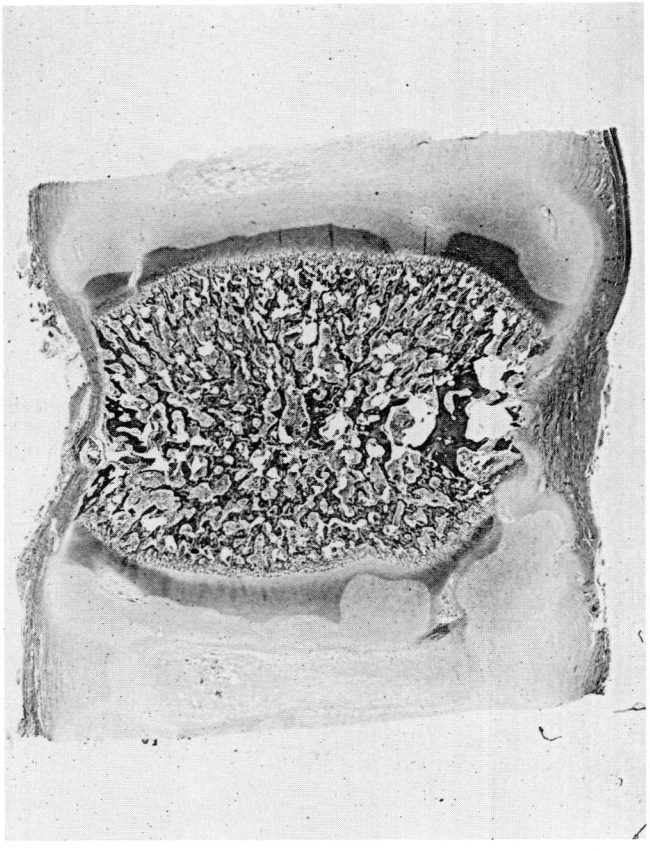

Figure 2-22 ■ Photomicrograph of a primary ossification center of a vertebra.

centers of ossification in the major long bones appear about the third month of fetal life and represent the first evidence of bone formation in the skeleton. Later in fetal life, primary centers of ossification appear in other bones.

Ossification in each primary center has several stages. First, chondrocytes in the center of the model begin to hypertrophy, the first stage of endochondral ossification. About the same time, the mesenchymal sleeve around the cartilage model ossifies, forming a peripheral shell of bone. This bone shell eventually becomes the diaphyseal cortex. Then, as the process of endochondral ossification proceeds, the center of the cartilage model becomes primary spongiosa. Subsequent remodeling hollows the center of the primary spongiosa to form a marrow cavity. The same perivascular tissue that differentiated into osteoblasts during endochondral ossification also differentiates into marrow precursor cells. As fetal development proceeds, the cartilage model grows and the ossification center enlarges (Fig. 2–22).

About the time of birth, secondary (or epiphyseal) ossification centers appear at the ends of the tubular bones (Fig. 2–23). At birth, six epiphyseal centers are already present: the proximal humerus, distal femur, proximal tibia, talus, calcaneus, and cuboid. Thereafter, other secondary centers appear in a specific sequence during infancy and childhood. Almost all are present by about age 17, at which point the secondary centers of ossification for the ischial tuberosity and iliac make their first appearance. The medial clavicle appears last, at about age 20.

The secondary centers of ossification also grow by endochondral ossification. However, the secondary centers, unlike the primary centers, lack a cuff of subperichondral bone. Also, their growth is centripetal rather than longitudinal. Some of the small epiphysioid bones, such as the carpal or tarsal bones, have only one ossification center, which ossifies in the same manner as the secondary center of a long bone.

As ossification continues, the primary and secondary centers grow closer. The outermost layer of cartilage in the

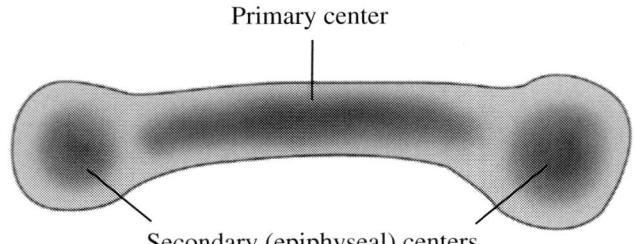

Figure 2-23 ■ A cartilage anlage of a long bone showing a primary ossification center and two secondary ossification centers. (Reprinted by permission of the publisher from THE HUMAN SKELETON by Pat Shipman, Alan Walker, and David Bichell, Cambridge, Mass.: Harvard University Press, Copyright © 1985 by the President and Fellows of Harvard College.)

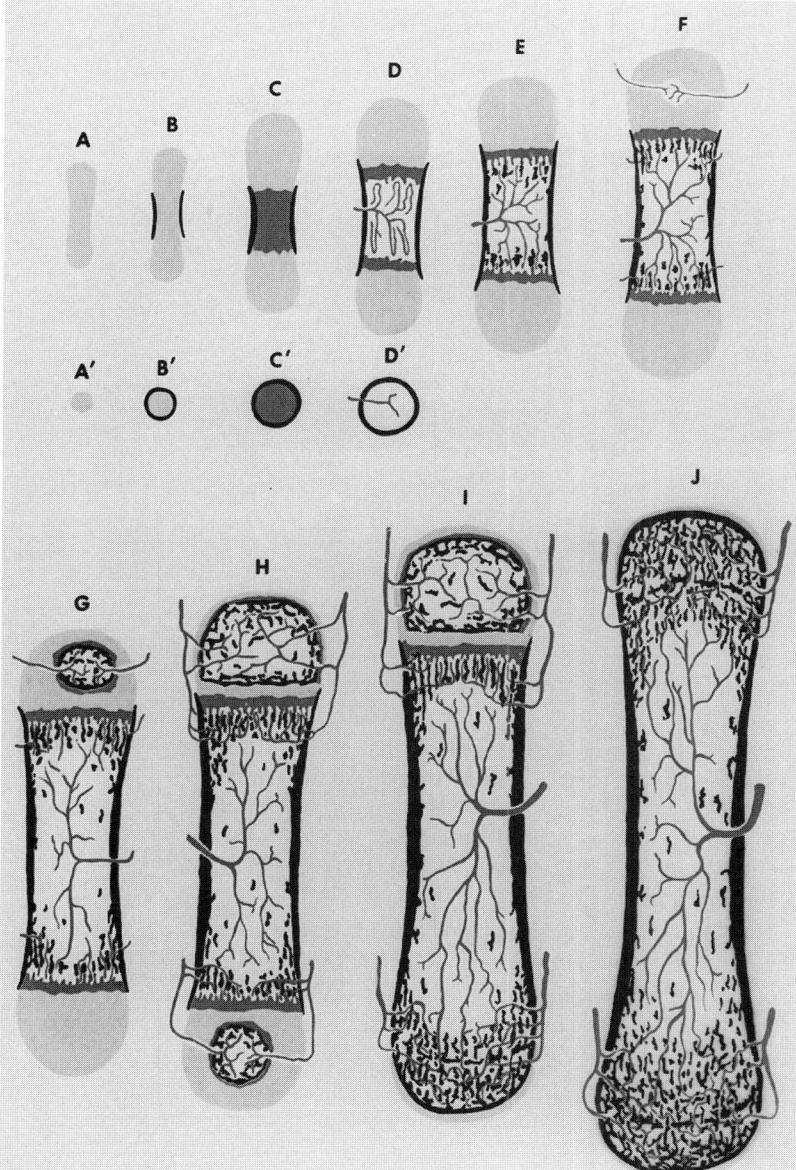

Figure 2-24 ■ The process of ossification. **A,** The cartilage anlage. **B,** A periosteal shell of bone forms. **C,** Cartilage encased in the periosteal bone shell becomes calcified. **D,** Vascular invasion of the calcified cartilage begins to form endochondral bone (shown in *panel E*). **F,** Blood vessels invade the epiphyseal zone of the bone. **G,** The secondary ossification center appears in the epiphyseal zone. **H** and **I,** Longitudinal growth of the bone occurs at the epiphyseal plate. **J,** The epiphyseal plate has fused uniting the epiphysis with the metaphysis. (From Bloom, W., and Fawcett, D. W.: *A Textbook of Histology,* 12th ed. New York, Chapman and Hall, 1994.)

epiphyseal center becomes the articular cartilage (Fig. 2–24). Also, a zone of cartilage persists between the primary and secondary ossification centers. This zone of cartilage, known as the epiphyseal plate (or physis) persists until completion of skeletal growth. Continuous, orderly endochondral ossification on the metaphyseal side of the epiphyseal plate is responsible for the longitudinal bone growth (Fig. 2–25).

The Epiphyseal Plate

Endochondral bone formation at the epiphyseal plate is highly regulated, as evidenced by four very distinct morphologic zones (Fig. 2–26). The first zone, closest to the epiphysis, is the reserve or resting zone. Chondrocytes in this zone are widely separated by cartilage matrix. In the next zone, the zone of proliferation, chondrocytes begin to divide. Mitotic figures are present, and the chondrocytes align in longitudinal columns. Cellular division in this zone is stimulated by various growth factors, one of which is growth hormone. The first two zones are the penetration by small blood vessels originating in the epiphysis. Disruption of these epiphyseal blood vessels results in death of the entire growth plate. In the next zone, the zone of hypertrophy, chondrocytes in their columns swell to five or six times their original size, and the intervening cartilage matrix becomes calcified. Therefore, this zone is also known as the zone of provisional calcification. In addition to type II collagen present in all hyaline cartilage, this zone contains a short-chained collagen not found anywhere else in the body. The function of this collagen, known as collagen X, is not known, although roles in calcification or vascular invasion have been suggested.

The last zone of the epiphyseal plate, closest to the metaphysis, is the zone of endochondral ossification. In this zone, there is chondrocyte death, vascular invasion, and bone

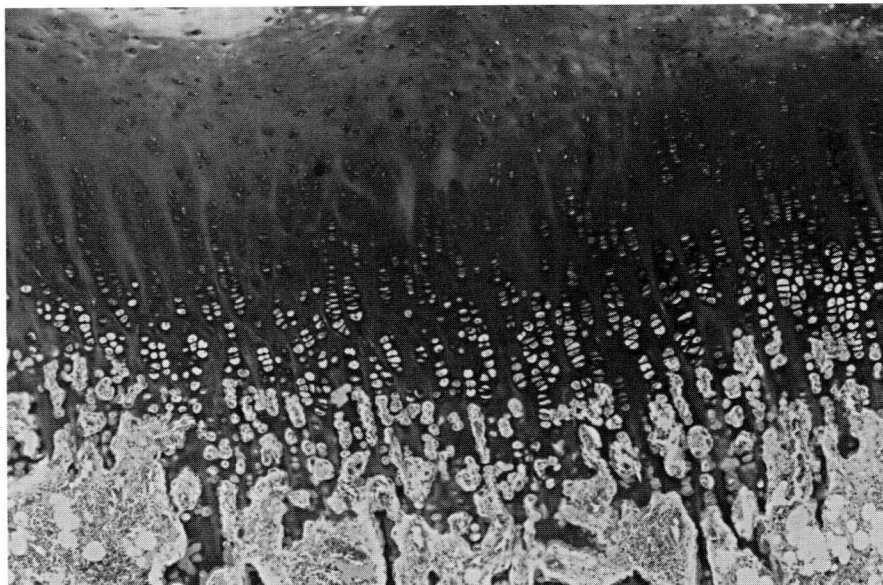

Figure 2-25 ■ Photomicrograph of an epiphyseal plate. On the metaphyseal side of the plate, orderly columns of hypertrophied chondrocytes are present. Beneath is the zone of endochondral ossification.

deposition on columns of calcified matrix. Osteoblasts that deposit the bone originate from the perivascular cells of small blood vessels on the metaphyseal side of the plate. Generally, blood vessels do not completely traverse the epiphyseal plate. The zone of bone deposition on calcified cartilage, known as primary spongiosa, is located between the diaphysis and the epiphyseal plate. This area becomes the metaphysis (Fig. 2–27).

Normal longitudinal growth of a bone is due to continuous chondrocyte proliferation and simultaneous endochondral ossification on the diaphyseal side of the plate. These processes are balanced so that thickness of the plate is constant during growth. However, with the cessation of growth hormone stimulation, the chondrocytes stop dividing. Endochondral ossification continues until the epiphyseal plate is completely ossified, an event known as closure of the physis. At this point, the epiphysis becomes fused to the metaphysis, and their respective marrow cavities become continuous. For a few years after closure of the epiphyseal plate, a radiodense line marks the zone of the former cartilage. This line, known as the *physeal scar*, consists of closely packed trabecular bone. Eventually, the physeal scar is removed by the remodeling process.

Depending on the bone, the epiphyseal plates close at different times during adolescence. When all the plates are closed, skeletal growth is complete. The epiphyseal plates of the distal femur and proximal tibia close between ages 16 and 19, marking the end of growth in height. The last plates to close are the iliac crest, the ischial tuberosity (age 20–21), and the medial clavicle (age 22–25).

The sequence of the appearance and fusion of the secondary centers of ossification has been tabulated for normal skeletal growth and maturation. Knowing the normal time sequence is useful in determining discrepancies between skeletal age and chronologic age.

Modeling

Modeling is a process by which a bone is sculpted to its proper shape while growing longitudinally. The diaphyses of most of the long bones, particularly the femur and tibia, are long narrow cylinders with dense cortices. However, the diameter of the epiphyseal plate is much greater than that of the diaphysis. Therefore, as bone formation progresses beneath the plate, organized teams of subperiosteal osteoclasts resorb bone from the outer surface of the cortex to narrow the shaft to the diameter of the diaphysis. At the same time, the cortical thickness is maintained by teams of osteoblasts depositing bone on the endosteal side of the cortex. This modeling process stops when the epiphyseal plate closes.

PHYSIOLOGY OF BONE

In addition to providing stability to the human frame, bones are a reservoir of calcium ions. This reservoir is a buffer in a complicated homeostatic system that precisely regulates the serum calcium level. Maintaining serum calcium in a narrow range is critical to the human organism. This range must be maintained, even at the expense of skeletal strength. For example, in extreme calcium loss or deprivation, the bones will dissolve in an effort to maintain the correct serum calcium levels.

Serum Calcium

Normal serum calcium levels range from 8.6 to 10.3 mg/dl, and during the day, variation is less than 10% within this range. Maintaining calcium levels precisely in this range is critical for many of the body's physiologic activities. For

ANATOMY AND PHYSIOLOGY OF BONE   43

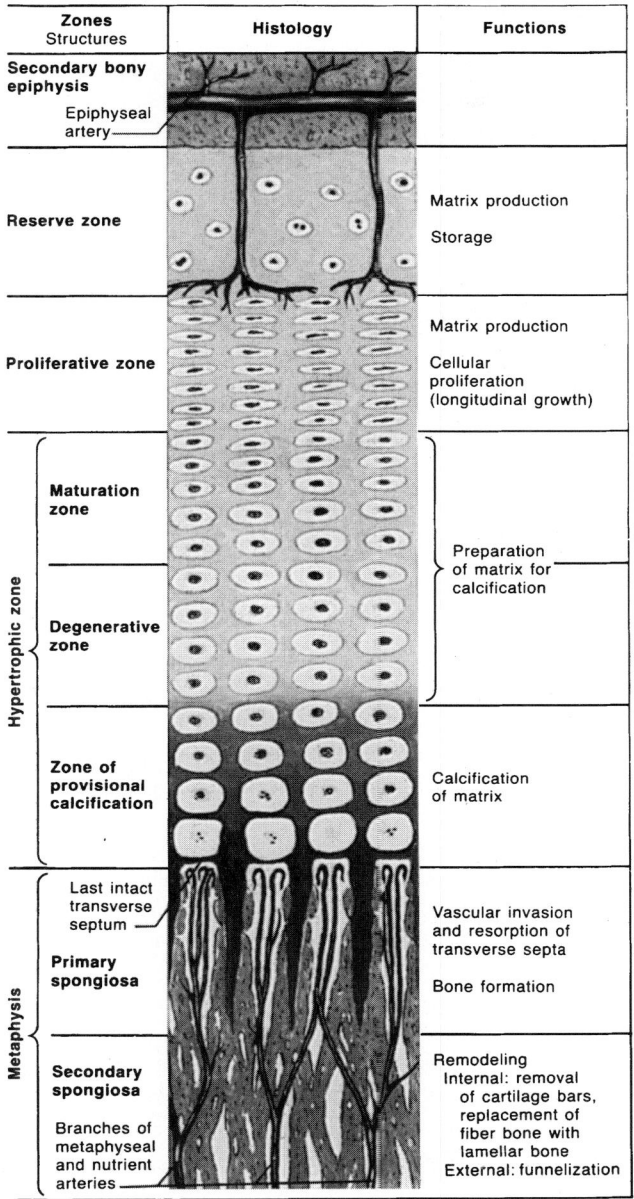

Figure 2-26 ▪ The zones of the epiphyseal plate. (Copyright 1987 Novartis. Modified with permission from *The Ciba Collection of Medical Illustrations,* illustrated by Frank H. Netter, MD. All rights reserved.)

example, correct serum calcium levels are necessary for many enzymatic reactions and for hormone secretion. In addition, neurotransmission and muscular contraction depend on correct serum calcium levels. Other functions, such as cell division, fertilization, and blood clotting also depend on regulated serum calcium. These functions are all adversely affected by large fluctuations in the serum calcium.

Hypocalcemia

When calcium ion concentration falls below normal, the neuromuscular system becomes excitable. Increased membrane permeability to sodium, a condition caused by low calcium ion concentration, allows easy initiation of action potentials. If the calcium ion concentration falls 35% below normal, peripheral nerves become so excitable that they discharge spontaneously and result in tetanus. More severe hypocalcemia causes seizures and even death. Hypocalcemia is rare in clinical practice. Most cases result from hypoparathyroidism.

Hypercalcemia

Elevated calcium ion concentration leads to the effect opposite that seen with hypocalcemia—depression of the nervous system. Although mildly elevated serum calcium levels (from 10.5–12.0) are often asymptomatic, higher levels usually lead to fatigue, mental confusion, nausea, and vomiting. Even higher levels (above 13 mg/dl) eventually lead to renal insufficiency and heterotopic calcification. Levels above 15 are a medical emergency because they can cause coma and death. Clinically, 80% of patients with hypercalcemia have either hyperparathyroidism or malignancy. Less common causes of hypercalcemia are vitamin D intoxication and sarcoidosis.

Distribution of Calcium in the Body

Depending on a person's size, the adult human body contains 1000 to 2000 g of calcium. About 99% of this calcium is in the bone, primarily as calcium hydroxyapatite crystals. The remainder of the calcium is located in two compartments. The first compartment is intracellular. Intracellular calcium is associated with mitochondria, the endo-

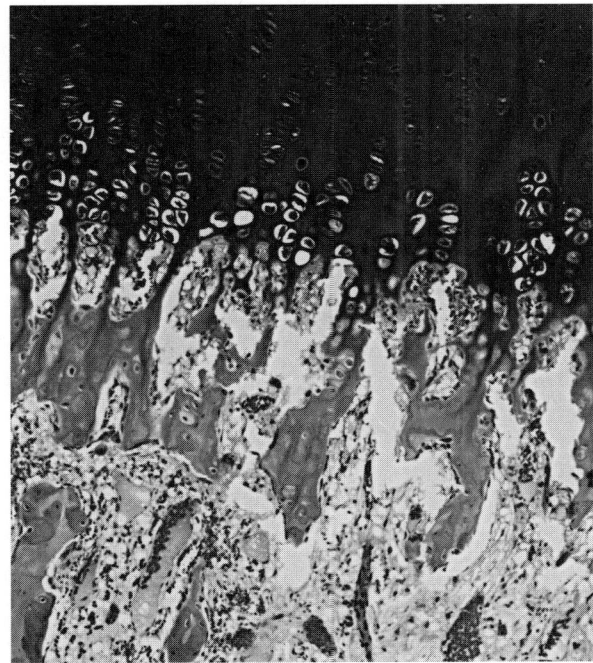

Figure 2-27 ▪ Photomicrograph showing the primary spongiosa on the metaphyseal side of the epiphyseal plate.

plasmic reticulum, and the plasma membranes. The other compartment is the extracellular fluid. This extracellular pool of calcium, about 1000 mg, is in several forms. About 40% is bound to albumin and remains in the blood. Ten percent of the extracellular calcium, although able to leave the blood, is bound to such anions as citrate or phosphate. The remaining 50% is ionized calcium, a critical fraction that is exchangeable and participates in skeletal mineralization.

Exchangeable Calcium

Although most of the calcium in bone is tightly bound in apatite crystals, some is less tightly bound and is available for passive exchange. This exchangeable calcium is in the form of amorphous calcium salts and calcium brushite, a poorly formed crystal. The extracellular pool of ionized calcium is in equilibrium with this exchangeable bone calcium via passage through the osteocytic membrane system.

The exchangeable calcium in bone is a much larger pool than the total extracellular calcium. Therefore, bone functions as a buffer against sudden changes in the calcium ion concentration. For example, after a large intravenous dose of calcium, the serum calcium rises steeply. However, levels return to normal within a half hour, before any hormones can be activated. This rapid return to normal is due to the passive flux of calcium into the bone, where it is precipitated as a calcium phosphate salt. Conversely, in a response to sudden hypocalcemia, calcium can flow from the bone to the extracellular space. In addition to the exchangeable calcium that is available as a buffer, about 500 mg of calcium is exchanged each day during normal bone turnover.

However, exchangeable calcium is available only for rapid buffering. Therefore, sustained perturbations of extracellular calcium require the assistance of the hormonal aspect of the homeostatic system.

Calcium Balance

Adults must be in calcium balance to maintain a constant serum calcium and solid bones. Calcium balance implies that the amount of calcium absorbed in the intestine equals the amount excreted in the feces and urine, processes regulated by parathormone and vitamin D. For example, the calcium intake in the United States varies from 200 to 2000 mg per day. An average intake is 1000 mg, the equivalent of about three glasses of milk. Calcium is absorbed in the small intestine, mostly in the proximal regions. With the average intake of 1000 mg, only about 450 mg is normally absorbed. About 300 mg of the amount absorbed is secreted back into the intestine, leaving a net absorption of 150 mg. This amount is eventually excreted in the urine (Fig. 2–28).

At certain times, calcium balance is shifted. For example, during skeletal growth or pregnancy, a net gain in the amount of calcium retained occurs. By contrast, in old age, when bone mass gradually diminishes, calcium is slowly lost from the body.

Phosphorus

Phosphorus is an integral part of the calcium hydroxyapatite crystal. Therefore, when calcium is deposited or mobilized, it is always accompanied by the phosphate ion (PO_4). In addition, phosphorus accompanies calcium during intestinal absorption. However, in contrast to regulated calcium absorption, almost all the dietary phosphorus (about 1000–1500 mg/d, mainly from dairy products) is absorbed in the intestine. However, despite great variations of phosphorus intake due to unregulated absorption, the serum level is maintained at a fairly constant level (between 2.4 and 4.5 mg/dl). This range is maintained by variations in renal excretion, a function controlled by parathyroid hormone. For example, states of extremely low phosphorus intake are

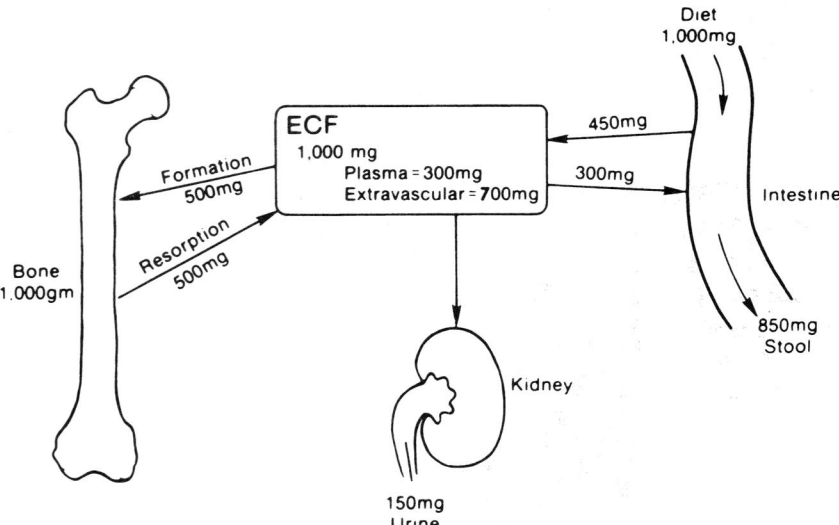

Figure 2-28 ■ Calcium balance. (From Albright, J. A., and Brand, R. A. (Eds.): *The Scientific Basis of Orthopaedics,* 2nd ed. East Norwalk, CT, Appleton & Lange, 1987.)

accompanied by renal tubular reabsorption rates as high as 100%.

Vitamin D

The main function of vitamin D is to get calcium into the extracellular fluid. Although vitamin D has a direct effect on bone, its main action is to promote intestinal absorption of calcium by stimulating the synthesis in the epithelial cells of a calcium transport protein. Vitamin D is needed because only a very small amount of calcium is passively absorbed by the intestinal mucosa. Therefore, lack of vitamin D leads to calcium depletion. Interestingly, vitamin D is a hormone, not a vitamin. A true vitamin is an exogenous substance that is a cofactor in a chemical reaction. However, vitamin D is synthesized in the body, binds to a receptor site, and stimulates the synthesis of another substance. These are the characteristics of a hormone.

Sources of Vitamin D

Vitamin D is synthesized in the skin or ingested in the diet. However, vitamin D must undergo a series of chemical reactions, first in the liver and then in the kidney, to become active.

The natural source of vitamin D is the skin, where it is synthesized by the energy of sunlight. This form of vitamin D, known as vitamin D_3 or cholecalciferol, results from the cleavage of a benzene ring in a cholesterol precursor. This precursor, 7-dehydrocholesterol, occurs naturally in the skin. Most of the synthesis occurs in the deep squamous cells of the epithelium, although a small amount is also synthesized in the dermis.

Active individuals usually receive enough sunlight to synthesize the recommended minimum daily requirement of 2.5 μm (100 units) to maintain calcium balance; the recommended daily intake, however, is 400 units.

Various factors influence the effectiveness of solar energy. First, sunscreens block the exact wavelengths (290–315 nm) needed for photoconversion. Second, melanin absorbs much solar energy. As a result, dark-skinned individuals require seven times the sun exposure that light-skinned people require. Third, indirect sunlight, at times constant in northern latitudes (north of Boston during winter), is extremely ineffective in the photosynthesis of vitamin D_3. Finally, aging skin, due to lack of sufficient precursor, synthesizes vitamin D_3 only one fourth as effectively as younger skin. Older people, therefore, require more sun exposure.

Inadequate sun exposure necessitates dietary intake of vitamin D. However, food sources of natural vitamin D are rare. Egg yolk and liver, particularly fish liver, are the only significant sources. Therefore, vitamin D is often added to foods during processing. For example, in the United States, vitamin D is added to milk products in the form of vitamin D_2, another form of vitamin D that differs slightly from vitamin D_3. Vitamin D_2 is produced artificially by irradiating ergosterol, a substance found in some foods (wheat germ, for example). Vitamin D_2 is also used in vitamin supplement tablets. Because vitamin D is a fat-soluble vitamin, adequate oral intake requires bile salts in the intestine to ensure fat absorption. Therefore, patients with malabsorption syndromes absorb vitamin D_2 poorly.

Activation of Vitamin D

After synthesis in the skin or absorption in the intestine, vitamin D_3 or D_2 enters the blood (Fig. 2–29). However, these forms of vitamin D are inert. Two activation steps are required. They must travel to the liver for the first stage of activation, the addition of a hydroxyl group to form 25 (OH) vitamin D. Hydroxylation is accomplished by hepatic microsomal and mitochondrial enzymes, which are NADP and O_2 dependent. Feedback inhibition of this hydroxylation is minimal. Therefore, serum levels of 25 (OH) vitamin D in the plasma can rise abnormally. Some feedback inhibition occurs, however, because the rise in serum 25 (OH) vitamin D is not proportional to large increases in vitamin D intake.

Excess vitamin D that is not converted to 25 (OH) vitamin D is stored in the liver and adipose tissue for future use. Storage ensures an adequate supply of vitamin D despite fluctuations in intake or sun exposure.

After the addition of the hydroxyl group, 25 (OH) vitamin D leaves the liver and enters the blood, where it has a half-

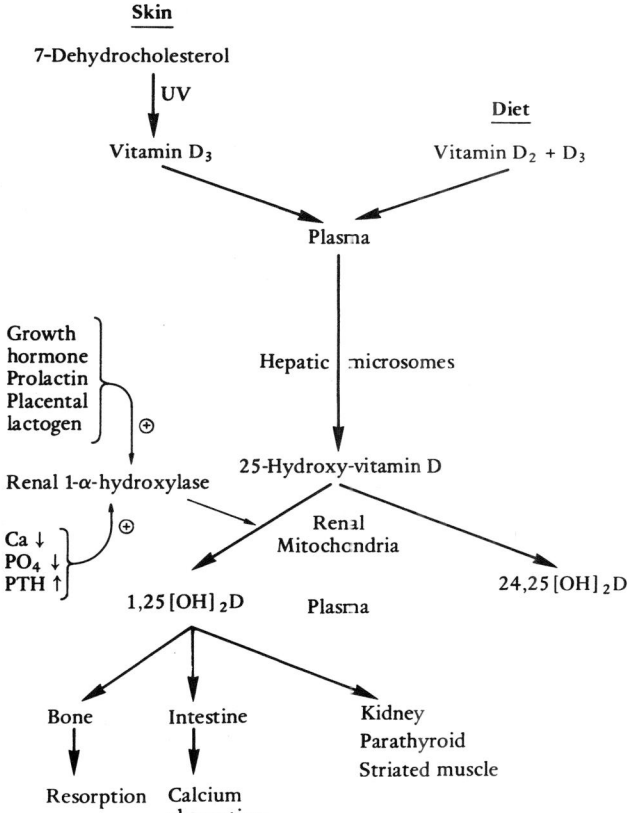

Figure 2-29 ■ The pathways of vitamin D activation. (From Woolf, A. D., and Dixon, A. S.: *Osteoporosis: A Clinical Guide.* London, Martin Dunitz Ltd, and Philadelphia, J. B. Lippincott, 1988.)

life of 14 to 21 days. Because of this long half-life, 25 (OH) vitamin D is the principal form of vitamin D in the blood. Measurement of serum levels, therefore, is a useful clinical monitor of vitamin D intake.

At normal serum levels 25 (OH) vitamin D has no significant physiologic activity. The second step of activation is required. This step occurs in the proximal convoluted tubules of the kidney, where another hydroxyl group is added. Thus, 25 (OH) vitamin D is changed to 1,25 $(OH)_2$ vitamin D, the active form of this substance. The hydroxylation responsible for this conversion is stimulated by parathyroid hormone.

Because of the extreme potency of 1,25 $(OH)_2$ vitamin D, also known as calcitriol, conversion is under tight feedback control. The feedback system is regulated by several mechanisms. First, increased serum levels of 1,25 $(OH)_2$ vitamin D shut off its own synthesis by negative feedback. Alternatively, low levels of serum calcium stimulate parathormone secretion, which in turn increases the synthesis of 1,25 $(OH)_2$ vitamin D. Low levels of serum phosphorus also stimulate the synthesis of 1,25 $(OH)_2$ vitamin D.

Another reaction that regulates the synthesis of 1,25 $(OH)_2$ vitamin D is an alternative pathway of hydroxylation. If the kidney is presented with too much 25 (OH) vitamin D, as might occur in excess vitamin D intake, 24,25 $(OH)_2$ vitamin D is synthesized instead of 1,25 $(OH)_2$vitamin D. Because 24,25 $(OH)_2$vitamin D is much less potent, this alternative pathway is a sluice for disposing of excess precursor.

Actions of Vitamin D

By its effect on both intestinal mucosa and bone, 1,25 $(OH)_2$ vitamin D ensures that enough calcium reaches the extracellular fluid. In the intestine, during its short serum half-life of 6 to 12 hours, 1,25 $(OH)_2$ vitamin D activates calcium absorption by stimulating the synthesis of a special protein in the intestinal epithelial cells. First, the serum 1,25 $(OH)_2$ vitamin D is bound at a receptor site in the cytoplasm of the villus epithelial cells in the small intestine. Then, by the stimulation of mRNA, several proteins are synthesized. The most important protein binds dietary calcium and transports it from the intestinal lumen into the cell against a concentration gradient. From the cell, calcium enters the blood. In addition to stimulating calcium absorption, 1,25 $(OH)_2$ vitamin D also stimulates phosphate absorption. However, the mechanism of phosphate transport is poorly understood.

Bone is also affected by 1,25 $(OH)_2$ vitamin D. However, the action on bone is paradoxical. The intestinal effect of 1,25 $(OH)_2$ vitamin D ensures that calcium is available to mineralize osteoid and thereby strengthen bone. By contrast, the effect of 1,25$(OH)_2$ vitamin D on bone is to stimulate osteoclastic resorption. However, large nonphysiologic levels of 1,25 $(OH)_2$ vitamin D are required for this effect. Interestingly, osteoclasts lack vitamin D receptors. Therefore, osteoclasts must be stimulated by osteoblasts, which have vitamin D receptors. The resorptive effect on bone is similar to the main action of parathyroid hormone on bone, as discussed later. The overlapping functions of these two compounds result in mutual potentiation. For example, it appears that vitamin D sensitizes the bone cells to parathormone.

Vitamin D also has an effect on the parathyroid gland. Increased levels of 1,25$(OH)_2$ vitamin D repress the gene directing parathyroid hormone synthesis. Conversely, low levels of 1,25 $(OH)_2$ vitamin D activate this gene, raising the set point for calcium levels. Thus, low levels of 1,25 $(OH)_2$ vitamin D can directly cause increased parathyroid hormone secretion.

Vitamin D has poorly understood functions in nonosseous tissues, particularly in the immune system. Macrophages, monocytes, and transformed lymphocytes can synthesize 1,25 $(OH)_2$ vitamin D from 25 (OH) vitamin D. In addition, T lymphocytes have receptors for 1,25 $(OH)_2$ vitamin D. Binding of vitamin D by these cells reduces the synthesis of various lymphokines. Also, proliferation of lymphocytes may be decreased by the action of vitamin D. For this reason, vitamin D may be useful for the chemotherapy of lymphomas.

Parathyroid Hormone

Parathyroid hormone, secreted by the four parathyroid glands in the neck, increases serum calcium and lowers serum phosphorus by its affects on bones and the kidneys. Its action to raise serum calcium is its most important function. Variation in secretion maintains the serum calcium in a very narrow physiologic range. Hyperactivity of these glands causes hypercalcemia, and by contrast, hypofunction causes hypocalcemia. Parathyroid hormone also increases the renal excretion of phosphorus.

Regulation of Parathyroid Hormone Secretion

Parathyroid hormone, synthesized in the chief cells of the parathyroid glands, is a polypeptide consisting of 84 amino acids. Initially, a polypeptide of 110 amino acids is synthesized; then, several cleavages occur before the hormone is packaged in secretory granules.

Parathyroid hormone is synthesized at a continuously high rate. However, most of the hormone undergoes intracellular degradation to inert products. Therefore, when the need for parathormone increases, less hormone is degraded and more is secreted. Calcium receptors are present in the plasma membrane of the parathyroid gland cells. Slight decreases in serum calcium result in an increased secretion of parathyroid hormone within minutes. If a low serum calcium level persists for months or more, the parathyroid glands, normally weighing 130 mg as a group, undergo hyperplasia, sometimes to more than five times normal size. By contrast, high levels of serum calcium decrease parathyroid hormone secretion. In this setting, the synthesis, packaging into secreting granules, and release of the hormone are all reduced. In addition, high levels of serum calcium stimulate intracellular degradation of parathyroid hormone. By contrast, prolonged hypoactivity of the glands in response to hypercalcemia ultimately reduces the total parathyroid mass.

Although the rate of secretion varies, parathyroid hormone is always present in the serum. Serum levels, therefore, reflect the activity of the glands. Because parathyroid hormone can be assayed, serum levels are useful clinical indicators of parathyroid activity. For example, increased levels indicate parathyroid overactivity.

The Effect of Parathyroid Hormone on Bone

Bones release calcium in response to parathyroid hormone. Both a rapid response and a delayed response occur. In the rapid response, observable within only 2 to 3 hours, calcium is released from bone without degradation of organic matrix. This process, called osteocytic osteolysis, results from the activity of osteocytes and osteoblasts. These cells, which are interconnected by the osteocytic membrane system, have receptors for parathyroid hormone. Binding with parathyroid hormone activates a calcium pump in these cells and rapidly moves some of the exchangeable bone calcium into the extracellular fluid. The exchangeable calcium in bone, as mentioned previously, is poorly crystallized brushite or amorphous calcium salts. In osteocytic osteolysis, phosphate does not appear to be mobilized, and bone matrix is not digested.

In the delayed response, beginning after 12 hours of parathyroid hormone stimulation, calcium is released from bone by osteoclastic resorption. Not only are both calcium and phosphate released in this late response, but also bone matrix is removed. Osteoclasts, however, have no parathyroid hormone receptors. The increased osteoclastic activity is initiated by local signals from the osteoblasts, which have these receptors. This signal, as yet unidentified, causes increased activity of existing osteoclasts as well as recruitment of new osteoclasts. Because bone is resorbed in this delayed mechanism of calcium release, continuous hyperactivity of the parathyroid glands weakens the skeleton. Eventually, severe osteopenia and fractures result.

Interestingly, parathyroid hormone also has a paradoxical anabolic effect on bone. The administration of intermittent, low doses of parathyroid hormone causes woven bone formation and fibrosis in areas adjacent to resorption cavities. This anabolic effect is probably mediated by local growth factors activated when parathyroid hormone binds to osteoblasts. Also, the amount of bone formed as a result of this anabolic effect depends on other factors, such as levels of calcium, phosphate, and vitamin D.

The Effect of Parathyroid Hormone on the Kidney

Parathyroid hormone decreases the renal excretion of calcium and increases the renal excretion of phosphate. Normally, about two thirds of the calcium in the glomerular filtrate is reabsorbed in the proximal renal tubules. However, in a response mediated by cyclic adenosine monophosphate (cAMP), increased parathyroid hormone levels cause additional calcium reabsorption in the distal parts of the nephron. Thus, parathyroid hormone acts to retain as much calcium as possible in response to hypocalcemia.

Although parathyroid hormone stimulation of the distal nephron can markedly reduce calcium excretion, its effect on bone to release calcium floods the kidney with calcium. As a result, the net amount of excreted calcium rises, despite increased reabsorption.

In addition to promoting calcium reabsorption, parathyroid hormone dramatically increases phosphate excretion. This phosphaturic effect prevents simultaneous elevations of both plasma calcium and phosphate. Otherwise, heterotopic calcification in critical tissues would result. Although parathyroid hormone lowers serum phosphate, serum phosphate levels do not influence the amount of parathyroid hormone secreted because the parathyroid cells have no receptors for phosphate.

Another action of parathyroid hormone on the kidney, and perhaps the most important, is the stimulation of $1,25(OH)_2$ vitamin D synthesis. Parathyroid hormone stimulates the 1-hydroxylase enzyme in a response mediated by cAMP (Fig. 2–30).

Parathyroid Hormone–Related Protein

Some human cancers, particularly squamous carcinoma and renal cell carcinoma, cause hypercalcemia without bone metastasis. Previously, this effect was thought to be caused by ectopic parathyroid hormone synthesized by the tumor cells. However, this effect is now known to be caused by another polypeptide. This polypeptide, called *parathyroid hormone–related protein* (PTHrP), is quite different from parathyroid hormone except for a few regions of structural homology. Due to this homology, PTHrP affects the bone and kidney in a way identical to parathyroid hormone. In addition to carcinomas, a few normal cells synthesize PTHrP. These include squamous epithelial cells in the skin and lactating mammary epithelium. Synthesis by normal squamous cells carries over in neoplastic squamous cells. This explains the hypercalcemia seen in about 20% of squamous cell carcinomas.

Calcitonin

Calcitonin, a short polypeptide (32 amino acids) synthesized in the thyroid gland, lowers the serum calcium. Calcitonin, therefore, provides a defense against hypercalcemia and has an effect opposite that of parathyroid hormone. Calcitonin lowers calcium by two mechanisms. First, calcitonin reverses the process of osteocytic osteolysis by promoting a flux of ionized calcium into the bone. Second, calcitonin decreases the number and the activity of osteoclasts.

Calcitonin is synthesized by the parafollicular C cells of the thyroid, cells that are vestigial remnants of the ultimobranchial glands. Interestingly, the ultimobranchial glands are prominent in lower animals that changed their habitat

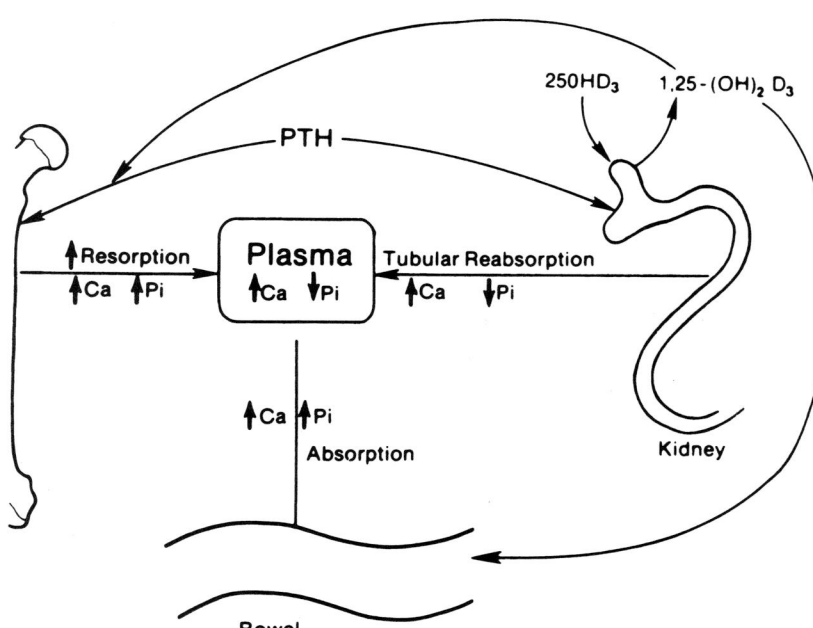

Figure 2–30 ■ The effects of parathyroid hormone. A fall in the serum calcium results in increased parathyroid hormone synthesis by the parathyroid glands. This results in an increase in the serum calcium and a decrease in the serum phosphorus. (From Albright, J. A., and Brand, R. A. (Eds.): *The Scientific Basis of Orthopaedics,* 2nd ed. East Norwalk, CT, Appleton & Lange, 1987.)

from fresh water to sea water. This change required them to adapt to large fluctuations in serum calcium.

Calcitonin is not an important regulator of serum calcium levels in the human adult. Two observations support this. First, the daily absorption and deposition of calcium in bone vary little. Therefore, the body rarely needs to handle huge doses of calcium, and the protective effect of calcitonin against hypercalcemia is usually not needed. Moreover, if hypercalcemia is caused by increased parathyroid hormone, the calcium-lowering effect of calcitonin is quickly overwhelmed by the continuous release of calcium from bone. Second, the effects of calcitonin are short lived. Although osteoclast activity is reduced, a coupled reduction in osteoblastic activity also occurs. Therefore, over a short period, calcitonin results only in a decreased rate of bone turnover. A final observation that supports the idea that calcitonin is relatively unimportant in calcium homeostasis is evident after total thyroidectomy. This procedure, which removes the source of calcitonin, results in no disturbance in calcium homeostasis.

Although calcitonin plays little role in calcium homeostasis in the adult, its effects are probably more important in childhood. During childhood, bone modeling and remodeling result in much larger serum calcium fluctuations. Sometimes the amount of calcium released in the remodeling process is 10 times the amount of exchangeable calcium. Thus, the calcium-lowering effect of calcitonin may be necessary.

Integrated Regulation of Calcium and Phosphate

Calcium balance and proper serum calcium levels are maintained by a complex interaction of parathyroid hormone, vitamin D, and the kidneys. Parathyroid hormone maintains the serum calcium in a normal range, and vitamin D brings calcium into the system. In conditions of hypocalcemia and hypercalcemia, these two hormones act in concert to restore serum calcium to the normal range. Calcitonin probably plays a role only in childhood.

Response to Hypocalcemia

Calcium balance cannot be maintained without the dietary intake of calcium. Although renal excretion of calcium can be limited, some calcium is always excreted. In addition, calcium is lost in the intestinal secretions. Therefore, to maintain a balance, calcium must be ingested in the diet. If dietary intake is low, the body must respond to a hypocalcemic challenge. First, the parathyroid glands, being extremely sensitive to even small decreases in serum calcium, promptly increase their secretion. The most immediate effect of this hormone, evident in about an hour, is on the kidney. An increased amount of calcium is reabsorbed in the distal nephron, causing serum calcium to rise. Bone also responds rapidly to parathyroid hormone by releasing calcium in the process of osteocytic osteolysis. Thus, a transient hypocalcemic episode may be corrected by these rapid mechanisms.

If the hypocalcemic challenge continues, additional actions of parathyroid hormone are required. First, after about a day, the increased levels of parathyroid hormone begin to stimulate the kidney to increase production of $1,25\ (OH)_2$ vitamin D in the proximal tubules. Then, the increased levels of $1,25\ (OH)_2$ vitamin D act to maximize calcium absorption from the intestine. Second, after a few days, parathyroid hormone begins to activate osteoclasts, which degrade bone. Once bone degradation begins, a huge source of calcium is available to the extracellular fluid to maintain the serum calcium. However, if continued for a year or more, bone resorption leads to weak bones.

Response to Hypercalcemia

Hypercalcemia usually indicates overactivity of the parathyroid glands. However, in the absence of parathyroid disease, hypercalcemia occasionally complicates such conditions as sarcoidosis or metastatic carcinoma. In these states, the parathyroid glands reduce the secretion of parathyroid hormone. Although lowering parathyroid hormone levels reduces bone resorption and osteocytic osteolysis, calcium levels are reduced most efficiently by increased renal excretion, also a result of reduced parathyroid hormone secretion. Finally, reduction in parathyroid hormone reduces the synthesis of 1,25 $(OH)_2$ vitamin D, and less calcium is absorbed in the intestine.

Any prolonged abnormality in calcium homeostasis leads to a wide range of clinical symptoms that are regarded as metabolic bone disease. These diseases, discussed in Chapter 4, also include conditions in which the maintenance bone matrix is impaired.

BIBLIOGRAPHY

Bone and Bone Cells

1. Athanasou, N. A.: Current concepts review. Cellular biology of bone-resorbing cells. *J Bone Joint Surg* 78A:1096–1107, 1996.
2. Cooper, R. R., Milgram, J. W., and Robinson, R. A.: Morphology of the osteon. *J Bone Joint Surg* 48A:1239–1271, 1966.
3. Marks, S. C., and Popoff, S. N.: Bone cell biology: The regulation of development, structure and function in the skeleton. *Am J Anat* 183:1–44, 1988.
4. Martin, T. J., Wah, K., and Suda, R.: Bone cell physiology. *Endocrinol Metab Clin North Am* 18:833–858, 1989.
5. Nijweide, P. J., Burger, E. H., and Feyen, J. H.: Cells of bone: Proliferation, differentiation and hormonal regulation. *Physiol Rev* 66:885, 1986.
6. Ninomiya, J. T., Tracy, R. P., Calore, J. D., Gendreau, M. A., Kelm, R. J., and Mann, K. G.: Heterogeneity of human bone. *J Bone Miner Res* 5:933–938, 1990.
7. Recker, R. R.: Embryology, anatomy and microstructure of bone. Coe, F. L., and Favus, M. J., Eds. *Diseases of Bone and Mineral Metabolism.* New York, Raven Press, 1992, pp. 219–240.
8. Roodman, G. D.: Advances in bone biology: The osteoclast. *Endocrine Rev* 17:308–327, 1996.

Organic Matrix: Collagen

1. Leblond, C. P.: Synthesis and secretion of collagen by cells of connective tissue, bone and dentin. *Ant Rec* 224:123–138, 1989.
2. Miller, A.: Collagen: The organic matrix of bone. *Philos Trans R Soc Lond Biol Sci* 304:455–477, 1984.
3. Miller, E. J., and Gay, S.: The collagens: An overview and update. *Methods Enzymol* 144:3–41, 1987.

Organic Matrix: Noncollagenous Proteins

1. Boskey, A. L.: Noncollagenous matrix proteins and their role in mineralisation. *Bone Miner* 6:111–123, 1989.
2. Calvo, M. S., Eyre, D. R., and Gundberg, C. M.: Molecular basis and clinical application of biological markers of bone turnover. *Endocr Rev* 17:333–358, 1996.
3. Canalis, E., McCarthy T. L., and Centrella, M.: Growth factors and cytokines in bone cell metabolism. *Annu Rev Med* 42:17–24, 1991.
4. Centrella, M., Horowitz, M. C., Wozney, J. M., and McCarthy, T. L.: Transforming growth factor-β gene family members and bone. *Endocrine Rev* 15:27–39, 1994.
5. Centrella, M., McCarthy, T. L., and Canalis, E.: Transforming growth factor-beta and remodeling of bone. *J Bone Joint Surg* 73A:1418–1428, 1991.
6. Epstein, S.: Serum and urinary markers of bone remodeling: Assessment of bone turnover. *Endocr Rev* 9:437, 1988.
7. Fisher, L. W., and Termine, J. D.: Noncollagenous proteins influence the local mechanisms of calcification. *Clin Orthop* 200:362–385, 1985.
8. Reddi, A. H.: Bone morphogenetic proteins, bone marrow stromal cells, and mesenchymal stem cells. *Clin Orthop* 313:115–119, 1995.
9. Schulz, A., Jundt, G., Berghauser, K. H., Gehron-Robey, P., and Termine, J. D.: Immunohistochemical study of osteonectin in various types of osteosarcoma. *Am J Pathol* 132:233–238, 1988.
10. Serra, M., Morini, M. C., Scotlandi, K., Fisher, L. W., Zini, N., Colombo, M. P., Campanacci, M., Maraldi, N. M., Olivari, S., and Baldini, N.: Evaluation of osteonectin as a diagnostic marker of osteogenic bone tumors. *Hum Pathol* 23:1326–1331, 1992.
11. Yamashita, H., Ten Dijke, P., Heldin, C. H., and Miyazono, K.: Bone morphogenetic protein receptors. *Bone* 19:569–574, 1996.
12. Young, M. F., Kerr, J. M., Ibaraki, K., Heegaard, A. M., and Robey, P. G.: Structure, expression, and regulation of the major noncollagenous matrix proteins of bone. *Clin Orthop* 281:275–294, 1992.

Mineralization

1. Anderson, H. C.: Mechanism of mineral formation in bone. *Lab Invest* 60:320–330, 1989.
2. Anderson, H. C.: Molecular biology of matrix vesicles. *Clin Orthop* 314:266–280, 1995.
3. Fisher, L. W., and Termine, J. D.: Noncollagenous protein influencing the local mechanisms of calcification. *Clin Orthop* 200:362–385, 1985.
4. Glimcher, M. J.: Mechanism of calcification: Role of collagen fibrils and collagen-phosphoprotein complexes in vitro and in vivo. *Anat Rec* 224:139–153, 1989.
5. Posner, A. S.: The mineral of bone. *Clin Orthop* 200:87–99, 1985.

Bone Remodeling

1. Dempster, D. W.: Bone remodeling. Coe, F. L., and Favus, M. J., Eds. *Disorders of Bone and Mineral Metabolism.* New York, Raven Press, 1992, pp. 355–380.
2. Hattner, R., Epker, B. N., and Frost, H. M.: Suggested sequential mode of control of changes in cell behaviour in adult bone remodelling. *J NIH Res* 7:54–59, 1995.
3. Kerley, E. R.: The microscopic determinates of age in human bone. *Am J Phys Anthrop* 23:149–163, 1965.
4. Manolagas, S. C., and Jilka, R. L.: Bone marrow, cytokines, and bone remodeling: Emerging insights into the pathophysiology of osteoporosis. *N Engl J Med* 332:305–311, 1995.
5. Mundy, G. R.: Bone resorption and turnover in health and disease. *Bone* 8(Suppl 1):S9–S16, 1987.

Electrical Activity of Bone

1. Otter, M. W., Palmieri, V. R., and Cochran, G. V. B.: Transcortical streaming potentials are generated by circulatory pressure gradients in living canine tibia. *J Ortho Res* 8:119–126, 1990.
2. Pollack, S. R., Petrov, N., Salzstein, R., Brankov, G., and Blagoeva, R.: An anatomical model for streaming potentials in osteons. *J Biomechanics* 17:627–636, 1984.
3. Pollack, S. R., Salzstein, R., and Pienkowski, D.: The electric double layer in bone and its influence on stress-generated potentials. *Calcif Tissue Int* 36:S77–S81, 1984.

Growth Plate

1. Hanaoka, H.: The fate of hypertrophic chondrocytes of the epiphyseal plate. An electron microscopic study. *J Bone Joint Surg* 58A:226–229, 1976.
2. Howell, D. S., and Dean, D. D.: The biology, chemistry and biochemistry of the mammalian growth plate. Coe, F. L., and Favus, M. J., Eds. *Disorders of Bone and Mineral Metabolism.* New York, Raven Press, 1992, pp. 313–353.
3. Poole, A. R.: The growth plate: Cellular physiology, cartilage assembly and mineralisation. Hall, B. K., and Newman, S. A., Eds. *Molecular Aspects.* Boca Raton, FL, CRC Press, 1991, pp. 179–211.

Calcium Homeostasis

1. Belanger, L. F.: Osteocytic osteolysis. *Calcif Tissue Res* 4:1–12, 1969.
2. Parfitt, A. M.: Bone and plasma calcium homeostasis. *Bone* 8(Suppl 1):S1–S8, 1987.

Parathyroid Hormone

1. Fukayama, S., Bosma, T. J., Goad, D. L., et al.: Human parathyroid hormone (PTH)-related protein and human PTH: Comparative biologi-

cal activities on human bone cells and bone resorption. *Endocrinology* 123:2841–2848, 1988.
2. Ishimi, Y., Russell, J., and Sherwood, L. M.: Regulation by calcium and 1,25(OH)$_2$-D$_3$ of cell proliferation and function of bovine parathyroid cells in culture. *J Bone Miner Res* 5:755–760, 1990.
3. Orloff, J. J., Wu, T. L., and Stewart, A. F.: Parathyroid hormone-like proteins: Biochemical responses and receptor interactions. *Endocr Rev* 10:476–495, 1989.
4. Parfitt, A. M.: The actions of parathyroid hormone on bone: Relation to bone remodeling and turnover, calcium homeostasis, and metabolic bone disease. I. Mechanisms of calcium transfer between blood and bone and their cellular basis: morphologic and kinetic approaches to bone turnover. *Metabolism* 25:809–844, 1976.
5. Parfitt, A. M.: The actions of parathyroid hormone on bone: Relation to bone remodeling and turnover, calcium homeostasis, and metabolic bone disease. II. PTH and bone cells: bone turnover and plasma calcium regulation. *Metabolism* 25:909–955, 1976.

Vitamin D

1. Bickel, D. D., Nemanic, M. V., Gee, E., et al.: 1,25-Dihydroxyvitamin D$_3$ production by human keratinocytes: kinetics and regulation. *J Clin Invest* 78:557–566, 1986.
2. Kanis, J. A.: Vitamin D metabolism and its clinical application. *J Bone Joint Surg* 64B:542–560, 1982.
3. Norman, A., Roth, J., and Orci, L.: The vitamin D endocrine system: Steroid metabolism, hormone receptors, and biological response (calcium binding proteins). *Endocr Rev* 3:331–366, 1982.
4. Reichel, H., Koeffler, H. P., and Norman, A. W.: The role of the vitamin D endocrine system in health and disease. *N Engl J Med* 320:980–991, 1989.
5. Silver, J., Navel-Many, T., Mayer, H., et al.: Regulation by vitamin D metabolites of parathyroid hormone gene transcription in vivo in the rat. *J Clin Invest* 78:1296–1301, 1986.
6. Stern, P. H.: Vitamin D and bone. *Kidney Int* 38(Suppl 29):S17–S21, 1990.

CHAPTER 3
Genetic Diseases of Bones and Joints

Genetic constitution is a factor in the development of most diseases, including those of bones and joints. Evidence for the influence of genes in disease development is expressed in two ways. First, some diseases occur in families at higher rates than in the general population. Second, other diseases are passed from one generation to the next. In the first group of diseases, known as polygenic disorders, the genetic influence is weak and indirect. In the second group, an abnormal gene is directly responsible for the disease, and the gene is passed on to subsequent generations in one of the patterns of mendelian inheritance. Skeletal diseases in the second group, those resulting from single gene mutations, are the primary focus of this chapter. However, before turning to these, we first offer a brief discussion of polygenic disorders of bones and joints.

Polygenic disorders cluster in families. It may be said that members of these families are "predisposed" to develop these diseases. Usually, these diseases result from the interaction of two or more genes, none of which causes a disease by itself. Also, an environmental factor, such as infection, is often needed to initiate the disorder. For instance, nonorthopedic polygenic disorders are coronary heart disease, hypertension, and obesity. An example of an orthopedic disorder with probable polygenic inheritance is reactive arthritis. In this disease, a microbial infection, such as gonorrhea, initiates chronic arthritis in a genetically susceptible person—one who has the gene that encodes the human leukocyte antigen B27 protein. Other examples of orthopedic polygenic disorders are ankylosing spondylitis and Paget's disease. In infants, orthopedic disorders with polygenic inheritance include spina bifida, congenital club foot, and congenital dislocation of the hip. All polygenic disorders have an unpredictable pattern of inheritance but tend to recur in families in the range of 7 to 9%.

In contrast to the unpredictable inheritance of polygenic disorders, diseases resulting from single gene mutations follow patterns of mendelian inheritance: autosomal dominant, autosomal recessive, and X-linked. However, these diseases also appear spontaneously as a result of new mutations, and if reproductive capacity is maintained, the abnormal gene is passed on. The mechanism by which a mutant gene causes disease is that gene's inability to correctly encode a protein. In these diseases, either an abnormal protein is synthesized, or a normal protein is synthesized in decreased amounts. Depending on the gene, the affected protein may be a growth factor, an enzyme, a receptor, or a structural protein. Because proteins have such varied functions, single gene mutations result in a vast range of phenotypic expression. In fact, over 5000 disorders are produced by single gene mutations, and at least 500 affect the bones and joints.[1]

Skeletal disease caused by single gene mutations can be divided into two categories: mutations that affect other tissues and involve the skeleton indirectly and those that manifest almost exclusively in the skeleton. The most common diseases in the first category include neurofibromatosis, Gaucher disease, the mucopolysaccharidoses, and alkaptonuria. The second group of genetic diseases, those that affect the skeleton directly, are known as the *skeletal dysplasias* or constitutional disorders of bone. Almost 170 skeletal dysplasias have been recognized, and most are extremely rare. Only the most common are discussed in this book.

Although most constitutional disorders of bone are caused by abnormal genes, several developmental bone diseases have no known genetic basis. However, because they manifest as abnormalities of skeletal growth, two of these disorders, melorheostosis and dysplasia epiphysealis hemimelica, are discussed in this chapter. Because diseases of single gene mutations follow mendelian inheritance, a brief discussion of these basic patterns is in order.

MENDELIAN INHERITANCE

Autosomal dominant disorders are expressed in the heterozygous state, i.e., when only one allele is affected. Therefore, if either parent is affected, each child has a 50% chance of having the disorder. Some autosomal dominant disorders, however, result from new mutations—the parents do not carry the gene. Depending on the reproductive capability of patients affected by new mutations, the abnormal gene may or may not be passed on. For example, patients with fibrodysplasia ossificans progressiva, an autosomal dominant disorder, usually do not live long enough to reproduce (see Chapter 14). Therefore, most cases of this disorder result from new mutations.

Occasionally, a person with a gene for an autosomal dominant disorder may not have the disease. This is known as *nonpenetrance,* a situation that can be deduced from the family tree. In addition, autosomal dominant disorders sometimes show *variable expressivity.* One patient with the abnormal gene may be severely affected, whereas another may show only mild changes. For example, neurofibromatosis is a disease characterized by marked variable expressivity. Usually, autosomal disorders affect structural proteins or protein receptors.

The next group of mendelian disorders, *autosomal recessive disorders,* are expressed only in the homozygous state; both alleles of a gene must be abnormal. Therefore, both parents must carry the abnormal gene for a child to express the disorder. However, only one in four children will have the disease, and two of three nonaffected children will be carriers. These diseases appear sporadically in populations because they are expressed only when the carrier of one abnormal allele (heterozygote) mates by chance with another carrier. The incidence of autosomal recessive diseases, therefore, depends on the number of carriers in a population. As a result, these diseases occur more often in close-knit cultural groups and in populations with frequent consanguineous marriages.

Autosomal recessive disorders differ from autosomal dominant disorders in several ways. First, the protein affected in most autosomal recessive disorders is an enzyme. Therefore, most autosomal recessive disorders are inborn errors of metabolism. This contrasts with autosomal dominant disorders in which the abnormal proteins are usually receptors, growth factors, or structural proteins. Second, unlike autosomal dominant disorders, autosomal recessive disorders rarely show variable expressivity; all patients are uniformly affected. Finally, unlike autosomal dominant disorders, penetrance is usually complete in autosomal recessive disorders.

The smallest group of mendelian disorders consists of those linked to the X chromosome. Almost all of these disorders are recessive. Therefore, only a male child who receives the gene will express the disease, because no paired normal allele is present. A woman is carrier because she has one normal allele, and she will pass the abnormal allele to one half of her offspring. A man with the disorder will not pass the gene to his sons, but all of his daughters will be carriers.

An X-linked disorder having important orthopedic complications is hemophilia. Others include X-linked hypophosphatemic rickets and chronic granulomatous disease, a disorder often complicated by inflammatory bone lesions.

GENETIC DISEASES INDIRECTLY AFFECTING THE SKELETON

Neurofibromatosis

Neurofibromatosis 1, a disease caused by a mutation in a tumor suppressor gene, is characterized by the development of cutaneous neurofibromas and café au lait spots. Patients also develop plexiform neurofibromas of nerve trunks, macrocephaly, local gigantism, and central nervous system neoplasms. In addition to these features, skeletal changes occur in many patients. Neurofibromatosis 1 is the most common single gene disorder in humans. Over 100,000 people in the United States are affected.[2] It is usually diagnosed in infancy or childhood and progressively worsens throughout the patient's life.

Another genetic disease, called neurofibromatosis 2, has similar features but is genetically unrelated. The characteristic feature of this disease is bilateral acoustic schwannomas. Because neurofibromatosis 2 is very rare and usually lacks orthopedic complications, it is not discussed here.

Neurofibromatosis 1 is also called von Recklinghausen's disease after the German surgeon who described the disorder in 1882.[3] Earlier reports date from the 17th century.[4] A great public interest in this disorder resulted from the play (and subsequent movie) entitled *The Elephant Man.*[5] This play is based on the true story of Joseph Merrick, an Englishman who, with great dignity, suffered a disease that was most probably severe neurofibromatosis.

General Features

Neurofibromatosis 1 results from a mutation in the *nf1* gene, a tumor suppressor gene located on the long arm of chromosome 17. This very large gene encodes a protein called neurofibromin, which downregulates the function of the p21 ras oncoprotein. Neurofibromin is present throughout the body but is in high concentrations in the nervous system. Therefore, defects in this protein predispose to the characteristic neural neoplasms of neurofibromatosis 1.

Neurofibromatosis 1 is transmitted as an autosomal dominant disorder. However, 50% of patients lack a family history of the disease, suggesting that new mutations are common. The disease exhibits a broad range of expressivity. Some patients have mild disease with only a few neurofibromas and café au lait spots. Other patients, almost 30%, have severe deforming disease. Despite variable expressivity, penetrance is 100%.

Because neurofibromas and café au lait spots occur in patients who do not have neurofibromatosis, rigorous criteria, established in 1987, are necessary to be certain of the diagnosis (Table 3–1).[6] Some individuals with café au lait spots or neurofibromas limited to one or more zones in the body do not meet the diagnostic criteria. However, because

Table 3–1 ■ **DIAGNOSTIC CRITERIA FOR NEUROFIBROMATOSIS 1 (TWO OR MORE OF THE FOLLOWING CRITERIA MUST BE MET)**

1. Six or more café au lait macules over 5 mm in greatest diameter in prepubertal persons and over 15 mm in postpubertal persons
2. Two or more neurofibromas of any type or one plexiform neurofibroma
3. Freckling in the axillary or inguinal regions
4. Optic glioma
5. Two or more Lisch nodules (pigmented iris hamartomas)
6. A distinctive osseous lesion such as congenital pseudoarthrosis
7. A first-degree relative (i.e., parent, sibling, or offspring) with neurofibromatosis 1 by the above criteria

some of their children develop unequivocal disease, these individuals may have segmental neurofibromatosis.[7] Presumably, segmental neurofibromatosis results from a somatic (rather than germ cell) mutation in the *nf1* gene. This results in somatic and germ cell mosaicism and causes limited expression of neurofibromatosis. Thus, even one or two café-au-lait spots or neurofibromas may indicate that the individual carries, and may transmit, the *nf1* gene.

Osseous Abnormalities

Although the skeleton is not the main target of neurofibromatosis, 30 to 60% of patients have osseous abnormalities.[8] The most common abnormality, affecting almost 50% of patients, is *scoliosis*.[9] Most cases of scoliosis in neurofibromatosis are due to osseous abnormalities of the vertebrae, particularly vertebral body wedging or scalloping. Scoliosis is usually detected in patients between ages 8 and 10 years, and the most common curve pattern is a single thoracic curve, although other patterns also occur.

Another orthopedic disorder, affecting 13% of patients with neurofibromatosis, is congenital bowing and pseudarthrosis.[8] Most cases involve the tibia, especially the distal third (Fig. 3–1). Other reported sites are the fibula, ulna, femur, clavicle, and humerus. *Congenital pseudoarthrosis of the tibia* usually presents within the first year of life. Mild lesions present as thinning or bowing of the tibial shaft. In severe cases, a fracture occurs at the site of narrowing. Although congenital pseudoarthrosis of the tibia may occur as an isolated orthopedic condition, 50% of patients with this disorder have neurofibromatosis. However, many of the remaining patients ultimately develop other features of neurofibromatosis.

Congenital pseudarthrosis, especially of the tibia, is often resistant to therapy. Despite bracing and bone grafting, many of the fractured lesions never heal, and amputation is sometimes necessary. The poor healing of these lesions suggests a segmental field defect in the fracture site. Histologic study of the tissue in the fracture site reveals mature fibrous tissue with little osteoid or cartilage formation. Ultrastructural studies fail to demonstrate schwannian differentiation in this tissue, disproving an earlier theory that congenital pseudarthrosis is secondary to an intraosseous neurofibroma.[10,11]

Another characteristic, osseous manifestation of neurofibromatosis 1, is the subperiosteal hemorrhagic cyst, which is rare.[12–14] This lesion is initiated by an episode, often spontaneous, of subperiosteal hemorrhage and bone erosion. Then reactive bone proliferates, and gradually the cyst ossifies until it is incorporated into the cortex as a smoothly contoured bony excrescence. The histologic features of an early lesion are similar to a post-traumatic aneurysmal bone cyst.

In addition to scoliosis, pseudarthrosis, and hemorrhagic cysts, other less common osseous abnormalities occur in neurofibromatosis. For example, macrodactyly, a result of a subcutaneous fibroadipose tissue proliferation, occurs in a small percentage of patients.[15] A similar problem, local gigantism, results in massive overgrowth of skin and subcutaneous tissue due to diffuse dermal and subcutaneous proliferation of neurofibromatous tissue. Other orthopedic problems include myelocele, bone erosion by a neurofibroma, and malignant transformation of a neurofibroma. This last complication occurs in about 2% of patients with severe, long-standing neurofibromatosis.

Lysosomal Storage Diseases

General Features

Lysosomal storage diseases are a large group of genetic disorders, some of which cause secondary osseous abnormal-

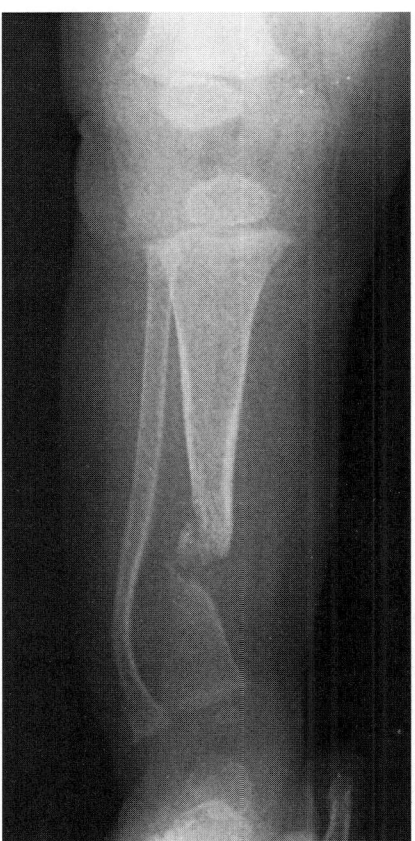

Figure 3–1 ■ Congenital pseudarthrosis of the tibia in a child with neurofibromatosis.

ities due to the intraosseous accumulation of insufficiently catabolized cellular products. These diseases are characterized by defective synthesis of lysosomal enzymes necessary for the intracellular digestion of either cellular breakdown products or phagocytized extracellular material. Depending on the gene affected, specific lysosomal enzymes are not synthesized or do not function properly. As a result, the product usually digested by that enzyme accumulates inside the lysosomes and greatly interferes with cellular function. In addition, the distorted cells often interfere with the function of adjacent unaffected cells.

Most lysosomal storage diseases are autosomal recessive, i.e., the disease is expressed only in the homozygous state. Heterozygotes (carriers) are not phenotypically affected because one normal allele synthesizes enough enzyme for adequate lysosomal function. However, heterozygotes can be identified by assays that demonstrate reduced levels of the enzyme.

Approximately three dozen well-defined lysosomal storage diseases exist.[16] Each disease targets the organs rich in the product that cannot be degraded properly. The affected cells in each organ are those that contain lysosomes, and macrophages, having many lysosomes, are most vulnerable. Therefore, tissues rich in macrophages, such as the bone marrow, lymph nodes, spleen, and liver are usually severely affected in the lysosomal storage diseases.

Bones and joints are secondarily affected in some lysosomal storage diseases. For example, two diseases, Gaucher disease and a group of disorders known as the mucopolysaccharidoses, are complicated by severe bone or joint involvement. Bone changes of Gaucher disease are due to the accumulation of abnormal macrophages in the bone marrow. The mucopolysaccharidoses result from accumulation of insufficiently degraded glycosaminoglycans.

Gaucher Disease

Gaucher disease is an autosomal recessive disorder characterized by the accumulation of glucocerebrosides in macrophages throughout the body. Glucocerebrosides are breakdown products of senescent blood cell membranes and are normally digested by glucocerebrosidase, a lysosomal enzyme that cleaves glucose from cerebroside. Gaucher disease is caused by a mutation in the gene, located on chromosome 1q21, which synthesizes this enzyme. As a result, patients have low levels of glucocerebrosidase.

Abnormal macrophages are the principle pathologic feature of Gaucher disease. These abnormal macrophages, known as Gaucher cells, accumulate in the bone marrow, liver, spleen, and lymph nodes. Their cytoplasm is engorged with material that, with routine histologic preparation, resembles "crumpled tissue paper" and reacts strongly with a periodic acid-Schiff stain (Fig. 3–2). With the electron microscope, this intracellular material corresponds to stacks of bilayered membrane within elongated lysosomes.

Gaucher disease is not rare. A genetics clinic at a university hospital may see two or three new cases per year.

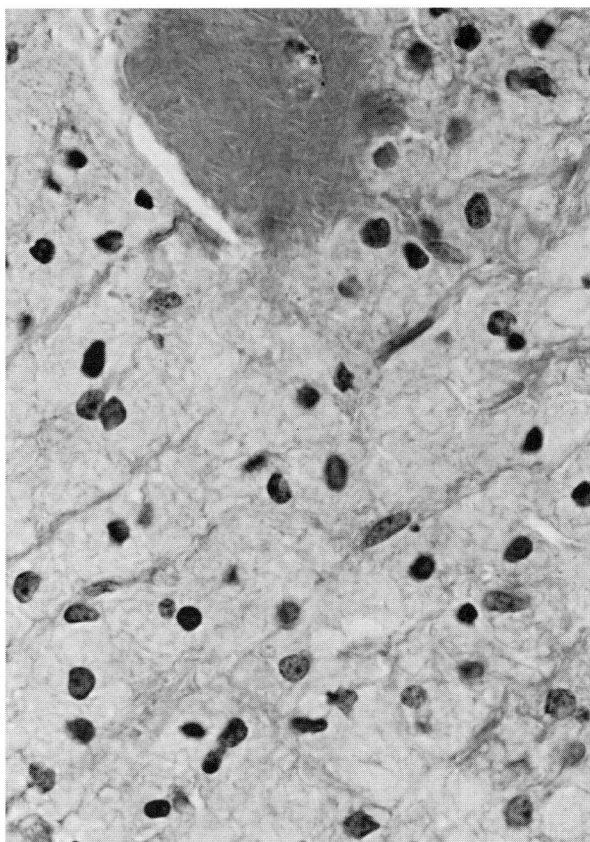

Figure 3-2 ▪ Gaucher cells in the marrow.

Although the abnormal gene has a high frequency in Jews of European origin, the disease occurs in all racial and ethnic groups.

Clinical Features. Gaucher disease is characterized by a wide range of clinical severity, a reflection of different point mutations in the glucocerebrosidase gene. However, three major phenotypes are recognized. Most patients (99%) have type I Gaucher disease. In this form of the disease, signs and symptoms do not appear until adult life. Types II and III are infantile and juvenile presentations. These patients have severe disease, and many die with neurologic involvement.

The clinical features of Gaucher disease are caused by the accumulation of Gaucher cells in organs rich in macrophages: the liver, spleen, and bone marrow. As a result, patients present with hematologic problems and bone lesions. The hematologic problems, pancytopenia or thrombocytopenia, are usually mild and are the result of bone marrow replacement and hypersplenism. However, the bone lesions, caused by marrow infiltration by Gaucher cells, may lead to severe complications.

Skeletal Manifestations. There are three principal skeletal manifestations of Gaucher disease.[17,18] First, Gaucher cells compress the intraosseous vasculature and cause osteonecrosis in 55% of patients. Usually the femoral head is affected. However, the proximal humerus and proximal tibia are also frequently involved. The second way bone is affected in Gaucher disease is the development of modeling deformities due to the intraosseous accumulation of the abnormal macrophages. Modeling deformities are most evident in the long bones, particularly the femur, which resembles an Erlenmeyer flask. The third osseous manifestation is the development of large lytic defects filled with Gaucher cells (Fig. 3–3). These lytic lesions are often complicated by pathologic fracture or cystic degeneration. The extent of all these osseous manifestations is best visualized with the magnetic resonance imaging scan.[19, 20]

As with most inborn errors of metabolism, the treatment of Gaucher disease is supportive. Managing the orthopedic complications is one of the most important aspects of supportive care. In addition, promising results have been achieved in some patients by intravenous infusion of the missing enzyme, glucocerebrosidase.[21]

Mucopolysaccharidoses

Pathogenesis. The mucopolysaccharidoses are a group of lysosomal storage disorders caused by deficiencies in the enzymes that catabolize glycosaminoglycans (formerly known as mucopolysaccharides).[22] Because hyaline cartilage is rich in glycosaminoglycans, it is one of the tissues affected in these disorders, and skeletal deformities result.

Glycosaminoglycans are long-chained, unbranched molecules composed of repeating disaccharide units. Four major types exist: chondroitin sulfate, keratan sulfate, heparan sulfate, and dermatan sulfate. Multiple glycosaminoglycan molecules, when attached to a protein core, form a proteoglycan molecule (see Chapter 16). Proteoglycans are an important component of the extracellular matrix of various connective tissues for two reasons. First, they contribute to tissue resiliency by their ability to trap water. For example, the resiliency of articular cartilage is due to the high concentration of proteoglycans. Second, proteoglycans function as a medium for the transmission of cell to cell messages.

The integrity of the extracellular matrix is maintained by a constant turnover of proteoglycan molecules. New molecules are synthesized, and old molecules are degraded. Part of the degradation process of proteoglycans involves enzymatic cleavages in the various glycosaminoglycans chains. At least 10 steps (and therefore 10 enzymes) are required to catabolize glycosaminoglycans. Genetic deficiency in any of these 10 enzymes results in the accumulation of the substrate. Various clinical phenotypes depend on which substrate accumulates. Not only does the particular substrate accumulate in tissue, but excess amounts are excreted in the urine, a feature that aids in distinguishing the various phenotypes.

All the mucopolysaccharidoses share a common pathogenesis. The particular glycosaminoglycan (mucopolysaccharide) accumulates in lysosomes and causes cellular dysfunction, injury, and often cellular death. As with most lysosomal storage diseases, the cells most vulnerable are those rich in lysosomes, particularly mononuclear phagocytes. Other affected cells include granulocytes, endothelial cells, smooth muscle cells, and fibroblasts. The organs most severely affected in each phenotype are those richest in the particular glycosaminoglycan that cannot be degraded.

The mucopolysaccharidoses also share common pathologic features. The affected cells in all syndromes show cytoplasmic clearing and are called balloon cells. This feature results from numerous cytoplasmic vacuoles that, with the electron microscope, correspond to distended lysosomes.[23, 24]

Six major phenotypes of the mucopolysaccharidoses have been described: Hurler syndrome, Hunter syndrome, Sanfilippo syndrome, Morquio syndrome, Maroteaux-Lamy syndrome, and Sly syndrome.[25] All syndromes are autosomal recessive except for Hunter syndrome, which is X linked. Each syndrome is associated with specific enzymatic defects that result in the accumulation and excretion of either heparin sulfate, keratan sulfate, or dermatan sulfate. In addition, a few of these syndromes exhibit a spectrum of clinical severity, probably caused by different point mutations in the affected gene.

General Clinical Features. Although the phenotypes of the mucopolysaccharidoses are quite variable, they share numerous clinical features. First, infants appear normal at birth; abnormalities usually become apparent by age 2. Second, varying degrees of mental retardation are present in most syndromes. Third, cardiac anomalies are common, and hepatosplenomegaly usually is present. Fourth, coarse facial

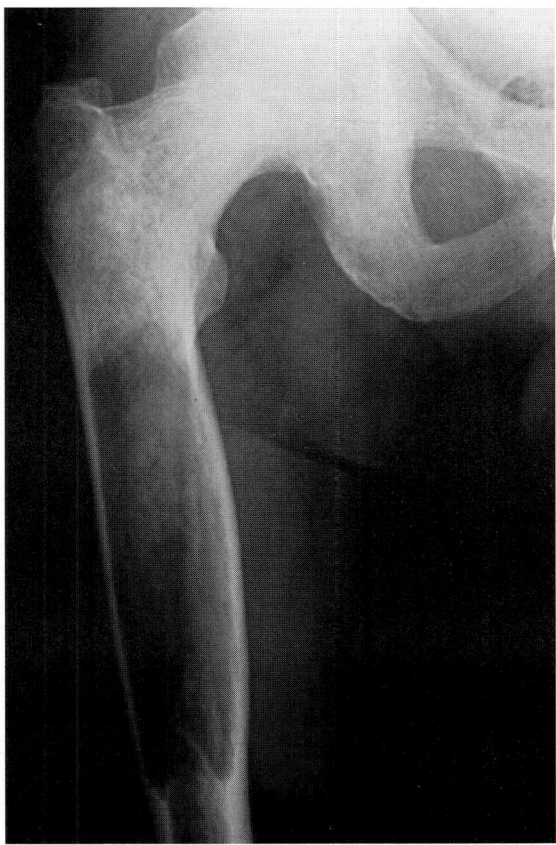

Figure 3-3 ■ A cystic lesion of Gaucher disease in the proximal femur.

features are present (except in the Morquio syndrome), and corneal clouding usually is seen. Fifth, growth retardation, sometimes severe, is present in all syndromes.

Skeletal Complications. Osteoarticular abnormalities are also present in the mucopolysaccharidoses. The common pathogenesis of these syndromes causes a shared pattern of skeletal changes known as *dysostosis multiplex*.[26] One feature of dysostosis multiplex is abnormality of the spine. The vertebral bodies are oval, and they are diminished in height or flattened. In addition, anterior beaking of the vertebral bodies often occurs. These vertebral abnormalities usually lead to kyphoscoliosis, sometimes with a pronounced gibbus. In the cervical spine, the dens is sometimes hypoplastic, a feature that may lead to instability.

Abnormality of the pelvis is another feature of dysostosis multiplex. The acetabular roof is poorly developed, and flaring of the wings of the ilium is present. Also, the femoral heads show varying degrees of dysplasia, and, because of the poorly formed acetabula, the femoral heads may dislocate. Coxa valga is very common (Fig. 3–4).[27]

Long bone changes, more severe in the upper extremity, also occur in dysostosis multiplex. The bones are expanded, and the cortices are thin. Usually, the epiphyseal ends are malformed, which, in the knees, results in genu valgum (Fig. 3–5). Also, a constriction of the humeral and femoral necks is often present.

Other bones are also involved. The phalanges of the hand are short and wide, and the metacarpals are tapered proximally. In the skull, the calvarium is thickened, and sclerotic changes occur in the mastoid bone.

Specific Phenotypes. Although the mucopolysaccharidoses share a common pathogenesis and many clinical features, each syndrome is distinctive. *Hurler syndrome*, or mucopolysaccharidosis, type I (MPS I) is one of the most severe disorders. A defect in alpha-L-iduronidase leads to the accumulation and increased urinary excretion of both dermatan sulfate and heparan sulfate. Children with Hurler syndrome have severe skeletal abnormalities, progressive neurologic deterioration, and cardiopulmonary disorders that almost always lead to death before age 10 years. In addition, these children have short stature and coarse facial features.

A different mutation in the same gene affected in the Hurler syndrome leads to a much milder disorder. This syndrome, known as *Scheie syndrome* (or MPS I S), is characterized by a normal life span and normal intelligence. Like Hurler syndrome, patients excrete both heparan and dermatan sulfate, although in much reduced amounts.

Hunter syndrome (MPS II) is the next major mucopolysaccharidosis and, with Charles Hunter's report in 1917, was the first to be described.[28] A mild and a severe form of this disease are recognized. Patients have clinical features similar to, but less severe than, Hurler syndrome. Nonetheless, most patients die between ages 10 and 20. Like Hurler syndrome, both heparan and dermatan sulfate are excreted in the urine. Unlike the other mucopolysaccharidoses, which are autosomal recessive, Hunter syndrome is X-linked recessive.

The third major mucopolysaccharidosis, and perhaps the most common, is the *Sanfilippo syndrome* (MPS III). Profound mental retardation characterizes this syndrome. In addition, the skeleton and heart may be mildly involved, but patients survive to adulthood. This phenotype is caused by a mutation in any one of four genes and leads to the accumulation of heparan sulfate. Clinical severity varies, depending on the gene affected.

The next phenotype, *Morquio syndrome* (MPS IV), is characterized, like most of the other mucopolysaccharidoses, by short stature and severe skeletal abnormalities. Because patients with this syndrome usually survive to adulthood, orthopedic surgery is often required to stabilize the spine and reconstruct joints. Other organs are also involved in this disease, particularly the heart and lungs. Unlike the other mucopolysaccharidoses, which are characterized by coarse facial features, fine facial features characterize Morquio syndrome. Morquio syndrome results from either of two differ-

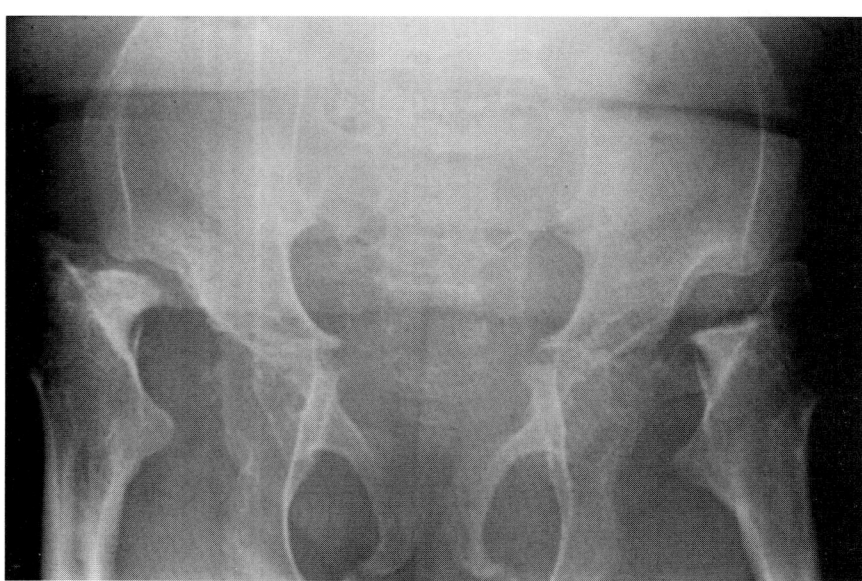

Figure 3–4 ■ Skeletal manifestation of dysostosis multiplex. This radiograph represents Morquio disease. Dysplastic femoral heads and marked coxa valga are present.

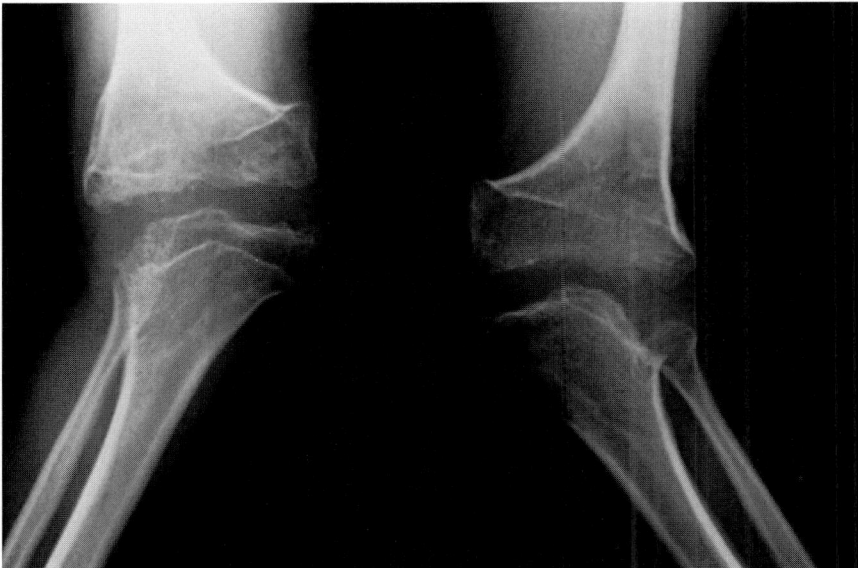

Figure 3-5 ■ Morquio disease of the knee showing dysplastic epiphyses and marked genu valgum.

ent enzyme defects, both of which lead to the accumulation of keratan sulfate.

The *Maroteaux-Lamy syndrome* (MPS VI) is the fifth important mucopolysaccharidosis. Patients with this syndrome excrete excessive amounts of dermatan sulfate. Like patients with Morquio syndrome, patients with Maroteaux-Lamy syndrome often survive until adulthood and therefore require management of dysostosis multiplex. Unlike the Morquio syndrome, however, coarse facial features are characteristic of the Maroteaux-Lamy syndrome.

The last mucopolysaccharidosis, *Sly syndrome* (MPS VII), is the rarest of this group of disorders. Patients have clinical features similar to the other mucopolysaccharidoses: short stature, hepatosplenomegaly, dysostosis multiplex, and mental retardation. Varying degrees of clinical severity characterize this disorder. A deficiency in β-glucosonidase leads to the inability to catabolize dermatan sulfate, heparan sulfate, and chondroitin sulfate.

Alkaptonuria (Ochronosis)

Alkaptonuria, also known as *ochronosis,* is another genetic disease that indirectly affects the skeleton. This disorder is characterized by black urine and, in later life, severe arthropathy due to pigment deposition. Alkaptonuria is caused by an enzyme deficiency resulting in the inability to catabolize homogentisic acid, an intermediary compound in the metabolism of tyrosine and phenylalanine. A genetic mutation at an unknown locus causes a deficiency of homogentisic acid oxidase. As a result, large amounts of homogentisic acid accumulate in tissue and are excreted in the urine. Thereafter, oxidation of homogentisic acid, both in the urine and tissue, leads to black pigmentation.[29]

History

Humans have long suffered from alkaptonuria. Although patients with black urine were reported as early as 1584,[30] even earlier evidence of this disease, both biochemical and radiographic, has been found in Egyptian mummies.[31, 32] This disease was named alkaptonuria in 1859 because alkalinization exaggerated the blackening of the urine.[33] Later, in 1866, Virchow called this disease ochronosis after noting an ochre color of the pigment.[34]

Alkaptonuria is historically significant because it was the first inborn error of metabolism to be characterized. Sir Archibald Garrod, the successor to William Osler as Regius Professor of Medicine at Oxford, postulated in 1901 that this disease was due to an enzyme defect.[35] Garrod's study of alkaptonuria led him to formulate the "one disease—one enzyme deficiency" theory. Unfortunately, this theory was ignored for many years.

General Features

Alkaptonuria is rare, but a very high incidence in the Dominican Republic and in the former Czechoslovakia is likely due to frequent consanguineous marriages in these regions. Alkaptonuria may be diagnosed shortly after birth because diapers are discolored by black urine. Other clinical features are usually delayed until adulthood. These features are the result of deposition of pigment in three major areas: the joints, the cardiovascular system, and the urinary tract. After the onset of symptoms, this disease progressively worsens throughout life. Although patients usually have a normal life span, the symptoms can be crippling.[36]

The cardiovascular and urinary systems are involved in alkaptonuria, but clinical problems are not severe. Pigment is deposited in cardiac valves and in the intima of blood vessels. The latter often leads to premature atherosclerosis. In the urinary tract, calcified ochronotic pigment leads to renal or prostatic calculi; sometimes these calculi cause urinary tract obstruction.

Skeletal Changes

Orthopedic problems usually begin in early adulthood and cause the most severe symptoms.[37, 38] The spine is usually the first region to be affected by pigment deposition in the intervertebral discs and paravertebral soft tissues. Patients present with low back pain, stiffness, and nerve root compression. The radiographic features are characteristic.[39] The disc spaces are narrowed and are usually calcified. In addition, traction or extension of the spine often produces a radiolucent vacuum in the disc space anterior to the disc calcification. The intraarticular vacuum, a consistent finding in alkaptonuria, is best seen on lateral plain radiographs.[40]

Involvement of large joints, such as the hips and knees, usually begins later than spinal involvement. Dark brown or black ochronotic pigment is extensively deposited in articular cartilage, which grossly appears dark brown or black. The pigment renders the cartilage extremely brittle, and large fragments are shed into the joint and become embedded in the synovial membrane (Fig. 3–6).[41] An intense synovitis often results. Ultimately, patients develop severe secondary osteoarthritis, often with extensive intraarticular calcified loose bodies.[42] Although severe arthropathy of peripheral joints may be successfully treated by total joint arthroplasty, spinal involvement produces severe disability; patients often require long periods of bed rest.

GENETIC DISEASES DIRECTLY AFFECTING THE SKELETON—THE SKELETAL DYSPLASIAS

Some single gene mutations manifest primarily or exclusively as generalized disorders of the skeleton. These diseases are collectively known as skeletal dysplasias or constitutional disorders of bone. Patients with these disorders usually have short stature, and many have abnormally shaped bones. In some dysplasias, the bones are fragile. Patients with short stature due to skeletal dysplasia have been called "dwarfs," but many prefer the designation *little people*. A support organization called Little People of America has over 10,000 members.

Although short stature poses no health problems, patients with skeletal dysplasias often have orthopedic disabilities and require medical care. In a population of 10,000 patients with skeletal dysplasia in Great Britain, 6000 required substantial orthopedic care and were handicapped throughout life. About half of these were severely handicapped.[43] Orthopedists must manage the complications of skeletal fragility, and they must treat the arthropathies and nerve impingements resulting from abnormally shaped bones.[44]

Many types of skeletal dysplasia exist, and systematic attempts to classify them began in 1941. Since then, newly discovered dysplasias have been studied both pathologically and radiographically. As a result, many additional classification systems have appeared, but most have been cumbersome and confusing. Most recently, in 1991, the International Nomenclature of Constitutional Diseases of Bone was proposed.[45] This nomenclature, the most comprehensive to date, includes about 170 skeletal dysplasias.

All classification systems are based primarily on the radiographic appearance of the bones. For example, dysplasias are classified according to which parts of the bones are involved, e.g., epiphyseal or metaphyseal, and whether the spine is involved. Other classification systems incorporate age of onset, inheritance, and histopathologic features.

Recent progress in medical genetics has led to the identification of many mutations that cause skeletal dysplasia. For example, the mutations causing osteogenesis imperfecta, achondroplasia, and spondyloepiphyseal dysplasia have been identified. This genetic information may be the basis of future classification systems. Indeed, many dysplasias once thought to be different disorders are now known to be examples of variable expression of the same gene defect. Conversely, some disorders with similar phenotypes are now known to result from mutations in different genes.

Once the mutation in a skeletal dysplasia has been identified, the abnormal encoded protein can be deduced and its effect on the skeleton elucidated. Therefore, understanding

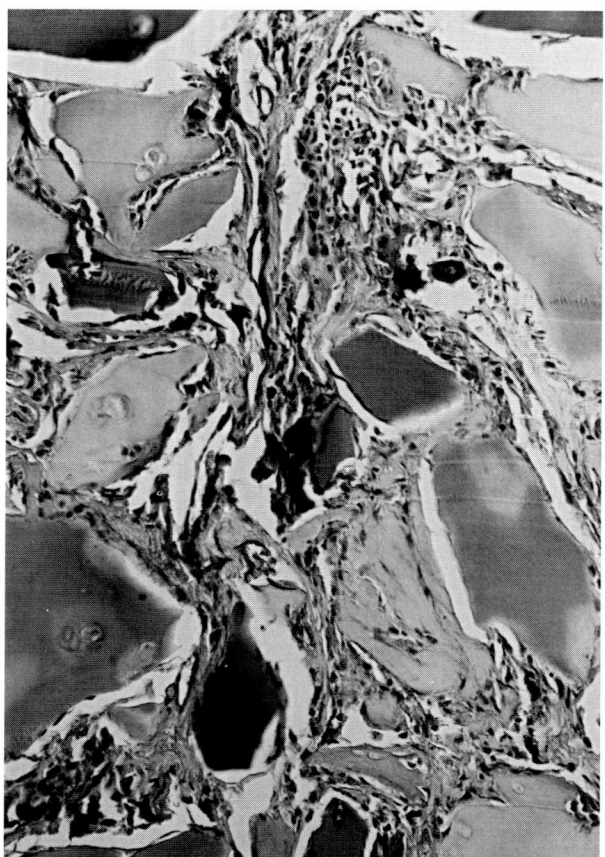

Figure 3-6 ▪ Ochronotic pigment and articular cartilage fragments in the synovial membrane. (Courtesy of Professor René Lagier, Geneva, Switzerland.)

Table 3-2 ■ **CONSTITUTIONAL DISORDERS OF BONE**

Disease	Clinical Defect	Inheritance	Molecular Defect
Heritable Disorders			
Osteogenesis imperfecta	Brittle bones	AD and AR	Type I collagen synthesis
Osteopetrosis	Radiodense bones	AD and AR	Osteoclast function
Osteopoikilosis	Spotted bones	AD	Remodeling disorder?
Achondroplasia	Short stature due to short tubular bones	AD	Fibroblast growth factor receptor
Pseudoachondroplasia	Spinal and epiphyseal abnormalities	AD	Core protein secretion
Spondyloepiphyseal dysplasia	Spinal and epiphyseal abnormalities	AD and AR	Type II collagen synthesis
Multiple epiphyseal dysplasia	Epiphyseal abnormalities	AD	Proteoglycan secretion
Metaphyseal chondrodysplasia	Metaphyseal rickets-like changes	AD and AR	Unknown
Multiple hereditary osteochondromas*	Many osteochondromas	AD	Unknown
Fibrodysplasia ossificans progressiva†	Progressive heterotopic bone formation	AD	Overexpression of *BMP4* gene
Sporadic Disorders			
Multiple enchondromatosis*	Many enchondromas	Sporadic	Unknown
Progressive diaphyseal dysplasia	Painful diffuse periosteal new bone deposition	Sporadic	Unknown
Epiphysealis hemimelica	Osteochondroma-like epiphyseal lesions	Sporadic	Unknown
Melorheostosis	Painful limited periosteal new bone deposition	Sporadic	Unknown
Polyostotic fibrous dysplasia*	Multiple fibroosseous lesions	Sporadic	Oncogene overexpression

* See Chapter 12.
† See Chapter 14.
AD = autosomal dominant; AR = autosomal recessive.

---

the causes of the skeletal dysplasias will undoubtedly lead to new insights about the growth and development of the normal skeleton. For example, the large number and variety of skeletal dysplasias attest to the large number of genes necessary for skeletal structure and function.

We turn now to more specific discussion of the most common skeletal dysplasias (Table 3-2).

Osteogenesis Imperfecta

Osteogenesis imperfecta (OI) is the most common genetic disease of the skeleton, affecting between 15,000 and 20,000 patients in the United States. In this disorder, defective synthesis of type I collagen leads to brittle bones, osteopenia, and varying degrees of skeletal deformity. A characteristic feature of most patients is blue sclerae.

History

Osteogenesis imperfecta was present in ancient times. Skeletal changes in an Egyptian mummy dating from 1000 BC are consistent with this disease.[46] Reports of patients with brittle bones begin to appear in medical treatises in the 17th century. Probably the first case was described by Malebranche in 1674.[47] The hereditary nature of skeletal fragility was recognized in 1788 by Ekman, a Swedish military surgeon.[48] He noted four generations of a family in Sweden who suffered fractures with little trauma. Over 100 years later, in 1896, Spurway first noted the association of blue sclerae with fragile bones.[49] A few years later, in 1900, Eddowes suggested that the association of blue sclerae with brittle bones indicated a "poorly quality of connective tissue" in affected patients.[50] However, it was not until 1975 that specific abnormalities in bone collagen were first identified.[51]

Type I Collagen

Type I collagen, the most abundant collagen in the body, composes 90% of the proteins in osteoid. Type I collagen is also present in many other sites, such as skin, tendons, and fascia. However, these tissues are not seriously affected in OI; patients have only mild to moderate ligamentous laxity. Type I collagen is synthesized by two genes, *COL1A1* and *COL1A2*, which are located on chromosome 17 and chromosome 7, respectively. These genes code for the proalpha$_1$ (I) and proalpha$_2$ (I) chains. Because the triple helix of type I collagen contains two alpha$_1$ chains and one alpha$_2$ chain, twice as much alpha$_1$ procollagen is synthesized, a ratio governed by the amount of mRNA available (see Chapter 2).

A mutation in either *COL1A* gene interferes with type I collagen synthesis. However, depending on the site of the mutation, collagen synthesis is disrupted in varying degrees of severity. Over 150 different mutations in these genes have been identified in OI.[52] As a result, the disease exhibits a wide range of clinical severity.

Clinical Spectrum

The spectrum of severity in OI is broad and ranges from neonatal death with multiple fractures to patients who present in middle age with mild osteopenia and a history of only a few fractures. This clinical heterogeneity was recognized in 1906 by Looser, who used the terms *congenita* and *tarda* for the severe and mild forms of the disease.[53] Since 1978, clinicians have adopted the Sillence classification, which assigns patients to one of four major phenotypes.[54] However, approximately 20% of patients resist classification because of overlapping clinical features. Unfortunately, attempts to classify patients by biochemical criteria have not been successful.

Type I OI, the most common phenotype, accounts for 60% of cases. It is also the mildest form of this disease. Patients have fewer fractures, less severe osteopenia, and little or no skeletal deformity. However, even within this phenotype, patients are variably affected. In some, the first fractures occur in infancy, but the rate of fracture decreases in adolescence and adulthood. Some patients have even milder disease. They present in adulthood with unexplained osteopenia and a history of only a few fractures during their lifetime. Because an estimated 10% of patients with type I disease never fracture, some patients go undiagnosed.[55]

The clinical features of type I OI may help establish the diagnosis. All patients have blue sclera. This feature is due to decreased collagen in the sclerae, allowing for visualization of the underlying choroid. About 25% of patients also have hearing impairment. In addition, some patients have mild scoliosis and by adulthood, about 50% have some stunting of stature. Type IB patients, a more specific subtype, also have dentinogenesis imperfecta.

The radiologic features of type I OI are nonspecific; only osteopenia is present. However, sometimes the osteopenia is subtle and can only be recognized by dual-energy x-ray absorptiometry. Skeletal deformity is usually absent.

Type I OI is transmitted as an autosomal dominant disorder. However, as many as 20 to 30% of patients have apparently normal parents, indicating new mutations.

The *type II* phenotype is the most severe form of OI and accounts for 20% of patients. This phenotype is invariably lethal. Intrauterine fractures are common, and many infants are stillborn (Fig. 3–7). Liveborn infants usually die within the first weeks. Infants have shortened, deformed extremities, and radiographs show multiple fractures with varying amounts of callus. The cranium is large and soft, and sometimes multiple fractures cause fatal intracranial bleeding. Patients may also die of pulmonary insufficiency due to a small chest cavity and multiple rib fractures. This disorder, also characterized by blue sclerae, is autosomal dominant.

Type III patients have severe, progressive disease that, however, is compatible with survival into adulthood. This phenotype accounts for 20% of cases. Patients may have blue or white sclerae. Type III OI presents at birth with bowing of the limbs, and patients commonly sustain over 200 fractures by adulthood. As a result, adults are extremely short, often under 4 ft, and their limbs are markedly deformed. Many patients never walk and are confined to a wheelchair. However, some are able to propel themselves along the floor. Spinal deformities, such as scoliosis and vertebral compression, also occur. In addition, thoracic cage deformity causes cardiorespiratory insufficiency in some patients.

Radiographic examination of patients with type III disease reveals deformed bones with very thin cortices (Fig. 3–8). The diaphysis of the long bones is very slender, and an abrupt widening of the metaphysis and epiphysis is present. Often, the epiphyseal and metaphyseal regions contain stippled radiodensities consistent with intramedullary islands of calcified cartilage. Some patients with type III OI have another radiographic pattern of bone involvement—broad, osteopenic long bones with little cortical-medullary differentiation. In the spine, the osteopenic vertebrae usually show a "cod fish" deformity due to compression of the vertebral body by the intervertebral disc.

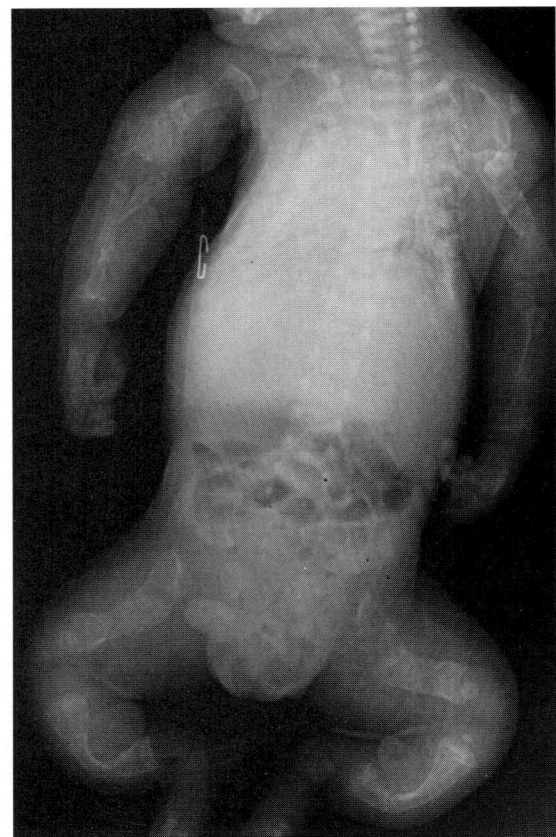

Figure 3-7 ■ Fetus with type II osteogenesis imperfecta. Fractures in all of the long bones are present.

Although most cases of type III OI are due to autosomal dominant mutations, approximately 6% are transmitted in a manner that suggests germ cell mosaicism.

Type IV OI is intermediate in severity between types I and III. This autosomal dominant phenotype is the least common form of OI, representing about 5% of cases. Characteristically, the blue sclerae are present in childhood, but they gradually whiten as the patient ages. Also, patients with this phenotype usually have a large calvarium with a high forehead and an occipital overhang.

Pathogenesis

The most common mutations in OI, those responsible for the type I phenotype, cause a *null allele effect*.[56] This effect results in the synthesis of normal collagen but in one half the normal amount. With a null allele effect, either the mutant gene, almost always the *COL1A1* gene, is not transcribed, or the mutant proalpha (I) chains are degraded intracellularly. Therefore, no abnormal collagen fibers are excreted. However, the paired normal allele encodes its share of normal proalpha 1 (I) chains. These combine with half the normally synthesized proalpha 2 (I) chains. As a result,

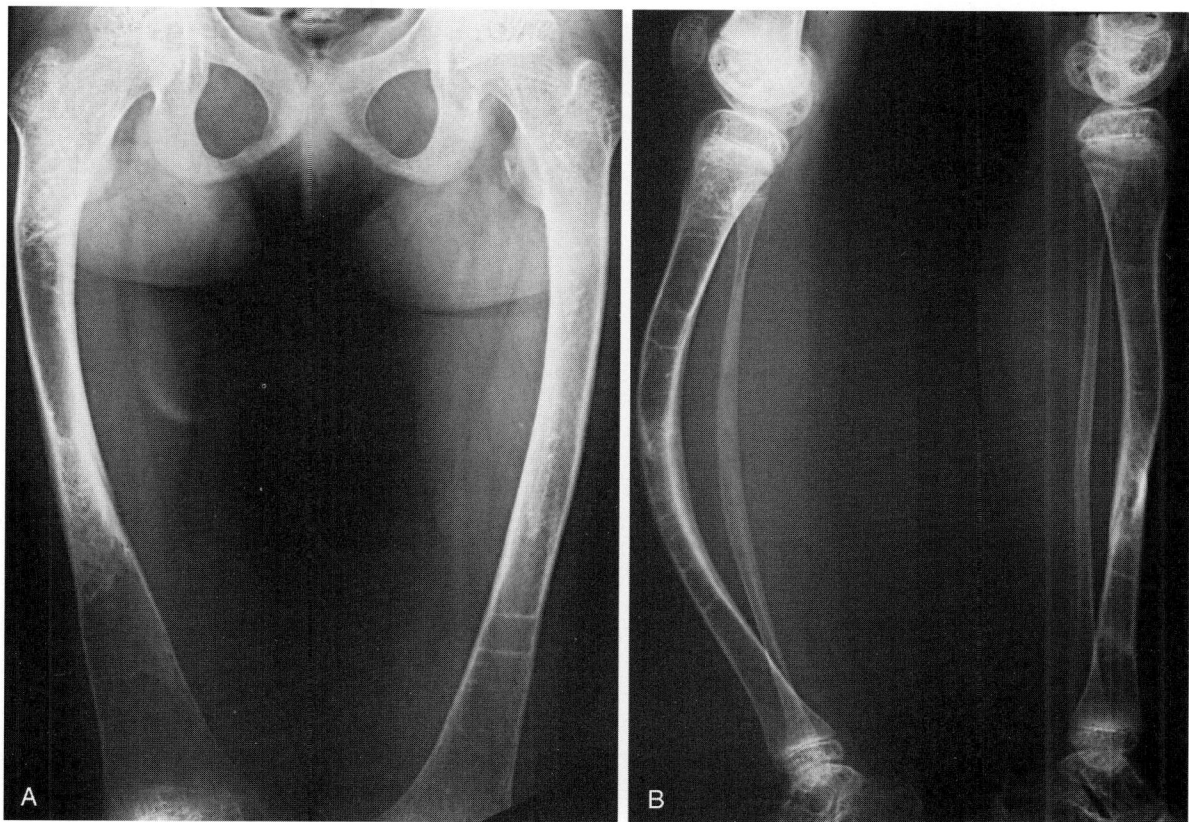

Figure 3-8 ■ **A,** Osteogenesis imperfecta, type III. The femurs show osteopenia with bone deformities. **B,** Osteogenesis imperfecta, type III. The tibia shows marked bowing bone deformity and extreme osteopenia.

synthesis of normal type I collagen is reduced. This results in reduced bone volume, but because the bone is qualitatively normal, the phenotype expression of the disease is mild.

In contrast to mutations that cause a null allele effect, expressed mutations lead to the excretion of abnormal collagen chains. These mutations cause the more severe forms of OI and are known as *dominant negative* because the abnormal chains compromise the function of the normal chains. Several types of mutations lead to the excretion of abnormal collagen. The most common are point mutations substituting another amino acid for a glycine in the proalpha 1 (I) chain. Glycine, the smallest amino acid, occurs in every third position in the collagen amino acid chain. This arrangement allows the three alpha (I) chains to form the triple helix. Therefore, substitutions for glycine either inhibit coiling or disrupt the helical stability. Because the helix formation begins at the C terminal ends of the alpha chains, the closer the substitution to this end, the more disrupted the collagen molecule and the more severe the phenotype. Thus, glycine substitution within the triple helix may produce different phenotypes of OI, depending on the location of the mutation.

Pathology

The pathologic features of type I OI, although nonspecific, reflect the biochemical defect that collagen is qualitatively normal but quantitatively reduced by one half. Osteopenia is the only significant finding. Both cortical thickness and trabecular volume, measured by histomorphometry, are diminished. However, the architecture is normal, the bone is lamellar, and haversian systems are present (Fig. 3–9). Bone turnover is normal or slightly reduced.[57]

Several important histopathologic features characterize the more severe forms of OI.[58,59] These features are present in types II, III, and IV in varying degrees of severity. The first feature, an increased number of osteocytes (hyperosteocytosis) is present in both cortical and trabecular bone. For the most part, the hyperosteocytosis is relative to the decreased volume of the extracellular matrix.

The next important pathologic feature is the persistence of woven bone. Woven bone is most abundant in type II OI. In fact, almost no lamellar bone is present. In types III and IV OI, most bone is lamellar, although some woven bone persists.

A third important histopathologic feature, seen in the more severe forms of OI, is the absence of mature cortical haversian systems. Although remodeling lines are present, a finding indicating bone turnover, a purposeful pattern is not recognizable.

In addition to the features described here, the cortices and trabeculae are thin, and the orientation of trabeculae is haphazard. These histologic features—purposeless remodeling, absence of mature cortical haversian systems, and trabecular disorientation—suggest that the genetic mutation

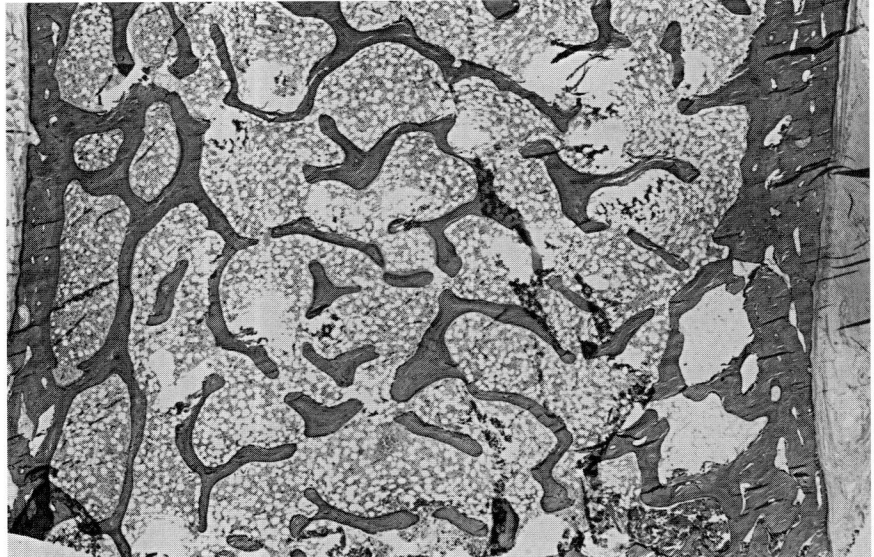

Figure 3-9 ■ Low-power photomicrograph of type I osteogenesis imperfecta. This transiliac crest biopsy shows mild osteopenia. However, bone architecture and trabecular connectedness are normal.

affects not only the quality and quantity of collagen synthesis, but also the bone organization.

The growth plate is also affected in OI. The growth plate is thin, the zones of columnation and hypertrophy are disorganized, and the amount of primary spongiosa is scant (Fig. 3–10). In addition, islands of hyaline cartilage persist in the metaphysis and epiphysis, presumably due to decreased endochondral ossification of cartilage. These entrapped islands of unossified cartilage account for the stippled radiodensities seen in the epiphyseal and metaphyseal zones.

Osteopetrosis

Unlike many skeletal dysplasias that lead to osteopenia, some genetic diseases, the most common being *osteopetrosis*, result in radiodense bones.[60] Osteopetrosis is a group of disorders characterized by decreased osteoclastic bone resorption. As a result, the bones become extremely dense, a feature that has led to the name "marble bone disease."

Pathogenesis

A spectrum of clinical severity in osteopetrosis indicates that bone resorption can be inhibited in varying degrees and reflects the complex origin of functional osteoclasts.[61] Indeed, osteoclast differentiation and activation is multifactorial and depends on hematopoietic stem cell competence as well as signals from osteoblasts and the extracellular microenvironment. Because of these complex interactions, osteoclast function can be blocked at a number of points, thereby inhibiting bone resorption in varying degrees of severity. For example, in some forms of osteopetrosis, osteoclasts are present (even in large numbers) but cannot resorb bone. In other forms, osteoclasts are markedly reduced in number or absent.[62] In those cases in which osteoclasts are absent, excellent therapeutic results have been achieved with bone marrow transplantation, a procedure that delivers competent stem cells. This effect, first noted in 1975, when osteopetrotic rats were cured by bone marrow transplantation, established that osteoclasts are derived from hematopoi-

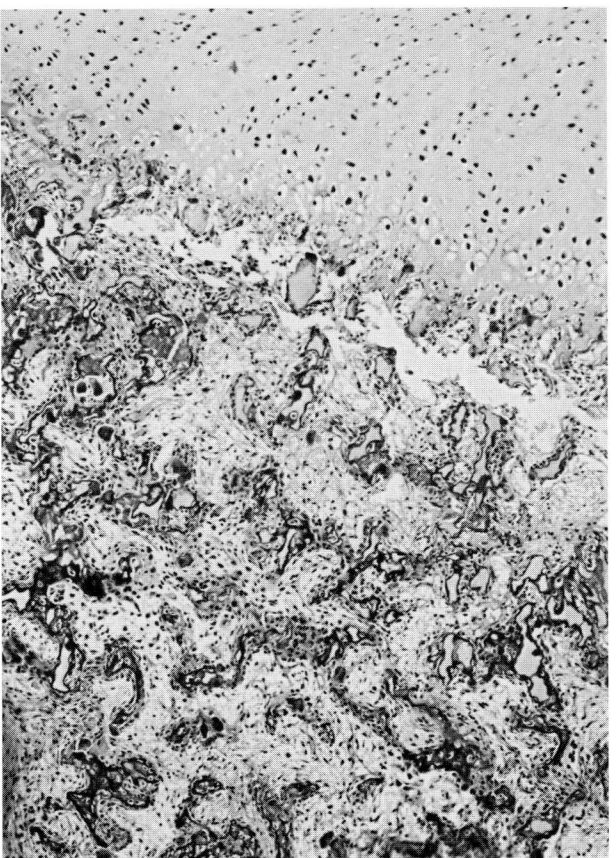

Figure 3-10 ■ Growth plate of osteogenesis imperfecta. Near total disorganization of the primary spongiosa has occurred.

etic stem cells.[63] By contrast, bone marrow transplantation is ineffective in those cases in which osteoclasts are present but paralyzed. In these cases, osteoclast dysfunction is probably the result of inefficient signals from the microenvironment.

The molecular genetics of osteopetrosis is poorly understood. Unlike OI, in which different point mutations in a single gene result in different phenotypes, the varying clinical severity in osteopetrosis is likely due to mutations in different genes. However, the exact mutation in most forms of the disease has not been identified. In some patients or animal models, a defect in the *C-src*[64] or *C-fos*[65] gene has been identified. Other investigators have demonstrated a defect in osteoblasts.[66] Specifically, osteoblasts are unable to synthesize macrophage colony factor, an important cytokine that stimulates the differentiation of osteoclasts. Finally, some patients with osteopetrosis encode reverse transcriptase, a viral protein, suggesting that in these patients' families, the mutation originated with a viral infection.[67]

Radiographic Features

The radiographic features of osteopetrosis reflect defective bone resorption, although changes vary in severity in different patients. The bones show diffuse, symmetric sclerosis. The long bones frequently show transverse metaphyseal sclerotic bands (Fig. 3–11). They also show modeling deformities, a feature particularly evident in the femurs, which are shaped like Erlenmeyer flasks. In addition, the vertebrae frequently have a "rugger jersey" appearance due to sclerosis beneath the endplates (Fig. 3–12). Other bones, such as the ilium, show a "bone within a bone" pattern. The bones of the skull are also thickened and sclerotic, a feature most marked at the base.

Pathologic Features

The pathologic features of osteopetrosis are also a result of the osteoclast's inability to resorb bone. Changes are most evident in the metaphyseal region. Unresorbed primary spongiosa fills the metaphysis and diaphysis with broad streams of calcified cartilage encased by bone. The bone is usually woven, although in some instances, lamellar features are present. In severe cases, the marrow cavity is entirely effaced by unresorbed bone. In those cases in which osteoclasts are abundant, they are not, like functional osteoclasts, present in Howship's lacunae. Electron microscopic study of these osteoclasts reveals the absence of a ruffled border.[68]

Clinical Presentation

Three important clinical features of osteopetrosis result from resorptive failure and the disordered bone architecture. First, despite very dense bones, the disordered architecture leads to bone fragility. Therefore, fractures are a frequent complication of osteopetrosis. Second, obliteration of the marrow cavity causes anemia. Third, impingement of neural foramina in the skull often causes cranial nerve palsies. In

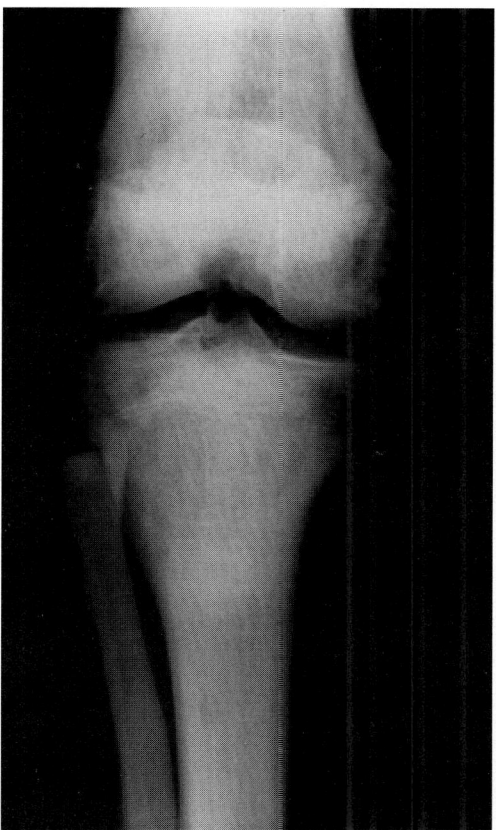

Figure 3-11 ■ Osteopetrosis of the femur and tibia. Intense radiodensity with transverse radiodense bands is present.

addition to the clinical features related to failure of resorption, patients are also susceptible to osteomyelitis. This feature, caused by a degree of immune incompetence, is probably due to the same defect that inhibits osteoclast differentiation.

At least nine forms of osteopetrosis exist, each exhibiting a different pattern of osteoclast dysfunction. However, most patients can be classified as one of four phenotypes. The largest category includes patients with mild autosomal dominant disease. The mild form of osteopetrosis was the first to be recognized. In 1907, Albers-Schönberg, a German radiologist, described a 24-year-old man with dense bones and multiple fractures (osteopetrosis is sometimes called Albers-Schönberg disease).[69] Even within this category of mild disease, variations in severity and varying patterns of skeletal involvement indicate genetic heterogeneity.[70] For example, serum acid phosphatase is elevated in some patients and not in others. The general health and life span of patients with mild autosomal dominant osteopetrosis is normal. Indeed, some patients are asymptomatic and are diagnosed only incidentally when radiographs are taken for other reasons. Other patients have mild anemia and a history of a few fractures. More severely affected patients may develop osteomyelitis or suffer cranial nerve palsies.[71]

At the other end of the clinical spectrum, an autosomal recessive form of osteopetrosis, known as malignant os-

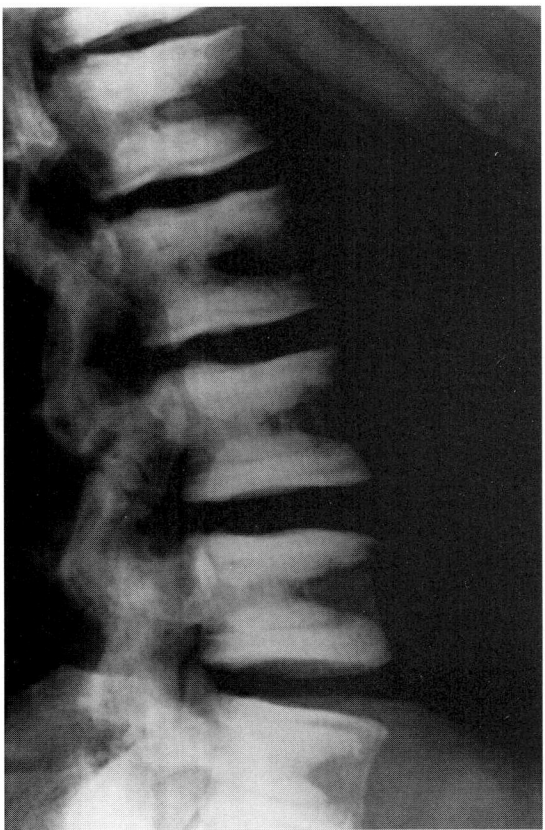

Figure 3-12 ■ Osteopetrosis of the spine. Radiodensity beneath the endplates causes a "rugger jersey" pattern.

teopetrosis, causes severe disease. Patients present in infancy and usually die before age 10.[72] Severe pancytopenia, hepatosplenomegaly, and cranial nerve palsies are common. In addition, patients sustain multiple fractures and are prone to develop osteomyelitis.

A third clinical pattern of osteopetrosis, an autosomal recessive disorder, is intermediate in severity between the mild autosomal dominant pattern and the malignant form.

A rare fourth pattern of osteopetrosis is associated with renal tubular acidosis. To date, this phenotype is the only form of osteopetrosis understood at the genetic level. Patients have a genetic mutation resulting in very low levels of carbonic anhydrase II, an enzyme necessary for bone resorption. In addition to sclerotic bones, patients with carbonic anhydrase II deficiency have dense cerebral calcifications (marble brain disease), a complication that frequently causes mental retardation.[73]

Treatment

Osteopetrosis has been treated in various ways. Bone marrow transplantation has been used in young patients with severe disease. However, an acceptable donor can be found for only 40% of patients. Following this procedure, 45% of patients survive, and half of these are cured of the disease. Alternatively, some patients (about 25%) respond to high doses of calcitriol (1,25 vitamin D), a compound known to stimulate osteoclasts. Finally, some therapeutic success has been achieved with interferon-γ, a compound that stimulates osteoclast superoxide.[74]

Progressive Diaphyseal Dysplasia

Progressive diaphyseal dysplasia, also known as Camurati-Engelmann disease, is another skeletal dysplasia that causes dense bones. The genetic abnormality in progressive diaphyseal dysplasia is unknown, and both sporadic and familial cases occur. The familial cases suggest an autosomal dominant mode of inheritance. Unlike the increased bone density of osteopetrosis, which is caused by paralysis of osteoclastic resorption, the dense bones of progressive diaphyseal dysplasia are the result of excessive periosteal osteoblastic activity. The characteristic feature of this disease is fusiform thickening of the diaphyseal cortex, which symmetrically involves the long bones of the skeleton (Fig. 3-13). The bones most frequently involved are the tibia, femur, fibula, humerus, radius, and ulna. The cortical thickening, caused by both periosteal and endosteal bone deposition, narrows but does not obliterate the marrow cavity. In addition, the skull is sometimes hyperostotic.

Progressive diaphyseal dysplasia usually begins in the first decade of life.[75, 76] Patients present with bone pain, muscular weakness, and sometimes with muscular wasting. Blood chemistries, including indices of bone turnover, are normal. Although the disease progresses in severity for a number of years, the process is self-limited and generally resolves by age 30.

The pathologic features of diaphyseal dysplasia are nonspecific and offer no clue to the genetic defect. In the diaphyseal portions of the long bones, the periosteum is thickened, and there is a zonal pattern of new bone, which, in the deeper layers, is transformed into lamellar bone. This lamellar bone blends with the outer cortex in successive layers.[77]

Osteopoikilosis

Osteopoikilosis is another hereditary bone disease that causes increased bone density. However, unlike the diffuse or fusiform radiodensity of most other sclerosing bone dysplasias, osteopoikilosis, also known as spotted bone disease, is characterized by multiple discrete round or oval radiodensities. Each locus is an enostosis (bone island), a common isolated lesion of bone. However, in osteopoikilosis, hundreds of these lesions are symmetrically clustered in epiphyseal and metaphyseal regions throughout the skeleton.

Osteopoikilosis is transmitted as an autosomal dominant condition. Although not understood at the molecular level, osteopoikilosis seems to be a result of focal disordered bone remodeling. This disorder is asymptomatic; cases are usually discovered incidentally during radiographic examination for other reasons. In addition to bone lesions, some patients with

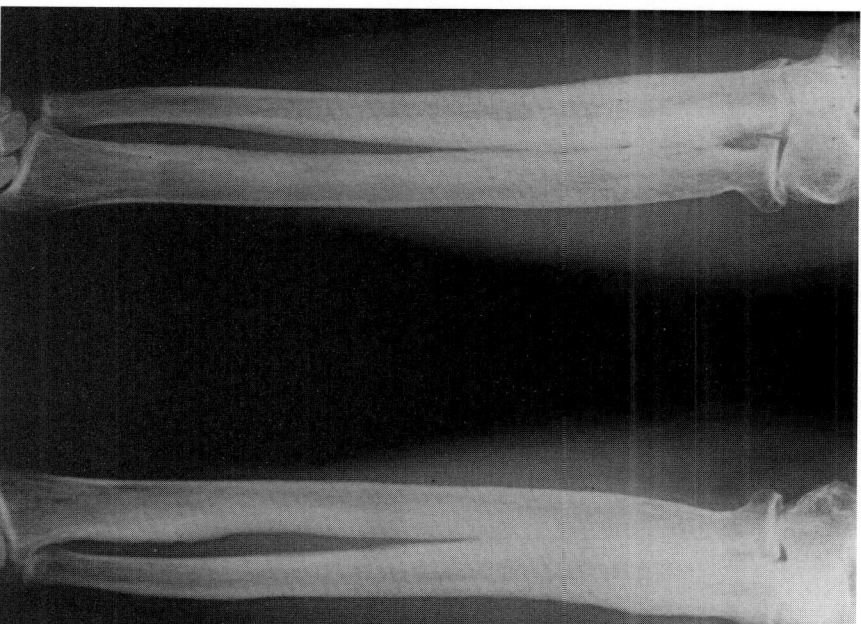

Figure 3-13 ■ Progressive diaphyseal dysplasia. Irregular periosteal new bone is present along the entire shafts of both the ulna and radius.

osteopoikilosis have a hereditary dermatologic condition called dermatofibrosis lenticularis disseminata.[78] This skin condition is characterized by multiple small subcutaneous or dermal fibromas. The association of these skin lesions with osteopoikilosis suggests an underlying connective tissue disorder.

Radiographically, each osteopoikilotic focus is an oval or lenticular density that is 0.5 to 1.0 cm in maximal diameter. Like a bone island (see Chapter 12), each focus is either sharply circumscribed or has radiating bone spicules that blend with the surrounding trabeculae. Usually, each focus is confluent with the endosteal cortex. Importantly, the radiodensities are scattered symmetrically throughout the skeleton, a feature that helps distinguish this disease from metastatic osteoblastic carcinoma (Fig. 3–14).

The histologic features of each osteopoikilotic focus are identical to an isolated enostosis. A condensation of dense compact bone is present in the spongiosa. The bone is lamellar and shows evidence of remodeling. Also, haversian systems may be present.[79]

Achondroplasia

Osteogenesis imperfecta and the sclerosing bone dysplasias are disorders of the formation or remodeling of bone. However, the largest group of skeletal dysplasias, known as the *chondrodysplasias,* are disorders of the structure or growth of cartilage. Achondroplasia is one of the most common chondrodysplasias. However, because many chondrodysplasias are erroneously classified as achondroplasia, this disorder is not as common as previously thought.[80]

Pathogenesis

Achondroplasia is a disease of retarded cartilage growth, a problem most manifested at the growth plate. As a result, bones formed by endochondral ossification, particularly the long bones, are short and abnormally shaped. Achondroplasia is diagnosable at birth, and by adulthood, patients have a markedly short stature.

Although achondroplasia is inherited as an autosomal dominant disorder, 87% of cases are caused by a new mutation (patients have normal parents). At the molecular level, cartilage in achondroplasia lacks a receptor for a growth factor. Specifically, the disease is a result of mutation in the gene encoding fibroblast growth factor receptor 3, located at the p16.3 locus of chromosome 4.[81] The transcript of this gene is abundant in the cartilage anlage of all bones as well as in the resting zone of the epiphyseal plate. The mutation, which affects the transmembrane domain of the receptor, substitutes an arginine for a glycine in the amino acid chain. Because this mutation is constant in almost all patients with achondroplasia, very little phenotypic variation occurs in this disorder.

Pathology

The pathologic features of achondroplasia reflect a quantitative rather than qualitative abnormality of cartilage growth and endochondral ossification, although bones are abnormally shaped very early in development (Fig. 3–15). The organization of the growth plate is normal, but in some cases the various zones are shortened (Fig. 3–16).[82] The articular cartilage is normal; therefore, premature arthritic change is not a feature of achondroplasia. Membranous bone formation is also normal, so bones have a normal width.

Radiographic Features

The radiographic features of achondroplasia correlate with the clinical features. First, the skull is affected. The head is large, and frontal bossing is prominent. Children with this

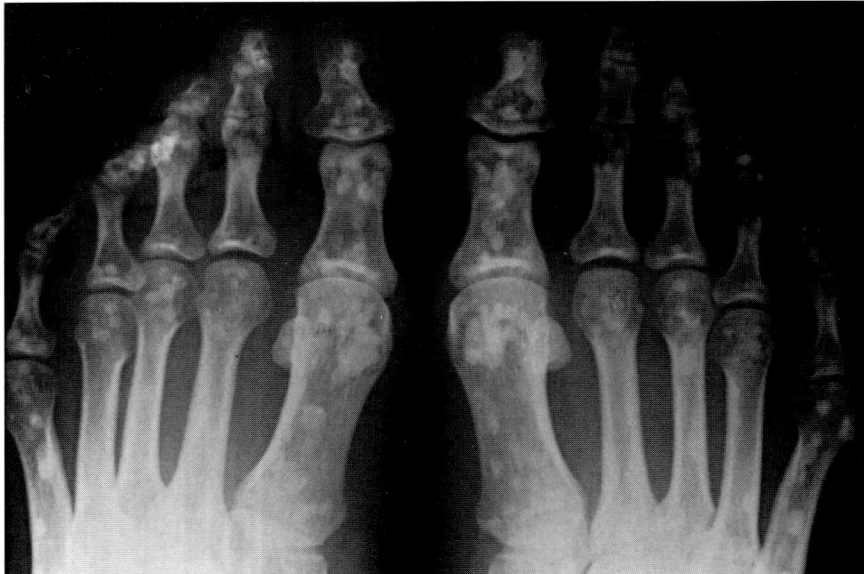

Figure 3-14 ■ Osteopoikilosis. The radiodense foci are symmetrically distributed throughout the feet.

disorder often have macrocephaly and a mild hydrocephalus. Also, the facial bones, particularly the bridge of the nose, are hypoplastic. The base of the skull, because of its origin in cartilage, is underdeveloped. As a result, the foramen magnum is small throughout the patient's life. This feature may lead to spinal cord compression and perhaps accounts for hypotonia present in affected infants.

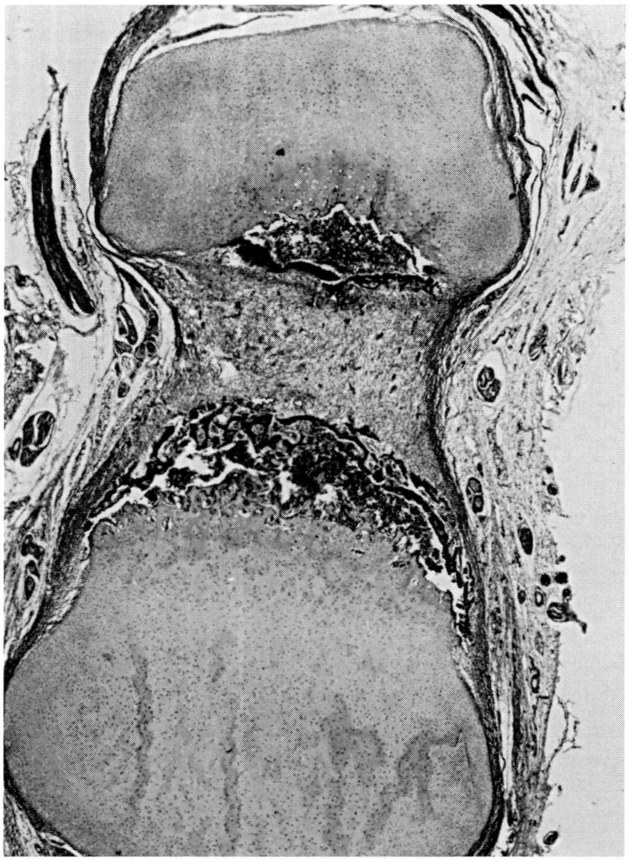

The spine is the second important area to be affected in achondroplasia. The height of the vertebral bodies, and therefore the trunk length, is relatively normal. However, the posterior elements are underdeveloped, a problem that causes narrowing of the spinal canal and neural foramina. Spinal stenosis, the most common orthopedic problem in achondroplasia, results from this narrowing.[83]

The third important manifestation of achondroplasia is shortening of the tubular bones, most severe in the femur and humerus (Fig. 3–17). Although the bones are short, they are quite broad, a reflection of normal membranous bone formation. The fibula is less affected than the tibia. Therefore, the proportionately longer fibula causes tibial bowing and contributes to the genu varum usually seen in this disorder.

Patients with achondroplasia have normal intelligence. With proper management of the orthopedic complications, patients may lead full and productive lives.

Related Disorders

Although very little phenotypic variation occurs in patients with achondroplasia, another disorder, known as *hypochondroplasia* is very similar but less severe.[84] The mutation in this disorder has been mapped to the same locus on chromosome 4. However, the mutation causes a less severe abnormality in fibroblast growth factor receptor 3 protein. The skeleton is affected in a similar way to achondroplasia, but the changes are mild.

At the severe end of the spectrum of skeletal abnormality, a disorder known as *thanatophoric dysplasia,* also shares features with achondroplasia. Due to a much more severe mutation in the achondroplasia gene, this syndrome is in-

Figure 3-15 ■ Achondroplasia. This section through a phalanx of an infant demonstrates the abnormally shaped long bones characteristic of achondroplasia.

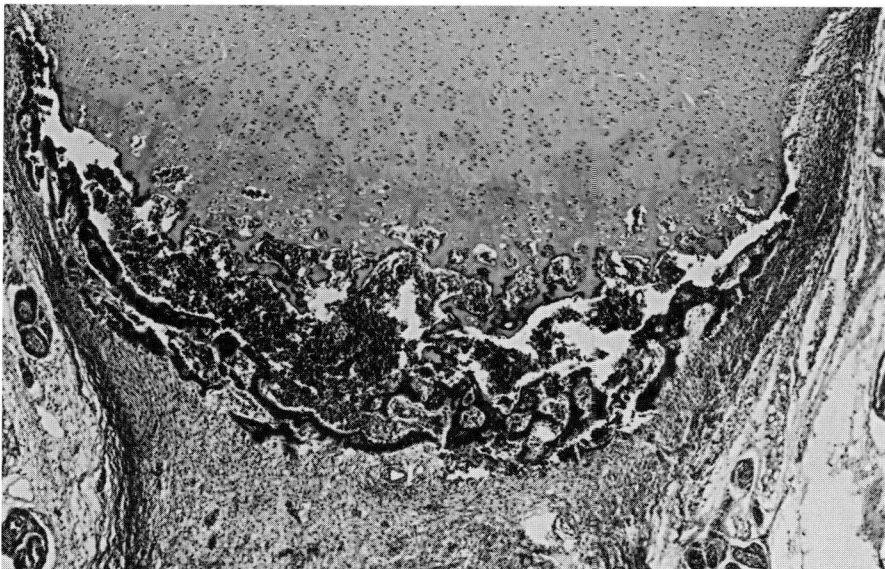

Figure 3-16 ■ Achondroplasia growth center. Disorganization of the primary spongiosa is present.

compatible with life. Thanatophoric dysplasia resembles homozygous achondroplasia, a lethal condition that affects 25% of the children of two achondroplastic parents. In both of these severe dysplasias, death usually occurs in infancy because of respiratory insufficiency.

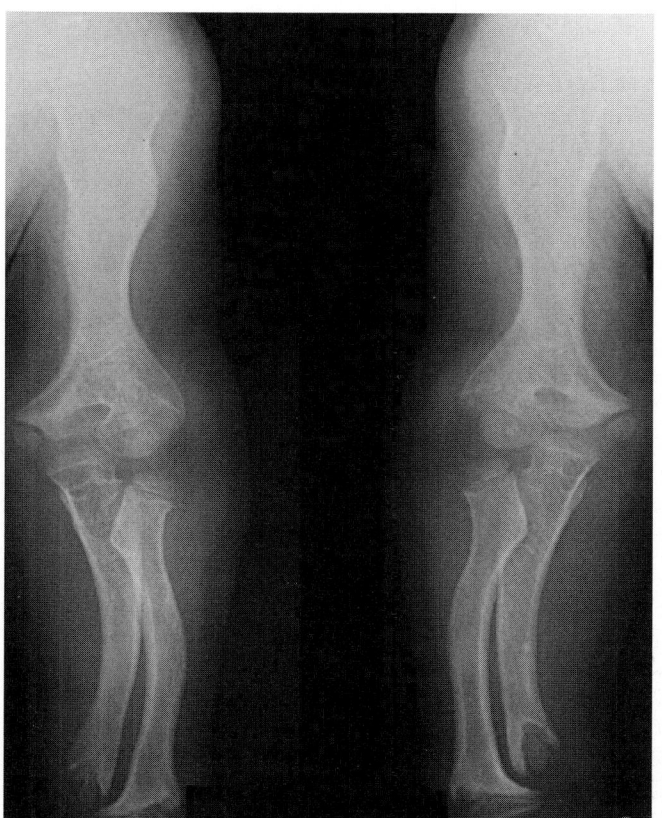

Figure 3-17 ■ Achondroplasia. The long bones of the arm are shortened and broad.

Spondyloepiphyseal Dysplasia

The spondyloepiphyseal dysplasias are a heterogeneous group of disorders characterized radiographically by an abnormal spine and dysplastic epiphyses. Genetically, however, these disorders are heterogeneous. Although they share radiographic features, the various manifestations of spondyloepiphyseal dysplasia are caused by mutations in different genes. One particular mutation, responsible for a number of chondrodysplasias in this group, occurs in the *COL2A1* gene on chromosome 12.[85, 86] This gene encodes the proalpha 1 (II) chains of type II procollagen.[87] As a result, patients have defective type II collagen, the major collagen of cartilage.

Spondyloepiphyseal dysplasias resulting from mutations in the *COL2A1* gene vary in clinical severity, depending on the site of mutation. Therefore, the phenotypic variation in this family of skeletal dysplasia is similar to that in OI. For example, the *Stickler syndrome,* a mild form of spondyloepiphyseal dysplasia, is caused by a null mutation.[86] Type II collagen is structurally normal but is synthesized in one half the normal amount, paralleling the pathogenesis of type I OI. Another mutation, one that causes defective collagen XI synthesis, also causes the Stickler syndrome.[88] At the severe end of the spondyloepiphyseal dysplasia spectrum, *achondrogenesis type II* results in death in the perinatal period. In this syndrome, a severe dominant negative mutation results in almost no type II collagen synthesis.

Clinical Features

The prototype of this family, *spondyloepiphyseal dysplasia congenita,* is a syndrome of intermediate severity.[89] This autosomal dominant syndrome, although diagnosable at birth, is compatible with survival into adulthood. The principal features are short stature with a proportionally short trunk and joint deformity caused by dysplastic epiphyses.

Premature osteoarthritis inevitably results, a feature that distinguishes this syndrome from achondroplasia. In addition, because the vitreous of the eye also contains type II collagen, patients almost always suffer severe visual impairment.

Radiographic Features

The radiographic features of spondyloepiphyseal dysplasia, most prominent in the spine and major joints, correlate with clinical problems. In the spine, the vertebrae are small and wedged (Fig. 3–18). Progressive kyphoscoliosis, often requiring fusion, usually develops in late childhood. Also in the spine, a hypoplastic odontoid leads to atlantoaxial instability. This feature poses the constant threat of neurologic catastrophe and often requires cervical fusion.

The joints, particularly the hips and knees, are also severely affected. The ossification centers are delayed. As a result, the epiphyseal ends of the bones are flattened and irregular. Severe coxa vara and genu valgum are common. Proximal femoral and tibial osteotomies sometimes forestall the development of osteoarthritis. Ultimately, however, patients usually require total joint arthroplasty.

Pathology

The pathologic study of cartilage in patients with spondyloepiphyseal dysplasia congenita reveals chondrocyte inclusions, which, when seen with the electron microscope, correspond to dilated endoplasmic reticulum. Cartilage changes are otherwise nonspecific. For example, the growth plates show only minimal disorganization.

Pseudoachondroplasia

Pseudoachondroplasia, one of the more common skeletal dysplasias, is a group of disorders that are members of the spondyloepiphyseal dysplasia family.[90] Although the name *pseudoachondroplasia* suggests a similarity to achondroplasia, these disorders are easily distinguished. First, unlike achondroplasia, the face and skull are normal in pseudoachondroplasia. Therefore, this disorder is not generally recognized at birth. However, by age 2 or 3 years, growth retardation calls attention to the osseous abnormalities. Second, the vertebral bodies in pseudoachondroplasia show mild flattening and anterior wedging, features not seen in achondroplasia. Third, although both dysplasias are characterized by short stature, the epiphyses are dysplastic in pseudoachondroplasia. Joint surface incongruity leads to deformity and the development of premature osteoarthritis. The joint deformities may be exaggerated by generalized ligamentous laxity, a prominent feature of pseudoachondroplasia.

Four subtypes of pseudoachondroplasia, based on modes of inheritance and severity, are recognized. Most cases are autosomal dominant, and the gene for this subtype has been mapped to chromosome 19.

Unlike some of the other spondyloepiphyseal dysplasias, defective type II collagen synthesis is not a feature of pseudoachondroplasia. Instead, pseudoachondroplasia is caused by ineffective proteoglycan synthesis. The pathogenesis appears to be an inability to secrete core protein, and as a result, proteoglycans cannot be assembled. Electron microscopic study of chondrocytes in pseudoachondroplasia reveals distinctive laminated cytoplasmic inclusions (Fig. 3–19).[91] These inclusions stain with antibodies to core protein, a finding supporting the theory of defective core protein secretion.[92, 93]

Multiple Epiphyseal Dysplasia

Multiple epiphyseal dysplasia, another of the more common skeletal dysplasias, is characterized by malformed epiphyses and relatively normal vertebrae. Although exhibiting a broad spectrum of clinical severity, multiple epiphyseal dysplasia is one of the milder skeletal dysplasias. Therefore, this disorder is usually not diagnosed until patients are between ages 5 and 10.[94] A few do not present until early adulthood. Usually, joint pain or an abnormal gait calls attention to this disorder. Because the vertebrae are minimally involved, shortening of stature is not severe. In fact, many patients are over 5 ft tall.

Multiple epiphyseal dysplasia is almost always transmitted as an autosomal dominant disorder. In families with this disorder, multiple affected members are common.

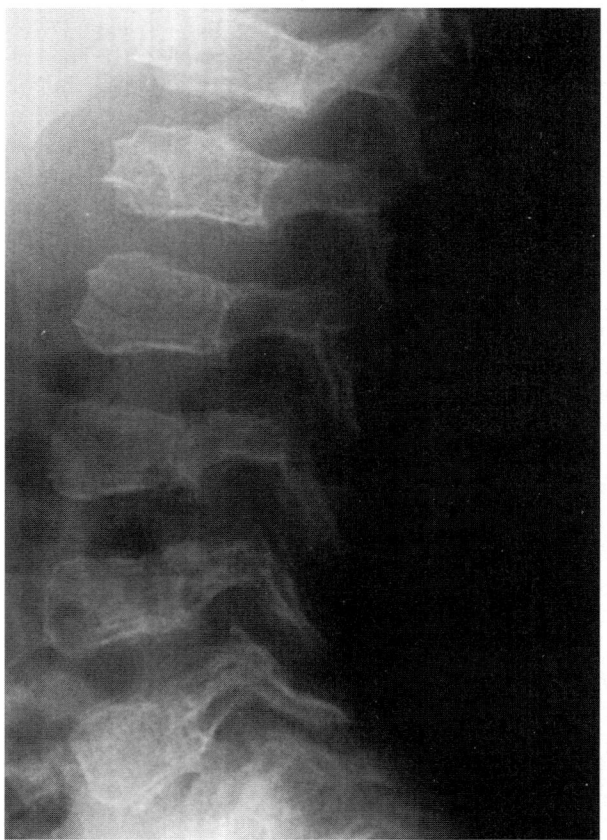

Figure 3–18 ▪ Spondyloepiphyseal dysplasia. The vertebral bodies are flattened and show typical step-off deformities.

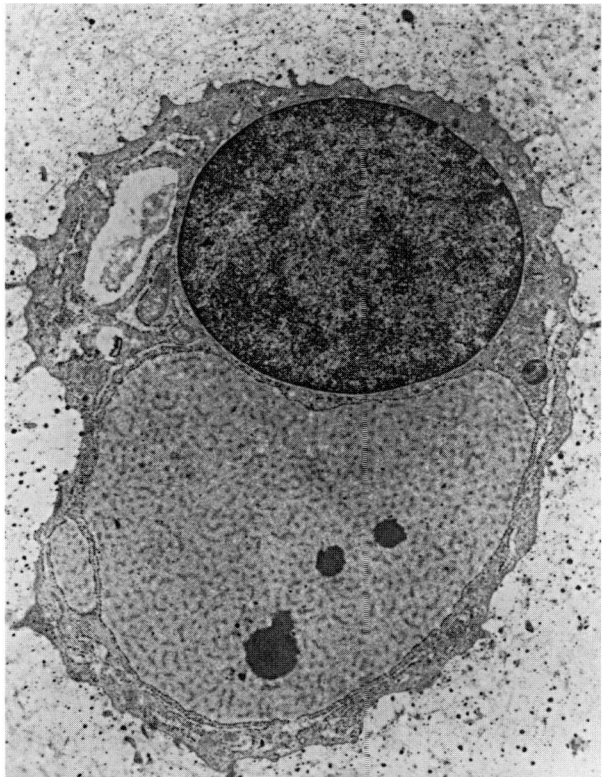

Figure 3-19 ■ A chondrocyte from the growth plate of a patient with pseudoachondroplasia. A large perinuclear inclusion containing laminated particles. This inclusion, which is larger than the nucleus, is a dilated portion of endoplasmic reticulum. (Courtesy of Dr. Jerry Maynard, Department of Exercise Science, University of Iowa, Iowa City.)

Radiographic Features

The radiographic changes are most evident in the epiphyses of the tubular bones. The first sign of this disorder is a generalized delay in the appearance of the epiphyseal ossification centers. When the centers do appear, they are irregular and mottled; often they appear fragmented. After completion of skeletal growth, the epiphyses are flattened and malformed (Fig. 3–20). Joint involvement is symmetric, although the hips, knees, and ankles are more severely affected. Because of apparent epiphyseal fragmentation, hip involvement may be misdiagnosed as bilateral Perthes disease. Multiple epiphyseal dysplasia does in fact predispose to secondary osteonecrosis.[95] However, a skeletal survey, disclosing other sites of epiphyseal dysplasia, confirms the diagnosis of multiple epiphyseal dysplasia. The malformed epiphyses often lead to joint deformity, such as coxa vara and genu valgum. As a result, severe osteoarthritis, particularly of the hips, is common before age 30. Therefore, the diagnosis of multiple epiphyseal dysplasia should be considered in any patient with precocious osteoarthritis.

Pathology

The histologic features of this disorder, like those of most other skeletal dysplasias, are not specific. The growth plates are mildly irregular, and, like many of the chondrodystrophies, cytoplasmic inclusions have been demonstrated in the chondrocytes by electron microscopy. Large accumulations of core protein have been demonstrated by immunohistochemical methods in these inclusions, a finding that suggests a kinship to pseudoachondroplasia.[96]

Metaphyseal Chondrodysplasia

Metaphyseal chondrodysplasia refers to a heterogeneous group of disorders characterized by abnormalities in the metaphyseal regions of the long bones and short tubular bones. At least seven distinct entities belong to this family of chondrodysplasias. In general, the metaphyseal changes in these disorders are caused by growth plate abnormalities.

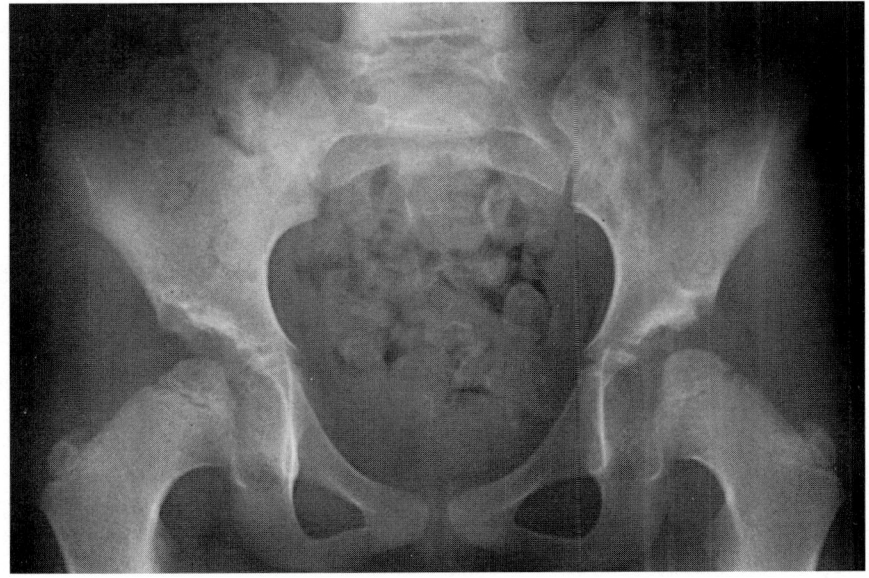

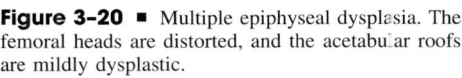

Figure 3-20 ■ Multiple epiphyseal dysplasia. The femoral heads are distorted, and the acetabular roofs are mildly dysplastic.

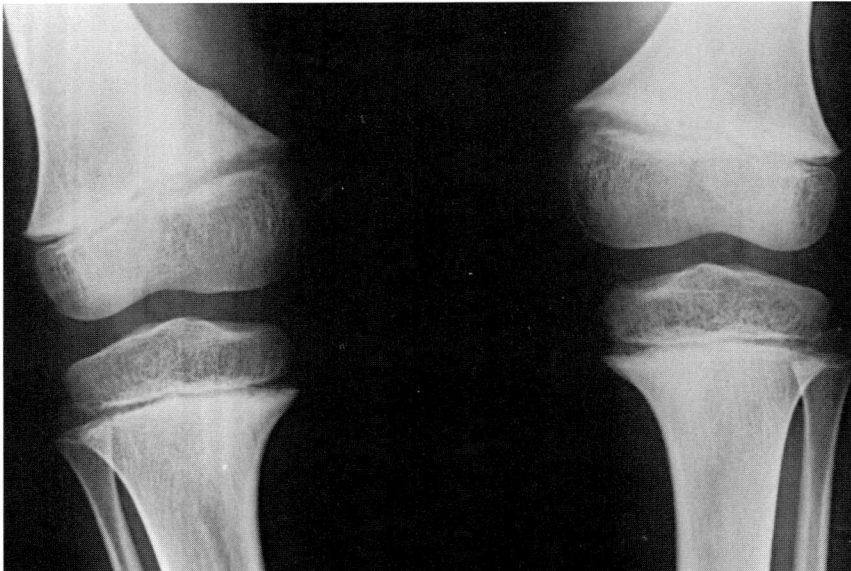

Figure 3–21 ▪ Metaphyseal chondrodysplasia, McKusick type. Irregularity and focal widening of epiphyseal plates is seen. This pattern may be mistaken for rickets.

Specifically, instead of normal columnation, the chondrocytes are arranged in clusters and nests. These changes result in widened and irregular growth plates that are often mistaken for evidence of rickets[97] (Fig. 3–21). With the electron microscope, chondrocytes in some forms of metaphyseal chondrodysplasia can be seen to contain granular precipitates in the endoplasmic reticulum.[98, 99]

Two of the more common forms of metaphyseal chondrodysplasia are the Schmid type and the McKusick type, originally called cartilage-hair hypoplasia. Children with the Schmid type, an autosomal dominant disorder, present with mildly shortened stature, varus deformities of the knees, and mild lordosis. The face and head are normal.[100]

The McKusick type of metaphyseal chondrodysplasia involves the spine as well as the metaphyseal regions of tubular bones. This autosomal recessive disorder is distinctive in its high rate of occurrence in two population groups—the Amish and the Finnish. In addition to growth plate abnormalities, patients with this disorder have the characteristic feature of sparse, lightly colored hair. Microscopically, the hair diameter is smaller than normal, and it often lacks pigment. Many patients with the McKusick type of metaphyseal chondrodysplasia suffer other problems that indicate that the genetic defect affects tissues other than bone.[101] For example, in over half of the patients, cellular immunity is diminished, a problem predisposing them to viral infections. In addition, intestinal malabsorption or megacolon sometimes occurs. Most patients have some degree of generalized ligamentous laxity.

FOCAL DEVELOPMENTAL DISORDERS

Dysplasia Epiphysealis Hemimelica

Dysplasia epiphysealis hemimelica, also known as Trevor's disease, is a developmental disorder characterized by bony overgrowth of the epiphyseal region of one or a few bones.[102] A resulting protuberance resembles a sessile osteochondroma. When more than one epiphysis is involved, lesions are usually confined to one side of one extremity, usually the medial side. Often, bones on both sides of a joint are involved. Although a family has been described with this disease, there is no known genetic cause.[103]

Patients with dysplasia epiphysealis hemimelica usually present before age 14 with a painless lump adjacent to a joint. Occasionally, mild limitation of joint motion or joint deformity occurs. The distal femur, proximal tibia, talus, and tarsal navicular are, in that order, the most commonly involved sites.[104] Other common sites include the distal tibial epiphysis, the carpal bones, and the scapula. In general, the upper extremities are less commonly involved than the lower extremities.

Radiographically, a bony protuberance is present on one side of the epiphysis (Fig. 3–22). Early lesions contain multiple centers of ossification that later fuse with the epiphysis.

Histologically, the bony mass resembles an osteochondroma. Mature cortical and cancellous bone is covered by a cartilage cap. This cap undergoes endochondral ossification, which increases the size of the lesion until skeletal maturity is reached. Usually, lesions are separated from the true epiphysis by a cartilage boundary. However, when skeletal maturation is achieved, this boundary disappears and the lesion fuses to the epiphysis.

Melorheostosis

Melorheostosis is a disorder characterized by irregular cortical hyperostosis that follows the long axis of a bone, often for its entire length (Fig. 3–23). Usually, multiple bones in the same extremity are involved.[105] In addition, the skull, spine, pelvis, and ribs are sometimes affected.

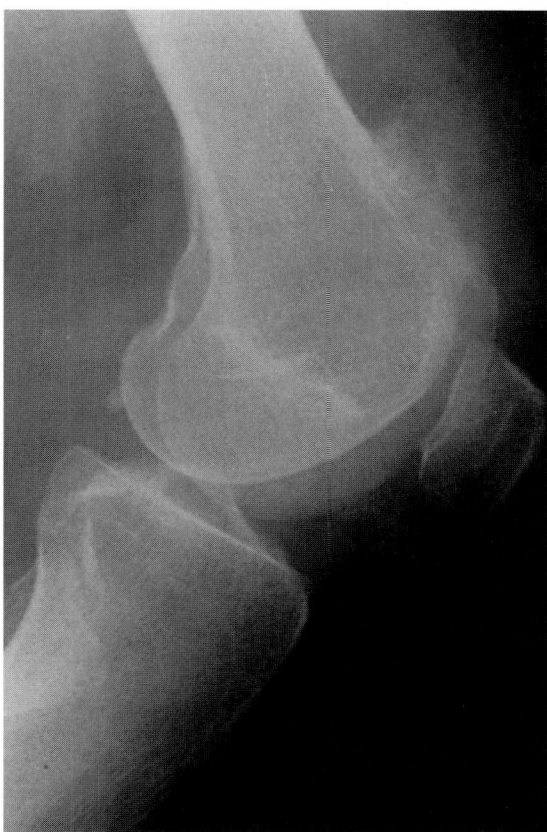

Figure 3-22 ■ Dysplasia epiphysealis hemimelica showing a bony protrusion from the epiphysis of the distal femur.

Sometimes ossification even occurs in the skin and soft tissue overlying involved bones. In addition to periosteal ossification, the patient's skin is often tight and shiny, and soft tissue fibrosis results in joint contractures. This disorder occurs sporadically, and no genetic factors have been identified. Because the hyperostosis appears to follow dermatomes, a neuropathic etiology has been postulated.

Melorheostosis occurs in both children and adults. The usual presentation in childhood is a painless contracture before age 6.[106] Pain does not develop until late adolescence. Flexion contracture of the knee is most common, followed by that of the ankle, hip, and fingers. Children may also present with leg length discrepancy due to premature closure of the epiphyseal plate on the affected side.

Pathologically, the cortical hyperostosis is the result of the deposition of periosteal new bone, which gradually matures into mature lamellar bone with haversian systems. Endosteal hyperostosis also occurs.

Treatment of melorheostosis is supportive. Surgery to release flexion contractures is often unsuccessful because of the severity of the soft tissue fibrosis. The pain responds somewhat to analgesics.

ROLE OF THE PATHOLOGIST IN THE SKELETAL DYSPLASIAS

The diagnosis and management of the skeletal dysplasias requires teamwork among the radiologist, the geneticist, the orthopedic surgeon, and the pathologist. The pathologist's role is to insure that tissues removed at surgery or at autopsy are correctly collected and processed. Although the histologic features of bone and cartilage in most skeletal dysplasias are nonspecific and nondiagnostic, the pathologist must carefully study these specimens to correlate changes with radiographs and clinical information. Occasionally, morphologic features do aid in the diagnosis of a dysplasia or help clarify its pathogenesis. In addition, tissues can be used for DNA analysis, which may identify mutations.

Surgical Specimens

The pathologist studies tissues that have been removed during autopsy or surgical procedures from a skeletal dysplasia. These latter tissues require special attention. The pathologist must study the articular surface, growth plate, and bone marrow. In addition, bone marrow and cartilage from the epiphyseal plate and articular surface should be processed for electron microscopic study. Electron microscopy is necessary to characterize the cytoplasmic inclusions seen in many skeletal dysplasias. Finally, cartilage and marrow should be frozen at $-70°C$ for future genetic or biochemical studies.

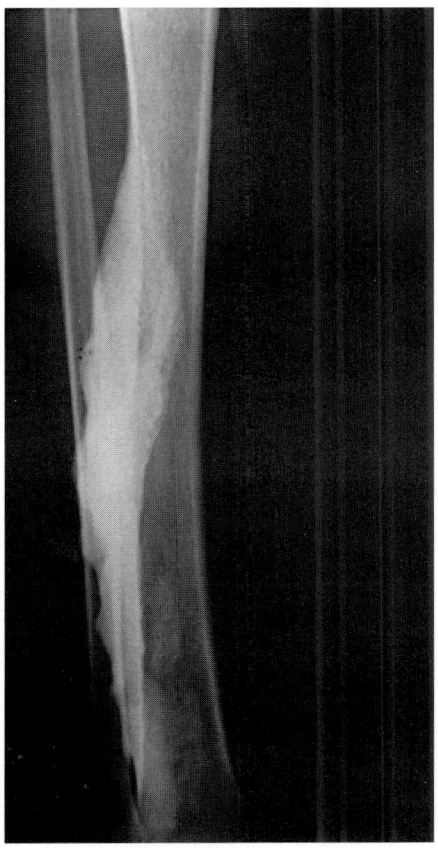

Figure 3-23 ■ Melorheostosis. A stream of periosteal new bone flows down the shaft of the tibia.

The Autopsy

The autopsy provides unique opportunities to study the skeletal dysplasias. Abundant tissues can be studied with radiographic correlation. For stillborns, neonates, and children, proper procedure is necessary to insure the correct diagnosis, critical to genetic counseling.

Autopsy services should have a protocol to direct the examination of deceased infants and children with congenital bone disease. The autopsy protocol should be centered around *photographic and radiographic documentation.* Photographs, both black and white and color, should be taken of the whole body. Anterior, posterior, and lateral views should be taken of the face, head, and hands. In addition to photographs, high-quality radiographs should be taken in the autopsy suite. An anteroposterior and a lateral view of the full body are a minimum. As with photographs, close-up radiographs of the head and hands should also be taken.

For microscopic study, sections of the long bones and vertebral bodies are most informative. Ideally, the whole femur and tibia should be removed and bivalved coronally with a gentle saw or, preferably, with a knife. Care should be taken to preserve the articular surface, epiphysis, growth plate, and metaphysis en bloc. An entire vertebral body should be studied or, preferably, several contiguous vertebrae with intervertebral discs. As with surgical specimens, samples of articular cartilage, growth plate, and bone marrow should be preserved for electron microscopic study. Also, samples of the tissues should be frozen for genetic analysis. Finally, sterile sections of skin and bone should be placed in tissue culture media for future study.

REFERENCES

1. McKusick, V. A.: *Mendelian Inheritance in Man. Catalogue of Autosomal Dominant, Autosomal Recessive, and X-Linked Phenotypes,* 10th ed. Baltimore, Johns Hopkins University Press, 1992.
2. Mulvihill, J. J., Parry, D. M., Sherman, D. L., Pikus, A., Kaiser-Kupfer, M. I., and Eldridge, R.: Neurofibromatosis 1 (Recklinghausen disease) and neurofibromatosis 2 (bilateral acoustic neurofibromatosis). An update. *Ann Int Med* 113:39–52, 1990.
3. von Recklinghausen, F. D.: *Ueber die in multiplen Fibrome der Haut und ihre Beziehung zu den multiplen Neuromen.* Berlin, Hirschwald, 1882.
4. Madigan, P., and Masello, M. J.: Report of a neurofibromatosis-like case: Monstrorum Historia, 1642. *Neurofibromatosis* 2:53–56, 1989.
5. Pomerance, B.: *The Elephant Man.* New York, Grove Press, 1979.
6. Neurofibromatosis Conference Statement: National Institutes of Health Consensus Development Conference. *Arch Neurol* 45:575–578, 1988.
7. Moss, C., and Green, S. H.: What is segmental neurofibromatosis? *Br J Dermatol* 130:106–110, 1994.
8. Crawford, A. H., and Bagamery, N.: Osseous manifestations of neurofibromatosis in childhood. *J Pediatr Orthop* 6:72–88, 1986.
9. Winter, R. B., Moe, J. H., Bradford, D. S., Longstein, J. E., Pedras, C. V., and Weber, A. H.: Spine deformity in neurofibromatosis. A review of one hundred and two patients. *J Bone Joint Surg* 61A:677–694, 1979.
10. Brown, G. A., Osebold, W. R., and Ponseti, I. V.: Congenital pseudoarthrosis of long bones. A clinical, radiographic, histologic and ultrastructural study. *Clin Orthop* 128:228–242, 1977.
11. Briner, J., and Yunis, E.: Ultrastructure of congenital pseudoarthrosis of the tibia. *Arch Pathol* 95:97–99, 1973.
12. Sane, S., Yunis, E., and Greer, R.: Subperiosteal or cortical cyst and intramedullary neurofibromatosis—uncommon manifestations of neurofibromatosis. *J Bone Joint Surg* 53A:1194–1200, 1971.
13. Locht, R. C., Huebert, H. T., and McFarland, D. F.: Subperiosteal hemorrhage and cyst formation in neurofibromatosis: A case report. *Clin Orthop* 155:141–146, 1981.
14. Hooper, G., and McMaster, M. J.: Neurofibromatosis with tibial cyst caused by recurrent hemorrhage. *J Bone Joint Surg* 61A:274–276, 1979.
15. Dennyson, W. G., Bear, J. N., and Bhoola, K. D.: Macrodactyly in the foot. *J Bone Joint Surg* 59B:355–359, 1977.
16. Neufeld, E. F.: Lysosomal storage diseases. *Ann Rev Biochem* 60:257–280, 1991.
17. Greenfield, G. B.: Bone changes in chronic adult Gaucher's disease. *Am J Roentgenol Radium Ther Nucl Med* 110:800–807, 1996.
18. Goldblatt, J., Sachs, S., and Beighton, P.: The orthopedic aspects of Gaucher disease. *Clin Orthop* 137:208–214, 1978.
19. Cremin, B. J., Davey, H., and Goldblatt, J.: Skeletal complications of type I Gaucher disease: The magnetic resonance features. *Clin Radiol* 41:244–247, 1990.
20. Hermann, G., Shapiro, R. S., Abdelwahab, I. F., and Grabowski, G.: MR imaging in adults with Gaucher disease type I: Evaluation of marrow involvement and disease activity. *Skeletal Radiol* 22:247–251, 1993.
21. Beutler, E.: Gaucher's disease. *New Engl J Med* 325:1354–1360, 1991.
22. Muenzer, J.: Mucopolysaccharidoses. *Adv Pediatr* 33:269–302, 1986.
23. Anderson, C. E.: Morquio's disease and dysplasia epiphysealis multiplex: A study of epiphyseal cartilage in seven cases. *J Bone Joint Surg* 44A:295–306, 1962.
24. McClure, J., Smith, P. S., Sorby-Adams, G., et al.: The histological and ultrastructural features of the epiphyseal plate in Morquio type A syndrome (mucopolysaccharidosis type IVA). *Pathology* 18:217–221, 1986.
25. Hopwood, J. J., and Morris, C. P.: The mucopolysaccharidoses: diagnosis, molecular genetics and treatment. *Mol Biol Med* 7:381–404, 1990.
26. Hubeny, M. J., and Delano, R. J.: Dysostosis multiplex. *Am J Roentgenol* 46:336–342, 1941.
27. Langer, L. O., and Carey, L. S.: The roentgenographic features of the KS-mucopolysaccharidosis of Morquio (Morquio-Brailsford's disease). *Am J Roentgenol* 97:1–20, 1966.
28. Hunter, C.: A rare disease in two brothers: Evaluation of scapula, limitation of movement of joints and other abnormalities. *Proc R Soc Med* 10:104–116, 1917.
29. O'Brien, W. M., La Du, B. N., and Bunim, J. J.: Biochemical, pathologic and clinical aspects of alkaptonuria, ochronosis and ochronotic arthropathy: Review of world literature (1584–1962). *Am J Med* 34:813–838, 1963.
30. Garrod, A. E.: The Croonian lectures on inborn errors of metabolism. Lecture II. Alkaptonuria. *Lancet* 2:73–79, 1908.
31. Lee, S. L., and Stenn, F. F.: Characterization of mummy bone ochronotic pigment. *JAMA* 240:136–138, 1978.
32. Stenn, F. F., Milgram, J. W., Lee, S. L., et al.: Biochemical identification of homogentisic acid pigment in an ochronotic Egyptian mummy. *Science* 197:566–568, 1977.
33. Boedeker, C.: Ueber das Alcapton; ein neuer Beitrag zur Frage; welche Stoffe des Harns Konnen Kupferreduction bewirken? *Z Rat Med* 7:130–145, 1859.
34. Virchow, R.: Ein Fall von allgemeiner Ochronose der Knorpel und knorpelahnlichen Teile. *Arch Pathol Anat* 37:212–219, 1866.
35. Garrod, A. E.: About alkaptonuria. *Lancet* 2:1484–1486, 1901.
36. Coodley, E. L., and Greco, A. J.: Clinical aspects of ochronosis, with report of a case. *Am J Med* 8:816–822, 1950.
37. Laskar, F. H., and Sargison, K. D.: Ochronotic arthropathy. A review with four case reports. *J Bone Joint Surg* 52B:653–666, 1970.
38. Mueller, M. N., Sorensen, L. B., Strandjord, U., et al.: Alkaptonuria and ochronotic arthropathy. *Med Clin North Am* 49:101–115, 1965.
39. Justesen, P., and Andersen, P. E., Jr.: Radiologic manifestations in alcaptonuria. *Skeletal Radiol* 11:204–208, 1984.
40. Deeb, Z., and Frayha, R. A.: Multiple vacuum discs; an early sign of ochronosis: Radiologic findings in two brothers. *J Rheumatol* 3:82–87, 1976.
41. Gaines, J. J., Jr.: The pathology of alkaptonuric ochronosis. *Hum Pathol* 20:40–46, 1989.
42. Lagier, R., Baud, C.-A., Lacotte, D., and Cunningham, T.: Rapidly progressive osteoarthrosis of ochronotic origin. A pathologic study. *Am J Clin Pathol* 90:95–102, 1988.

43. Wynne-Davies, R., and Gormley, J.: The prevalence of skeletal dysplasias: An estimate of their minimum frequency and the number of patients requiring orthopaedic care. *J Bone Joint Surg* 67B:133–137, 1985.
44. Kopits, S. E.: Orthopedic complications of dwarfism. *Clin Orthop* 114:153–179, 1976.
45. Beighton, P., Giedion, A., Gorlin, R., Hall, J., Horton, B., Kozlowski, K., Lachman, R., Langer, L. O., Maroteaux, P., Poznanski, A., Rimoin, D. L., Sillence, D., and Spranger, J.: International classification of osteochondrodysplasias. *Am J Med Genet* 44:223–229, 1992.
46. Gray, P. H. K.: A case of osteogenesis imperfecta associated with dentinogenesis imperfecta, dating from antiquity. *Clin Radiol* 21:106–108, 1970.
47. Malebranche, N.: *Traite de la recherche de la verite*. Paris, 1674.
48. Ekman, O. J.: Descriptionem et casus aliquot osteomalaciae sistens [abstract]. J. Edman, Upsala, 1788.
49. Spurway, J.: Hereditary tendency to fracture. *Br Med J* 2:845, 1896.
50. Eddowes, A.: Dark sclerotics and fragilitas ossium. *Br Med J* 2:222, 1900.
51. Penttinen, R. P., Lichtenstein, J. R., Martin, G. R., and McKusick, V. A.: Abnormal collagen metabolism in cultured cells in osteogenesis imperfecta. *Proc Natl Acad Sci* 72:586–589, 1975.
52. Cole, W. G.: Osteogenesis imperfecta as a consequence of naturally occurring and induced mutations of type I collagen. Heersche, J. K. J., Ed. *Bone and Mineral Research*. Amsterdam, Elsevier Science, 1994, pp. 67–204.
53. Looser, E.: Zur Erkenntniss der Osteogenesis imperfecta congenita und tarda (sogenannte idiopathische Osteopsathyrosis). *Mitt Grenzgeb Med Chir* 15:161–207, 1906.
54. Sillence, D. O., Senn, A. S., and Danko, D. M.: Genetic heterogeneity in osteogenesis imperfecta. *J Med Genet* 16:101–116, 1979.
55. Sillence, D.: Osteogenesis imperfecta: An expanding panorama of variants. *Clin Orthop* 159:11–25, 1981.
56. Barsh, G. S., David, K. E., and Byers, P. H.: Type I osteogenesis imperfecta: A nonfunctional allele for pro $a_1(1)$ chains of type I procollagen. *Proc Natl Acad Sci U S A* 79:3838–3842, 1982.
57. McCarthy, E. F., Earnest, K., Rossiter, K., and Shapiro, J.: Bone histomorphometry in adults with type IA osteogenesis imperfecta. *Clin Orthop* 336:254–262, 1997.
58. Bullough, P. G., Davidson, D., and Lorenzo, J. C.: The morbid anatomy of the skeleton in osteogenesis imperfecta. *Clin Orthop* 159:42–57, 1981.
59. Milgram, J. W., Flick, M. R., and Engh, C. A.: Osteogenesis imperfecta: A histopathological case report. *J Bone Joint Surg* 55A:506–515, 1973.
60. Greenspan, A.: Sclerosing bone dysplasias—a target-site approach. *Skeletal Radiol* 20:561–583, 1991.
61. Popoff, S. N., and Marks, S. C. J.: The heterogeneity of the osteopetroses reflects the diversity of cellular influences during skeletal development. *Bone* 17:437–445, 1995.
62. Lian, J. B.: Mysterious cross talk between bone cells. *J Clin Invest* 98:1697–1698, 1996.
63. Walker, D. G.: Bone resorption restored in osteopetrotic mice by transplants of normal bone marrow and spleen cells. *Science* 190:784–785, 1975.
64. Soriano, P. C., Montgomery, C., Geske, R., and Bradley, A.: Targeted disruption of the c-src proto-oncogene leads to osteopetrosis in mice. *Cell* 64:693–702, 1991.
65. Grigoriadis, A. E., Wang, A. Q., Cecchini, W., Hofstetter, W., Felix, R., Fleisch, H. A., and Wagner, E. F.: C-Fos: A key regulator of osteoclast-macrophage lineage determination and bone remodeling. *Science* 266:443–448, 1994.
66. Lajeunesse, D., Busque, L., Menard, P., Brunette, M. G., and Bonny, Y.: Demonstration of an osteoblast defect in two cases of human malignant osteopetrosis. Correction of the phenotype after bone marrow transplant. *J Clin Invest* 98:1697–1698, 1996.
67. Labat, M. L., Bringuier, A. F., Chandra, A., et al.: Retroviral expression in mononuclear blood cells isolated from a patient with osteopetrosis (Albers-Schönberg disease). *J Bone Miner Res* 5:425–435, 1990.
68. Shapiro, F., Glimcher, M. J., Holtrop, M. E., Tashjian, A. H., Jr., Brickley-Parson, D., and Kenzora, J. E.: Human osteopetrosis: A histological, ultrastructural, and biochemical study. *J Bone Joint Surg* 62A:384–399, 1980.
69. Albers-Schönberg, H.: Eine bisher nicht beschriebene Allgemeinerkrankung skelettes im Rontgenbild. *Forschr Geb Rontgenstr* 11:261, 1907.
70. El-Tawil, T., and Stoker, D. J.: Benign osteopetrosis: A review of 42 cases showing two different patterns. *Skeletal Radiol* 22:587–593, 1993.
71. Johnston, C. C., Jr., Lavy, N., Lord, T., Vllios, F., Merritt, A. D., and Deiss, W. P.: Osteopetrosis: A clinical, genetic, metabolic, and morphologic study of the dominantly inherited, benign form. *Medicine* 47:149–167, 1968.
72. Tips, R. L., and Lynch, H. T.: Malignant congenital osteopetrosis resulting from a consanguineous marriage. *Acta Paediat* 51:585–588, 1962.
73. Ohlsson, A., Cummings, W. A., Paul, A., et al.: Carbonic anhydrase II deficiency syndrome: Recessive osteopetrosis with renal tubular acidosis and cerebral calcification. *Pediatrics* 77:371–381, 1986.
74. Key, L. L., Jr., Rodriguiz, R. M., Willi, S. M., Wright, N. M., Hatcher, H. C., Eyre, D. R., Cure, J. K., Griffin, P. P., and Ries, W. L.: Long-term treatment of osteopetrosis with recombinant human interferon gamma. *N Engl J Med* 332:1594–1599, 1995.
75. Naveh, Y.: Progressive diaphyseal dysplasia: Genetics and clinical and radiologic manifestations. *Pediatrics* 74:399–405, 1984.
76. Sparkes, R. S., and Graham, C. B.: Camurati-Engelmann disease: genetics and clinical manifestations with a review of the literature. *J Med Genet* 9:73–85, 1972.
77. Fallon, M. D., Whyte, M. P., and Murphy, W. A.: Progressive diaphyseal dysplasia (Engelmann's disease): Report of a sporadic case of the mild form. *J Bone Joint Surg* 62A:465–472, 1980.
78. Verbov, J.: Buschke-Ollendorff syndrome (disseminated dermatofibrosis with osteopoikilosis). *Br J Dermatol* 96:87–90, 1977.
79. Lagier, R., Mbakop, A., and Bigler, A.: Osteopoikilosis: A radiological and pathological study. *Skeletal Radiol* 11:161–168, 1984.
80. Andersen, P. E., Jr., Hauge, M.: Congenital generalised bone dysplasias: A clinical, radiological, and epidemiological survey. *J Med Genet* 26:37–44, 1989.
81. Shiang, R., Thompson, L. M., Zhu, Y.-Z., Church, D. M., Fielder, T. J., Bocian, M., Winokur, S. T., and Wasmuth, J. J.: Mutations in the transmembrane domain of FGFR3 cause the most common genetic form of dwarfism, achondroplasia. *Cell* 78:335–342, 1994.
82. Rimoin, D. L., Hughes, G. N., Kaufman, R. L., Rosenthal, R. E., McAlister, W. H., and Silberberg, R.: Endochondral ossification in achondroplastic dwarfism. *N Engl J Med* 283:728–735, 1970.
83. Bailey, J. A.: Orthopaedic aspects of achondroplasia. *J Bone Joint Surg* 52A:1285–1301, 1970.
84. Scott, C. I., Jr.: Achondroplastic and hypochondroplastic dwarfism. *Clin Orthop* 114:18–30, 1976.
85. Cole, W. G.: Collagen genes: Mutations affecting collagen structure and expression. *Prog Nucleic Acid Res Mol Biol* 47:29, 1994.
86. Spranger, J., Winterpacht, A., and Zabel, B.: The type II collagenopathies: A spectrum of chondrodysplasias. *Eur J Pediatr* 153:56, 1994.
87. Murray, L. W., Bautista, J., and James, P. L.: Type II collagen defects in the chondrodysplasias. *Am J Med Genet* 45:5–15, 1989.
88. Vikkula, M., Mariman, E. C. M., Lui, V. C. H., Zhidkova, N. I., Tiller, G. E., Goldring, M. B., van Beersum, S. E. C., de Waal Malefijt, M. C., van den Hoogen, F. H. J., Ropers, H. H., Mayne, R., Cheah, K. S. E., Olsen, B. R., Warman, M. L., and Brunner, H. G.: Autosomal dominant and recessive osteochondrodysplasias associated with the COL11A2 locus. *Cell* 80:431–437, 1995.
89. Cole, W. G., Hall, R. K., and Rogers, J. G.: The clinical features of spondyloepiphyseal dysplasia congenita resulting from the substitution of glycine 997 by serine in the alpha 1(II) chain of type II collagen. *J Med Genet* 30:27, 1993.
90. Heselson, N. G., Cremin, B. J., and Beighton, P.: Pseudoachondroplasia, a report of 13 cases. *Br J Radiol* 50:473–482, 1977.
91. Cooper, R. R., Ponseti, I. V., and Maynard, J. A.: Pseudoachondroplastic dwarfism: A rough-surfaced endoplasmic reticulum storage disorder. *J Bone Joint Surg* 55:475–484, 1973.
92. Finklestein, J. E., Doege, K., Yamada, Y., et al.: Analysis of the chondroitin sulfate proteoglycan core protein (CSPGCP) gene in achondroplasia and pseudoachondroplasia. *Am J Hum Genet* 48:97–102, 1991.
93. Stanescu, V., Maroteaux, P., and Stanescu, R.: The biochemical defect of pseudoachondroplasia. *Eur J Pediatr* 138:221–225, 1982.
94. Ingram, R. R.: Early diagnosis of multiple epiphyseal dysplasia. *J Pediatr Orthop* 12:241–244, 1992.
95. MacKenzie, W. G.: Avascular necrosis of the hip in multiple epiphyseal dysplasia. *J Pediatr Orthop* 9:666–671, 1989.

96. Stanescu, R., Stanescu, V., Muriel, M. P., et al.: Multiple epiphyseal dysplasia, Fairbank type: Morphologic and biochemical study of cartilage. *Am J Med Genet* 45:501, 1993.
97. Evans, R., and Caffey, J.: Metaphyseal dysostosis resembling vitamin D-refractory rickets. *Am J Dis Child* 95:640, 1958.
98. Cooper, R. R., and Ponseti, I. V.: Metaphyseal dysostosis: Description of an ultrastructural defect in the epiphyseal plate chondrocytes. Case report. *J Bone Joint Surg* 55A:485–495, 1973.
99. Maynard, J., Ippolito, E. G., Ponseti, I. V., et al.: Histochemistry and ultrastructure of the growth plate in metaphyseal dysostosis: Further observations on the structure of the cartilage matrix. *J Pediatr Orthop* 1:161, 1981.
100. Dent, C. E., and Normano, I. C. S.: Metaphyseal dysostosis, type Schmid. *Arch Dis Child* 39:444, 1958.
101. Vander-Burgt, I., Haraldsson, A., Oosterwijk, J. C., et al.: Cartilage hair hypoplasia, metaphyseal chondrodysplasia type McKusick: Description of seven patients and review of the literature. *Am J Med Genet* 41:371, 1991.
102. Kettelkamp, D. B., Campbell, C. J., and Bonfiglio, M.: Dysplasia epiphysealis hemimelica. *J Bone Joint Surg* 48A:746–765, 1966.
103. Hensinger, R. N., Cowell, H. R., Ramsey, P. L., and Leopold, R. G.: Familial dysplasia epiphysealis hemimelica, associated with chondromas and osteochondromas. *J Bone Joint Surg* 56A:1513–1516, 1974.
104. Keret, D., Spatz, D. K., Caro, P. A., and Mason, D. E.: Dysplasia epiphysealis hemimelica: Diagnosis and treatment. *J Pediatr Orthop* 12:365–372, 1992.
105. Campbell, C. J., Papademetriou, T., and Bonfiglio, M.: Melorheostosis. A report of the clinical, roentgenographic, and pathological findings in fourteen cases. *J Bone Joint Surg* 50A:1281–1304, 1968.
106. Younge, D., Drummond, D., Herring, J., and Cruess, R. L.: Melorheostosis in children. Clinical features and natural history. *J Bone Joint Surg* 61B:415–418, 1979.

CHAPTER 4
Metabolic Bone Diseases

Metabolic bone diseases are disorders of the skeleton resulting from abnormalities in the chemical milieu of the body. With rare exceptions, these diseases cause a generalized decrease in bone mass and a tendency to fracture. The diagnosis and treatment of the specific metabolic bone diseases is usually the province of endocrinologists. However, because the initial presentation of these diseases is often a fracture, especially following little or no trauma, orthopedic surgeons are usually the first physicians to see affected patients. Therefore, orthopedic surgeons must be able to recognize the presence of a metabolic bone disease alerted by the clue of bones that fracture easily. Orthopedists who recognize these diseases get better results from their treatment and are less likely to make the metabolic bone disease worse.

Surgical pathologists, like orthopedists, depend on the endocrinologist to diagnose specific metabolic bone diseases, because the morphologic features of these diseases are best studied by undecalcified bone histomorphometry, and this modality is usually the province of bone biologists or endocrinologists. However, pathologists must also recognize the presence of metabolic bone disease, especially when studying tissue specimens removed by orthopedic surgeons. They may then initiate dialogue with endocrinologists, and bone specimens may find their way to the hard tissue laboratory.

Because metabolic bone diseases usually result in decreased bone mass, two terms must be defined at this point. Decreased bone mass, when described radiographically or histologically, is known as *osteopenia*. Symptomatic osteopenia (with bone pain or fractures) is the clinical syndrome known as *osteoporosis*. In an alternative definition, osteopenia is a decrease in bone mass greater than 2.0 standard divisions below normal (as measured by densitometry techniques), and osteoporosis is a decrease greater than 2.5 standard deviations below normal.

Metabolic bone diseases may be grouped in three major categories. The first category includes diseases caused by specific endocrine abnormalities, particularly those that disturb calcium homeostasis. Because parathyroid hormone and vitamin D are critical for calcium homeostasis, excess or deficiency of these compounds has a profound effect on the skeleton. The effect on the skeleton in these cases is specific, and the cause can be diagnosed histologically or biochemically. The second category of metabolic bone disease includes the osteopenic syndromes without specific endocrine abnormalities, particularly age-related osteoporosis. Although humoral abnormalities are etiologic factors in these syndromes, laboratory studies usually produce normal results, and the osteopenia is caused primarily by a gradual decrease in the organic matrix of bone. The third category of metabolic bone disease represents the osteopenic syndromes due to disuse. Bone health is dependent on the stress and strain of physical activity. Absence of stress somehow results in nonphysiologic bone remodeling and gradual bone loss.

SPECIFIC ENDOCRINE DISORDERS

Primary Hyperparathyroidism

The presentation of hyperparathyroidism has changed in recent times. Formerly, primary hyperparathyroidism was a rare disease with florid skeletal complications. However, today primary hyperparathyroidism is common. As many as 1 in 500 to 1000 persons are affected.[1] In fact, after diabetes and hyperthyroidism, hyperparathyroidism is the most common endocrine disorder. Also today, the skeleton is rarely involved—less than 5% of patients have clinical bone disease.[2]

This change in the incidence (a four- to fivefold increase) and presentation of hyperparathyroidism began in the early 1970s with the use of the autoanalyzer. This laboratory machine routinely screens serum calcium levels in patients being evaluated for other reasons.[3] As a result, hyperparathyroidism can be diagnosed very early in its long natural history. At this point in the disease, patients are asymptomatic and the skeleton is not yet affected. Many of these patients probably would have gone undiagnosed in their lifetime.

Primary hyperparathyroidism is caused by oversecretion of parathyroid hormone by the parathyroid glands. The effects of increased parathyroid hormone secretion on the bones, kidneys, and, indirectly, on the intestine result in hypercalcemia. In 80% of cases, a parathyroid adenoma in one gland causes this disease. The other three glands are normal. In most of the remaining cases, the hypersecretion of parathyroid hormone results from hyperplasia of all four glands, a condition that occurs in the multiple endocrinopathy syndromes. Parathyroid carcinoma, another cause of primary hyperparathyroidism, accounts for fewer than 0.5% of cases.

The causes of parathyroid hormone hypersecretion are not fully understood. Ordinarily, rising serum calcium levels turn off parathyroid hormone secretion. However, this function is modulated in the cells of a parathyroid adenoma, and the result is a higher "set point" for sensing serum calcium levels. Thus, an adenoma is less sensitive to high calcium levels and continues to secrete parathyroid hormone. A clonal origin of the adenoma cells suggests genetic defect in the control of parathyroid hormone secretion, and in some patients, a gene rearrangement at the site of the PRAD-1 oncogene has been demonstrated.[4]

History

In 1891, von Recklinghausen described a generalized affectation of the skeleton that he called *osteitis fibrosa cystica generalisata*.[5] For several decades, this term was used to describe a variety of bone disorders that included Paget's disease, osteomalacia, and other lesions characterized by skeletal deformity and cysts.

The origin of osteitis fibrosa began to be elucidated at the turn of the century. By 1901, Askanazy had shown that the parathyroid glands influenced the calcium metabolism of the skeleton.[6] Then, in 1925, Collip demonstrated that parathyroid extract prevented parathyroid tetany and regulated serum calcium.[7] A year later, Mandl performed the first parathyroidectomy for an adenoma and successfully ameliorated the skeletal changes of osteitis fibrosa.[8] The relationship of the parathyroid gland to skeletal disease was confirmed in 1931. In that year, Jaffe, Blair, and Bodansky, working at the Hospital for Joint Diseases in New York, experimentally produced osteitis fibrosa in rabbits by the injection of parathyroid hormone.[9]

Clinical Features

Primary hyperparathyroidism occurs in any age group. However, it is most common in the 6th decade of life, and women are affected more than men by a ratio of three to one. Therefore, the majority of patients with primary hyperparathyroidism are postmenopausal women.

Asymptomatic hypercalcemia is the most common clinical presentation. However, calcium values rarely exceed 1 mg/dl over the upper limits of normal. These patients are usually discovered with routine screening studies and have no complaints referable to parathyroid hormone target organs. The diagnosis is confirmed by an elevated serum parathyroid hormone level, a finding present in over 90% of patients. In addition, serum phosphorus may be low and alkaline phosphatase elevated, although these changes are inconstant.

Although most patients with primary hyperparathyroidism are asymptomatic, some have vague symptoms, including easy fatigability, muscular weakness, and a sense of being ill at ease. In more advanced cases, target organ complications occur. Nephrolithiasis, affecting 20% of patients, is the most common complication.[10] As with skeletal complications, nephrolithiasis was formerly more common (33% of cases in the 1960s). In addition to nephrolithiasis, nephrocalcinosis also occurs.

The gastrointestinal tract may also be affected in hyperparathyroidism. Complications include peptic ulcer disease and pancreatitis. However, these complications are also now rare because of early diagnosis.

Skeletal Manifestations

Radiographic Features. Plain radiographic changes are rare in primary hyperparathyroidism. When present, the most characteristic feature is subperiosteal bone resorption. This change first occurs in the tufts of the distal phalanges (Fig. 4–1) or along the radial border of the middle phalanges (Fig. 4–2). However, these early skeletal changes are seen in only 17% of cases of hyperparathyroidism. In more advanced cases, erosion of the distal clavicles and a faint salt and pepper appearance of the calvarium may be seen. Lytic bone lesions, known as brown tumors, are a result of extensive bone resorption caused by hyperparathyroidism. However, they are rarely seen in primary hyperparathyroidism. Today, brown tumors occur almost exclusively in advanced secondary hyperparathyroidism.

Although plain radiographic changes are rare in primary hyperparathyroidism, densitometry studies are much more sensitive. Approximately 50% of patients show demineralization with x-ray absorptiometry studies. This modality demonstrates that the loss of bone is predominately cortical.[11,12] Because of the high level of sensitivity, densitometry is an important tool in evaluating therapy for all cases of primary hyperparathyroidism.

Pathologic Changes. Because primary hyperparathyroidism is usually diagnosed early, tissue samples removed from affected patients rarely show significant pathologic changes with routine microscopic techniques. A few resorption cavities may be noticed in trabecular bone. The bone changes are best evaluated with histomorphometry techniques. This modality demonstrates an increase in both bone resorption and bone formation, a so-called "high-turnover state." The number of resorption surfaces and osteoid surfaces is increased. Mineralizing surfaces, as indicated by the extent of

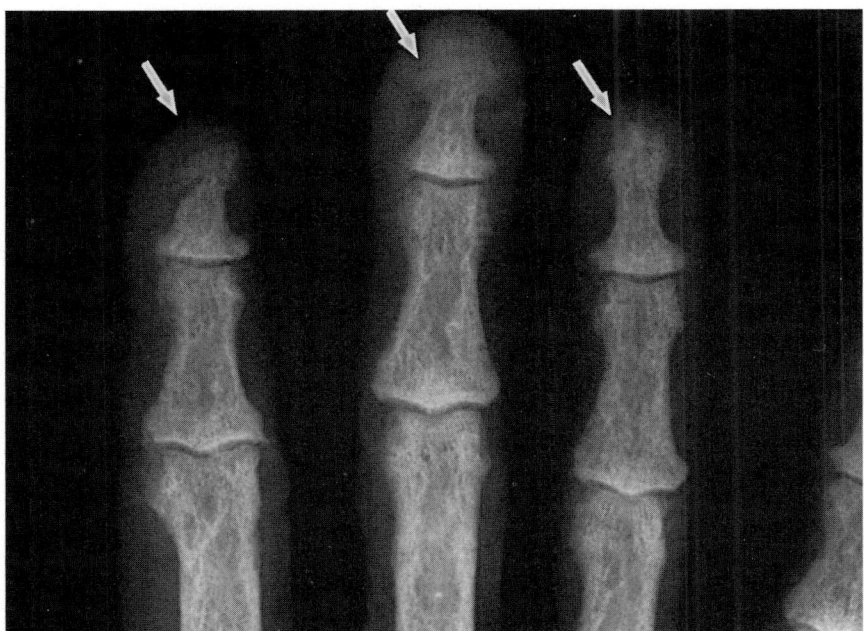

Figure 4-1 ■ The earliest radiographic changes in hyperparathyroidism. Erosion of the tufts of the distal phalanges is present *(arrows)*.

tetracycline labels, are also increased. The high turnover of primary hyperparathyroidism is generally balanced—bone formation equals bone resorption. Therefore, cancellous bone volume is usually normal, and trabecular connectivity is maintained.[13,14] However, a distinctive change present in the majority of patients is a reduced amount of cortical bone.[15] Reduced cortical bone is reflected histomorphometrically in both a decreased cortical thickness and an increased cortical porosity.

In the advanced cases of parathyroid hormone excess, usually seen only in secondary hyperparathyroidism, extensive osseous changes occur. The most characteristic feature is *tunneling resorption* (Fig. 4–3). This unusual pattern of resorption occurs because osteoclasts cannot penetrate the seams of unmineralized osteoid that covers trabecular surfaces. Therefore, they must tunnel into the center of trabeculae where they have access to a mineralized surface. In addition to tunneling resorption, other changes of advanced hyperparathyroidism include extensive woven bone deposition and paratrabecular fibrosis.

Treatment

Primary hyperparathyroidism can be cured by surgical removal of the gland containing the adenoma. In cases caused by parathyroid hyperplasia, a three and one half gland parathyroidectomy usually results in restoration of normal calcium balance. After surgery, bone mass improves substantially in 2 to 4 years.[16]

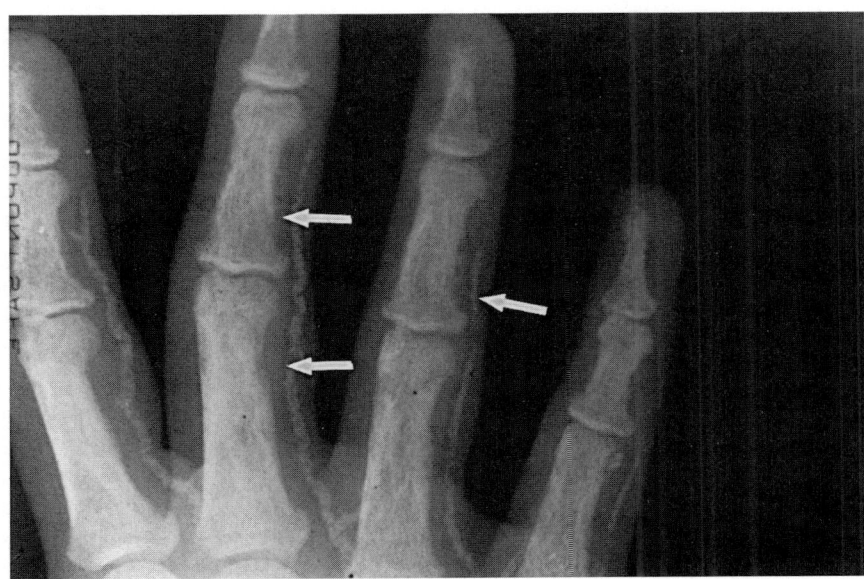

Figure 4-2 ■ Another early radiographic change in hyperparathyroidism. Erosion of the ulnar aspect of the phalanges is present *(arrows)*. The digital arteries are calcified.

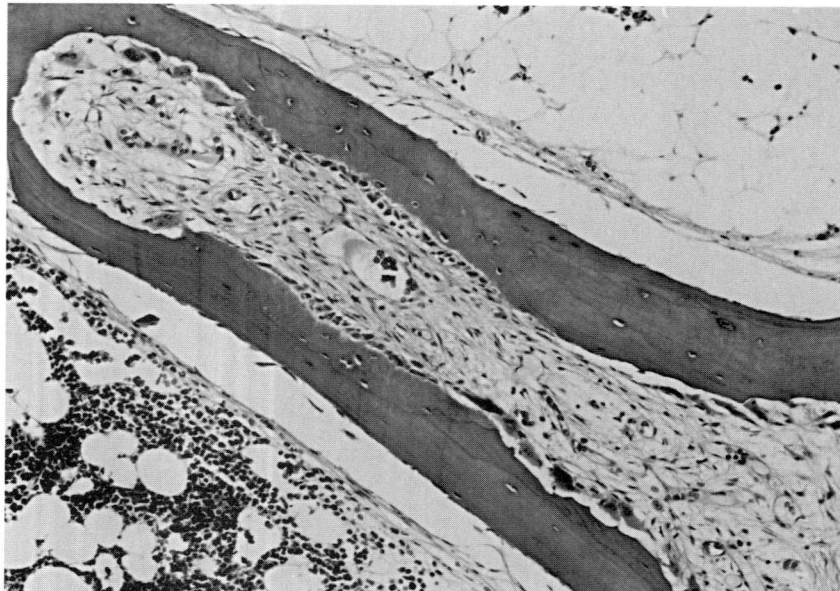

Figure 4-3 ■ Photomicrograph showing tunneling resorption of a trabecula.

About 50% of patients with primary hyperparathyroidism can be managed medically. These patients are usually asymptomatic and have no evidence of bone or renal disease. Also, mildly symptomatic older patients who are poor surgical risks can be treated conservatively. Conservative treatment consists of adequate hydration and low calcium. Regimens may also include drugs that inhibit osteoclasts, such as estrogen or a bisphosphonate.

Disorders of Mineralization: Rickets and Osteomalacia

Both serum calcium and serum phosphorus must be at sufficient levels to mineralize growing cartilage and bone. If either is low, mineralization is inhibited and patients develop rickets or osteomalacia (Table 4–1). Rickets is due to ineffective mineralization of the growth plate and causes deformity and growth retardation. By contrast, osteomalacia (literally "soft bones") is due to poor mineralization of osteoid. As a result, unmineralized osteoid accumulates on trabecular and cortical surfaces. Because growing bones undergo extensive modeling and appositional bone formation, children with mineralization defects develop both rickets and osteomalacia. Adults can only develop osteomalacia.

Because bone mineral is composed of both calcium and phosphorus, it is convenient to classify rickets and osteomalacia according to the particular deficiency: calcium or phosphate.[17] Calcium-deficient (calcipenic) conditions are more common and include low calcium intake and vitamin D deficiency (either primary or secondary). These calcipenic disorders are usually complicated by secondary hyperparathyroidism, and the clinical, radiographic, and pathologic features are similar.

Hereditary disorders of vitamin D metabolism also cause rickets. Two well-characterized hereditary disorders are type I and type II vitamin D–dependent rickets. In type I vitamin D–dependent rickets, a hereditary deficiency of the 1α-hydroxylase enzyme limits the formation of 1,25 $(OH)_2$ vitamin D. Type II vitamin D–dependent rickets is a hereditary end-organ failure of the vitamin D receptor. In this condition, the intestinal mucosa does not respond to vitamin D. Therefore, calcium absorption is limited. Both types I and II vitamin D–dependent rickets are autosomal recessive disorders.

Phosphorus-deficient conditions also cause rickets and osteomalacia. However, because serum calcium is usually normal in these conditions, secondary hyperparathyroidism does not occur. Phosphate-deficient states include renal disorders with phosphorus leakage and oncogenic osteomalacia. Loss of phosphorus also occurs in the genetic syndrome X-linked hypophosphatemic rickets. Patients with this syndrome not only have rickets but also have radiodense bones, a feature

Table 4–1 ■ **CAUSES OF OSTEOMALACIA AND RICKETS**

Vitamin D deficiency
  Inadequate sun exposure
  Low dietary intake
Vitamin D malabsorption
  Gastrointestinal surgery
    Gastric bypass
    Billroth II gastrectomy
  Small intestinal disease
    Sprue
    Celiac disease
  Liver disease
Vitamin D metabolism abnormalities
  Renal failure
  Dilantin therapy
Oncogenic osteomalacia
Congenital diseases
  Vitamin D–dependent rickets, type I
  Vitamin D–dependent rickets, type II
  X-linked hypophosphatemic rickets

possibly related to an additional defect in bone-forming cells.[17]

History

Although uncommon in recent years, rickets was formerly a major cause of childhood illness. It reached its peak during the Industrial Revolution, when many children lived in the squalid slums of cities. However, the disease was well documented in medical treatises before the Industrial Revolution. In 1645, Whistler published his medical thesis (in Latin), *The Disease of English Children Which Is Popularly Termed the Rickets.*[18] Five years later, Glisson wrote the classic text on this disease that offers the still unsurpassed clinical description. Although the origin of the term *rickets* is obscure, Glisson suggested that the term derives from the Greek *rachitis,* meaning spine, because affected children often had kyphosis.[19]

It was not until 1890, however, that the etiologic understanding of rickets began to unfold. In that year, Theobald Palm gathered worldwide data and concluded that lack of sunlight was a causal factor.[20] In that era, rickets was widespread. In 1899, Escherich reported that in Vienna, 97% of infants between 9 and 15 months of age had clinical evidence of rickets.[21] However, by 1929, Alfred Hess and L. J. Unger described the prevention of rickets by using cod liver oil or by ultraviolet irradiation.[22]

Nutritional Rickets

Nutritional rickets is almost always due to an inadequate supply of vitamin D, although a low calcium intake can also cause this disease. Inadequate sun exposure was formerly the main cause of low vitamin D levels. Food supplementation with vitamin D_2 has greatly reduced the incidence of rickets in developed countries. By contrast, in certain cultural groups, both in developed and developing countries, consumption of unfortified foods and inadequate exposure to sunlight still cause vitamin D deficiency. For example, nearly 30% of children in an Ethiopian clinic showed evidence of rickets. These children had been swaddled as infants to avoid the "evil eye."[23] Also, the Middle East tradition of *purdah,* which requires that female children be totally covered outdoors, is likely to result in rickets. A study of Moslem girls in India showed that 40% had skeletal evidence of this disease.[24] In addition, because breast milk is low in vitamin D, breast-fed infants among these cultural groups are especially at risk.[25]

Pathogenesis and Pathology of Calcipenic Rickets

Calcipenic rickets is caused by inadequate serum levels of ionizable calcium. As a result, the growing epiphyseal plate fails to mineralize properly. Usually, calcium is low because of poor intestinal absorption due to low levels of vitamin D. Although compensatory rise in parathyroid hormone secretion raises the serum calcium, increased parathyroid hormone causes phosphaturia and high-turnover bone resorption. This sequence explains the usual biochemical features of rickets: a normal (or low) serum calcium, low serum phosphorus, low 25(OH) vitamin D, elevated parathyroid hormone levels, and an elevated serum alkaline phosphatase.

Pathologic changes are apparent in the growth plates and in the bones. Inadequate mineralization causes marked distortion of the growth plate.[26,27] The zone of provisional calcification is poorly defined due to scant mineral deposition. Because a well-mineralized zone of provisional calcification normally provides a feedback inhibition to the zone of proliferation, poor mineralization leads to unregulated chondrocyte proliferation. As a result, the growth plate thickens, sometimes 5 to 15 times normal. In addition, gross distortion in the orderly zone of chondrocyte columnation and hypertrophy occur. Therefore, the epiphyseal plate is soft, and mechanical forces squash it into the metaphysis.

In addition to epiphyseal plate distortion, the rachitic bones show abnormalities consistent with osteomalacia. Wide osteoid seams are present around thin spicules of irregular trabeculae. Also, the cortices are thin and show increased resorption as a result of secondary hyperparathyroidism.

Clinical and Radiological Features

Today, the clinical features of florid nutritional rickets are rarely seen in developed countries. However, in rare cases, the changes are striking. The rachitic child is apathetic and irritable. A generalized weak musculature is especially prominent in the abdomen and results in a characteristic potbelly appearance. Severely rachitic children show marked changes in the axial skeleton. Flattening of the skull with frontal bossing usually occurs. The spine is also deformed. A characteristic dorsal kyphosis causes the so-called "rachitic catback." The chest is also deformed with enlargement of the costal cartilages (the "rachitic rosary"), and indentations of the lower ribs occur at the insertion of the diaphragm (Harrison grooves).

The extremities are also severely affected in rickets. The long bones are shortened, and the lower extremities are bowed. In addition, the hypertrophic cartilage of the epiphyseal plates causes swelling of the wrists, knees, and ankles.

The most characteristic radiographic feature of rickets is a *widened epiphyseal plate* (Fig. 4–4). Also, a cup-shaped deformity of the metaphysis (metaphyseal flaring) is usually present due to squashing of the epiphysis into the metaphysis. These changes in the epiphyseal plate, present in all forms of rickets, are pathognomonic. In addition to the epiphyseal plate changes, other radiographic changes occur in rickets. The weight-bearing bones are often bowed, and generalized osteopenia, which is particularly prominent in the metaphyses, occurs. Also, many bones show transverse radiodense lines, known as Looser lines. These lines, present in 20% of patients with all forms of rickets, represent stress fractures and are most prominent on the concave side of

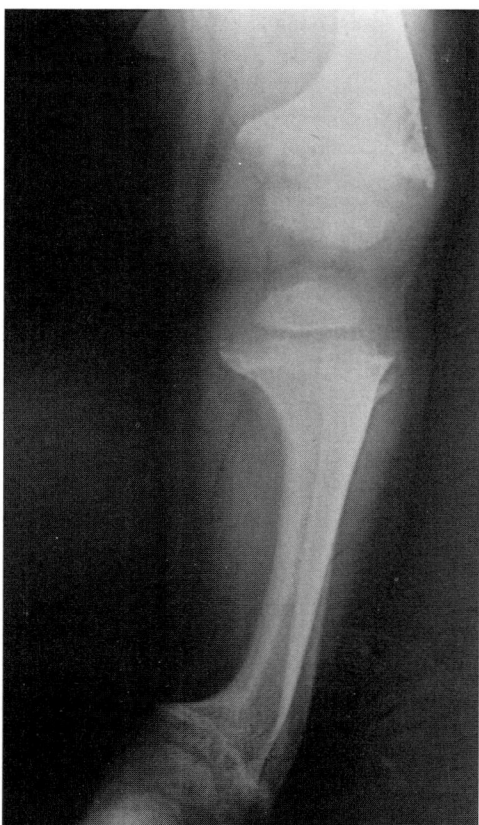

Figure 4-4 ■ Plain radiograph of the knee from a child with rickets. The epiphyseal plates are widened, and flaring of the metaphysis has occurred. These changes are diagnostic of rickets.

long bones.[28] Looser lines also occur in the scapulae, ribs, clavicles, and pubic rami.

Hereditary Forms of Childhood Rickets

Three genetic causes of rickets exist. Two, type I and type II vitamin D–dependent rickets, are calcipenic diseases. The third, X-linked hypophosphatemic rickets, is caused by phosphorus loss.

Type I vitamin D–dependent rickets, an autosomal recessive disorder, is caused by a deficient or biologically inactive form of the 1α-hydroxylase enzyme. Therefore, children with this disorder cannot synthesize $1,25(OH)_2$ vitamin D in the kidney.[29] Affected children are normal at birth but show signs of rickets by age 1 year. Like nutritional rickets, calcium is low normal, phosphorus is normal, and both serum parathyroid hormone and alkaline phosphatase are elevated. However, unlike nutritional rickets, 25(OH) vitamin D is normal, indicating that the intake of vitamin D is adequate. This disorder may be cured by administration of $1,25(OH)_2$ vitamin D.

Type II vitamin D–dependent rickets, also an autosomal recessive disorder, is caused by mutations in the vitamin D receptor gene. A clinical heterogeneity seen in this disorder is caused by at least five different mutations in this gene.[30] Usually, the defect causes abnormal binding of calcitriol to the receptor. As a result, no cellular response to $1,25(OH)_2$ vitamin D occurs.[31] Before the genetic defect was identified, this disease was called vitamin D–resistant rickets because patients were not cured with the usual doses of vitamin D. Although end-organ resistance to vitamin D occurs in all cells in this disorder, the effects on the intestinal mucosa greatly limit calcium absorption and produce the bone changes. Children with this syndrome develop rickets any time between infancy and adolescence. Management of type II vitamin D–dependent rickets is difficult. Some patients show partial response to massive doses of vitamin D.

The third genetic cause of rickets, X-linked hypophosphatemic rickets, is caused by phosphate loss. This disease, also called phosphate diabetes or familial hypophosphatemia, is X linked dominant. One component of X-linked hypophosphatemic rickets is a renal tubular defect, which causes continuous loss of phosphorus. Children have normal serum vitamin D levels and normal serum calcium, but they become rachitic because of the marked decrease in phosphorus available for skeletal mineralization. Another component of this syndrome is a defect in osteoblasts to control mineral deposition.[17] This defect may be the cause of the generalized increased bone density that characterizes this disorder (Fig. 4–5). The absence of secondary hyperparathyroidism, a feature of phosphaturic rickets, may also be a factor that causes

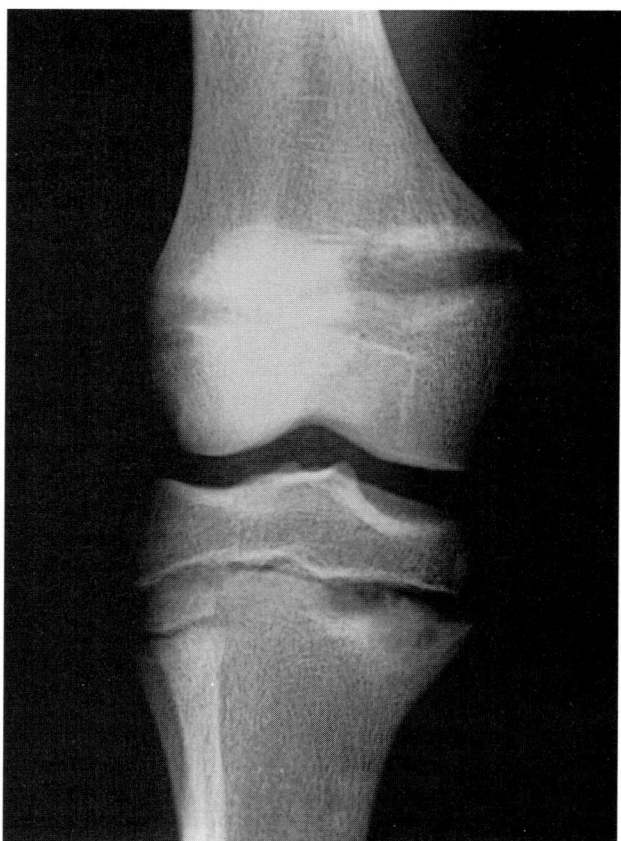

Figure 4-5 ■ Radiograph of X-linked hypophosphatemic rickets. The widened epiphyseal plates are consistent with rickets. However, the bones are radiodense, a typical feature of X-linked hypophosphatemic rickets.

radiodense bones (see Fig. 4–6 on color plate). As is characteristic of X-linked dominant mutations, hypophosphatemic rickets is fully expressed in male patients and variably expressed in female patients. Onset occurs in the second year of life, and children often present with abnormal dentition. Older children with this disorder are short and stocky, and they usually have bowed legs. Hypophosphatemia is the principal chemical manifestation of this disorder. Treatment of X-linked hypophosphatemic rickets is the lifelong administration of phosphate and $1,25(OH)_2$ vitamin D. This therapy usually reverses the rickets but can cause hyperparathyroidism and nephrocalcinosis.

Osteomalacia in Adults

Vitamin D deficiency in adults causes osteomalacia. In this disease, new bone, deposited during normal remodeling cycles, fails to mineralize. As a result, osteoid accumulates at the expense of bone, and the skeleton softens.

The rarity of nutritional childhood rickets in developed countries may lead to the conclusion that osteomalacia in adults is also rare. Unfortunately, however, it is common. There are several reasons for this. First, today, more people are living into old age, and old people often get inadequate sun exposure and eat poorly. Second, vitamin D metabolism is abnormal in the elderly. Third, gastrointestinal surgery, common in developed countries, may result in poor vitamin D absorption. Finally, some drugs cause osteomalacia.

Because older adults are the most commonly affected, osteomalacia is usually engrafted on involutional or postmenopausal bone loss. Bones become even weaker. Therefore, in caring for any patient with osteoporosis, the clinician must always ask, "Could this patient also have osteomalacia?" Answering this question is crucial because osteomalacia responds to vitamin D therapy, and treatment may reduce the incidence of fractures.

Epidemiology. In developed countries, as just indicated, osteomalacia is a disease of the elderly. Three causal factors contribute to this age predilection. First, because aging skin has low levels of vitamin D precursors, the elderly require at least three times the sun exposure to synthesize enough vitamin D.[32] This is difficult to achieve because older people are often immobile and spend less time outdoors. A second factor contributing to osteomalacia in the elderly is a poor diet. Although vitamin D is added to dairy and grain products, the elderly may eat few of these fortified foods. This problem is exaggerated when they have little choice of meals, such as with institutionalized patients or the homebound elderly. The third contributing factor is elderly patients' impaired hepatic synthesis of $25(OH)$ vitamin D and impaired renal synthesis of $1,25(OH)_2$ vitamin D. These three factors conspire to make osteomalacia a common disease of old people. For example, almost one third of institutionalized patients and 54% of the homebound elderly are vitamin D deficient.[33] In addition, a fourth of elderly patients with hip fracture show histologic evidence of osteomalacia,[34] and a third of these patients are vitamin D deficient, as determined by laboratory studies.[35]

In addition to elderly patients, osteomalacia affects patients of certain ethnic and dietary traditions. For example, the custom of *purdah* in the Middle East, which causes rickets in girls, also causes osteomalacia in adult women. This tradition of covering the body persists even among Asian women in Western countries. These women frequently remain indoors or wear traditional clothing that limits sun exposure.[36] A culturally related dietary practice, which may worsen osteomalacia among Indian and Pakistani women, is their consumption of large quantities of chupatti flour. This wheat flour contains phytates that bind calcium and inhibit calcium absorption. Lignin, also a component of the wheat fiber, binds to bile acids and further inhibits calcium absorption.[37]

Although nutritional and cultural practices can lead to osteomalacia, the most common cause of this disease in the United States is intestinal malabsorption.[38] Because vitamin D is a fat-soluble vitamin, gastrointestinal surgical procedures, such as gastric bypass surgery[39] or Billroth II partial gastrectomy,[40] often lead to osteomalacia. In addition to surgical procedures, primary diseases of the small intestine, such as celiac disease, Crohn's disease, and scleroderma, also result in poor vitamin D absorption. Hepatobiliary disease also reduces vitamin D absorption. For example, biliary obstruction not only diminishes bile release but also impairs the hepatic synthesis of $25(OH)$ vitamin D.

Some patients receiving anticonvulsant therapy, particularly phenobarbital and Dilantin, develop osteomalacia or rickets.[41] Approximately 25% of children on long-term Dilantin therapy for epilepsy develop skeletal features of rickets.[42] However, the incidence of abnormal laboratory values is higher. Patients usually have mildly reduced serum calcium levels and mild reductions in serum $25(OH)$ vitamin D. Although poor nutrition, seen occasionally in epileptic patients, may contribute to calcium imbalance, anticonvulsants have been shown in experimental animals to cause mineralization abnormalities, even with controlled vitamin intake.[43]

The anticonvulsant effect on mineral metabolism is not fully understood. Apparently, these medicines result in a reduced sensitivity to vitamin D. In animals, phenytoin inhibits the intestinal absorption of calcium, and both phenytoin and phenobarbital inhibit the mobilization of calcium from bone in vitro. In addition, mild hepatic injury caused by these drugs decreases the release of $25(OH)$ vitamin D. Treatment with vitamin D reduces the incidence of osteopenia and fractures in these patients.[44]

Clinical and Radiographic Features. On rare occasions, osteomalacia is asymptomatic. However, 94% of patients have at least one symptom.[45] Usually, they complain of vague muscular aches, particularly in the back and legs. Muscle weakness and atrophy may also be present.[46] In addition, bone pain and tenderness may occur, even when no obvious stress fractures are present.

The biochemical abnormalities associated with osteomalacia are highly characteristic. Patients have an elevated serum parathyroid hormone level (due to secondary hyperparathyroidism) and a low or normal serum calcium. The normal serum calcium level distinguishes osteomalacia from primary hyperparathyroidism. In addition, some patients with osteomalacia have low levels of serum 25(OH) vitamin D.

Although the laboratory features are characteristic, some patients with osteomalacia lack the diagnostic laboratory profile. Therefore, evaluation of a patient by laboratory studies alone may be inaccurate.[45] For example, only 47% of patients have a low serum calcium, and only 29% have a low serum 25(OH) vitamin D. Also, elevated serum parathyroid hormone levels are present in only 41%. A consistent finding, however, is an elevated serum alkaline phosphatase, present in 94% of cases. However, this laboratory finding is nonspecific and could indicate any high-turnover bone disease.

Radiographically, the most characteristic feature of osteomalacia is osteopenia, and changes may be indistinguishable from those of involutional osteoporosis. The presence of stress fractures, or *Looser zones,* favors a diagnosis of osteomalacia. However, these zones are present in only 18% of patients. Looser zones, transverse bands of mottled radiodensity and radiolucency, occur most commonly in the femur and tibia (Fig. 4–7). With the more highly sensitive bone scan, occult stress fractures appear as discrete lines of increased technetium uptake.[47] Looser zones are typically bilateral and symmetric (Fig. 4–8). The presence of florid symmetric Looser zones is known as Milkman syndrome after the radiologist who described these features in 1934.[48] If severe secondary hyperparathyroidism is engrafted on osteomalacia, subperiosteal resorptive changes are also present.

Pathologic Features. Because the laboratory studies are variable and the radiographic features often nonspecific, the unequivocal diagnosis of osteomalacia can be made only with the undecalcified bone biopsy.[49, 50]

The accumulation of unmineralized osteoid[51] is the most important pathologic feature of osteomalacia (see Fig. 4–9 on color plate). Using histomorphometric techniques, several characteristic features are usually present. First, total osteoid thickness is increased. Also, because mineralization is diminished, the amount of tetracycline labeling is reduced. Typically, tetracycline labels in osteomalacia are broad and ill defined, unlike the typical crisp labels seen in normal mineralization. The dynamic indices of bone metabolism are also abnormal in osteomalacia. A low mineralization rate and a low bone formation rate are present. Most characteristically, the mineralization lag time, an index of the efficiency of mineralization, is elevated, often to many times the normal value.

Treatment of Osteomalacia and Rickets

Rickets and osteomalacia can be cured with vitamin D therapy. Nutritional osteomalacia and rickets respond to oral vitamin D, usually 1500 to 5000 units daily. Also, exposure to an ultraviolet lamp or increased sun exposure may be effective. For malabsorption-related osteomalacia, treatment with 25(OH) vitamin D (20–30 μg/d) may be more efficacious. In addition to vitamin D therapy, calcium supplementation may be necessary, although care must be taken to avoid hypercalcemia.

Oncogenic Osteomalacia

An unusual and rare presentation of osteomalacia results from the paracrine effect of a localized bone or soft tissue neoplasm. In this syndrome, known as *oncogenic osteomalacia,* a neoplasm synthesizes and secretes a circulating compound, known as phosphatonin, which acts on the kidney in two ways. First, the substance diminishes the tubular reabsorption of phosphate and leads to phosphate wasting. This effect mimics the pathophysiology of X-linked hypophosphatemic rickets. Second, the substance diminishes the renal activity of 1α-hydroxylase, resulting in the decreased synthesis of 1,25(OH)$_2$ vitamin D. Evidence for these two effects has been demonstrated in nude mice bearing transplants of these neoplasms and in kidney cell cultures exposed to the serum of affected patients.[52, 53]

Oncogenic osteomalacia can be caused by a wide variety of neoplasms, although they are usually primary soft tissue or bone tumors. Most commonly, the causative neoplasm is a benign or low-grade malignant vascular or fibrous tissue

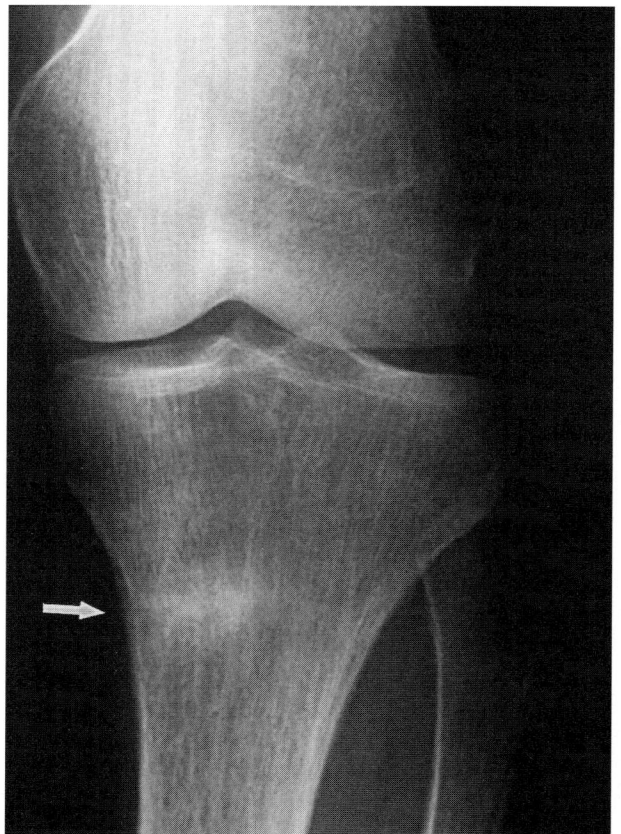

Figure 4-7 ■ Osteomalacia. Osteopenia and a stress fracture of the proximal tibia are present *(arrow).*

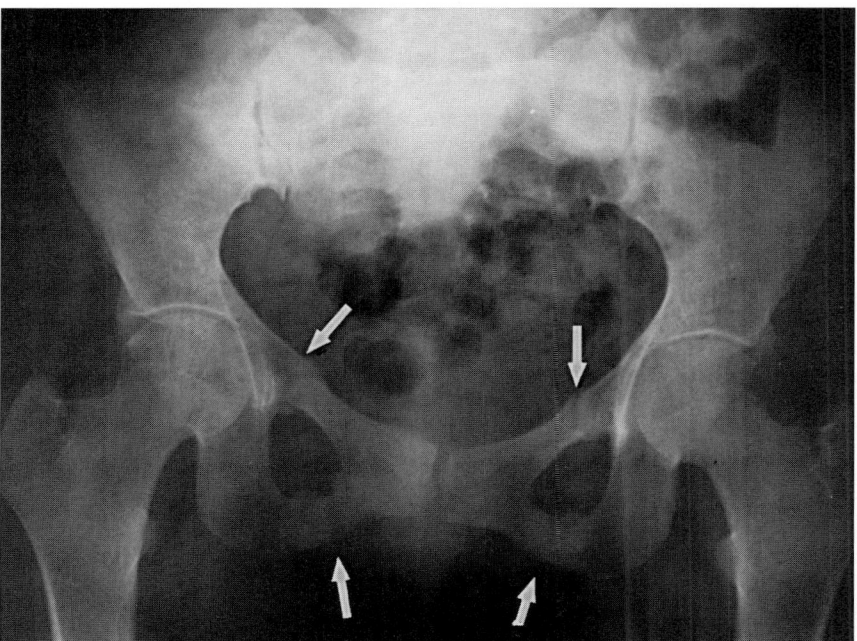

Figure 4-8 ■ Osteomalacia. Symmetric stress fractures are present in the pubic and ischial rami (*arrows*).

tumor. In addition, polyostatic fibrous dysplasia,[54] neurofibromatosis,[55] and metastatic prostate carcinoma may produce this syndrome.[56]

Patients with oncogenic osteomalacia present with unexplained muscular aches and hypophosphatemia. Bone pain and skeletal demineralization may also be present. Stress fractures are sometimes present (Fig. 4-10). In addition, serum $1,25(OH)_2$ vitamin D is always low in these patients, and serum calcium may also be low. By contrast, serum $25(OH)$ vitamin D and serum parathyroid hormone levels are normal. In the absence of renal disease, this constellation of abnormalities is almost diagnostic of oncogenic osteomalacia, even if the patient has no obvious neoplasm. Thorough clinical and radiographic examination usually uncovers a tumor. Occasionally, however, patients present with the clinical and laboratory features of oncogenic osteomalacia, but a neoplasm cannot be found with extensive clinical and radiographic studies. Sometimes it takes months or years to discover the causative neoplasm.

Complete removal of the offending neoplasm completely reverses the osteomalacia. If successful, the osteomalacia resolves. However, incomplete removal of the neoplasm necessitates treatment with phosphate and $1,25(OH)_2$ vitamin D to ameliorate the skeletal disease.

RENAL OSTEODYSTROPHY

Because of the importance of the kidney in calcium and phosphorus metabolism, renal disease adversely affects the skeleton. However, clinically significant bone changes, known as renal osteodystrophy, usually are delayed until end-stage renal disease. Therefore, prior to the use of renal dialysis, renal osteodystrophy was rare—patients died before severe skeletal changes appeared. Today, however, renal dialysis or renal transplantation supports the estimated 300,000 Americans with end-stage renal disease long enough for them to develop clinically significant bone disease.[57] Renal osteodystrophy may, therefore, be considered an iatrogenic disorder.

Although symptoms of renal osteodystrophy are delayed until end-stage renal failure, abnormalities in calcium and phosphorus metabolism appear early in the course of kidney disease. For example, elevated parathyroid hormone levels occur in patients with only 20% reduction in renal function. Therefore, to prevent the late development of severe bone disease, management of mineral abnormalities is a concern for the clinical nephrologist beginning early in the course of renal disease.

Pathophysiology

Renal osteodystrophy is a combination of secondary hyperparathyroidism and, to a lesser extent, osteomalacia.[58] Secondary hyperparathyroidism is the most important factor contributing to bone disease. The principal factor stimulating the parathyroids in renal failure is the ever-present tendency for the serum calcium to fall. As a result, the constantly elevated serum parathyroid hormone levels remove calcium from the bone.

Although secondary hyperparathyroidism causes the bone changes, the principal driving factor in renal osteodystrophy—the factor that causes the serum calcium to fall—is *hyperphosphatemia*. Hyperphosphatemia is a result of a reduced glomerular filtration rate and a failure of damaged tubules to excrete phosphorus. Also, as renal disease continues, the hyperphosphatemia is enhanced by the failure of the

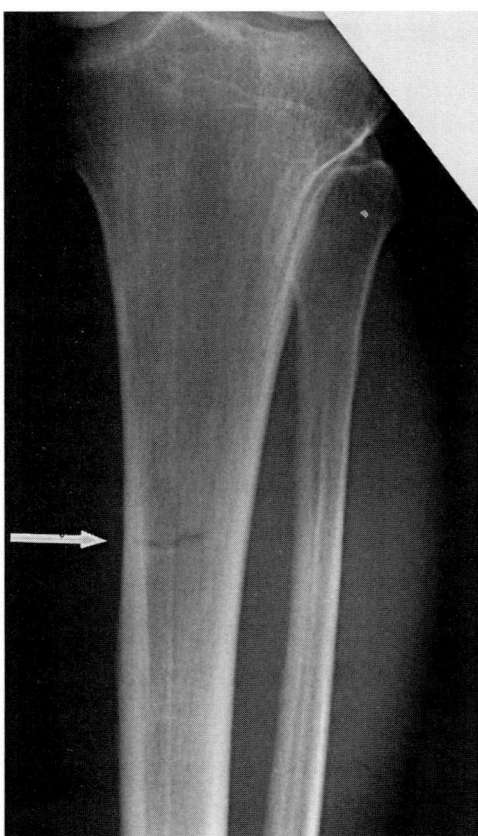

Figure 4-10 ■ Oncogenic osteomalacia. Osteopenia is not apparent on plain radiographs. However, a stress fracture is present *(arrow)*.

Clinical Features

Although abnormalities of mineral metabolism appear early in renal insufficiency, the symptoms of renal osteodystrophy are usually delayed until advanced renal failure. Bone pain is the most common symptom. Usually the bone pain is vague and localized to the back and legs. However, sometimes the pain may be severe enough to require bed rest. The severe pain is usually due to pathologic fractures, particularly in the ribs and vertebrae. Patients with renal osteodystrophy also develop multiple stress fractures in weight-bearing bones, further enhancing the generalized bone pain. Additional clinical features are muscle weakness, resulting from a myopathy, and itching, caused by deposition of calcium in the skin. In children with renal osteodystrophy, growth retardation is common, a problem usually caused by a combination of malnutrition, acidosis, and osteomalacia. Because of growth retardation, renal osteodystrophy in children has been called *renal rickets*.

Radiologic Features

Bone changes of hyperparathyroidism dominate the radiologic features of renal osteodystrophy.[61] The changes are similar to those in primary hyperparathyroidism, but in renal osteodystrophy they are more pronounced. Subperiosteal and subchondral resorption is characteristic. The earliest and most common osseous abnormality is resorption of the tufts of the distal phalanges. This change may be recognized early in the course of renal failure using high-grain radiographic film or direct magnification radiography. Another site of early subperiosteal resorption is along the radial aspect of the middle phalanges. Other than in the hands, the most frequent site of resorption is the distal end of the clavicle. In advanced cases, subperiosteal resorptive changes may be seen in the femoral and humeral necks, the distal radius and ulna, and the pelvis (Fig. 4–11).

Osteosclerosis, present in 20% of patients, is a striking radiographic feature of renal osteodystrophy.[62] This change, caused by extensive woven bone deposition, is paradoxical because osteopenia and cortical thinning are present in other parts of the skeleton (see Fig. 4–12 on color plate). The osteosclerosis is most prominent in areas of the skeleton with a high proportion of cancellous bone; the spine, therefore, is the most common site. In each vertebra, the radiodensity is most prominent beneath the endplates, a pattern that imparts a "rugger-jersey" appearance to the spine (Fig. 4–13). The osteosclerosis of renal failure is usually pronounced in children.

Brown tumors also occur in renal osteodystrophy. In fact, they occur more commonly in end-stage renal failure than in primary hyperparathyroidism. Brown tumors, which may often be multiple in renal failure, are well-defined lytic lesions that usually occur in the metaphysis (Fig. 4–14). Cortical expansion is sometimes present. Management of the secondary hyperparathyroidism usually leads to healing of the brown tumors by progressive lesional sclerosis.

tubule to respond to the phosphaturic effect of parathyroid hormone. Hyperphosphatemia can lower serum calcium directly. In addition, hyperphosphatemia impairs renal 1α-hydroxylase, thereby diminishing the synthesis of 1,25 $(OH)_2$ vitamin D.[59] As a result, calcium absorption in the gut is dramatically reduced, further increasing the tendency of the serum calcium to fall. Thus, the inefficient entry of calcium into the homeostatic system, caused by vitamin D deficiency, is responsible for the osteomalacia component of renal osteodystrophy.

In addition to the adverse effect of low levels of 1,25$(OH)_2$ vitamin D on gut and bone, diminished levels can also directly cause oversecretion of the parathyroid glands. Because 1,25$(OH)_2$ vitamin D is a potent regulator of parathyroid secretion, low levels increase parathyroid secretion by raising the set point for sensing calcium.[60] As a result, higher levels of calcium are required to turn down parathyroid secretion. In addition to regulating secretion of parathyroid hormone, 1,25$(OH)_2$ vitamin D regulates the growth of parathyroid cells by altering the expression of oncogenes. Thus, low levels of 1,25$(OH)_2$ vitamin D directly result in both parathyroid hypersecretion and hyperplasia. Conversely, administration of 1,25$(OH)_2$ vitamin D reduces parathyroid secretion, an effect that has important therapeutic implications.

Figure 4-11 ■ Advanced renal osteodystrophy. Erosion of the medial surface of the proximal humerus has occurred *(arrow)*. Erosion of the distal clavicle and tumoral calcinosis also is present.

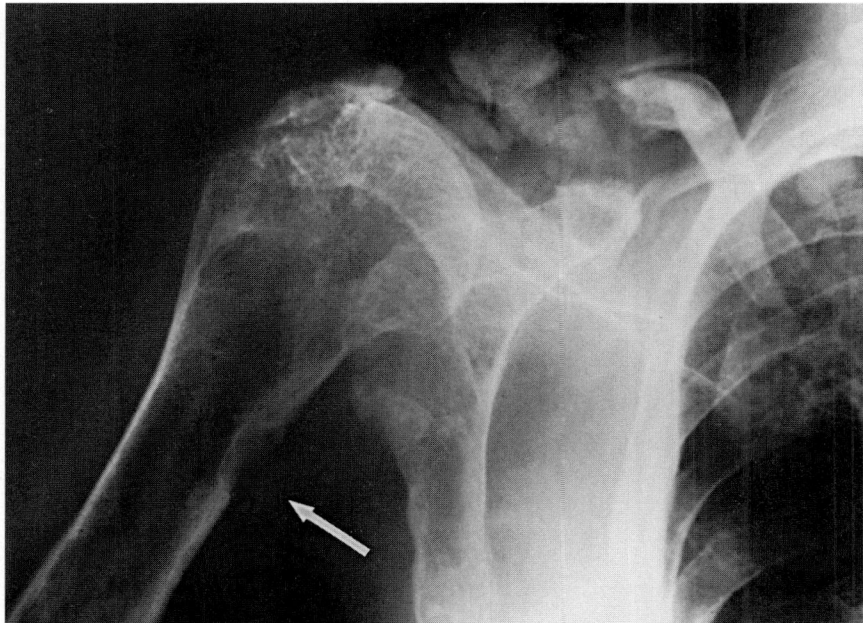

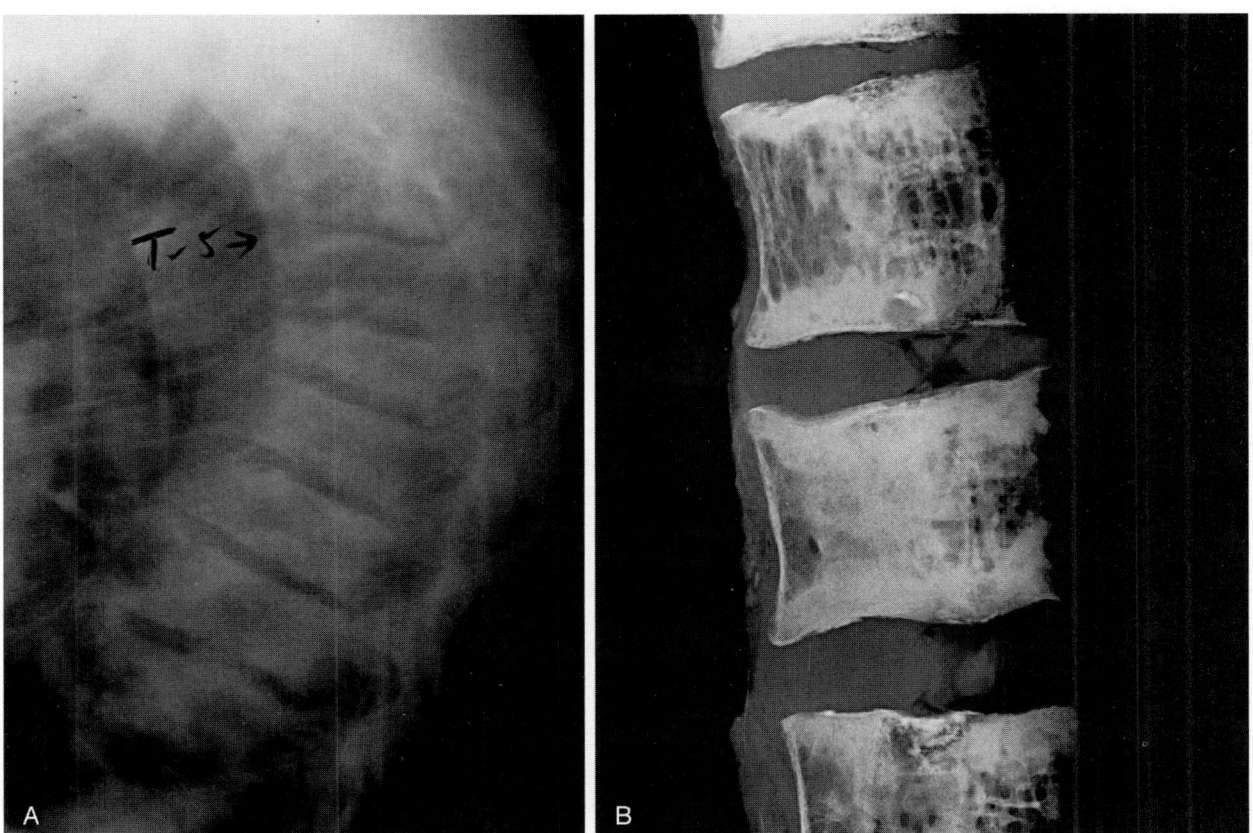

Figure 4-13 ■ The manifestations of renal osteodystrophy in the spine. **A,** Plain radiograph showing radiodensities beneath the subchondral plates. **B,** Specimen radiograph of a slab of a spine showing dense bone beneath the endplates. This pattern of radiodensity imparts a "rugger jersey" pattern to the plain radiographs.

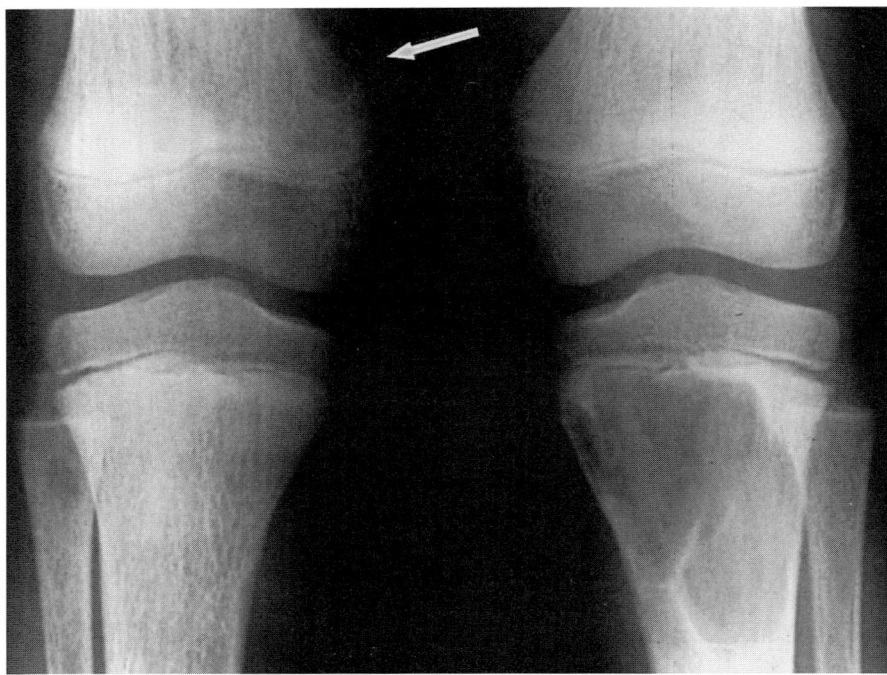

Figure 4–14 ■ Renal osteodystrophy in a child. Plain radiographs show multiple brown tumors. A large brown tumor (lytic area) is present in the tibial metaphysis. Another is present in the contralateral distal femoral metaphysis (arrow). (From McCarthy, E. F.: *Differential Diagnosis in Pathology. Bone and Joint Disorders.* New York and Tokyo, Igaku-Shoin, 1996. With permission from Williams & Wilkins.)

In addition to radiographic changes of hyperparathyroidism, features of osteomalacia are present in some patients with renal osteodystrophy. These changes are most prominent in aluminum related bone disease. The bones are severely osteopenic, and stress fractures (Looser zones) may be numerous.

Histopathologic Features

General Features

Two overlapping histopathologic patterns of renal osteodystrophy—high-turnover disease and low-turnover disease—exist.[63] In most cases, the predominant histopathologic features are the result of the effects of secondary hyperparathyroidism, and bone turnover is high. An additional feature that may be engrafted on the changes of hyperparathyroidism in some patients is a mineralization defect resulting in osteomalacia. This change is usually not present until the late stages of renal failure or until patients have begun dialysis. In some treated patients, particularly those undergoing peritoneal dialysis, high turnover may be shut down. In fact, these patients show almost no bone turnover, a condition known as low-turnover (adynamic) renal osteodystrophy.

High-Turnover Renal Osteodystrophy

Excessive osteoclastic and osteoblastic activity, caused by secondary hyperparathyroidism, characterizes high-turnover renal osteodystrophy. Increased osteoclastic activity is evident by many irregular resorption cavities cut deeply into trabeculae, a process known as *tunneling resorption* (see Fig. 4–15 on color plate). Increased osteoblastic activity is manifested by an increased number of osteoblasts and an increased amount of osteoid, known as *hyperosteoidosis* (see Fig. 4–16 on color plate). Unlike the regular array of osteoblasts that characterize normal bone remodeling, the osteoblasts in high-turnover renal osteodystrophy are irregularly arranged. As a result, the newly deposited osteoid is woven rather than lamellar. In high-turnover renal osteodystrophy, osteoid covers most of the trabecular surfaces, but the thickness of the osteoid seams is not increased. In addition to tunneling resorption and hyperosteoidosis, histomorphometric data also indicate high-turnover bone disease. For example, tetracycline-labeled surfaces are increased and the bone formation rate is elevated.

The osteosclerosis seen radiographically is the result of extensive woven bone formation (see Fig. 4–17 on color plate). The additional woven bone is added almost exclusively to cancellous bone, thereby increasing trabecular thickness. As a result, osteosclerosis is most prominent in skeletal areas with a high proportion of cancellous bone, principally the spine. The extent of woven bone deposition parallels the severity of the hyperparathyroidism and the duration of chronic renal failure. The cause of the osteosclerosis is unclear. Most likely, the encasement of trabeculae by osteoid inhibits the osteoclasts.

In addition to increased bone resorption and bone formation, marrow fibrosis, the most characteristic feature of high-turnover renal osteodystrophy, is also prominent. A feature of all high-turnover states, marrow fibrosis results from the stimulation by parathyroid hormone of osteoblast precursors to synthesize collagen. Initially this process occurs adjacent to trabeculae (Fig. 4–18). As bone changes worsen, the typical paratrabecular fibrosis spreads to involve much of the marrow space, a condition known as *osteitis fibrosa* (Fig. 4–19).

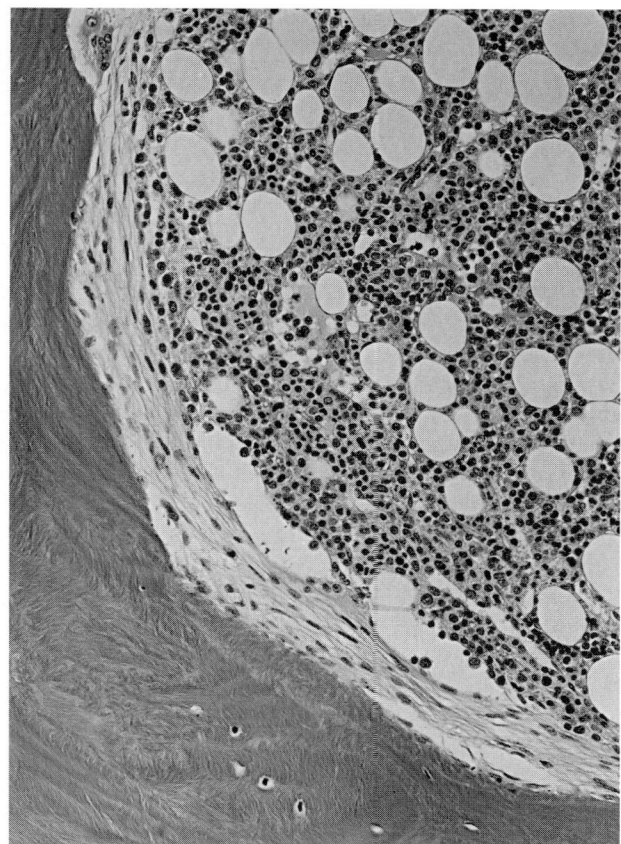

Figure 4-18 ■ Photomicrograph showing paratrabecular fibrosis of early secondary hyperparathyroidism.

Low-Turnover Renal Osteodystrophy

Although high bone turnover of hyperparathyroidism is characteristic of most cases of renal osteodystrophy, 5 to 25% of patients on renal dialysis show low bone turnover. This pattern, known as low-turnover uremic osteodystrophy, represents the other end of the spectrum of bone changes. Because this pattern of bone involvement is rarely seen before commencing dialysis, low turnover most likely results from the shutdown of parathyroid hyperactivity due to therapy. For example, patients may have been treated with calcitriol or calcium salts, both substances that decrease parathyroid function. Histomorphometric studies of low-turnover renal osteodystrophy reveal a marked reduction in the number of osteoblasts and osteoclasts. In addition, resorption surfaces are decreased, and tetracycline labels, indicating mineralizing surfaces, are scanty.

A number of patients with low-turnover disease also have a degree of osteomalacia. In addition to low turnover, patients have wide osteoid seams and an elevated mineralization lag time. In almost all cases, the osteomalacia associated with renal osteodystrophy is caused by aluminum deposition in bone.[64]

Aluminum Bone Disease

Aluminum bone disease is an iatrogenic form of osteomalacia. This metal inhibits bone mineralization and may enter the body in four ways. First, patients may acquire aluminum from the dialysate fluid during renal dialysis. Formerly, this often occurred in geographical areas with high levels of aluminum in the water (some communities add aluminum to drinking water to clear turbidity). Second, phosphate binders, used to treat the hyperphosphatemia of renal failure, often utilize aluminum as the binding agent. Third, patients on total parenteral nutrition (TPN) inadvertently receive aluminum in the form of casein hydrolysate in the TPN solution. Fourth, on rare occasions, frequent use of aluminum-containing antacids results in an increased body load of this metal.

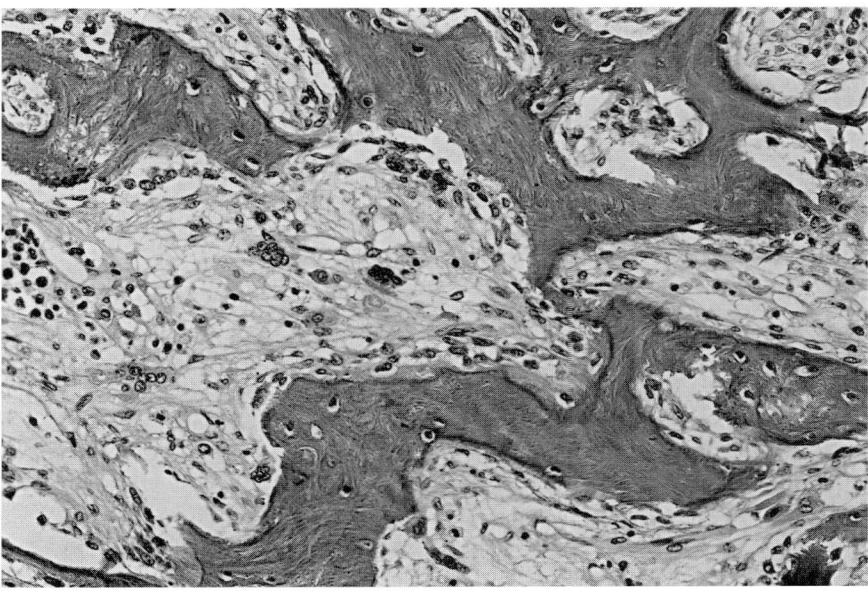

Figure 4-19 ■ Photomicrograph of more advanced osteitis fibrosa. Woven bone is irregularly present in a fibrous tissue background.

Aluminum adversely affects bone in several ways. Most importantly, aluminum is deposited at the mineralization front, where it disrupts the rate of formation and growth of the hydroxyapatite crystals.[65] As a result, mineralization is inhibited and osteomalacia develops. In addition, aluminum also inhibits bone turnover—it directly inhibits osteoblastic activity and it inhibits the release of parathyroid hormone from the parathyroid cells.[66, 67]

Aluminum may be diagnosed by special stains performed on undecalcified bone biopsies[68, 69] (see Fig. 4–20 on color plate). Usually, aluminum is present on the trabecular surface, but it may also be present within bone trabeculae. Aluminum positivity on 30% of the bone surface is considered clinically significant. Aluminum bone disease, first recognized in 1979, was a frequent complication of renal dialysis in the 1980s. Today, awareness of this complication has reduced the incidence of this disease. However, in 1991, 30% of dialysis patients were still aluminum positive.[70]

Aluminum-induced bone disease may be successfully treated with desferoxamine, a chelating agent. Provided that the source is eliminated, aluminum is also removed (although gradually) by normal bone turnover over several years.

Amyloidosis in Patients with Chronic Renal Failure

A wide variety of proteins deposited in tissues in various diseases have the characteristics of amyloid. One form of amyloid, β_2-microglobulin, is unique to renal dialysis patients. In this setting, amyloid is deposited in bones and periosteal soft tissues and is another manifestation of renal bone disease.

Beta$_2$-microglobulin is a low–molecular weight protein normally produced by lymphoid cells and other cells with high turnover. In these cells, β_2-microglobulin stabilizes the structure of the major histocompatibility complex antigens located on cell surfaces. Approximately 180 to 250 mg of this protein are generated each day as complexes are shed from cell membranes. Normally, almost all β_2-microglobulin is filtered by the glomerulus and catabolized in the renal tubules. However, this protein does not filter well through dialysis membranes and, as a result, accumulates in tissue.[71] This disorder is common in long-term renal dialysis patients. After 10 or more years of dialysis, 70 to 80% of patients are affected.

The clinical features of amyloid deposition are usually delayed until after at least 5 years of dialysis therapy. Although amyloid is deposited throughout the body, osteoarticular manifestations are the most severe. Carpal tunnel syndrome, a common presentation of many forms of amyloidosis, is the most frequent clinical picture.[72] In this presentation, amyloid is deposited in tenosynovial tissue. Numerous other clinical manifestations may occur. Deposition of amyloid around major joints, particularly the shoulder joint, causes soft tissue masses. Subchondral bone cysts are another presentation.[73] In this presentation, amyloid accumulates in the marrow spaces beneath the articular cartilage and leads to an erosive arthropathy. The humeral and femoral heads are most commonly involved, but the hand and spine are also affected.

OSTEOPOROSIS

Osteoporosis is a general term indicating a symptomatic, generalized decrease in bone mass. Three varieties occur: primary, secondary, and idiopathic. *Primary osteoporosis* is a decrease in bone mass due to aging, often resulting in painful fractures and deformities. Primary osteoporosis may be subdivided into senile and postmenopausal varieties. *Senile osteoporosis* is the gradual loss of bone mass that begins in middle adulthood and proceeds relentlessly until death. This gradual reduction in bone mass occurs in both men and women in all ethnic groups and cultures. *Postmenopausal osteoporosis* is a rapid bone loss engrafted on the process of senile osteoporosis. This form of osteoporosis is experienced by women whose bones are extremely sensitive to estrogen withdrawal. These women suffer a rapid reduction in bone mass in the years following the menopause.

Secondary osteoporosis is a premature bone loss or an exaggerated age-related bone loss caused by a wide variety of endogenous or exogenous factors not related to age. These factors include corticosteroid therapy, diabetes, and secondary amenorrhea. Identification and removal of these deleterious factors slows the rate of bone loss and often restores bone mass.

On rare occasions, young adults or even children become osteoporotic. In the absence of an identifiable endocrine abnormality or risk factor, this clinical syndrome is called *idiopathic osteoporosis.*

Skeletal Failure

In any of the syndromes of osteoporosis, the loss of bone mass may become so severe that the structural function of the skeleton is lost. Fractures occur spontaneously or with only the slightest trauma. As a result, patients live with constant pain and disability. This condition, known as *skeletal failure,* is a concept akin to renal failure or heart failure.

Peak Bone Mass

An important factor determining whether a person's skeleton fails in late adulthood is the amount of bone present before the reduction in bone mass begins. During skeletal growth, the point of maximal bone development is known as *peak bone mass*. Bone mass, measured by dual energy x-ray absorptiometry (DEXA), is the amount of bone per unit area and is independent of bone size. The amount of bone present at peak bone mass is the starting point from which bone loss begins. Bone mass increases dramatically throughout puberty and, in girls, plateaus about 2 years after the menarche. Boys plateau at about age 17.[74] At this plateau, about 95% of bone mass is present.[75] However, additional bone mass accumulates when men and women are in their 20s, even after skeletal growth is complete. Healthy women may gain additional bone even until age 29.[76] In sum, people usually reach peak bone mass in their mid- to late 20s.

Many factors govern the amount of bone present at the time of peak bone mass. About 80% of the variance in peak bone mass is due to genetic factors.[77] For example, African-American women generally reach a higher peak bone mass than white women.[78] By contrast, Asians and Hispanics have a lower peak bone mass than whites.[79]

Environmental factors also contribute to peak bone mass variation. Among these factors, childhood nutrition is particularly important. For example, low calcium intake during adolescence is associated with a lower peak bone mass.[80] Although the recommended daily calcium intake for adolescents and young adults is 1200 mg, one survey discovered that only 15% of girls and 53% of boys meet this requirement.[80] Protein consumption is probably also important. Malnourished children in some low socioeconomic groups are likely to have lower peak bone mass and, as a result, are more likely to have weak bones in old age.

Malnutrition is not unique to low socioeconomic groups, however. In affluent populations, adolescents, obsessed with the desire to be slender, are also probably malnourished. Especially at risk of malnutrition and therefore of low peak bone mass, are those training for a sport or a career requiring a thin body (e.g., fashion modeling, gymnastics, ballet, and figure skating).

Acquiring maximal peak bone mass in the first three decades of life is the initial step in preventing primary osteoporosis. The quote "Senile osteoporosis is a pediatric disease"[81] emphasizes the importance of this concept.

Primary Osteoporosis

Primary osteoporosis is a major public health problem because it causes pain and disability in many people and because it costs so much (Table 4–2). It is a common disease. As many as 54% of white postmenopausal women show evidence of decreased bone mass, and another 30% have clinical osteoporosis. Thus, white women alone account for 26 million of those suffering from weak bones.[82]

Fractures

Osteoporotic bones are weak and fracture easily. Not only are they weak because of the decrease in bone mass, but also they are brittle because of changes in the organic matrix.[83] Patients with osteoporosis commonly suffer vertebral compression fractures, hip fractures, and fractures of the distal radius (i.e., Colles' fractures). These fractures are common in the elderly, not only because their bones are weak but also because they fall more often. This may be due to cerebrovascular disease, muscular weakness, or medi-

Table 4–2 ■ **THE BURDEN OF OSTEOPOROSIS IN THE UNITED STATES**

- Osteoporosis affects more than 26 million women and leads to 1.5 million fractures each year.[159]
- A total of 54% of postmenopausal women are osteopenic. Another 30% are osteoporotic.[82]
- A total of 54% of women at age 50 will sustain at least one osteoporotic fracture during the remainder of their lifetime.[160]
- A total of 27% of women have sustained a vertebral compression fracture by age 65.[85]
- An estimated 300,000 hip fractures occur in the United States each year.[161] Ninety percent of these occur in patients older than age 70, and 90% are related to osteoporosis.
- The fatality rate after a hip fracture is 24% within 1 year.[86]
- In 1995, the per patient expenditure for a hip fracture averaged $32,000.[87]
- In 1995, the total estimated expenditure for treating osteoporotic fractures was $13.8 billion. Hip fractures alone account for $7.1 billion.[87]
- In the next 10 years, an estimated 5.2 million hip, spine, and forearm fractures will result in medical costs exceeding $45 billion.[162]

cations. For example, over a third of institutionalized patients have a history of a fall. Even without a fall, osteoporotic bone may fracture spontaneously. For example, an elderly woman may report that she felt her hip "snap" and then she fell. Likewise, almost half of vertebral compression fractures occur spontaneously.[84]

Vertebral fractures are the most common complication of osteoporosis. More than 25% of all women over 65 years of age have sustained a crush fracture.[85] Most commonly, the thoracic or lumbar vertebrae are involved. Two clinical patterns of vertebral fractures occur. The first pattern is the acute vertebral crush fracture (Fig. 4–21). Patients present with the acute onset of severe pain and muscle spasm. Occasionally, an acute osteoporotic compression fracture is very difficult to distinguish clinically and radiologically from metastatic carcinoma. A biopsy may be the only way to make the correct diagnosis. The second pattern of vertebral fracture is the asymptomatic anterior wedge fracture. Usually, multiple vertebrae are involved, a pattern that causes kyphosis and a gradual reduction in height. Presumably, the anterior wedging occurs in small, asymptomatic increments.

Although vertebral fractures are the most common complication of low bone mass, hip fractures are associated with the highest mortality. In addition, they cause the most financial strain on the health care system. Approximately 300,000 hip fractures occur in the United States each year. The mortality rate following hip fracture is 24% during the first year.[86] Most survivors are disabled, many seriously. The staggering annual cost to treat hip fractures in the United States exceeds 7 billion dollars.[87]

History

People in ancient times also suffered from osteoporosis. This disease has been documented in two populations of Native Americans (2600–2500 BC).[88] One of the first medical descriptions of this syndrome was offered in 1824 by Sir

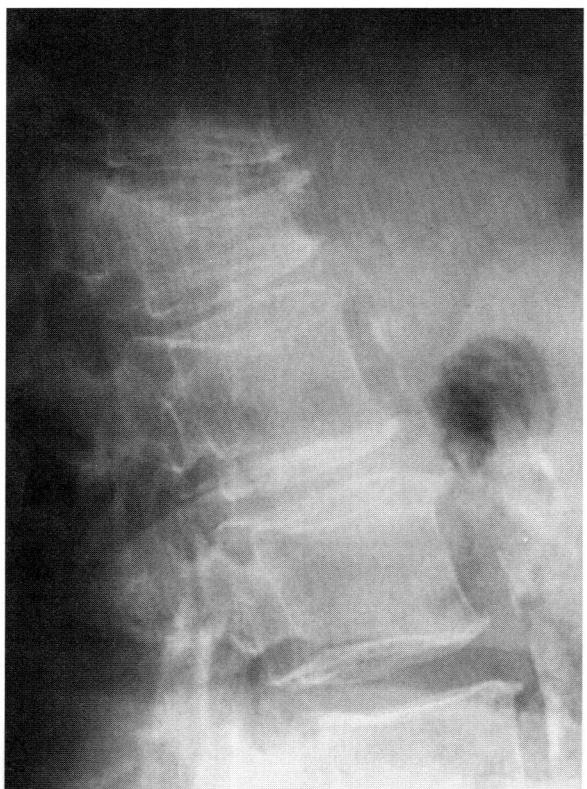

Figure 4-21 ■ An acute vertebral compression fracture due to osteoporosis.

Astley Cooper (p. 123): "That regular decay of nature which is called old age, is attended with changes which are easily detected in the dead body; and one of the principal of these is found in the bones, for they become thin in their shell, and spongy in their texture."[89] About 60 years later, Pommer noted that the bone loss of osteoporosis differed from that of osteomalacia and rickets.[90] However, it was not until 1948 that osteoporosis was recognized as a distinct clinical syndrome. In that year, Fuller Albright and Edward Reifenstein delineated the specific patterns of bone loss in postmenopausal and senile osteoporosis.[91]

Pathogenesis

Similar to all forms of osteoporosis, primary osteoporosis results from an excess of osteoclastic activity over osteoblastic activity, although this discrepancy in cellular activity is usually not apparent in routine histologic preparations. The bone loss occurs in tiny increments during each remodeling cycle.[92] In the normal skeleton, bone mass is maintained because remodeling is balanced. The amount of bone deposited by a team of osteoblasts equals the amount removed by a team of osteoclasts. However, in osteoporosis, osteoblasts deposit a little less bone than the amount that was removed. Therefore, with each remodeling cycle, skeletal mass becomes slightly less. Furthermore, any condition leading to an increased activation of remodeling cycles speeds up the reduction in skeletal mass.

The discrepancy in the remodeling cycle begins in the fourth decade of life. At this point, osteoblasts synthesize less bone at each remodeling site, and skeletal mass begins to decrease very gradually.[93] Bone loss occurs at a rate of 0.3% per year in men and 0.5% per year in women.[94] The reason why osteoblasts synthesize less bone, although not fully understood, is probably because of osteoblast senescence or a decrease in osteoblast longevity. In addition, the message sent to recruit osteoblasts after the resorption phase of the remodeling cycle may be deficient, perhaps a result of decreased synthesis of growth factors, such as transforming growth factor-β or insulin-like growth factor. Finally, decreased stress on bones due to the reduced physical activity of older people probably also contributes to decreased bone synthesis.

In addition to osteoblast senescence, hormonal factors are probably active in reducing bone mass in osteoporosis. For example, parathyroid hormone levels, a response to low serum calcium, are increased in many elderly patients. The lowered serum calcium is due to a combination of several factors: a decreased calcium intake, decreased calcium absorption, and a renal calcium leak.[95]

In addition to minimally increased parathyroid secretion, a decreased serum $1,25(OH)_2$ vitamin D level, noted in some patients with osteoporosis, is another possible factor leading to bone loss.[96] Decreased sun exposure or dietary intake, both common problems in the elderly, could be responsible for the low $1,25(OH)_2$ vitamin D levels. Also, the renal synthesis of $1,25(OH)_2$ vitamin D is impaired in some elderly patients.[97] Another possible cause for low serum calcium is the genetically acquired defect in the receptor for vitamin D that has been demonstrated in some patients. Two alleles for the vitamin D receptor gene have been isolated—b and B. Patients who are homozygous for b have a higher bone density, whereas patients who are homozygous for B have a lower bone density.[98] Identifying children with unfavorable vitamin D receptor genotypes may lead to early preventative measures.

Senile Osteoporosis

Primary osteoporosis encompasses two patterns of bone loss: senile (type II) osteoporosis and postmenopausal (type I) osteoporosis.[99] Senile osteoporosis is the pattern of skeletal loss that naturally occurs with aging. This pattern of bone loss, which begins in the fourth decade and continues throughout life, occurs in men and women of all racial and ethnic groups. The process usually becomes clinically apparent at about age 70, and patients often present with painless vertebral wedge deformities. Senile osteoporosis equally affects cortical and cancellous bone. However, because the volume of cortical bone in the skeleton is greater, senile osteoporosis has its greatest effect on the cortex. As a result, patients commonly suffer fractures of the femoral neck, an area consisting mainly of cortical bone. Asymptomatic vertebral wedge fractures also occur. Because increased osteoclastic activity is not a major factor in this pattern of

Table 4-3 ■ OSTEOPOROSIS RISK FACTORS

Genetic Factors	Behavioral Factors
Female	Inactivity
White	Smoking
Northern European descent	Alcohol abuse
Asian	Malnutrition
Fair hair and skin	
Tall, thin body habitus	

the bone loss, senile osteoporosis is also known as *low-turnover osteoporosis*.

Postmenopausal Osteoporosis

In addition to the gradual age-related bone loss, some women at the time of menopause develop a rapid increase in bone loss. This pattern of postmenopausal osteoporosis lasts from 3 to 6 years and appears to be self-limited. This process primarily affects trabecular bone, where the rate of loss is three times normal. Because of their greater proportion of trabecular bone, vertebrae may lose 5% of their mass per year.[100] Therefore, women with this syndrome often present with an acute vertebral crush fracture in contrast to the asymptomatic wedge fractures that occur in senile osteoporosis. Distal radius fractures are also common.

The biochemical abnormalities underlying postmenopausal osteoporosis are complex. One established factor is that estrogen withdrawal increases osteoclastic activity, and, therefore, bone turnover is increased. Estrogen normally inhibits osteoclastic activity indirectly by inhibiting interleukins, cytokines known to be potent osteoclast activators. For example, estrogen inhibits the production of interleukin-1 by peripheral blood monocytes.[101] Also, after estrogen withdrawal, interleukin-1 enhances the production of interleukin-6, a powerful osteoclast stimulator. Experimental observation confirms that estrogen withdrawal stimulates osteoclasts. For example, in a mouse model, oophorectomy increases in-terleukin-6 activity. Moreover, in this model, antibodies against interleukin-6 prevent any bone loss.[102]

The rapidity of bone loss in postmenopausal osteoporosis is due to the high bone turnover. The decreased increment of bone formed in the remodeling cycle, a feature of senile osteoporosis, is exaggerated by the high turnover. For this reason, postmenopausal osteoporosis is also known as *high-turnover osteoporosis*.

Clinical and Radiographic Features

The usual patient is a tall, thin, fair-haired white woman of Northern European descent. She is likely to have lax ligaments. Small Asian women are also prone to develop osteoporosis (Table 4–3). By contrast, osteoporosis is uncommon in African-Americans and in obese people of any ethnic group. Obesity protects against osteoporosis for two reasons. Increased weight stresses the bones, a factor that helps maintain balanced remodeling. More importantly, obese women have higher levels of protective serum free-estrogen. Free-estrogen results from the peripheral conversion of adrenal androgens to estrogen, a conversion that occurs in adipose tissue.[103]

In patients with primary osteoporosis, bone loss is insidious and asymptomatic until fractures occur. Vertebral fractures beginning in the sixth decade are the most common clinical manifestation. They may be painful or asymptomatic. A typical clinical feature of patients with long-standing osteoporosis is dorsal kyphosis, the so-called "dowager's hump." This kyphosis, a result of successive anterior vertebral wedging, leads to a loss of as much as a foot of the patient's original height (Fig. 4–22).

In the early phases of primary osteoporosis, changes are not apparent with plain radiographs; a 30% loss of bone mass is required before osteoporosis is apparent.[104] By this time, bones have lost 50% of their strength. In the advanced stages of osteoporosis, bones are diffusely osteopenic. Changes are most evident in the spine (Fig. 4–23). Preferen-

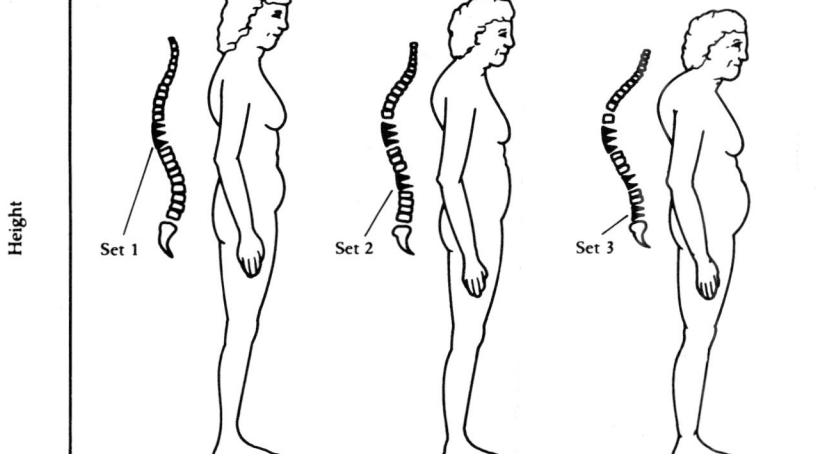

Figure 4–22 ■ Changes following menopause. Successive vertebral wedge fractures cause a dorsal kyphosis and a loss in height. (From Urist, M. R.: Orthopaedic management of osteoporosis in postmenopausal women. *Clin Endocrinol Metab* 2:159–176, 1973.)

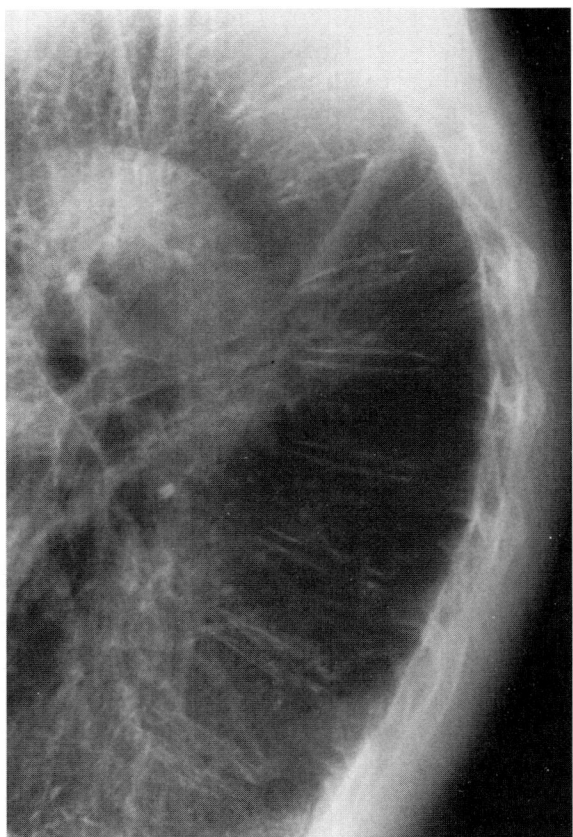

Figure 4-23 ■ Severe osteoporosis showing dorsal wedging of most vertebrae and mild kyphosis.

tial loss of horizontal trabeculae makes vertical trabeculae more prominent, but sometimes the vertebral bodies appear empty. In addition, a cod fish appearance is often present as the result of collapsed endplates and bulging of the disc into the vertebral body. In the appendicular skeleton, the cortices are markedly thin, and the trabecular pattern is lost. In the femoral neck, the pattern of trabecular bone loss may be used to assess the severity of the osteoporosis.[105]

Histopathology

With routine histopathologic techniques, only a diminished quantity of bone is present. Trabeculae are thin and disconnected, a feature manifested by "free-floating trabeculae" in histologic sections (see Fig. 4–24 on color plate). In some cases, trabecular plates are replaced by thin rods.[106] Cortices are also thin, especially the subchondral cortex adjacent to large joints. In addition, cortical porosity is increased by enlargement of haversian canals and by endosteal erosion.

Architectural changes are an important pathologic feature of osteoporosis. These changes are most prominent in the vertebral bodies, where the number of horizontal trabeculae is markedly diminished. Normally, the horizontal trabeculae are cross-bracing struts that support the load-bearing vertical trabeculae. In osteoporosis, unsupported vertical trabeculae result in a high prevalence of microfractures within the vertebral body. Typically, 200 to 450 healing or healed trabecular microfractures can be identified in autopsy specimens of osteoporotic women.[107] If the rate of trabecular microfracture exceeds the reparative remodeling process, vertebral collapse occurs.

Histomorphometric analysis of undecalcified bone of osteoporotic patients has demonstrated low-, normal-, and high-turnover states.[108] The increased osteoclastic and osteoblastic activity of high-turnover osteoporosis is rarely recognizable with routine histologic examination. Therefore, histomorphometric studies, which accurately quantify the rate of turnover, may be important in planning therapy and monitoring the results. In addition, histomorphometric studies may demonstrate a component of osteomalacia, a condition very responsive to treatment.

Secondary Osteoporosis

Although most cases of osteoporosis are caused by age-related factors, some are caused by identifiable exogenous or endogenous agents (Table 4–4). These agents may cause premature skeletal failure or they may exacerbate the normal rate of bone loss, a condition known as *secondary osteoporosis*. Identification and treatment of the causes of secondary osteoporosis may arrest or even reverse bone loss. Many causes of secondary osteoporosis exist. Some causes, such as neoplastic infiltration of bone or genetic disorders, are discussed in other parts of this book. The three most common causes are discussed in this chapter: glucocorticoid excess, secondary amenorrhea, and diabetes. In addition, two risk factors are discussed. These risk factors, smoking and alcohol abuse, while not direct causes of osteoporosis, contribute to its development.

Glucocorticoid Excess

Glucocorticoid excess is the most common cause of secondary osteoporosis. Excess endogenous glucocorticoids are occasionally the result of adrenal hyperplasia or neoplasia. More commonly, excess glucocorticoids are caused by steroid therapy. For example, patients receiving large doses of steroids for diseases such as lupus erythematosus, chronic lung disease, or multiple sclerosis or for post-transplant immunosuppression commonly develop secondary osteoporosis. As many as 50% of these patients experience bone loss.[109] In addition, 30 to 35% of patients on long-term steroids experience vertebral crush fractures, and the risk of hip fracture is increased by 50%.[110] In an individual patient,

Table 4-4 ■ CAUSES OF SECONDARY OSTEOPOROSIS

Steroid excess (endogenous or iatrogenic)
Diabetes
Hypogonadism
Hyperparathyroidism
Hyperthyroidism

bone loss, which is most pronounced in the first 6 months of therapy, may be as high as 40%. Even low doses of steroids cause osteoporosis. Regimens as low as 8 to 10 mg of prednisone per day have been shown by DEXA to cause spinal bone loss. Although the degree of bone loss is proportional to the cumulative dose, the effect of steroids on the skeleton is almost immediate. An acute administration of 10 mg of prednisone suppresses osteocalcin levels, an index of osteoblast activity, by as much as 80%.[111]

The major impairment in bone physiology caused by glucocorticoids is suppression of osteoblast activity. Most probably, a block in cell-to-cell signaling inhibits osteoblast differentiation. The diminished productivity of osteoblasts is probably caused by a decrease in their longevity.[112]

Histomorphometric data support the hypothesis of depressed osteoblast function.[113, 114] First, the dynamic data show depressed indices of bone formation, particularly a low mineral apposition rate. Also, the number of osteoid seams is reduced. Second, trabecular thickness is markedly decreased. However, unlike the disconnected trabeculae seen in senile osteoporosis, trabeculae remain connected in corticosteroid-induced osteoporosis.[115] Trabecular attenuation without disruption supports the hypothesis that depressed bone formation, rather than increased resorption, reduces bone mass. Third, the trabecular volume is markedly reduced because of the thinness of trabeculae. Because the cortex is less affected in this syndrome, bone loss is most prominent in areas with a high proportion of trabecular bone, particularly the spine.

Glucocorticoids may also enhance resorption, although to a lesser degree than they suppress osteoblasts. Glucocorticoids reduce the efficiency of calcium absorption by a direct effect on intestinal mucosa and also by modulation of $1,25(OH)_2$ vitamin D receptors.[116, 117] As a result, increased parathyroid hormone secretion, responding to low calcium, enhances bone resorption.

Treating corticosteroid-induced osteoporosis is problematic because the steroids usually cannot be discontinued. However, a shift to alternating-day regimens may be beneficial.[118] In addition, calcium and vitamin D supplementation may minimize the steroid effect on bone.

Secondary Amenorrhea

Secondary amenorrhea, another cause of secondary osteoporosis, is a common syndrome in the United States in young women with anorexia nervosa and in young female athletes. Unfortunately, many of these women develop complications of osteoporosis while they are young. Moreover, they fail to develop peak bone mass and are therefore at great risk of developing severe senile and postmenopausal osteoporosis.

Anorexia nervosa, a psychiatric condition affecting 0.4% of female adolescents, is characterized by self-imposed starvation. Girls with this disorder have a 20 to 25% reduction in mean lumbar spine density,[119] and some even sustain compression fractures.[120] Significant bone loss occurs rapidly in these patients; sometimes within 1.5 years from the onset of the eating disorder. Two factors contribute to the development of osteoporosis. First, girls with this syndrome are malnourished and calcium deficient. Second, and more important, girls with anorexia nervosa are estrogen deficient, and usually they are amenorrheic.[121] Estrogen therapy, weight gain, and exercise have all been shown to restore some, but not all, bone mass.

Young female athletes also suffer from osteoporosis, as evidenced by a significant decrease in lumbar spine density in many of these women.[122, 123] As in anorexia nervosa, two factors contribute to osteoporosis in young female athletes. First, young female athletes tend to be malnourished because being thin is usually important to athletic performance. Second, as many as 50% of high-performance female athletes, particularly endurance runners, are amenorrheic. The incidence of osteoporosis in these athletes indicates that the ill effects of estrogen deprivation and malnutrition outweigh the beneficial effects of increased physical activity. Malnutrition is a particularly important factor because even high-performance male distance runners develop a high-turnover loss of bone mass.[124]

Diabetes

Insulin-dependent diabetes is also associated with osteoporosis.[125] However, the cause of reduced bone mass in diabetics is unclear. Insulin deficiency may be associated with deficient osteoid synthesis, and some patients may metabolize vitamin D abnormally. In addition, hypercalciuria is common in diabetes. However, serum parathyroid hormone and vitamin D levels are usually normal in these patients. The bone loss in diabetics is usually cortical and is often detectable as early as 2 to 3 years after the onset of clinical disease. Although osteoporosis complicates some cases of diabetes, the incidence of fractures is not increased.[126]

Smoking and Alcohol Abuse

Although not regarded as direct causes of osteoporosis, two behaviors, smoking and alcohol abuse, have a deleterious effect on the skeleton. Although people often engage in both of these bad habits simultaneously, each habit probably has independent (and additive) effects on bone. Heavy alcohol intake has been associated with reduced bone mass,[127, 128] but the reduction in bone mass is probably multifactorial. First, poor eating habits of alcoholics lead to malnutrition. Second, calcium and vitamin D absorption is diminished in alcoholics, a problem likely due to liver or pancreatic disease. Third, in addition to these indirect factors, alcohol appears to have a direct toxic effect on osteoblasts.

Heavy smoking also enhances bone loss. Female smokers have been shown to have a lower bone mass[129] and higher rates of vertebral fractures[130] than nonsmokers. The mechanism of this effect is not clear. One possibility is that smoking alters the metabolism of estrogen and reduces its biologic effectiveness.[131] However, the bones of men are also adversely affected by cigarette smoke.

Osteoporosis in Men

Although osteoporosis primarily affects women, men also suffer from this disorder.[132] Although they do not experience the same accelerated phase of bone loss due to estrogen withdrawal, men lose about 3 to 4% of their bone mass per decade after age 40. As a result, 30% of all hip fractures occur in men. Men also suffer vertebral fractures but at a rate of one half that of women.[133]

Factors causing bone loss in men are the same as those that cause senile osteoporosis in women. These include a negative calcium balance, a lack of exercise, and a reduction in osteoblast function. Also, similar to women, men suffer from secondary osteoporosis, particularly that caused by corticosteroids.

In addition to age-related and corticosteroid-induced bone loss, two additional osteoporotic syndromes occur in men: osteoporosis due to hypogonadism and idiopathic osteoporosis. About 30% of osteoporosis in men is due to long-standing testosterone deficiency.[134] This syndrome most commonly presents when men are in their 50s, and they usually have a long history of hypogonadal symptoms, such as decreased libido. Causes of hypogonadism in these men include castration, previous testicular inflammation, hyperprolactinemia, and pituitary dysfunction. This osteoporotic syndrome in men is readily diagnosed by low levels of serum testosterone. Histomorphometric studies suggest that osteoporosis in hypogonadal men is a high-turnover bone loss, similar to that seen in estrogen withdrawal in women.[134] Although hypogonadism leads to osteoporosis, a report of a 28-year-old man with osteoporosis due to an estrogen receptor mutation suggests that the effect of androgens is indirect.[135]

The second syndrome, *idiopathic osteoporosis,* is a premature or exaggerated involutional bone loss that occurs without an identifiable metabolic or genetic cause. This syndrome, which occurs almost exclusively in men, accounts for at least 30 to 40% of all cases of osteoporosis in men. Affected patients usually present between ages 20 and 50 with a vertebral fracture. By contrast, men with senile osteoporosis usually do not present until after age 70. Idiopathic osteoporosis shares some clinical and radiographic features with mild (type 1) osteogenesis imperfecta. Also, similar to type I osteogenesis imperfecta, histomorphometric studies show low bone turnover, a finding suggestive of depressed osteoblast function.[136] However, these diseases may be distinguished because men with idiopathic osteoporosis lack blue sclerae and a family history of fragile bones.

Juvenile Osteoporosis

Osteoporosis can also occur in children, but in most cases, an underlying cause is identifiable. These causes include rickets, glucocorticoid therapy, or an infiltrative neoplasm. In addition, genetic disorders, particularly osteogenesis imperfecta, cause osteoporosis in children. However, a few children develop osteoporosis with no identifiable metabolic or genetic abnormalities. This rare syndrome, known as *idiopathic juvenile osteoporosis,* affects children between ages 4 and 16.[137] The remarkable feature of idiopathic juvenile osteoporosis is its reversibility. Usually, children spontaneously regain bone mass after 1 to 4 years of illness.

The clinical features of idiopathic juvenile osteoporosis are characteristic. Typically, a previously healthy child, about 10 years old, presents with the insidious onset of pain in the back and legs. Physical examination is normal except for bone tenderness. More severely affected children may have a mild kyphosis or a pigeon chest deformity. All serum biochemical parameters are normal. Radiographic study demonstrates severe osteopenia and lower extremity metaphyseal impaction fractures. The distal tibia is particularly susceptible. In the spine, the vertebrae may be collapsed or wedged.

The cause of idiopathic juvenile osteoporosis is unknown. The reversibility of this syndrome and histomorphometric studies, which show increased bone resorption, suggest a similarity to disuse atrophy of bone.[138] This similarity suggests that idiopathic juvenile osteoporosis is caused by a temporary dissociation between mechanical forces and bone formation.

Supportive care is the most important therapy for juvenile osteoporosis. However, additional therapy, which includes sodium fluoride[139] and etidronate,[140] may hasten the return of bone mass.

Management

The management of osteoporosis presents numerous problems because, in most women, the disease is silent until fractures occur. By this time, the disease is advanced and restoration of bone mass is difficult, although some degree of bone density, as measured by photon absorptiometry, can be restored. Two factors at this late stage inhibit the therapeutic response. First, osseous architectural changes, particularly the loss of trabeculae, limit the amount of bone that can be restored. This is because bone volume can be increased only by adding osteoid to existing trabeculae, and once trabeculae are completely resorbed, templates for new bone deposition are permanently lost. The second factor limiting restoration of bone mass is physical inactivity, a result of painful fractures. Patients who have suffered osteoporotic fractures require immobilization and sometimes long periods of bed rest, further enhancing the tendency to lose bone.

Because advanced bone loss responds poorly to treatment, prevention of osteoporosis is the most important aspect of management. Prevention begins in childhood. Good nutrition, including adequate calcium and vitamin D intake, is necessary to reach the highest peak bone mass possible.

Therefore, parental awareness and public health policies are crucial. In addition, exercise programs for children and young adults are also important in attaining peak bone mass.

Throughout adulthood and into old age, adequate nutrition and physical activity are the mainstays in the prevention of osteoporosis. Adults need 800 IU of vitamin D and 1.2 g of elemental calcium per day. Exercise should be performed regularly and properly. Fast walking is effective and is the safest exercise. Impact exercises, such as aerobics, are the most effective.[141] Also, training with light weights maintains excellent muscle tone.

Screening with bone densitometry studies is another important aspect of osteoporosis prevention. Although screening all postmenopausal women is impractical, people at risk should be studied in the immediate postmenopausal period. These include fair-haired white women, women with a family history of osteoporosis, and men and women with risk factors, particularly glucocorticoid therapy. The DEXA scan can identify those who are "fast losers" of bone mass and who need drug therapy.

Currently, many drugs are available to arrest bone loss and restore some bone.[142] They may be divided into antiresorptive agents and formation-stimulating agents. Antiresorptive agents include estrogen, calcitonin, and the bisphosphonates. Theoretically, these drugs limit the amount of bone resorbed while not reducing the amount formed. In this way, they may increase bone mass. Of the antiresorptive agents, estrogen therapy is the mainstay in the prevention of osteoporosis[143] and has also been shown to even increase bone density.[144] For patients unable or unwilling to take estrogen, calcitonin has been recommended. Calcitonin decreases osteoclastic activity, and, in daily intranasal doses, can increase lumbar spine density.[145] Calcitriol (1,25[OH]$_2$ vitamin D) is another effective therapeutic agent. When used in addition to calcium supplementation, the incidence of fractures in women with established postmenopausal osteoporosis decreases, although the decrease is evident only after 3 years of therapy.[146] These drugs raise serum calcium levels which reduces parathyroid hormone secretion.

Recently, the bisphosphonates have been used to treat osteoporosis. These drugs are potent osteoclast inhibitors; therefore, they reduce bone resorption.[147] The bisphosphonates, analogs of pyrophosphate, adsorb to the surface of the hydroxyapatite crystal and render it less soluble. They also directly inhibit osteoclasts. Etidronate, a first-generation bisphosphonate, has been shown to stimulate significant vertebral bone formation.[148] Currently, alendronate (Fosamax), a third-generation bisphosphonate, is being used.

Of the bone-stimulating therapeutic agents, only sodium fluoride has shown promise. In some geographic areas, sodium fluoride has been added to drinking water to reduce dental caries. In these geographic areas, the incidence of hip fractures is lower,[149] an observation that suggested that sodium fluoride might be useful in the treatment of osteoporosis. Fluoride stimulates osteoblasts and has been shown to increase spinal and femoral condyle bone mass.[150]

Table 4–5 ■ **EVALUATION OF THE PATIENT WHO EASILY FRACTURES**

History to rule out
    Family history of fractures or blue sclerae
    Poor dietary habits
    Previous steroid therapy
    Previous gastrointestinal therapy
    Smoking and alcohol abuse
    History of bed rest
Laboratory studies
    Routine blood count
    Electrolytes
    Calcium, phosphorus, albumin
    Alkaline phosphatase, liver enzymes
    Serum 25(OH) vitamin D and 1,25(OH)$_2$ vitamin D
    Parathyroid hormone levels
    Indices of bone turnover
        Osteocalcin
        Tartrate-resistant acid phosphatase
        Urine hydroxyproline and pyridinium cross-links
Radiologic studies
    DEXA
    Quantitative computerized tomography
    Bone scan to rule out focal lesions

EVALUATING PATIENTS WHOSE BONES FRACTURE EASILY

Patients who suffer fractures with little or no trauma should be evaluated for metabolic bone disease, especially if the patient is age 50 or younger. First, if osteopenia is not apparent on plain radiographs, both young and old patients should have densitometry studies to establish if bone loss is present. If osteopenia is present, patients should be carefully evaluated with protocols (Table 4–5) to rule out specific causes of osteopenia, most of which are treatable (Table 4–6). Elderly patients should be similarly evaluated before assuming that their bones are weak because of old age.

The first step in evaluating a patient who fractures easily is to exclude a neoplastic or hereditary disorder. Multiple myeloma, the most common infiltrating disorder that causes osteopenia, can be excluded by a negative serum protein electrophoresis and a negative immune fixation electrophoresis. Leukemia may be excluded by a blood count. The principal hereditary disorder to be ruled out is undiagnosed type 1 (mild) osteogenesis imperfecta. Because all patients with type 1 osteogenesis imperfecta have blue sclerae and

Table 4–6 ■ **CAUSES OF OSTEOPENIA IN ADULTS**

Infiltrative (neoplastic) disorders
    Multiple myeloma
    Leukemia
    Metastatic carcinoma
Hereditary diseases
    Osteogenesis imperfecta, type I
Secondary osteoporosis (see Table 4–4)
    Endocrine disorders
    Osteomalacia
Primary osteoporosis

many have a family history of easy fracturability, this disease can usually be excluded.

After ruling out a neoplastic or hereditary disorder, the syndromes of secondary osteoporosis should be excluded (see Table 4–4). These include specific endocrine abnormalities such as hyperparathyroidism and osteomalacia. Only when these disorders are excluded can a diagnosis of idiopathic or senile osteoporosis be made.

LOCALIZED OSTEOPOROSIS

Unlike the generalized osteopenia that occurs in metabolic bone diseases, osteoporosis can occur in only part of the skeleton or even in only one bone. This pattern of bone loss, known as localized osteoporosis, is caused by local vascular, neurogenic, or mechanical disturbances rather than systemic conditions. There are three well-defined syndromes of localized osteoporosis: disuse atrophy, transient osteoporosis, and reflex sympathetic dystrophy.

Disuse Atrophy

Immobilization or non–weight bearing causes rapid bone loss, a condition known as *disuse atrophy*. The localized osteoporosis occurs in the bones that are not used, whether it be the bones of one limb or the entire skeleton. Disuse atrophy of bone affects people of any age or state of health.

Localized manifestations of this disorder accompany many forms of disuse. For example, non–weight bearing crutch walking or cast immobilization results in atrophy of the bones not stressed (Fig. 4–25). Particularly at risk are those patients with neuromuscular disorders or with paralysis following spinal cord injury. These patients lose as much as one third of their bone mass in 6 months. Thereafter, bone loss diminishes.[151] If immobilization is required after a fracture, disuse atrophy is often severe, and the pattern of bone loss may be mistaken for a malignant neoplasm. For example, patients with humeral fractures may develop diffuse disuse atrophy throughout the entire length of the humerus, a response evident from 7 months to 2 years after injury.[152] Following fractures, reflex hyperemia and neural injury, in addition to immobilization, may be contributing factors to bone loss.

In addition to affecting isolated bones, disuse atrophy can involve the entire skeleton. Long-term bed rest, required in a severe illness or in the treatment of a prolapsed intervertebral disc, leads to generalized osteoporosis. Even in young patients, bone loss during bed rest begins early and occurs at a rate of 0.9% per week.[153] After only 1 week, hypercalciuria, which is evidence of bone resorption, is evident. Hypercalcemia, by contrast, is extremely rare in immobilization osteopenia. It does occur, however, in patients with Paget's disease or hyperparathyroidism who require bed rest. In these patients, the hypercalcemia may be severe and even life threatening.

The pathogenesis of disuse atrophy is unclear. Mechanical forces on the skeleton are necessary for the homeostasis of bone. These mechanical forces deform bone and elicit streaming potentials and piezoelectric currents. Presumably, lack of this electrical activity in nonstressed bones causes the characteristic pathologic feature of disuse atrophy: increased osteoclastic activity. In addition, lack of bone deformation uncouples the remodeling process. As a result, osteoblasts fail to synthesize enough bone equal to the amount resorbed.

The pathologic features of disuse atrophy reflect this imbalance. A marked increase in osteoclastic activity results in numerous resorption cavities in both cortical and cancellous

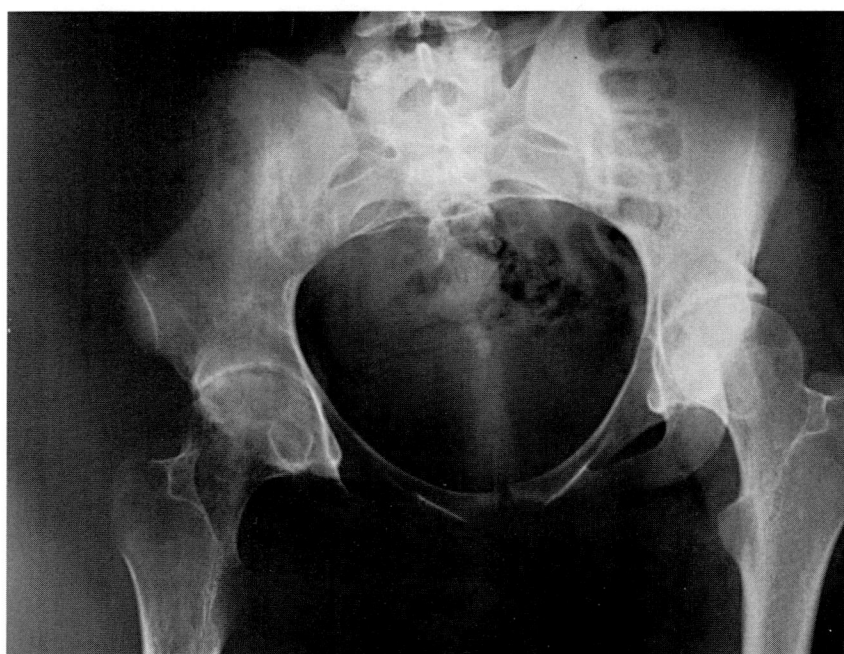

Figure 4-25 ■ Radiograph showing disuse atrophy of the right hemipelvis and the right proximal femur. This woman was non–weight bearing because of acute chondrolysis of her femoral head.

METABOLIC BONE DISEASES   97

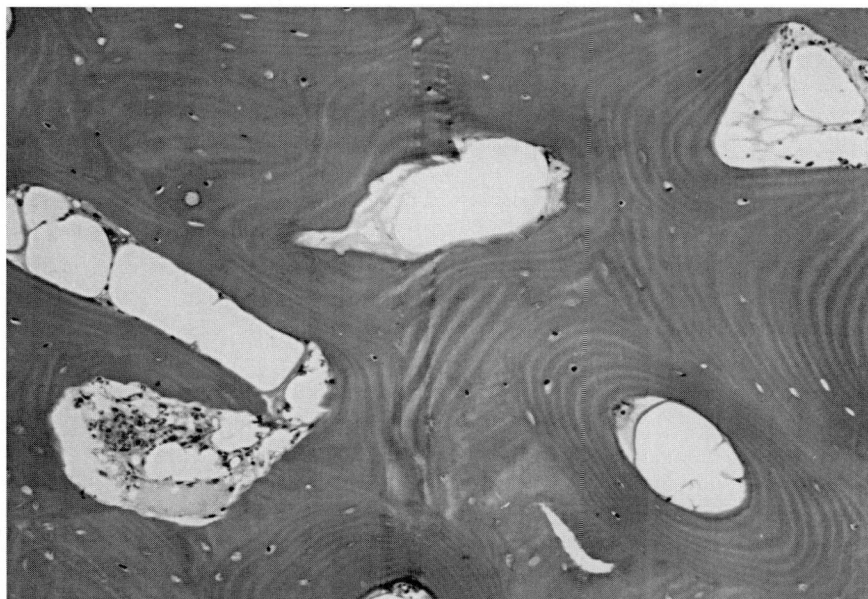

Figure 4-26 ■ Photomicrograph of cortex showing changes of disuse atrophy. The haversian canals are dilated.

bone (Fig. 4–26). Cortical bone is more severely affected. Characteristically, haversian canals in cortical bone are enlarged to 20 or 30 times their normal diameter.

Radiographically, "moth-eaten" radiolucencies are present diffusely and symmetrically in the immobilized bone. A characteristic feature of severe disuse atrophy is linear intracortical lucencies, a pattern that corresponds to the enlarged haversian canals seen histologically (Fig. 4–27). Endosteal cortical scalloping may also be present, but otherwise the cortex is intact.

Severe generalized disuse atrophy may simulate a malignant neoplasm, just as the localized form of this process can.[154] For example, disuse atrophy may be misdiagnosed as multiple myeloma or metastatic carcinoma. Several features of both local or generalized disuse atrophy help distinguish these processes from a malignant neoplasm. First, the history of immobilization or trauma should alert clinicians to the likelihood of disuse atrophy. Second, disuse atrophy tends to involve the bone uniformly. A malignant neoplasm, by contrast, usually has a central area of greater bone destruction. Third, the linear intracortical lucencies, a characteristic feature of disuse atrophy, are very rare in malignant neoplasms.

Fortunately, both localized and generalized disuse osteoporosis is reversible. Resumption of activity results in total restoration of bone mass, usually within 4 months.

Transient Osteoporosis

Transient osteoporosis is another syndrome of localized osteoporosis. But, unlike disuse atrophy, this syndrome is not associated with disuse or immobilization. The cause is unknown, although bone loss is probably initiated by marrow edema and possibly transient ischemia. Transient osteoporosis usually affects the hip, although the knee is another commonly involved site.[155] Patients with transient osteoporosis of the hip are usually men between the ages of 27 and 61 or women in the third trimester of pregnancy. Some patients have a history of trauma. They present with acute

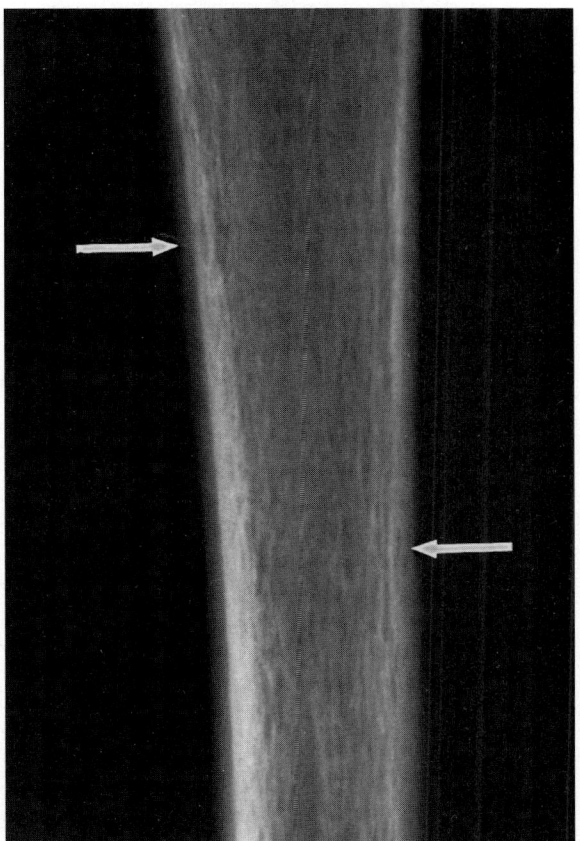

Figure 4-27 ■ Radiograph of a tibia showing disuse osteoporosis. A permeative pattern of radiolucency can be seen. Intracortical, linear lucencies are also present (arrows).

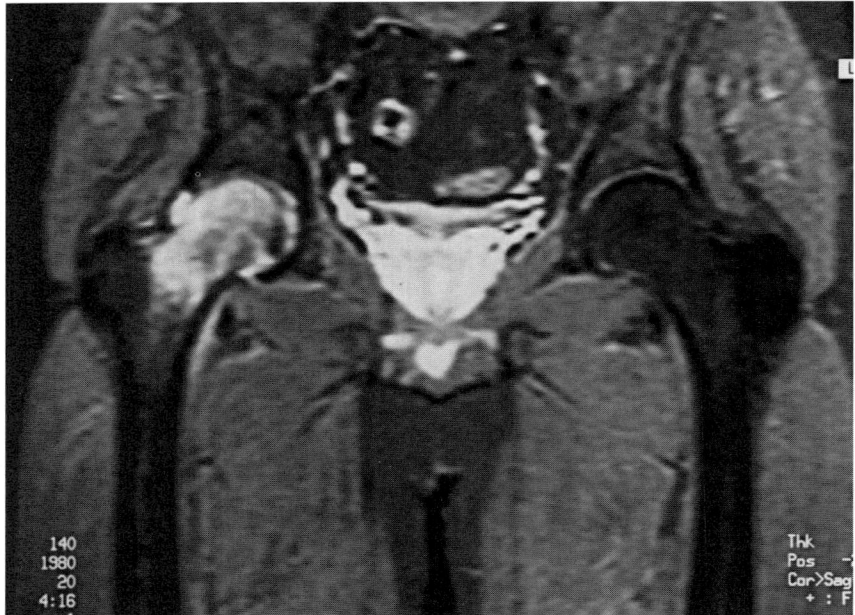

Figure 4-28 ■ T_2-weighted MRI of transient osteoporosis of the hip. The femoral head and femoral neck show increased signal secondary to bone marrow edema. (From McCarthy, E. F.: *Differential Diagnosis in Pathology. Bone and Joint Disorders.* New York and Tokyo, Igaku-Shoin, 1996. With permission from Williams & Wilkins.)

hip pain, a limp, and limitation of motion. Symptoms worsen for a few months and then begin to improve. Complete clinical resolution occurs in 4 to 11 months (mean, 6 months). Symptoms resolve in pregnant women after delivery. As many as 41% of patients have a recurrence in the same hip or in other sites, a syndrome known as *regional migratory osteoporosis.*

Plain radiographs in the early phases of this syndrome are unremarkable. However, magnetic resonance imaging (MRI) shows changes very early. T_1-weighted images show low signal intensity, and T_2-weighted images show high signal intensity, indicating bone marrow edema (Fig. 4–28). These changes involve the entire femoral head and often extend into the intertrochanteric region. Later in the evolution of this disease, the femoral head and intertrochanteric area show diffuse, ill-defined osteoporosis (Fig. 4–29).

Histologically, transient osteoporosis is characterized by bone marrow edema. The edema appears as an amorphous, faintly eosinophilic material between marrow fat cells (Fig. 4–30). Dilated, congested small vascular spaces are also

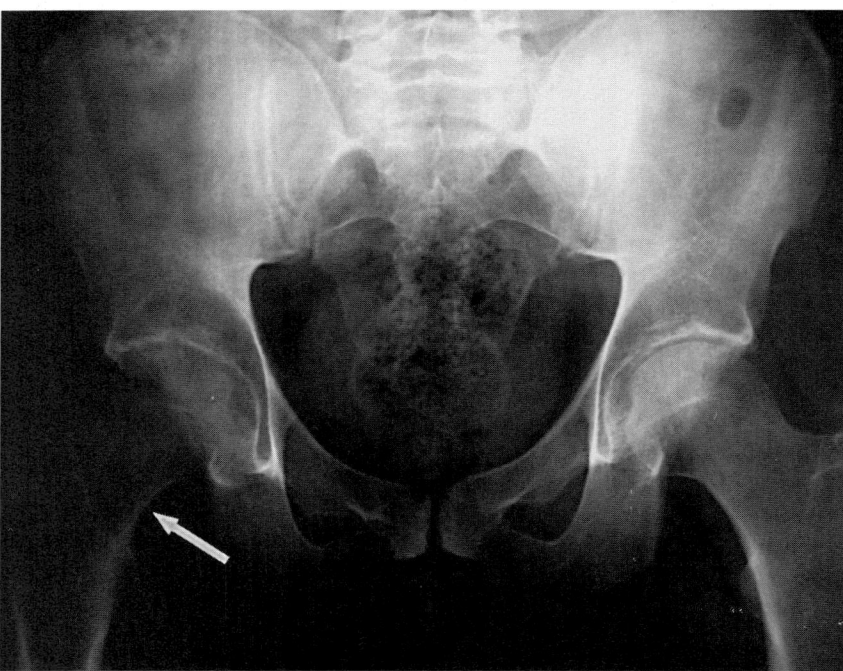

Figure 4-29 ■ Transient osteoporosis of the hip. The femoral head and neck show marked osteopenia *(arrows).*

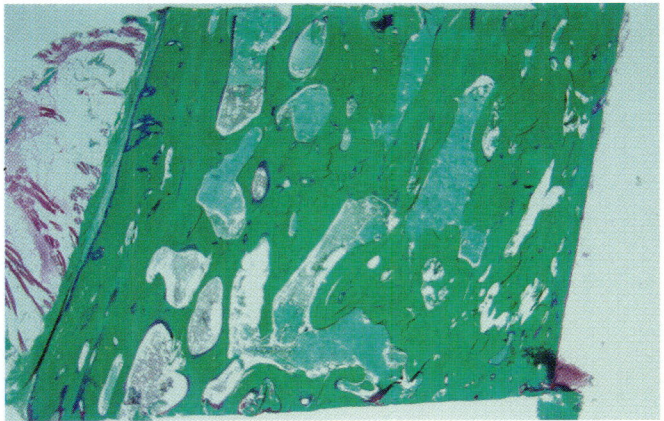

Figure 4-6 ■ Photomicrograph of an undecalcified iliac crest biopsy from a patient with X-linked hypophosphatemic rickets. Marked sclerosis is present (trichrome stain).

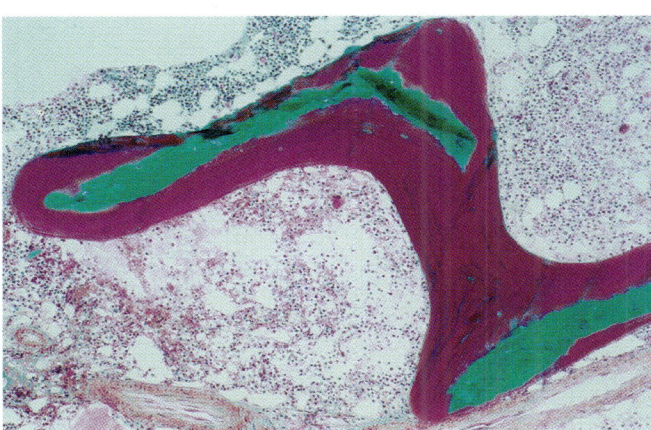

Figure 4-9 ■ Photomicrograph of an undecalcified bone biopsy stained with trichrome stain showing severe osteomalacia. Green bone is encased by very broad sheets of red osteoid.

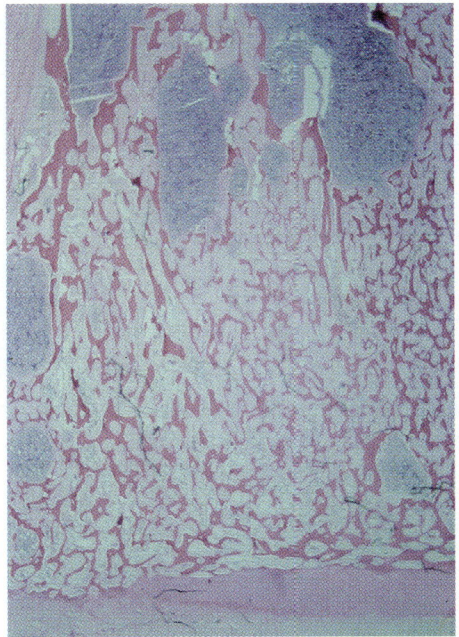

Figure 4-12 ■ Photomicrograph of tissue from a vertebral body. Extensive bone deposition is present beneath the endplate. This corresponds to the radiodense zone of the "rugger jersey" pattern seen on plain radiographs.

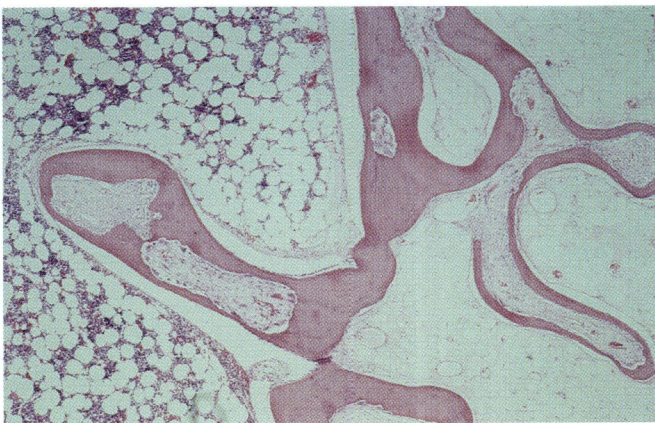

Figure 4-15 ■ Photomicrograph of cancellous bone with multiple sites of tunneling resorption.

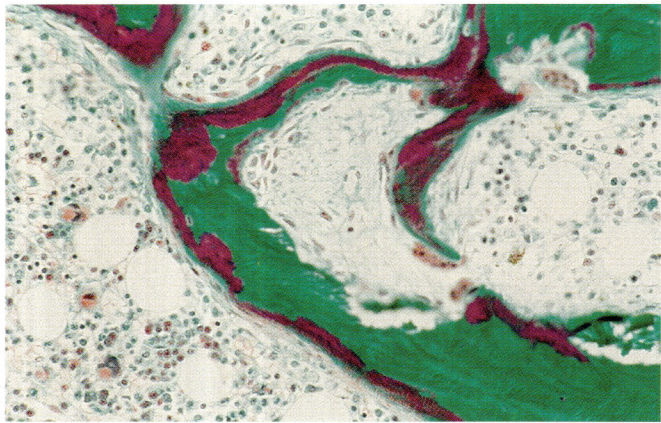

Figure 4-16 ■ Photomicrograph of specimen showing renal osteodystrophy. Extensive osteoclastic resorption and osteoid deposition are present. (Undecalcified section with a trichrome stain.)

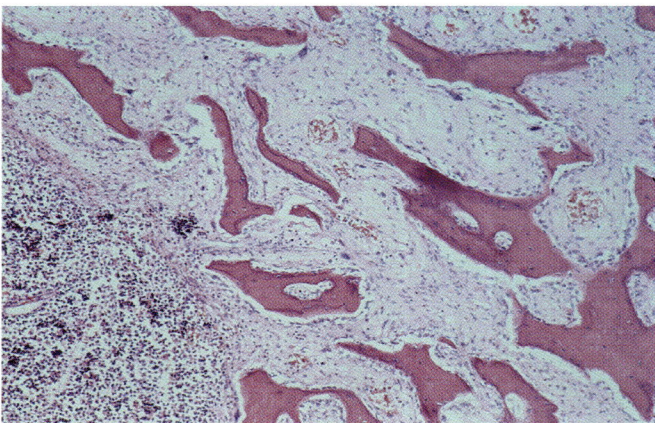

Figure 4-17 ■ Photomicrograph of a specimen with osteitis fibrosa. Woven bone and lamellar bone are present in the fibrous tissue background. This change is responsible for the osteosclerosis of renal osteodystrophy.

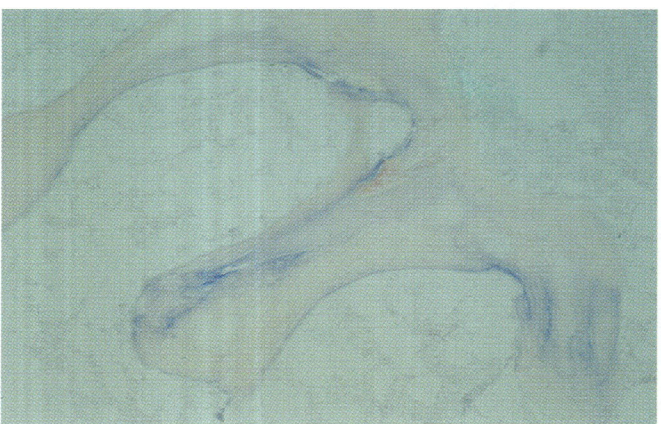

Figure 4-20 ■ Undecalcified bone biopsy sample stained for aluminum (acid solochrome azurine). Aluminum stains with blue.

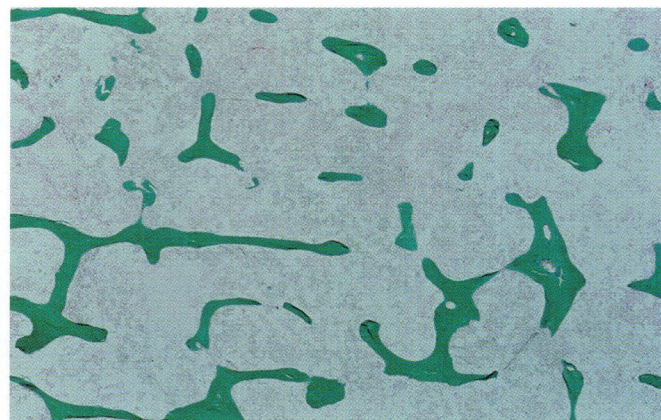

Figure 4-24 ■ Photomicrograph of severe osteoporosis with disconnected trabeculae. (Undecalcified section with trichrome stain.)

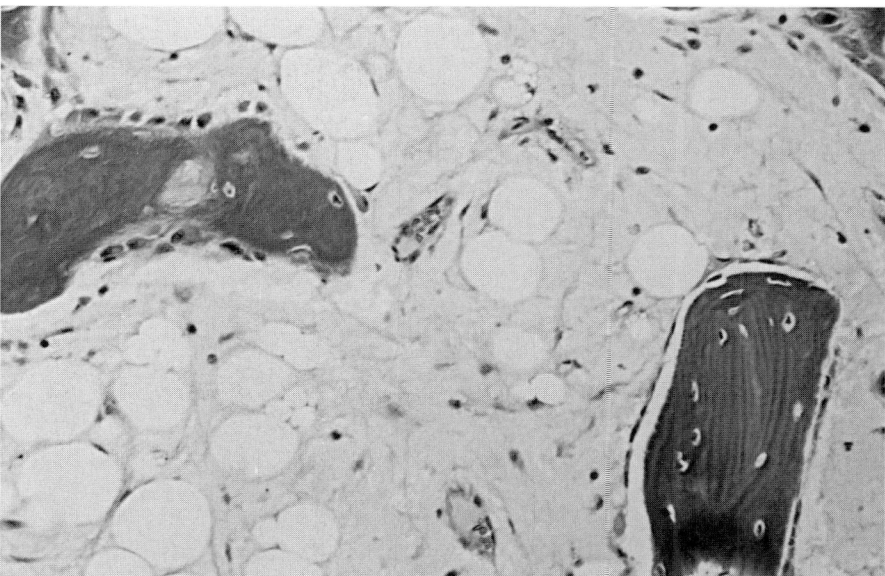

Figure 4-30 ■ Photomicrograph of a biopsy specimen from transient osteoporosis of a hip. Edema is present in the fatty marrow, as evidenced by amorphous material between fat cells. New, reactive bone is deposited in this zone.

present. Trabecular bone shows many resorption cavities, which in severe cases remove entire trabeculae. Seams of new woven bone are also present.

The treatment of transient osteoporosis is pain management and protection of the osteopenic bone. Lesions resolve spontaneously, although recurrence is possible. Some surgeons treat this disease with a decompression core biopsy.

Transient osteoporosis of the hip is often confused clinically with osteonecrosis.[156] However, in osteonecrosis, MRI demonstrates a discrete zone of signal change rather than a diffuse zone characteristic of transient osteoporosis. In addition, the bone shows histologic features of necrosis. Also, unlike transient osteoporosis, osteonecrosis does not resolve spontaneously. Despite these differences, transient osteoporosis of the hip may, after all, be a precursor process to osteonecrosis of the femoral head. If this hypothesis is correct, then only a rare severe case of transient osteoporosis progresses to osteonecrosis.

Reflex Sympathetic Dystrophy

Reflex sympathetic dystrophy, also known as *Sudeck's atrophy,* is regional osteoporosis in an extremity caused by an exaggerated vasomotor response to pain or injury. A resulting hyperemia leads to rapid bone resorption and painful soft tissue swelling. Most commonly, a hand or foot is involved, although the process occasionally affects an entire extremity. The knee is also a common site. This disorder occurs, although in varying degrees of severity, in as many as 5% of patients with limb trauma. Some studies report an incidence of 20% following Colles' fracture. Other initiating conditions are joint injuries, limb surgery, and spinal degenerative disease. Reflex sympathetic dystrophy may also involve the arm following myocardial infarction, a condition known as the *shoulder-hand syndrome.* Reflex sympathetic dystrophy is almost always bilateral, but one extremity is usually affected much more severely.

The clinical features of reflex sympathetic dystrophy are known as *causalgia.* Typically, a man or woman over age 50 develops this syndrome after trauma to a limb. A few

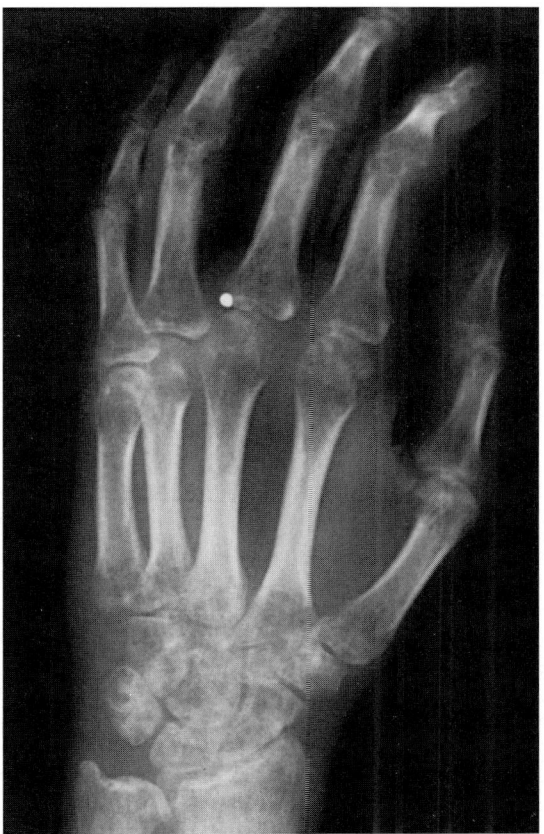

Figure 4-31 ■ Reflex sympathetic dystrophy. Diffuse symmetric, periarticular radiolysis is present around all the joints in the hand.

days to a few weeks after the injury, the hand or foot begins to swell, and intense burning pain and hyperesthesia occur. These symptoms usually continue for several months, during which time the involved area becomes stiff with flexion deformities. Also, atrophy of skin and muscle occur. In the late stages, from 6 months to 1 year after the onset, the skin is shiny and smooth, and pigmentary changes, hyperhidrosis, and hypertrichosis may be present.

Radiologically, all the bones in the affected portion of the extremity show patchy demineralization. The demineralization is ill defined and is most pronounced in the periarticular regions, particularly in the metaphysis (Fig. 4–31). Intracortical linear lucencies and endosteal scalloping are also characteristic. Bone scans show increased radionuclide uptake in the periarticular regions, a change that usually precedes any plain radiographic abnormalities.

Histologically, the bones show evidence of increased osteoclastic resorption and increased vascularity.[157] In addition, the synovial membranes from joints adjacent to involved bones show capillary dilation and proliferation, fibrosis, and foci of chronic inflammation.[158]

REFERENCES

1. Silverberg, S. J., Fitzpatrick, L. A., and Bilezikian, J. P.: Primary hyperparathyroidism. Becker, K. L., Ed. *Principles and Practice of Endocrinology and Metabolism*. Philadelphia, J. B. Lippincott, 1995, pp. 512–519.
2. Bilezikian, J. P., Silverberg, S. J., Gartenberg, F., Kim, T.-S., Jacobs, T. P., Siris, E. S., and Shane, E.: Clinical presentation of primary hyperparathyroidism. Bilezikian, J. P., Marcus, R., and Levine, M. A., Eds. *The Parathyroids. Basic and Clinical Concepts*. New York, Raven Press, 1994, pp. 457–470.
3. Heath, H. H., III, Hodgson, S. F., and Kennedy, M. A.: Primary hyperparathyroidism: Incidence, morbidity, and potential economic impact in a community. *N Engl J Med* 302:189–193, 1980.
4. Arnold, A.: Molecular genetics of parathyroid gland neoplasia. *J Clin Endocrinol Metab* 77:1108–1112, 1993.
5. von Recklinghausen, F. D.: Die Fibrose oder deformirende Osteitis, die Osteomalacia, und die osteoplastische Carcinose. *Festschrift fur R Virchow*. Berlin, G. Reimer, 1891.
6. Askanazy, M.: Hyperparathyroidism. *Arbeit Geb Path Anat Bact* 4:398, 1904.
7. Collip, J. B.: The extraction of a parathyroid hormone which will prevent or control parathyroid tetany and which regulates the level of the blood calcium. *J Biol Chem* 63:395–438, 1925.
8. Mandl, F.: Therapeutischer Versuch bei einem Falle von Osteitis Fibrosa generalisata mittles Extirpation eines Epithelkörperchen Tumors. *Zentralbl Chir* 53:260, 1926.
9. Jaffe, H. L., Bodansky, A., and Blair, J. E.: Fibrous osteodystrophy (osteitis fibrosa) in experimental hyperparathyroidism of guinea pigs. *Arch Pathol* 2:207–235, 1931.
10. Silverberg, S. J., Shane, E., Jacobs, T. P., Siris, E. S., Gartenberg, F., Seldin, D., Clemens, T. L., and Bilezikian, J. P.: Nephrolithiasis and bone involvement in primary hyperparathyroidism. *Am J Med* 89:327–334, 1990.
11. Genant, H. K., Vander Horst, J., Lanzl, L. H., Mall, J. C., and Doi, K.: Skeletal demineralization in primary hyperparathyroidism. Mazess, R. B., Ed. *International Conference on Bone Mineral Measurement*. U.S. Department of Health, Education, and Welfare, Public Health Service, National Institute of Arthritis, Metabolism, and Digestive Diseases, Bethesda, MD, 1975, p. 177.
12. Gryfe, C. I.: Bone loss in primary hyperparathyroidism. *Can Med Assoc J* 109:479, 1973.
13. Parisien, M., Mellish, R. W. E., Silverberg, S. J., Shane, E., Lindsay, R., Bilezikian, J. P., and Dempster, D. W.: Maintenance of cancellous bone connectivity in primary hyperparathyroidism: Trabecular strut analysis. *J Bone Miner Res* 7:913–919, 1992.
14. Parisien, M., Silverberg, S. J., Shane, E., De La Cruz, L., Lindsay, R., Bilezikian, J. P., and Dempster, D. W.: The histomorphometry of bone in primary hyperparathyroidism: Preservation of cancellous bone structure. *J Clin Endocrinol* 70:930–938, 1990.
15. Silverberg, S. J., Shane, E., De La Cruz, L., Dempster, D. W., Feldman, F., Seldin, D., Jacobs, T. P., Siris, E. S., Cafferty, M., Parisien, M., Lindsay, R., Clemens, T. L., and Bilezikian, J. P.: Skeletal disease in primary hyperparathyroidism. *J Bone Miner Res* 4:283–291, 1989.
16. Silverberg, S. J., Gartenberg, F., Jacobs, T. P., Shane, E., Siris, E. S., Staron, R. B., McMahon, D., and Bilezikian, J. P.: Increased bone mineral density after parathyroidectomy in primary hyperparathyroidism. *J Clin Endocrinol Metab* 80:729–734, 1995.
17. Glorieux, F.: Rickets, the continuing challenge. *N Engl J Med* 325:1875–1877, 1991.
18. Whistler, D.: *De morbo puerili Anglorum, quem patrio idiomate indigenae vocant The Rickets*. London, 1645.
19. Glisson, F.: Rachitide sive Morbo Puerili, qui vulgo. *The Rickets dicitur*. London, 1650.
20. Palm, T. A.: The geographical distribution and etiology of rickets. *Practitioner* 45:270–274, 1890.
21. Escherich, T.: Rickets [abstract]. *Comptes Rendu du XII*. Section 6, 1899.
22. Hess, A. F.: Rickets, including osteomalacia and tetany. Philadelphia, Lea and Febiger, 1929.
23. Mariam, T. W., and Sterky, G.: Severe rickets in infancy and childhood in Ethiopia. *J Pediatr* 82:876–878, 1973.
24. Madewell, J. E., Ragsdale, B. D., and Sweet, D. E.: Radiologic and pathologic analysis of solitary bone lesions. Part I: Internal margins. *Radiol Clin North Am* 19:715, 1981.
25. Sandstead, H. H.: Clinical manifestations of certain classical deficiency diseases. Goodhart, R. S., and Shils, M. E., Eds. *Modern Nutrition in Health and Disease*. Philadelphia, Lea & Febiger, 1980, pp. 693–696.
26. Dodds, G. S., and Cameron, H. C.: Studies on experimental rickets in rats. II. The healing process in the head of the tibia and other bones. *Am J Pathol* 14:273–305, 1938.
27. Dodds, G. S., and Cameron, H. C.: Studies on experimental rickets in rats. IV. The relation of rickets to growth, with special reference to the bones. *Am J Pathol* 19:169–185, 1943.
28. Steinbach, H. L., Kolb, F. O., and Gilfillan, R.: A mechanism of the production of pseudofractures in osteomalacia (Milkman's syndrome). *Radiology* 62:388, 1954.
29. Fraser, D., Kooh, S. W., Kind, H. P., et al.: Pathogenesis of hereditary vitamin D–dependent rickets (an inborn error of vitamin D metabolism involving defective conversion of 25-hydroxyvitamin D to 1,25-dihydroxyvitamin D). *N Engl J Med* 289:817–823, 1973.
30. Sone, T., Marx, S. J., Liberman, U. A., and Pike, J. W.: A unique point mutation in the human vitamin D receptor chromosomal gene confers hereditary resistance to 1,25-dihydroxyvitamin D_3. *Mol Endocrinol* 4:623–631, 1990.
31. Brooks, M. H., Bell, N. H., Love, L., and Stern, P. H.: Vitamin D–dependent rickets type II: Resistance of target organs to 1,25-dihydroxyvitamin D. *N Engl J Med* 298:996–999, 1978.
32. MacLaughlin, J., and Holick, M. F.: Aging decreases the capacity of human skin to produce vitamin D_3. *J Clin Invest* 76:1536–1538, 1985.
33. Gloth, F. M., III, Gundberg, C. M., Hollis, B. W., Haddad, J. G., and Tobin, J. D.: Vitamin D deficiency in homebound elderly persons. *JAMA* 274:1683–1686, 1995.
34. Sokoloff, L.: Occult osteomalacia in American (U.S.A.) patients with fracture of the hip. *Am J Surg Pathol* 2:21–30, 1978.
35. Rapin, C. H., Lagier, R., Boivin, G., et al.: Biochemical findings in blood of aged patients with femoral neck fractures: A contribution to the detection of occult osteomalacia. *Calcif Tissue Int* 34:465–469, 1982.
36. Holmes, A. M., Enoch, B. A., Taylor, J. L., and Jones, M. E.: Occult rickets and osteomalacia amongst the Asian immigrant population. *QJM* 42:125–149, 1973.
37. Eastwood, M. A., and Girdwood, R. H.: Lignin: A bile-salt sequestrating agent. *Lancet* 2:1170, 1968.
38. Coburn, J. W., Brickman, A. S., and Hartenblower, D. L.: Clinical disorders. Norman, A. W., and Schaeffer, P., Eds. *Vitamin D and Problems Related to Uremic Bone Disease*. New York, de Gruyter, 1975, p. 219.
39. Parfitt, A. M., Podenphant, J., Villanueva, A. R., and Frame, B.: Metabolic bone disease with and without osteomalacia after intestinal bypass surgery: A histomorphometric study. *Bone* 6:211, 1985.

40. Eddy, R. L.: Metabolic bone disease after gastrectomy. *Am J Med* 50:442–449, 1971.
41. Hahn, J. T.: Drug-induced disorders of vitamin D and mineral metabolism. *Clin Endocrinol* 9:107, 1980.
42. Tolman, K. G., Jubiz, W., Sannella, J., et al.: Osteomalacia associated with anticonvulsant drug therapy in a pediatric outpatient population. *Pediatrics* 56:52, 1975.
43. Villareale, M. E., Chirott, R. I., Berstrom, W. H., et al.: Bone changes induced by diphenylhydantoin in chicks on a controlled vitamin D intake. *J Bone Joint Surg* 60A:911–916, 1978.
44. Sherk, H. H., Cruz, M., and Stambaugh, J.: Vitamin D prophylaxis and the lowered incidence of fractures in anticonvulsant rickets and osteomalacia. *Clin Orthop Rel Res* 129:251–257, 1977.
45. Bingham, C., and Fitzpatrick, L.: Noninvasive testing in the diagnosis of osteomalacia. *Am J Med* 95:519–524, 1993.
46. Schott, G. D., and Wills, M. R.: Muscle weakness in osteomalacia. *Lancet* 1:626–629, 1976.
47. Steinbach, H. L.: Roentgen appearance of the skeleton in osteomalacia and rickets. *Am J Roentgenol* 91:955–972, 1964.
48. Milkman, L. A.: Multiple spontaneous idiopathic symmetrical fractures. *Am J Roentgenol* 32:622, 1934.
49. Malluche, H. H., and Faugere, M.-C.: Bone biopsies: Histology and histomorphometry of bone. Avioli, L. V., and Krane, S. M., Eds. *Metabolic Bone Disease and Clinically Related Disorders.* Philadelphia, W. B. Saunders, 1990, pp. 283–328.
50. Arnstein, A. R., Frame, B., and Frost, H. M.: Recent progress in osteomalacia and rickets. *Ann Intern Med* 67:1296–1330, 1967.
51. Teitelbaum, S. L.: Pathological manifestations of osteomalacia and rickets. *Clin Endocrinol Metab* 9:43–62, 1980.
52. Drezner, M. K.: Tumor associated rickets and osteomalacia. Favus, M. J., Christakos, S., Gagel, R. F., Kleerkoper, M., Langman, C. B., Stewart, A. F., and Shyte, M. P., Eds. *Primer on the Metabolic Bone Diseases and Disorders of Mineral Metabolism.* Boston, Raven Press, 1993, pp. 282.
53. Cai, Q., Hodgson, S. F., Kao, P. C., et al.: Brief report: Inhibition of renal phosphate transport by a tumor product in a patient with oncogenic osteomalacia. *N Engl J Med* 330:1645–1649, 1994.
54. Dent, C. E., and Gertner, J. M.: Hypophosphatemic osteomalacia in fibrous dysplasia. *QJM* 45:411, 1976.
55. Konishi, K., Nakamura, M., Yamakawa, H., et al.: Case report: Hypophosphaemic osteomalacia in von Recklinghausen neurofibromatosis. *Am J Med Sci* 301:322–420, 1991.
56. McMurtry, C., Godschalk, M., Malluche, H. H., et al.: Oncogenic osteomalacia associated with metastatic prostate carcinoma: Case report and review of the literature. *J Am Geriatr Soc* 41:983–985, 1993.
57. Malluche, H.: Uremic bone disease: Current knowledge, controversial issues, and new horizons. *Miner Electrolyte Metab* 17:281–296, 1991.
58. Sherrard, D. J., Hercz, G., Pei, Y., et al.: The spectrum of bone disease in end-stage renal failure—an evolving disorder. *Kidney Int* 43:436–442, 1993.
59. Portale, A. A., Booth, B. E., Halloran, B. P., and Morris, R. C., Jr.: Effect of dietary phosphorus on circulating concentrations of 1,25-dihydroxyvitamin D and immunoreactive parathyroid hormone in children with moderate renal insufficiency. *J Clin Invest* 73:1580–1589, 1984.
60. Dunlay, R., Rodriguez, M., Felsenfeld, A. J., and Llach, F.: Direct inhibitory effect of calcitriol on parathyroid function (sigmoidal curve) in dialysis. *Kidney Int* 36:1093–1098, 1989.
61. Sundaram, M.: Renal osteodystrophy. *Skeletal Radiol* 18:415–426, 1989.
62. Greenfield, G. B.: Roentgen appearance of bone and soft-tissue changes in chronic renal disease. *Am J Roentgenol* 116:749–757, 1972.
63. Teitelbaum, S. L.: Progress in pathology-renal osteodystrophy. *Hum Pathol* 15:306–322, 1984.
64. Romanski, S. A., McCarthy, J. T., Kluge, K., and Fitzpatrick, L. A.: Detection of subtle aluminum-related renal osteodystrophy. *Mayo Clin Proc* 68:419–426, 1993.
65. Talwar, H. S., Reddi, A. H., Menczel, J., Thomas, W. C., Jr., and Meyer, J. L.: Influence of aluminum on mineralization during matrix-induced bone development. *Kidney Int* 29:1038–1042, 1986.
66. Parisien, M., Charhon, S. A., Mainetti, E., et al.: Evidence for a toxic effect of aluminum on osteoblasts: A histomorphometric study in hemodialysis patients with aplastic bone disease. *J Bone Miner Res* 3:259, 1988.
67. Lieberherr, M., Grosse, B., Gourtnot-Witmer, G., Hermann-Erlee, M. P. M., and Balsan, S.: Aluminum action on mouse bone cell metabolism and response to PTH and 1,25(OH)$_2$D$_3$. *Kidney Int* 31:736–743, 1987.
68. Maloney, N. A.: Histological quantitation of aluminum in iliac bone from patients with renal failure. *J Lab Clin Med* 99:206–216, 1982.
69. Faugere, M.: Stainable aluminum and not aluminum content reflects bone histology in dialyzed patients. *Kidney Int* 30:717–722, 1986.
70. Malluche, H., and Monier-Faugere, M. C.: The role of bone biopsy in the management of patients with renal osteodystrophy. *J Am Soc Nephrol* 4:1631–1642, 1994.
71. Gejyo, F., Homma, N., Suzuki, Y., and Arakawa, K. M.: Serum levels of β-2-microglobulin as a new form of amyloid protein in patients undergoing long-term hemodialysis. *N Engl J Med* 314:585–586, 1986.
72. Bardin, T., Kuntz, D., Zingraff, J., Voisin, M.-C., Zelmar, A., and Lansaman, J.: Synovial amyloidosis in patients undergoing long-term hemodialysis. *Arthritis Rheum* 28:1052–1058, 1985.
73. Casey, T. T., Stone, W. J., DiRaimondo, C. R., Brantley, B. D., DiRaimondo, C. V., Gorevic, P. D., and Page, D. L.: Tumoral amyloidosis of bone of beta$_2$-microglobulin origin in association with long-term hemodialysis: A new type of amyloid disease. *Hum Pathol* 17:731–738, 1986.
74. Theintz, G., Buchs, B., Rizzoli, R., et al.: Longitudinal monitoring of bone mass accumulation in healthy adolescents: Evidence for a marked reduction after 16 years of age at the levels of lumbar spine and femoral neck in female subjects. *J Endocrinol Metab* 75:1060–1065, 1992.
75. Recker, R. R., Davies, K. M., Hinders S. M., Heaney, R. P., Stegman, M. R., and Kimmel, D. B.: Bone gain in young adult women. *JAMA* 268:2403–2408, 1992.
76. Bonjour, J. P., Theintz, G., Buchs, B. Slossman, D., and Rizzoli, R.: Critical years and stages of puberty for spinal and femoral bone mass accumulation during adolescence. *J Clin Endocrinol Metab* 73:555–563, 1991.
77. Krall, E. A., and Dawson-Hughes, B.: Heritable and lifestyle determinants of bone mineral density. *J Bone Miner Res* 8:1–9, 1993.
78. Cohn, S. H., Abesamis, C., Yasumura, S., Aloia, J. F., Zanzi, I., and Ellis, K. J.: Comparative skeletal mass and radial bone mineral content in black and white women. *Metabolism* 26:171–178, 1977.
79. Pollitzer, W. S., and Anderson, J. J.: Ethnic and genetic differences in bone mass: A review with a hereditary vs. environmental perspective. *Am J Clin Nutr* 50:1244–1259, 1989.
80. Chan, G. M.: Dietary calcium and bone mineral status of children and adolescents. *Am J Dis Child* 145:631–634, 1991.
81. Dent, C. E.: The keynote address: Problems in metabolic bone disease. Frame, B., Parfitt, M., Duncan, H., Eds. *Clinical Aspects of Metabolic Bone Disease (Proceedings of the International Symposium on Clinical Aspects of Metabolic Bone Disease. Henry Ford Hospital, Detroit, June, 1972).* Amsterdam, Excerpta Medica, 1973, pp. 1–7.
82. Melton, L. J.: How many women have osteoporosis now? *J Bone Miner Res* 10:175–177, 1995.
83. Burstein, A. H., Zika, H. M., Heiple, K. G., and Klein, L.: Contributions of collagen and mineral to the elastic plastic properties of bone. *J Bone Joint Surg* 57A:956–961, 1975.
84. Cooper, C., Atkinson, E. J., O'Fallon, W. M., and Melton, L. J., III: Incidence of clinically diagnosed vertebral fractures: A population based study in Rochester, Minnesota, 1985–1989. *J Bone Miner Res* 7:221–227, 1992.
85. Melton, L. J., III, Kan, S. H., Frye, M. A., et al.: Epidemiology of vertebral fractures in women. *Am J Epidemiol* 129:1000–1011, 1989.
86. Magaziner, J., Simonsick, E. M., Kashner, T. M., Hebel, J. R., and Kenzora, J. E.: Survival experience of aged hip fracture patients. *Am J Public Health* 79:274–278, 1989.
87. Ray, N. F., Chan, J. K., Thamer, M., and Melton, L. J., III: Medical expenditures for the treatment of osteoporotic fractures in the United States in 1995: Report from the National Osteoporosis Foundation. *J Bone Miner Res* 12:24–34, 1997.
88. Perzigian, A. J.: Osteoporotic bone loss in two prehistoric Indian populations. *Am J Phys Anthropo* 39:87–96, 1973.
89. Cooper, A. P.: *A Treatise on Dislocations and on Fractures of the Joints,* 4th ed. London, Longman, Hurst, Rees, Orme, and Browne, 1824.
90. Pommer, G.: Untersuchungen über Osteomalacie und Rachitis, neue Beitragen zur Kenntnis der Knochen-Resorption und Apposition in verschiedene Altersperioden und der durchbohrenden Gefässe. Leipzig, F. C. W. Vogel, 1885.
91. Albright, F., and Reifenstein, E. C., Jr.: Metabolic bone disease:

Osteoporosis. *The Parathyroid Glands and Metabolic Bone Disease.* Baltimore, Williams & Wilkins, 1948, pp. 145–204.
92. Burr, D. B., and Martin, R. B.: Errors in bone remodeling: Toward a unified theory of metabolic bone disease. *Am J Anat* 186:186–216, 1989.
93. Lips, P., Courpron, P., and Meunier, P. J.: Mean wall thickness of trabecular bone packets in human iliac crest: Changes with age. *Calcif Tissue Res* 26:13–17, 1978.
94. Riggs, B. L., and Melton, L. J., III: The prevention and treatment of osteoporosis. *N Engl J Med* 327:620–627, 1992.
95. Sakhaee, K., Nicar, M. J., Glass, K., and Pak, C. Y. C.: Postmenopausal osteoporosis as a manifestation of renal hypercalciuria with secondary hyperparathyroidism. *J Clin Endocrinol Metab* 61:368–373, 1985.
96. Tsai, K. S., Heath, H. H., III, Kumar, R., and Riggs, B. L.: Impaired vitamin D metabolism with aging in women: Possible role in pathogenesis of osteoporosis. *J Clin Invest* 73:1668, 1984.
97. Silverberg, S. J., Shane, E., de la Cruz, L., et al.: Abnormalities in parathyroid hormone secretion and 1,25-dihydroxyvitamin D formation in women with osteoporosis. *N Engl J Med* 320:277–281, 1989.
98. Morrison, N. A., Qi, J. C., Tokita, A., et al.: Prediction of bone density from vitamin D receptor alleles. *Nature* 367:284,1994.
99. Riggs, B. L., and Melton, L. J.: Involutional osteoporosis. *N Engl J Med* 314:1676–1684, 1986.
100. Riggs, B. L., Wahner, H. W., and Dunn, W. L.: Differential changes in bone mineral density of the appendicular and axial skeleton with aging; relationship to spinal osteoporosis. *J Clin Invest* 67:328–335, 1981.
101. Horowitz, M. C.: Cytokines and estrogens in bone: Anti-osteoporotic effects. *Science* 260:626, 1993.
102. Girasole, G., Jilka, R. L., and Passeri, G.: 17 β-Estradiol inhibits interleukin-6 production by bone marrow derived stromal cells and osteoblasts in vitro; a potential mechanism for the antiosteoporotic effect of estrogens. *J Clin Invest* 89:883–891, 1992.
103. Nisker, J. A., Hammond, G. L., Davidson, B. J., et al.: Serum sex hormone-binding capacity and the percentage of free estradiol in postmenopausal women with and without endometrial carcinoma: A new biochemical basis for the association between obesity and endometrial carcinoma. *Am J Obstet Gynecol* 138:637–642, 1980.
104. Steinbach, H. L.: The roentgen appearance of osteoporosis. *Radiol Clin North Am* 2:191–207, 1964.
105. Gallagher, J. C.: Epidemiology of fractures of the proximal femur in Rochester, Minnesota. *J Clin Orthop* 150:163, 1980.
106. Dempster, D. W., Shane, E., Horbett, W., and Linday, R.: A simple method for correlative light and scanning electron microscopy of human iliac crest bone biopsies: Qualitative observations in normal and osteoporotic subjects. *J Bone Miner Res* 1:15, 1991.
107. Kleerekoper, M., Villanueva, A. R., Stanciu, J., et al.: The role of three-dimensional trabecular microstructure in the pathogenesis of vertebral compression fractures. *Calcif Tissue Int* 37:594–597, 1985.
108. Whyte, M. P., Bergfeld, M. A., Murphy, W. A., Avioli, L. V., and Teitelbaum, S. L.: Postmenopausal osteoporosis. A heterogeneous disorder as assessed by histomorphometric analysis of iliac crest bone from untreated patients. *Am J Med* 72:193–202, 1982.
109. de Deuxchaisnes, C. N., Devogelaer, J. P., Esselinckx, W., et al.: The effect of low dosage glucocorticoids on bone mass in rheumatoid arthritis: A cross-sectional and a longitudinal study using single photon absorptiometry. *Adv Exp Med Biol* 171:210–239, 1984.
110. Lukert, B. P., and Raisz, L. G.: Glucocorticoid induced osteoporosis: Pathogenesis and management. *Ann Intern Med* 112:352–364, 1990.
111. Gosschalk, M. F., and Downs, R. W.: Effect of short-term glucocorticoids on serum osteocalcin in healthy young men. *J Bone Miner Res* 2:113–115, 1988.
112. Peck, W. A., Brandt, J., and Miller, I.: Hydrocortisone-induced inhibition of protein synthesis and uridine incorporation in isolated bone cells in vitro. *Proc Natl Acad Sci* 57:1599–1606, 1967.
113. Meunier, P. J., Dempster, D. W., Edouard, C., et al.: Bone histomorphometry in corticosteroid-induced osteoporosis and Cushing's syndrome. *Adv Exp Med Biol* 171:191–200, 1984.
114. Bressot, C., Meunier, P. J., Chapuy, M. C., Lejeune, E., Edourd, C., and Darby, A. J.: Histomorphometric profile, pathophysiology and reversibility of corticosteroid-induced osteoporosis. *Metab Bone Dis Rel Res* 1:303–319, 1979.
115. Aaron, J. E., Francis, R. M., Peacock, M. B., and Makins, N. B.: Contrasting microanatomy of idiopathic and corticosteroid-induced osteoporosis. *Clin Orthop* 243:294–305, 1989.
116. Klein, R. G., Arnaud, S. B., Gallagher, J. C., DeLuca, H. F., and Riggs, B. L.: Intestinal calcium absorption in exogenous hypercortisonism. Role of 25-hydroxyvitamin D and corticosteroid dose. *J Clin Invest* 60:253–259, 1977.
117. Hirst, M., and Feldman, D.: Glucocorticoids down-regulate the number of 1,25-dihydroxyvitamin D receptors in mouse intestine. *Biochem Biophys Res Commun* 105:1590–1596, 1982.
118. Gennari, C., Imbimbo, B., Montagnani, M., et al.: Effects of prednisone and deflazacort on mineral metabolism and parathyroid hormone activity in humans. *Calif Tissue Int* 36:245–252, 1984.
119. Bachrach, L. K., Guido, D., Katzman, D., Lin, I. F., and Marcus, R.: Decreased bone density in adolescent girls with anorexia nervosa. *Pediatrics* 86:440–447, 1990.
120. Rigotti, N. A., Nuesbaum, S. R., Herzog, W., et al.: Osteoporosis in women with anorexia nervosa. *N Engl J Med* 311:1601–1605, 1984.
121. Walsh, B. T.: The endocrinology of anorexia nervosa. *Psychoneuroendocrinol* 3:299–312, 1980.
122. Drinkwater, B. L., Nilson, K., Chestnut, C., III, Bremner, W. J., Shainholtz, S., and Southworth, M. B.: Bone mineral content of amenorrheic and eumenorrheic athletes. *N Engl J Med* 311:277–281, 1984.
123. Marcus, R., Cann, C., Madvig, P., et al.: Menstrual function and bone mass in elite women distance runners. *Ann Intern Med* 102:158–163, 1985.
124. Hetland, M. L., Haarbo, J., and Christiansen, C.: Low bone mass and high bone turnover in male long distance runners. *J Clin Endocrinol Metab* 77:770–775, 1993.
125. Soejima, K., and Landing, B. H.: Osteoporosis in juvenile-onset diabetes mellitus: Morphometric and comparative studies. *Pediatr Pathol* 6:289–299, 1986.
126. Heath, H. H., III, Melton, L. J., and Chu, C. P.: Diabetes mellitus and risk of skeletal fracture. *N Engl J Med* 303:567–570, 1980.
127. Bikle, D. D., Genant, H. K., and Cann, C.: Bone disease in alcohol abuse. *Ann Intern Med* 103:42, 1985.
128. Peris, P., Pares, A., and Guanabens, N.: Reduced spinal and femoral bone mass and deranged bone mineral metabolism in chronic alcoholics. *Alcohol Alcoholism* 27:619–625, 1992.
129. Slemenda, C. W., Hui, S. L., Longcope, C., and Johnston, C. C.: Cigarette smoking, obesity and bone mass. *J Bone Miner Res* 4:737–741, 1989.
130. Daniell, H. W.: Osteoporosis of the slender smoker. *Arch Intern Med* 136:298–304, 1976.
131. Michnovicz, J. J., Hershcopt, R. J., Naganuma, H., Bradlow, H. L., and Fishman, J.: Increased 2-hydroxylation of estradiol as a possible mechanism for the anti-estrogenic effect of cigarette smoking. *N Engl J Med* 315:1305–1309, 1986.
132. Kelepouris, N., Harper, K. D., Gannon, F., Kaplan, F. S., and Haddad, J. G.: Severe osteoporosis in men. *Ann Intern Med* 123:452–460, 1995.
133. Orwoll, E. S., and Klein, R. F.: Osteoporosis in men. *Endocr Rev* 16:87–116, 1995.
134. Jackson, J. A., Kleerekoper, M., Parfitt, A. M., Rao, D. S., Villanueva, A. R., and Frame, B.: Bone histomorphometry in hypogonadal and eugonadal men with spinal osteoporosis. *J Clin Endocrinol Metab* 65:53–58, 1987.
135. Smith, E., Boyd, J., Frank, G., Takahashi, H., Cohen, R., Specker, B., Williams, T., Lubahn, D., and Korach, K.: Estrogen resistance caused by a mutation in the estrogen-receptor gene in a man. *N Engl J Med* 331:1056–1061, 1994.
136. Reed, B. Y., Zerwekh, J. E., Sakhaee, K., Breslau, N. A., Gottschalk, F., and Pak, C. Y. C.: Serum IGF 1 is low and correlated with osteoblastic surface in idiopathic osteoporosis. *J Bone Miner Res* 10:1218–1224, 1995.
137. Smith, R.: Idiopathic osteoporosis in the young. *J Bone Joint Surg* 62B:417–428, 1994.
138. Jowsey, J., and Johnson, K. A.: Juvenile osteoporosis: Bone findings in seven patients. *J Pediatr* 81:511–517, 1972.
139. Harrison, J. E.: Fluoride treatment for osteoporosis. *Calcif Tissue Int* 46:287–288, 1990.
140. Hoekman, K., Papapoulos, S. E., Peters, A. C. B., and Bijvoet, O. L. M.: Characteristics and bisphosphonate treatment of a patient with juvenile osteoporosis. *J Clin Endocrinol Metab* 61:952–956, 1985.
141. Heinonen, A., Kannus, P., Sievanen, H., Oja, P., Pasanen, M., Rinne, M., Uusi-Rasi, K., and Vuori, I.: Randomised controlled trial of effect of high-impact exercise on selected risk factors for osteoporotic fractures. *Lancet* 348:1343–1347, 1996.

142. Riggs, B. L., and Melton, L. J.: The prevention and treatment of osteoporosis. *N Engl J Med* 327:620–627, 1992.
143. Harris, S. T., Genant, H. K., Baylink, D. J., Gallagher, J. C., Karp, S. K., McConnell, M. A., Green, E. M., and Stoll, R. W.: Effects of estrone (Ogen) on spinal bone density of postmenopausal women. *Arch Intern Med* 151:1980–1984, 1991.
144. Lufkin, E. G., Wahner, H. W., O'Fallon, W. M., Hodgson, S. F., Kotowicz, M. A., Lane, A. W., Judd, H. L., Caplan, R. H., and Riggs, B. L.: Treatment of postmenopausal osteoporosis with transdermal estrogen. *Ann Intern Med* 117:1–9, 1992.
145. Overgaard, K., Hansen, M. A., Jensen, S. B., and Christiansen, C.: Effect of calcitonin given intranasally on bone mass and fracture rates in established osteoporosis. *Br Med J* 305:556–561, 1992.
146. Tilyard, M. W.: Treatment of postmenopausal osteoporosis with calcitriol or calcium. *N Engl J Med* 326:357–361, 1992.
147. Papapoulos, S. E., Landman, J. O., Bijvoet, O. L. M., Lowik, W. G. M., Valkema, R., Pauwels, E. K. J., and Vermeij, P.: The use of bisphosphonates in the treatment of osteoporosis. *Bone* 13:S-41–S-49, 1992.
148. Storm, T.: Effect of intermittent cycline etidronate therapy on bone mass and fracture rate in women with postmenopausal osteoporosis. *N Engl J Med* 322:1265–1271, 1990.
149. Madans, J., Kleinman, J. C., and Cornoni-Huntley, J.: The relationship between hip fracture and water fluoridation: An analysis of national data. *Am J Public Health* 73:296–298, 1983.
150. Resch, H., Libanati, C., Farley, S., Bettica, P., Schulz, E., and Baylink, D. J.: Evidence that fluoride therapy increases trabecular bone density in a peripheral skeletal site. *J Clin Endocrinol Metab* 76:1622–1624, 1993.
151. Minaire, P., Meunier, P., Edouard, C., Bernard, J., Courpron, P., and Bourret, J.: Quantitative histological data on disuse osteoporosis. *Calcif Tissue Res* 17:57, 1974.
152. Kattapuram, S. V., Khurana, J. S., Ehara, S., and Ragozzino, M.: Aggressive posttraumatic osteoporosis of the humerus simulating a malignant neoplasm. *Cancer* 62:2525–2527, 1988.
153. Krolner, B., and Toft, B.: Vertebral bone loss: An unheeded side effect of therapeutic bed rest. *Clin Sci* 64:537–540, 1983.
154. Joyce, J. M., and Keats, T. E.: Disuse osteoporosis: Mimic of neoplastic disease. *Skeletal Radiol* 15:129–132, 1986.
155. Lakhanpal, S., Ginsburg, W. W., Luthra, H. S., and Hunder, G. G.: Transient regional osteoporosis. A study of 56 cases and review of the literature. *Ann Intern Med* 106:444–450, 1987.
156. Guerra, J. J., and Steinberg, M. E.: Current concepts review: Distinguishing transient osteoporosis from avascular necrosis of the hip. *J Bone Joint Surg* 77A:616–624, 1995.
157. Lenggenhager, K.: Sudeck's osteodystrophy: Its pathogenesis, prophylaxis and therapy. *Minn Med* 54:967–972, 1971.
158. Kozin, F., McCarty, D. J., Sims, J., and Genant, H. K.: The reflex sympathetic dystrophy syndrome. 1. Clinical and histologic studies: Evidence for bilaterality, response to corticosteroids and articular involvement. *Am J Med* 60:321–331, 1976.
159. Silver, J. J., and Einhorn, T. A.: Osteoporosis and aging. *Clin Orthop* 316:10–20, 1995.
160. Chrischilles, E. A., Butler, C. D., Davis, C. S., and Wallace, R. B.: A model of lifetime osteoporosis impact. *Arch Intern Med* 151:2026–2032, 1991.
161. Cummings, S. R., Kelsey, J. L., Nevitt, M. C., and O'Dowd, K. J.: Epidemiology of osteoporosis and osteoporotic fractures. *Epidemiol Rev* 7:178–208, 1985.
162. Chrischilles, E. A., Shireman, T., and Wallace, R.: Costs and health effects of osteoporotic fractures. *Bone* 15:377–386, 1994.

CHAPTER 5
The Pathophysiology of Fractures

In maintaining skeletal structure, healthy bones are able to withstand forces that greatly exceed those encountered in daily use. This ability is made possible by three factors. The first is the hardness of bone. Dense calcium crystals are embedded in a tough fibrous collagen, an arrangement with mechanical properties similar to those of steel-reinforced concrete. The second factor is the bone architecture. Each bone is shaped to sustain large forces, particularly those responsible for weight bearing. For example, the long bones are hollow tubes, a design that disperses forces more effectively than would solid cylinders. The third factor is the compliance of bone. It bends when forces act on it. This compliance allows bone to absorb much of the force that is applied. In addition to these factors, which give bones their strength, the skeleton is continuously remodeling itself. Old damaged bone is replaced by new bone. This process keeps the bones strong.

However, despite these properties, forces are occasionally great enough to cause bones to fracture. These forces may be delivered from outside the body, such as by an automobile bumper. They also may be generated from inside the body, such as from a hard muscle contraction. A femoral neck fracture in a patient undergoing electroshock therapy is an example of this mechanism. Fractures are by far the most common bone disease. Therefore, before discussing how fractures heal, a brief discussion of how they occur is necessary. The study of how fractures occur is known as *fracture mechanics*.[1]

FRACTURE MECHANICS

Stress and Strain

The skeleton is subjected to numerous kinds of forces in daily activity, such as walking, standing, dressing, bathing, eating. Because of their compliance, bones bend or deform during all of these activities. When a bone bends, a compression surface is present at the concave side of a bend, and a tension surface is present at the convex side. At the tension surface, the individual bone molecules are pulled apart, and at the compression surface, they are pushed together. Forces are generated during this deformation, which can be expressed in terms of stress and strain. *Stress* is defined as the internal force generated within a material as the result of the application of an external load (Fig. 5–1).[2] Stress is calculated by measuring the applied load and dividing it by the area on which the load acts. This is expressed either as pounds per square inch or as newtons per meter squared. Stress forces can be applied at 90° to a point in the bone (normal stress), or they can be applied parallel to a point in the bone (shear stress).[3] In contrast to stress, *strain* is a measure of deformation—how much the bone changes shape. Strain is expressed as a percentage of change relative to the original shape.

Forces on Bone

The mechanics of bone are similar to the mechanics of any deformable body. As forces are placed on the bone, deformation occurs, and a stress-strain curve can be developed (Fig. 5–2).[3] When a force is low, the deformation is extremely small, and when the force is removed, the bone returns to its normal shape. This zone of the curve is known as the linear portion. In contrast to a low force, a high force causes the bone to yield. The bone cannot absorb all the force without permanently changing its shape. This is the yield point on the stress-strain curve. As the force increases, the bone will continue to permanently deform. After an even further increase, the bone will fracture because the ultimate tensile strength has been surpassed. This pattern of failure is often called catastrophic failure. A nonmedical example of catastrophic failure is cracking a walnut or a lobster claw.

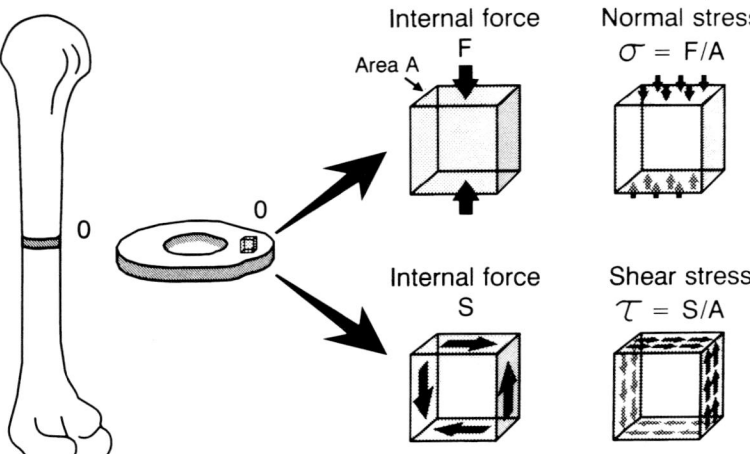

Figure 5-1 ▪ Both normal stress and shear stress in the diaphysis of the humerus. Normal stresses occur perpendicular to the bone whereas shear stresses occur parallel to a point on the surface of the bone. (From Chao, E., and Aro, H.: Biomechanics of fracture fixation. Mow, V. C., and Hayes, W. C., Eds. *Basic Orthopaedic Biomechanics*. New York, Raven Press, 1991. With permission from Lippincott-Raven.)

Direct Forces

The forces that fracture bones can be delivered directly (from outside the body) or from tension forces generated in the body (Fig. 5–3). External forces can be delivered by many mechanisms that may be divided into four categories: tapping forces, crushing forces, penetrating forces, and penetrating-explosive forces (Table 5–1).[3] An example of a tapping force is a blow to the forearm with a nightstick. A small force is applied over a small area. The ulna would fracture transversely, and the displacement would be minimal. The next force, a crushing force, is much more violent. An example would be an automobile bumper striking the leg in an auto-pedestrian accident. A high force (the car moving at 30 miles per hour) is delivered to the bones of the leg, and they would be crushed into multiple fragments. Severe soft tissue injury also would occur. The final type of force is a penetrating force, and two types can occur: moderate to high energy and extremely high energy. An example of moderate- to high-energy force would be a low-velocity gunshot wound to bone (muzzle velocity less than 2500 ft/s). In this example, a small entrance wound (1–2 cm) would be present, and the bone would shatter after being struck by the bullet. The muscle damage would be only minimal because the bone would receive most of the energy. In contrast, a high-velocity bullet (muzzle velocity greater than 2500 ft/s) would enter the body with a small entrance wound (1–2 cm) and then would shatter the bone and cause severe disruption of the soft tissues. In the low-velocity injury, the bone stops the bullet, and all the energy is dissipated. In contrast, the high-velocity bullet penetrates the bone and leaves the body through a large exit wound, which can be as large as 15 cm by 15 cm. As a result, the bone is comminuted into small fragments. The higher the velocity, the more destructive the injury. This is because velocity determines kinetic energy by the following equation: kinetic energy = mass times velocity squared.

Indirect Forces

In contrast to direct forces, indirect forces are tension or torsional forces generated within the body. Bones fracture in larger pieces, and the soft tissues are only minimally injured (Table 5–2).[3] Tension forces are usually generated by the forceful contraction of muscles. For example, a forceful muscle contraction can cause a transverse fracture through the patella or olecranon. Also, a pitcher or catcher can apply extremely high torsional forces to the humerus with a

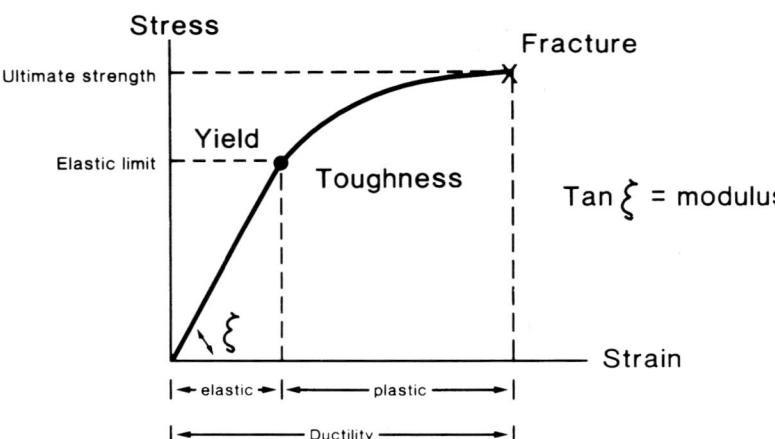

Figure 5-2 ▪ Typical stress-strain curve of a deformable body. In the linear elastic portion of the curve, stress and strain are directly proportional. At the yield point, the deformation changes from elastic to plastic. The slope of the stress strain curve is the modulus of the material and represents how stiff it is. If the forces applied to the bone exceed the ultimate strength, then the bone will fracture. (From Chao, E., and Aro, H.: Biomechanics of fracture fixation. Mow, V. C., and Hayes, W. C., Eds. *Basic Orthopaedic Biomechanics*. New York, Raven Press, 1991. With permission from Lippincott-Raven.)

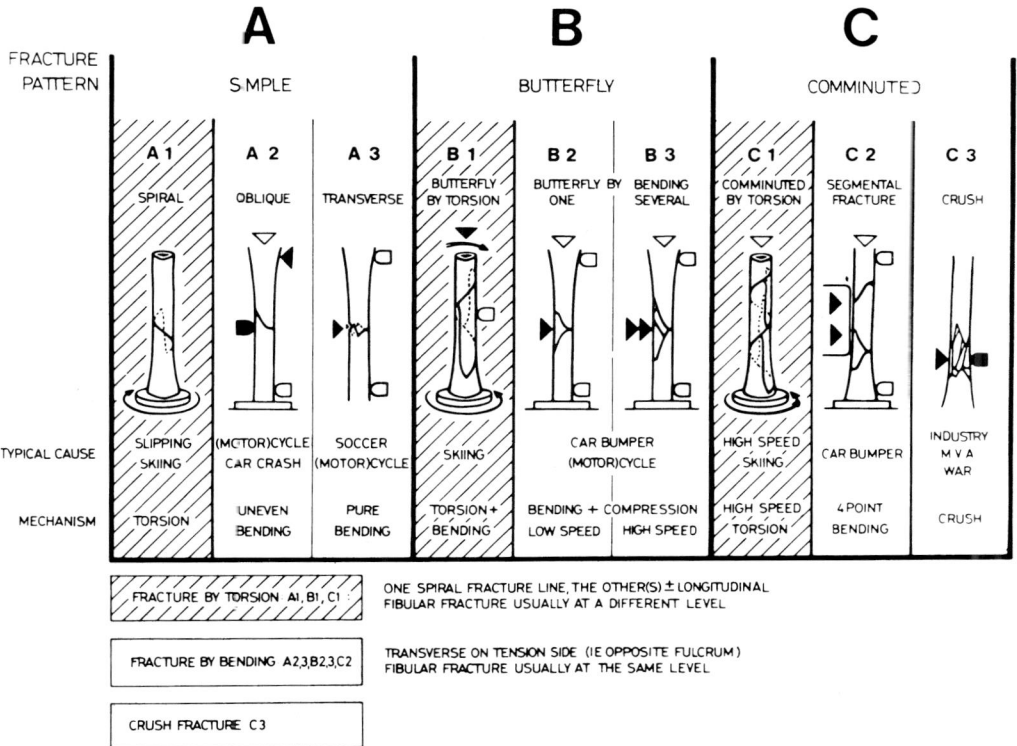

Figure 5-3 ■ Simple, butterfly, and comminuted fractures and the forces that produce them. (From Johner, R., and Wruhs, O.: Classification of tibial shaft fractures and correlation with results after rigid internal fixation. *Clin Orthop* 178:9, 1983.)

powerful throw. A midshaft spiral fracture may result. A third example of an indirect force is when an individual breaks a fall with an outstretched arm. A triceps contraction can drive the olecranon into the distal humerus, and this axial compression force causes a T or Y fracture of the distal humerus.

Failure Patterns

The failure patterns of long bones can be estimated by the appearance of the fracture lines (Fig. 5-4).[3] When a bending force is applied to a bone, the convex side is under tension, and the concave side is under compression. Because bone is weaker in tension than in compression, the tension side fractures first. If the external force continues, the fracture lines progress and create a transverse fracture line without comminution. If the cortex under compression also experiences shear stress, the fracture line will not be completely

Table 5-1 ■ **CLASSIFICATION OF FRACTURES CAUSED BY EXTERNAL FORCES**

Type of Force	Description of the Force	Fracture Characteristics
Tapping force	Small force acting on a small area	Nightstick fracture of ulna
Crushing force	High force acting on a large area	Crush fracture with comminution and severe soft tissue injury
Penetrating force	High force acting on a small area	Open fracture and minimal to moderate soft tissue disruption
Penetrating-explosive force	High force acting on a small area at a high or extremely high loading rate	Open fracture with severe soft tissue disruption and devitalized bone fragments

Modified from Chao, E., and Aro, H.: Biomechanics of fracture fixation. Mow, V. C., and Hayes, W. C., Eds. *Basic Orthopaedic Biomechanics*. New York, Raven Press, 1991, pp. 293–328.

Table 5-2 ■ **CLASSIFICATION OF FRACTURES CAUSED BY INDIRECT INJURY MECHANISMS**

Fracture Type	Example Fractures	Injury Force
Transverse	Transverse olecranon Transverse patella	Tension force
Oblique	Y or T fractures of the distal humerus or femur	Axial compressive force
Spiral	Spiral fracture of the humerus or tibia with intermittent longitudinal crack lines	Torsional force
Transverse	Transverse shaft fracture of the humerus or tibia, with butterfly fragment	Bending force
Transverse oblique	Transverse shaft fracture of the tibia with large butterfly fragment	Axial compression and bending

Modified from Chao E., and Aro, H.: Biomechanics of fracture fixation. Mow, V. C., and Hayes, W. C., Eds. *Basic Orthopaedic Biomechanics*. New York, Raven Press, 1991, pp. 293–328.

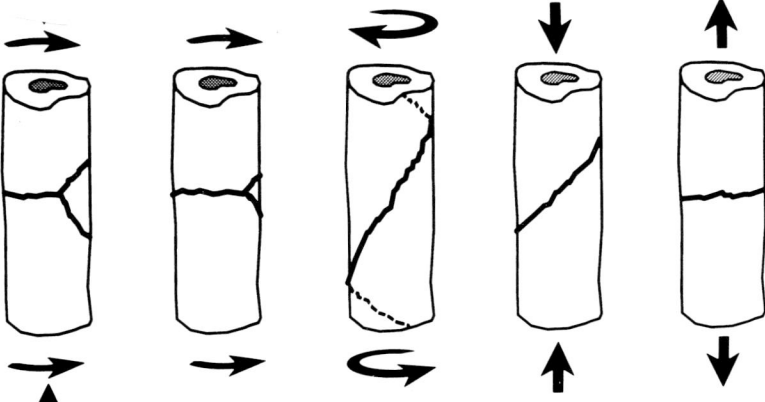

Figure 5-4 ■ The failure patterns under five different loading conditions. *From left to right,* axial loading and a bending moment producing a transverse fracture with a butterfly fragment; pure bending load with a transverse fracture with a small butterfly fragment; a torsional load producing a long spiral fracture; a pure axial load with shear forces producing a short oblique fracture; and a pure tension load producing a transverse fracture. (From Chao, E., and Aro, H.: Biomechanics of fracture fixation. Mow, V. C., and Hayes, W. C., Eds. *Basic Orthopaedic Biomechanics.* New York, Raven Press, 1991. With permission from Lippincott-Raven.)

transverse. This cortex will splinter and create a single butterfly fragment or multiple small fragments. When a torsional load is applied to the bone, a spiral fracture develops. With all torsional fractures, there is a component of bending forces that end the fracture line at a certain level rather than allowing an endless spiral through the entire bone shaft.

Bone or any material may also fail due to fatigue. A nonmedical example of fatigue is repetitive bending of a metal paper clip until it snaps. When metal is subjected to fatigue failure, small cracks develop and then propagate. A plot can be developed to show the relationship between the load applied and the number of cycles. When a large load is applied, the material may fail within a single cycle, or if the load is very small, thousands of cycles are necessary to cause failure. A common example of fatigue in bone is the stress fracture that develops in new military recruits. These recruits often march every day for up to 6 months, and many may have had sedentary lifestyles prior to entering military service. Stress fractures of the second metatarsal are very common in this setting (see later).

CLASSIFICATION OF FRACTURES

Numerous systems to classify fractures exist. One system classifies fractures as those occurring in normal bone and those occurring in abnormal bone. The latter are known as *pathologic fractures*. Fractures also may be classified as being closed or open. Closed fractures are those in which no violation of the overlying skin has occurred, whereas open fractures communicate with a skin wound. Three grades of open fractures exist (Table 5-3).[4] Grade 1 open fractures are the least severe, and grade III fractures involve very large soft tissue wounds and extensive periosteal stripping.

Common to most classification systems is an estimation of the degree of displacement and comminution. An incomplete fracture occurs when the break does not cross both cortices. By contrast, if both cortices are broken, the fracture is complete. Complete fractures may be nondisplaced or minimally displaced, or major displacement and angulation can occur. *Comminution* refers to the number of fracture fragments. When a fracture results in only two fragments, it is noncomminuted. However, a comminuted fracture may have three or more fragments. Segmental fractures may occur within a single bone, leaving an intervening nonfractured segment between two or more complete fractures.

In children, the fracture pattern may vary because their bones are less brittle and ductile. A single cortex may fracture while the opposite cortex bends, a pattern called a *greenstick fracture*. In children younger than 6 years old, the cortex may buckle; these are called buckle or *torus fractures*.

FRACTURE HEALING

Bone has remarkable healing activity. In fact, bone is one of the few tissues in which the healing process is so complete and the original structure is so well restored that evidence of injury is obliterated. Whereas other tissues, such as liver, brain, and kidney, heal with a fibrous scar, bone heals with bone.

The rate of fracture healing is dependent on many factors, such as the degree of adjacent soft tissue injury, the initial displacement of the fracture, the degree of comminution, the age of the patient, and the stability of the fractured ends. The simplest fractures may heal in 4 to 6 weeks, whereas the most severe require 6 to 12 months. Based on the factors

Table 5-3 ■ **GUSTILO/ANDERSON CLASSIFICATION OF OPEN FRACTURES**

Grade I	Small skin laceration < 1 cm. Usually one sharp point of the fractured bone has penetrated the skin and then returned below the skin.
Grade II	Soft tissue wound is greater than 1 cm, but the extent of soft tissue stripping is minimal.
Grade III	Large soft tissue wound with extensive periosteal stripping and bone damage.

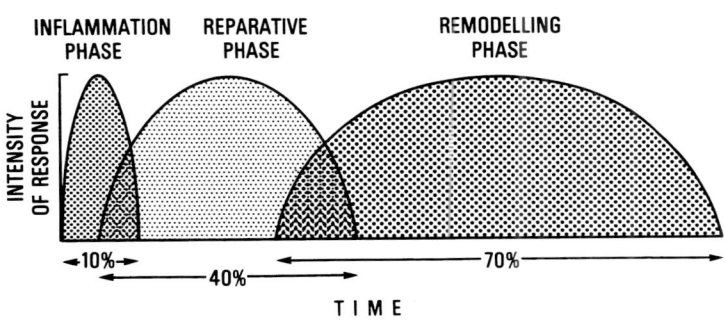

Figure 5-5 ■ The three phases of fracture healing. The inflammatory phase occurs first and is the shortest. At the end of the inflammatory phase, the reparative phase begins, and there is considerable overlap. The remodeling phase overlaps with the reparative phase and probably occurs for years after the fracture has healed. (From Rockwood, C., and Green, D., Eds. *Fractures in Adults*, 4th ed. Philadelphia, Lippincott-Raven, 1996, p. 268.)

discussed here, the clinician can often predict how long it will take a fracture to heal. In general, radiographs are taken every month to evaluate the healing process.

THE HISTOLOGY OF FRACTURE HEALING

Fracture healing may be divided into three phases: the inflammation phase, the reparative phase, and the remodeling phase (Fig. 5-5).

The immediate result of a fracture is bleeding. Bleeding originates from several sources: the marrow cavity, blood vessels in the cortex, and blood vessels in the torn periosteum. Bleeding also comes from torn blood vessels in damaged adjacent soft tissues. Bleeding is often extensive, and a hematoma encases the fractured bone ends. Because longitudinally arranged blood vessels in the haversian canals are ruptured, a small segment of cortex on each side of the fracture becomes necrotic (Fig. 5-6).

The first stage of healing, the inflammation phase, is the ingrowth of granulation tissue, which originates in the periosteum, the skeletal muscle, and possibly from the marrow space. Bone morphogenic proteins released from the damaged bone cause pluripotential cells in this granulation tissue to differentiate into osteoblasts and chondroblasts. These cells produce a mixture of cartilage, woven bone, and fibrous tissue, a mixture known as *fracture callus*. This is the reparative phase. The callus forms on the outside of the bone as well as in the medullary cavity (Fig. 5-7). Over a period of weeks, the amount of callus increases (Fig. 5-8). Mineralization of the new bone and cartilage occurs, and the callus can be seen on plain radiographs (Fig. 5-9).

Ideally, the fracture callus would consist entirely of bone-forming tissue. However, varying degrees of fibrous tissue

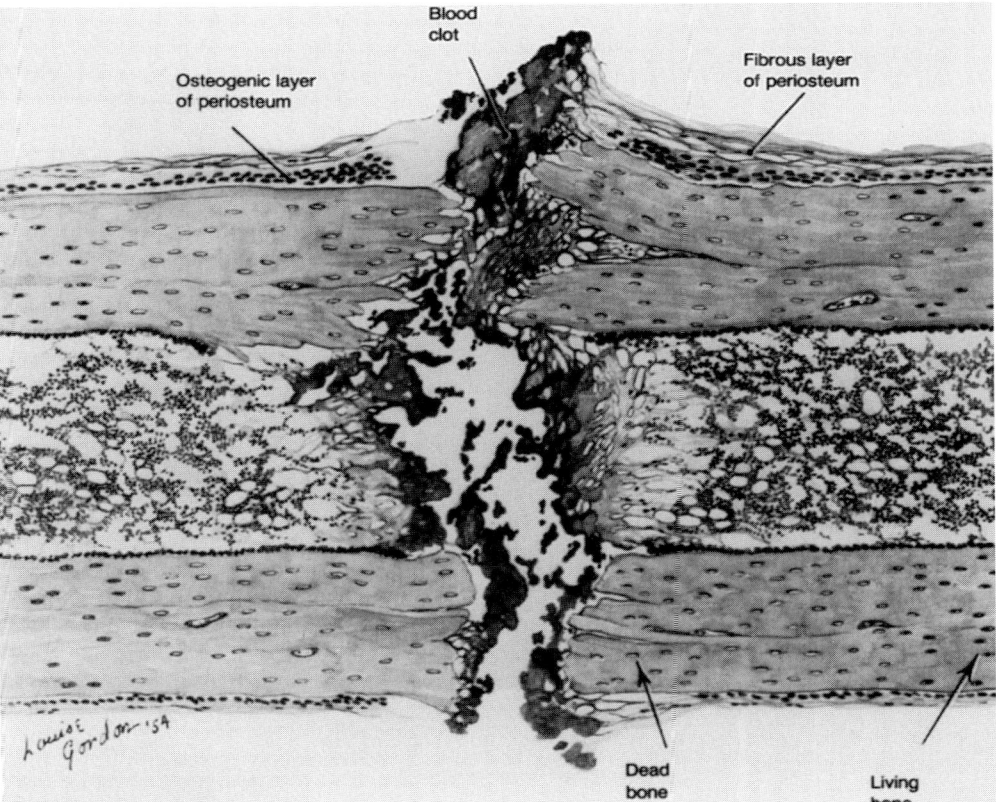

Figure 5-6 ■ A fresh fracture with disruption of the blood supply to the end of the bone and the formation of a hematoma between the bone ends. The inner layer of the periosteum is called the osteogenic layer, and the outer layer is called the fibrous layer. (From Ham, A. W., and Harris, W. R.: Bourne, G. H., Ed. *The Biochemistry and Physiology of Bone*, 2nd ed. Vol. 3. New York, Academic Press, 1971, p. 338.)

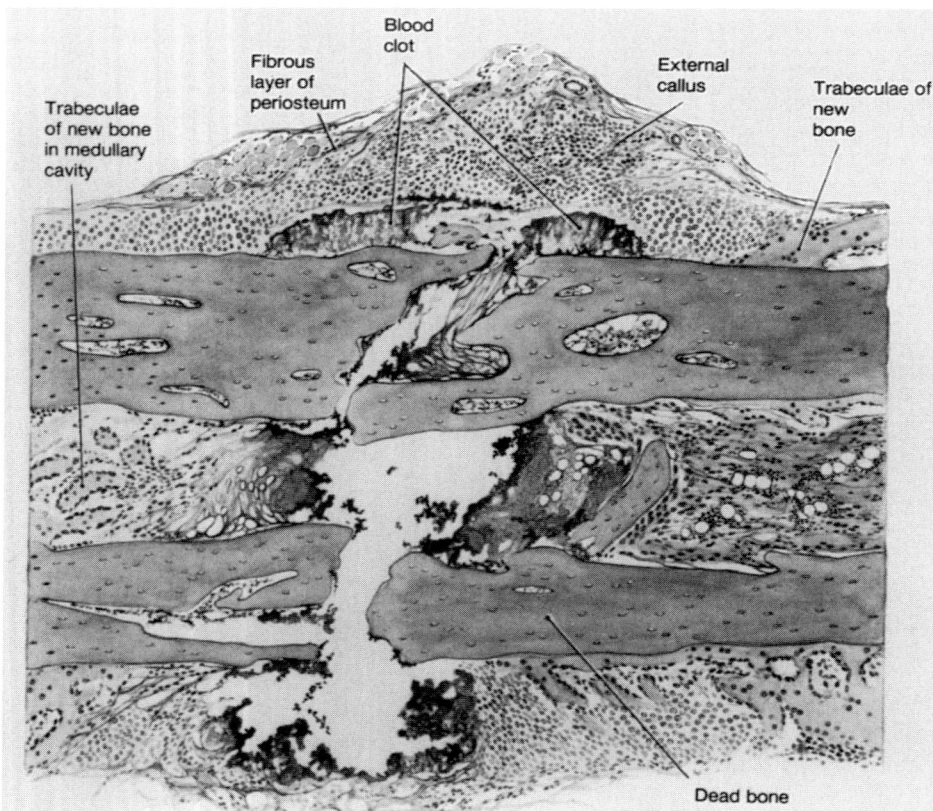

Figure 5-7 ▪ Fracture in the early reparative phase. Fracture callus is beginning in the medullary canal and on the cortical surface. (From Ham, A. W., and Harris, W. R.: Bourne, G. H., Ed. *The Biochemistry and Physiology of Bone*, 2nd ed. Vol. 3. New York, Academic Press, 1971, p. 338.)

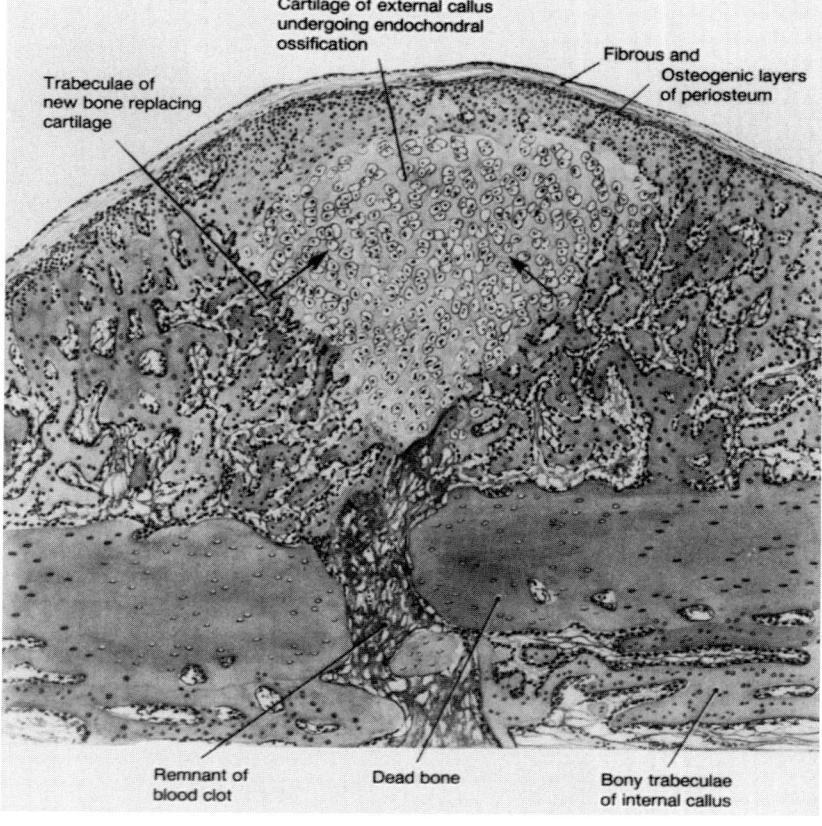

Figure 5-8 ▪ The reparative phase of bone healing with a large amount of external callus. The external callus welds the two ends of the bone together. The callus is made up of fibrous tissue, cartilage that undergoes endochondral ossification and fibrous tissue. (From Ham, A. W., and Harris, W. R.: Bourne, G. H., Ed. *The Biochemistry and Physiology of Bone*, 2nd ed. Vol. 3. New York, Academic Press, 1971, p. 338.)

and cartilage are present, depending on a number of factors, including oxygen tension, vascularity, and motion. The degree of electronegativity in the fracture site may also be a factor. For example, low oxygen tension and limited vascularity favor cartilage, rather than bone, formation. Alternatively, excessive motion favors fibrous tissue instead of bone. When the fracture gap is small, motion causes a high degree of strain on individual cells, a phenomenon called *strain intolerance*.[5,6] In this event, large amounts of fibrous tissue are produced, resulting in a delayed union or a nonunion.

In the remodeling phase of fracture healing, the cartilage of the callus undergoes endochondral bone formation, and the woven bone is converted into lamellar bone. Then, osteoblasts and osteoclasts sculpt the fracture callus to conform to the shape of the bone. Gradually, over a period of months, complete continuity of the cortices and medullary cavity is achieved (Fig. 5–10).

Fracture Reduction

The guiding principle of fracture care is to obtain and maintain a reduction. This means restoring the fractured bone ends to their original alignment and holding that alignment while the bone ends heal. Depending on the bone,

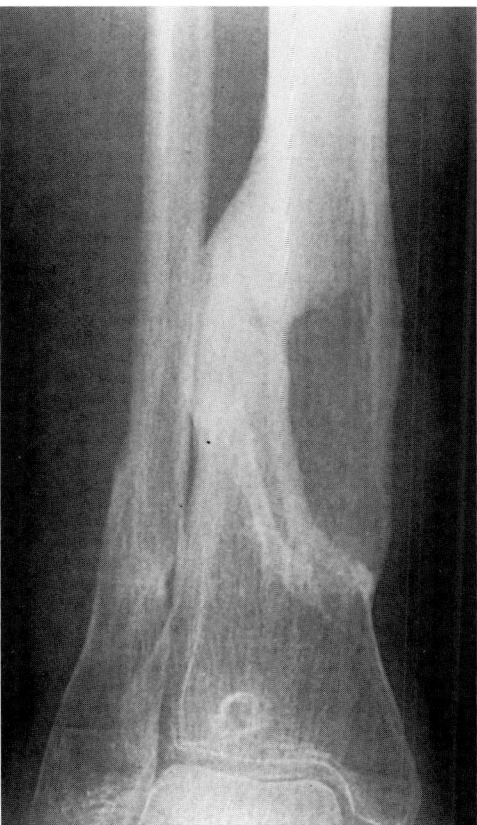

Figure 5–10 ■ An anteroposterior radiograph of the ankle in a patient with a distal tibial and fibular fracture treated with an external fixator. This method of treatment is nonrigid, and one can see the large amount of external callus.

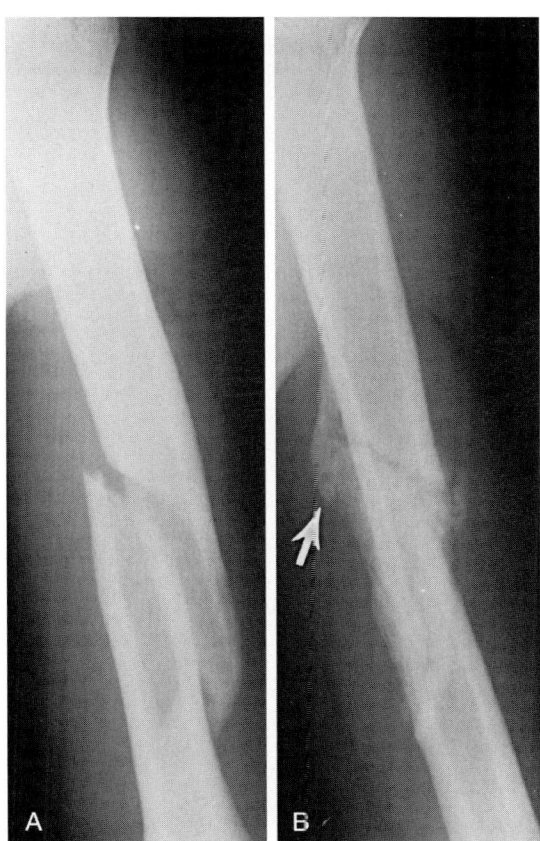

Figure 5–9 ■ A long spiral fracture occurred in the humerus while the patient was throwing a baseball. The fracture was treated with a fracture base. A large amount of periosteal callus can be seen on the outside of the bone 8 weeks following the fracture (arrow).

some degree of displacement and angulation is acceptable. Reduction can be maintained by either external or internal fixation.

External Fixation

External immobilization is accomplished with a cast, a traction device, a fracture brace, or an external fixation device. With these methods of immobilization, some motion occurs at the fracture site. This motion leads to large amounts of callus on the bone surface. This external callus stabilizes the two fracture ends—they become "sticky." The callus on the surface of the bone often contains large amounts of fibrocartilage. Once the fracture has become sticky, the environment in the endosteal cavity is then conducive to bone formation, and the fracture gap fills in with bone.

Internal Fixation

A surgical procedure is necessary to achieve internal fixation. The fractured bone ends are held together with metal plates and screws, rods, nails, or any combination of these. When a fracture is treated with internal fixation, virtually no motion in the fracture gap occurs. With the absence of motion, little or no periosteal callus forms, but healing occurs from the medullary cavity and between the cortices. At the cortical bone contact sites, remodeling cones cut across the fractured ends, and the osteoblasts lay down new bone to unite the fracture.

DELAYED UNION AND NONUNION

The impetus for healing is so strong that even fractures through abnormal bone heal normally. This includes even severely osteoporotic bone. Furthermore, fracture healing is seldom adversely affected by diseases of other organ systems. Only diabetes and smoking are associated with poor fracture callus formation.

However, complications occasionally occur at fracture sites. The two most common complications are delayed union and nonunion. A *delayed union* occurs when a fracture does not heal at a normal rate. Fracture callus is present, but its evolution is slower. Eventually, sometimes after a year or more, the fracture heals. If the healing process is arrested before union occurs, the fracture is called a *nonunion*. Instead of ossifying fracture callus, dense fibrous tissue forms between the bone ends. A special type of nonunion is called a *synovial pseudarthrosis*. If excessive motion is present at the nonunion site, a cavity develops in the dense fibrous tissue between the ununited bone ends. The cavity becomes lined by synovial membrane, which secretes synovial fluid. Nonunions occur in less than 5% of all fractures. They are most common in midshaft tibial fractures and fractures of the neck of the talus. Many factors can cause nonunion. They may be grouped as host-related factors, initial injury parameters, and method of treatment (Table 5–4).

Nonunions can be classified as atrophic or hypertrophic. In atrophic nonunions, the fracture callus is minimal, and the bone ends resorb (Fig. 5–11). Atrophic nonunions may occur when severe soft tissue injury, which removes the source of viable osteoprogenitor cells, has occurred. In hypertrophic nonunions, osteoprogenitor cells are present, and abundant fracture callus develops. However, the callus is not able to bridge the fracture site (Fig. 5–12).

Some nonunions heal with electric current applied across

Table 5–4 ■ **FACTORS THAT CONTRIBUTE TO NONUNIONS**

Type of Factor	Factor
Patient	Tobacco use
	Malnutrition
	Noncompliance with treatment regimens
Initial injury	Magnitude of initial injury
	Fracture displacement
	Soft tissue injury
	Open versus closed
	Comminution
	Presence of infection
	Vascular injury
Method of treatment	Poor surgical technique
	Inappropriate nonoperative treatment

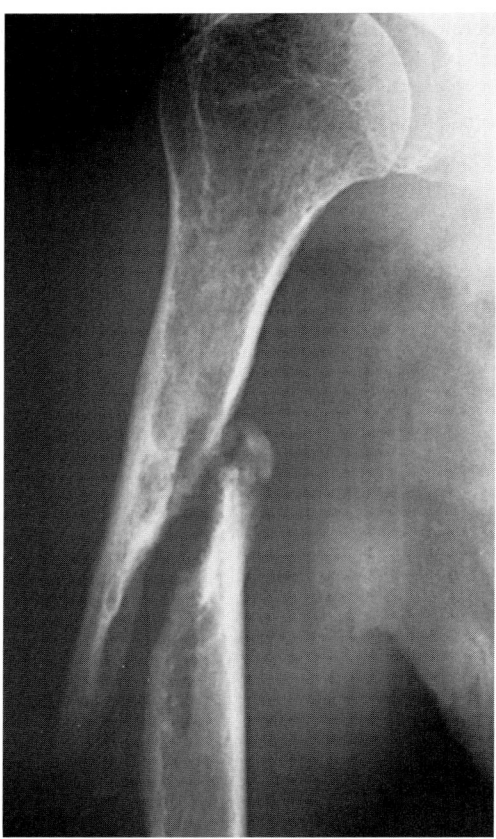

Figure 5–11 ■ An atrophic nonunion in a 70-year-old woman following a closed spiral fracture of the humerus. Nonunion can be caused by the interposition of soft tissues, such as muscle or tendon in the fracture gap. Note the lack of new bone formation.

the fracture site. An inductive coupling device is placed over the fracture site for 3 to 6 months. The electric current stimulates bone formation, probably by simulating normal bone electric activity, which regulates bone remodeling.[7-9] Most nonunions, however, require bone grafting. The fracture must be recreated by removing the fracture callus. Then the bones must be rigidly fixed and bone graft added. The bone graft has both osteoinductive and osteoconductive properties. Osteoinductive properties, due to the bone morphogenic proteins in the bone graft, induce new bone formation. Osteoconduction refers to the scaffold that the bone graft provides for new fracture callus.

SPECIAL TYPES OF FRACTURES

Although an occasional occult fracture may be missed on radiographic examination, typical fractures rarely present diagnostic problems. However, certain special types of fractures are frequently confused with other bone lesions. Most problematic are stress fractures or avulsion fractures.

Stress Fractures

Unlike a typical fracture, which is a complete break in a bone due to a single trauma, a stress fracture is a partial break secondary to repeated episodes of lesser trauma. The partial break is often accompanied by endosteal and periosteal new bone formation. If the repetitive stress continues, the lesion increases in size and may progress to a complete fracture. Diagnostic problems arise because the stress fracture may not be apparent on plain radiography or because the reactive bone changes mimic a more aggressive lesion.

Stress fractures occur in two settings. They may occur in normal bone subjected to unaccustomed stress (fatigue fractures), or they may occur in bone weakened by preexisting disease subjected to normal stresses (insufficiency fractures). Fatigue fractures are associated with a new, strenuous activity that is repeated regularly. Fatigue fractures may occur in any bone. At least 25 documented activities produce lesions at specific sites (Table 5–5). For example, fatigue fractures commonly occur in the metatarsals of military recruits who must march all day. Also, runners may develop fatigue fractures in almost any bone in the lower extremities, although the tibia and fibula are the most common sites.[10]

In contrast to fatigue fractures, insufficiency fractures develop in abnormal bone. Normal daily activities cause gradual fracturing through bone that is weak. Most commonly, this occurs in osteoporosis, and the bones affected are the pelvis, sacrum, and femur. Patients with osteomalacia also develop insufficiency fractures. In this setting, they are known as Looser zones (see Chapter 4).

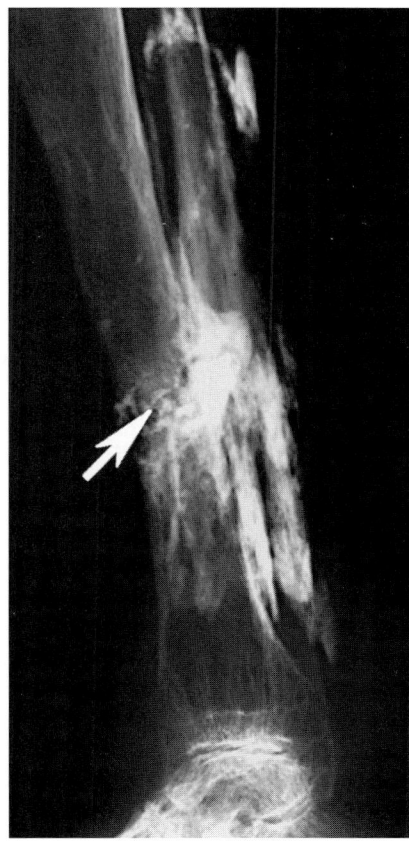

Figure 5–12 ■ Hypertrophic nonunion of the tibia. Extensive fracture callus can be seen, but the fracture line is still present (arrow).

Table 5–5 ■ **LOCATIONS OF STRESS FRACTURES BY INCITING ACTIVITY**

Location	Activity or Event
Sesamoids of metatarsal bones	Prolonged standing
Metatarsal shaft	Marching; standing on ground; prolonged standing; ballet
Navicular	Basketball; marching; long-distance running
Calcaneus	Jumping; parachuting; prolonged standing
Tibia	Long-distance running; baseball
Fibula	
Distal shaft	Long-distance running; jumping
Proximal shaft	Jumping; parachuting
Patella	Hurdling
Femur	
Shaft	Ballet; long-distance running
Neck	Long distance running; gymnastics; marching; ballet
Pelvis: Ischial and pubic rami	Stooping; bowling; gymnastics
Lumbar vertebra: pars interarticularis	Being an interior football lineman; gymnastics; ballet; lifting heavy objects; scrubbing floors
Lower cervical, upper thoracic spinous processes	Clay shoveling
Ribs	Carrying heavy packs; golf; coughing
Clavicle	Postoperative radical neck surgery
Coracoid of scapula	Trapshooting
Humerus: distal shaft	Throwing a ball
Ulna	
Coronoid	Pitching a ball
Shaft	Pitchfork work; propelling a wheelchair
Hook of the hamate	Striking a golf club; swinging a baseball bat or tennis racquet

Modified from Resnick, D., Goergen, T. G., and Niwayama, G.: Physical injury: Concepts and terminology. Resnick, D., Ed. *Diagnosis of Bone and Joint Disorders*, 3rd ed. Philadelphia, W. B. Saunders, 1995, p. 2590.

Stress fractures present with pain. Characteristically, the pain occurs with activity and is relieved by rest. In the early stages of a stress fracture, the pain is present only when the strenuous activity is performed. Later, pain is present even when normal stresses are applied.

Pathophysiology

The first stage in the development of a stress fracture is increased bone turnover, which is concentrated in the zone of maximum bone deformation.[11–15] This increased turnover, which is probably mediated by electric streaming potentials, is imbalanced—osteoblastic activity is less than osteoclastic activity. As a result, a thin zone of osteopenia develops. The trabeculae in this zone are thinner, and the cortex is porous. Next, a tiny crack develops in the porous cortex, and periosteal and endosteal reactive bone proliferates. If the activity continues, the crack lengthens to include trabecular bone, and reactive bone formation increases.

Radiologic Features

Early stress fractures may be completely inapparent on plain radiographs. As the lesion develops, however, a small

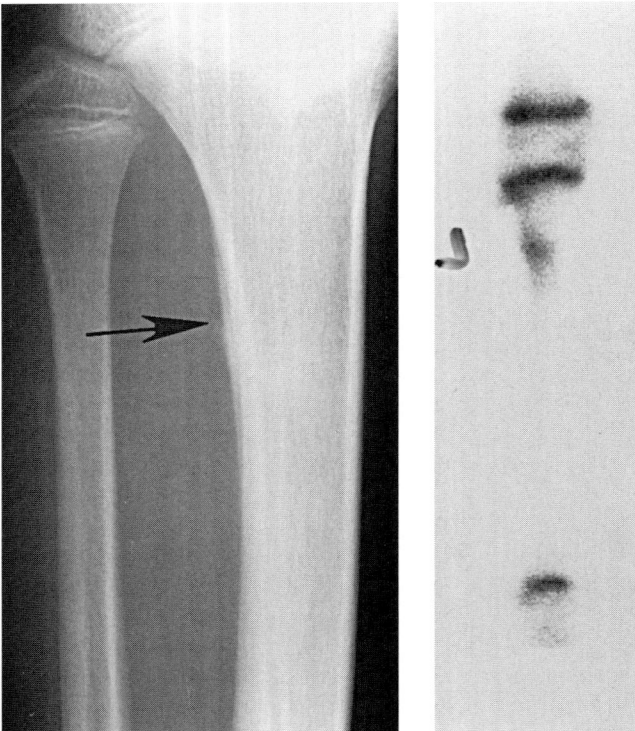

Figure 5-13 ■ An anteroposterior radiograph *(left panel)* demonstrates periosteal new bone formation along the lateral proximal cortex *(arrow)* in a 14-year-old boy with a stress fracture. The boy was a baseball player and developed pain at the beginning of the season. The technetium bone scan *(right panel)* demonstrates increased uptake as the osteoblasts lay down new bone.

amount of reactive periosteal new bone appears. At this stage, a bone scan is diagnostic—a linear zone of tracer accumulation is present (Fig. 5–13). As this process continues, plain radiographs show a linear zone of osteopenia or mixed osteopenia and sclerosis (Fig. 5–14). A magnetic resonance imaging scan is useful to delimit the osseous change (Fig. 5–15). The periosteal reaction is sometimes florid and can mimic a neoplasm. In late stress fractures and in healing lesions, the periosteal reaction consolidates into a smoothly contoured surface density.

Pathologic Features

Although the clinical history of pain associated with repeated activity should be a clue to the correct diagnosis, some stress fractures are misdiagnosed as infections or neoplasms and are biopsied. Histologically, a biopsy sample from a stress fracture shows fracture callus. Irregular seams of osteoid or woven bone are present in granulation tissue or a loose fibrovascular stroma. Islands of cartilage undergoing endochondral ossification are also present (Fig. 5–16). Sometimes, marked cellularity and abundant osteoid may mimic a bone-forming neoplasm. However, unlike a neoplasm, acute stress fractures show a zonal pattern—bone is denser and more mature at the periphery of the lesion. Also, pleomorphic cells are not present in a stress fracture. Chronic or healed stress fractures contain dense trabecular or cortical bone with an intervening fibrous stroma. The zonal pattern may no longer be present, and the bone is lamellar with mature haversian systems.

Avulsion Injury

An avulsion injury is another special type of fracture. Because tendon and the tendon insertion into bone often have stronger tensile strength than the bone itself, a violent muscle contraction or repetitive muscle contraction may pull off a portion of bone. This avulsion injury, which is occasionally seen in active young patients, causes cortical irregularity and periosteal reactive tissue proliferation. Sometimes a large fragment of bone is detached (Fig. 5–17). Common sites of avulsion include the ischial tuberosity, the greater or lesser trochanter, the iliac spines, and the humerus at the insertion of the pectoralis major. However, the two most common sites of avulsion are the tibial tuberosity, a disorder known as Osgood-Schlatter disease, and the medial distal

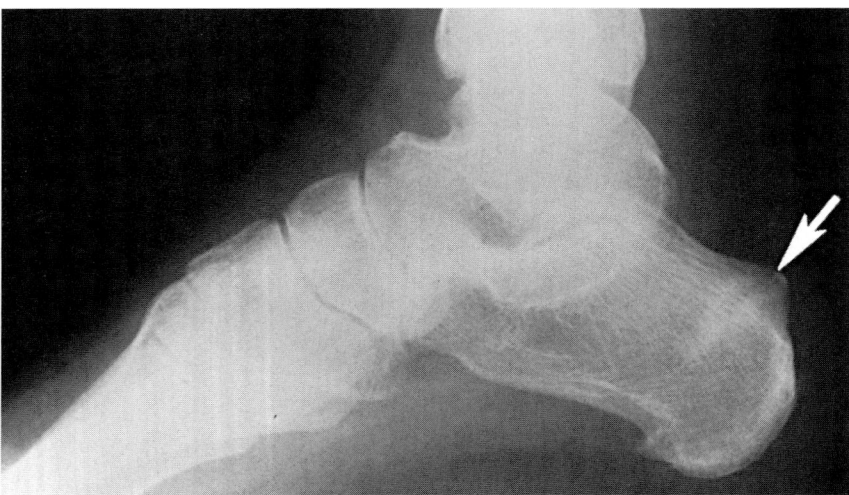

Figure 5-14 ■ Lateral radiograph of the calcaneus demonstrates a stress fracture with a lucent linear band with sclerotic borders *(arrow)*. Calcaneal stress fractures are common in runners.

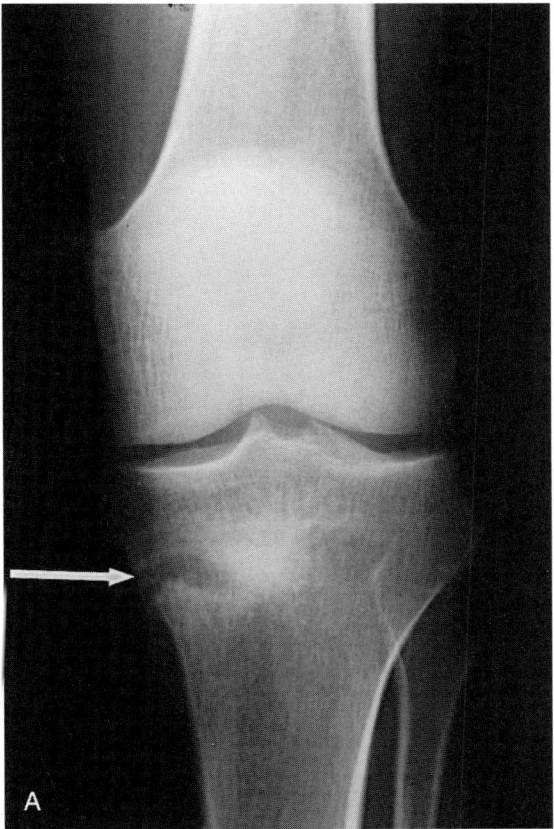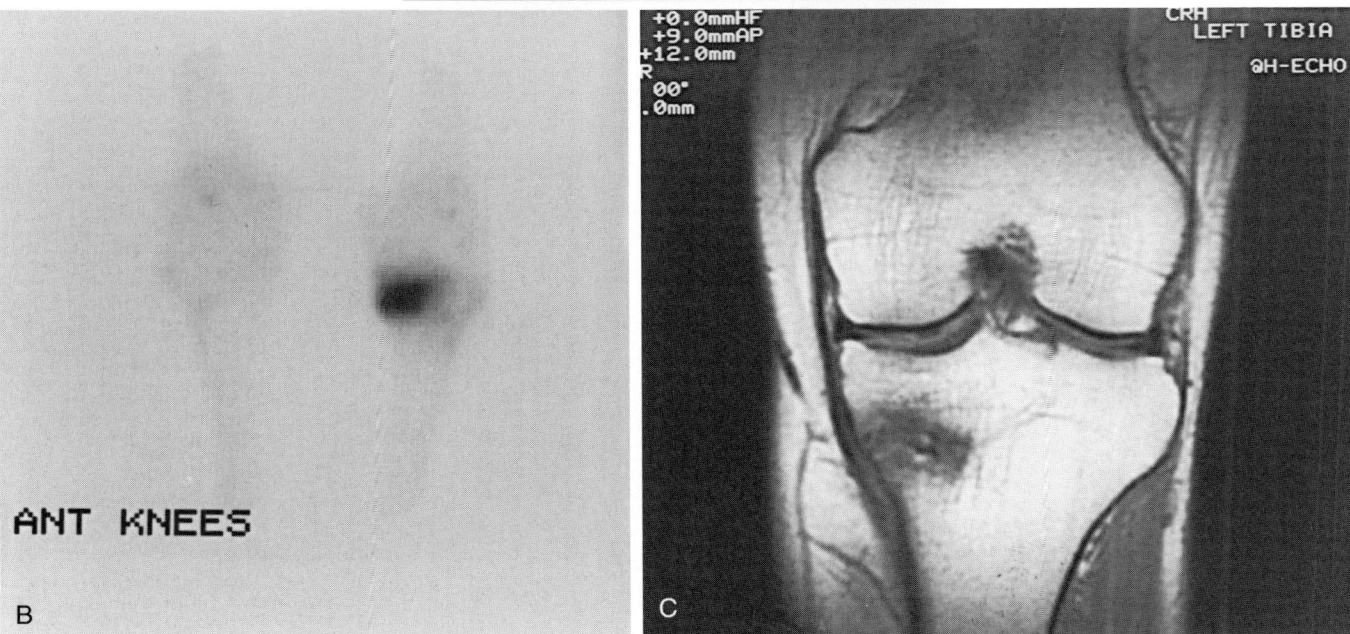

Figure 5-15 ■ Stress fracture of the proximal tibia. **A,** Anteroposterior radiograph of the knee in a 40-year-old man with knee pain following heavy activity. Because of the exuberant new bone formation seen in the metaphysis *(arrow),* he was referred with the diagnosis of osteosarcoma. **B,** The technetium bone scan demonstrates intense uptake over the medial tibial metaphysis. **C,** The T_1-weighted magnetic resonance imaging demonstrates the low signal associated with new bone formation. The normal marrow is demonstrated by the homogeneous high signal. No evidence of a malignant lesion is seen.

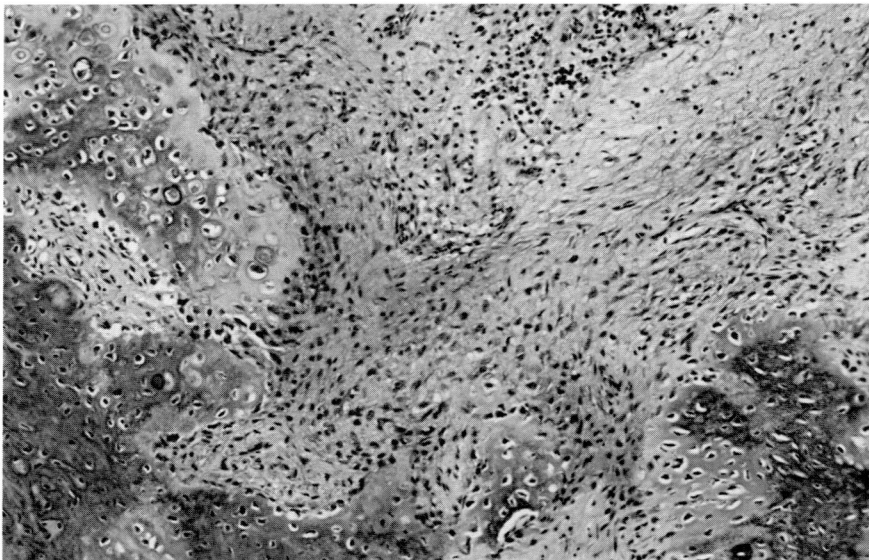

Figure 5-16 ■ Photomicrograph of a stress fracture showing fracture callus with a zonal arrangement of fibrous tissue, cartilage, and bone.

femoral metaphysis. Osgood-Schlatter disease is discussed in Chapter 7.

Distal Femoral Cortical Erosion Syndrome (Periosteal Desmoid)

An avulsion injury of the distal femoral metaphysis is known as the *distal femoral cortical irregularity syndrome*. Because fibrous tissue proliferation occurs in this lesion, it was formerly called "periosteal desmoid." This process characteristically occurs on the medial surface of the distal femoral metaphysis. Initiated by the pull of the adductor magnus tendon, periosteal reactive bone forms adjacent to a scalloped cortex.[16-24] This lesion occurs exclusively in children and adolescents, the reported age range being 3 to 22 years. Small cortical irregularities in this region are present in 11.5% of male patients and 3.5% of female patients, and as many as one third of patients have bilateral lesions. Although most patients are asymptomatic, some present with pain after strenuous physical activity, a symptom that prompts radiographic examination.

Radiographic Features. The plain radiographic features of most cases of the distal femoral cortical irregularity syndrome are characteristic. A 1- to 3-cm zone of cortical erosion is present on the posterior medial aspect of the distal femoral metaphysis (Fig. 5–18). Some lesions may cause a poorly defined lytic area, and in many cases, periosteal new bone is present. Occasionally, the reactive periosteal bone is extensive and has a sunburst appearance, a pattern simulating a malignant neoplasm. Magnetic resonance imaging is useful in florid cases to outline specific intramedullary reactive changes. This imaging modality shows a well-demarcated medullary lesion, which is hypointense on T_1-weighted images and hyperintense on T_2-weighted images. In both images, the lesion is surrounded by a dark rim.

Histologic Features. Like stress fractures, avulsion injuries are often accompanied by extensive reactive bone proliferation and therefore mistaken for malignant neoplasms. The distal femoral cortical erosion syndrome may be particularly problematic because it occurs in the same age group and most common location of osteosarcoma. Although awareness of the distal femoral cortical erosion syndrome

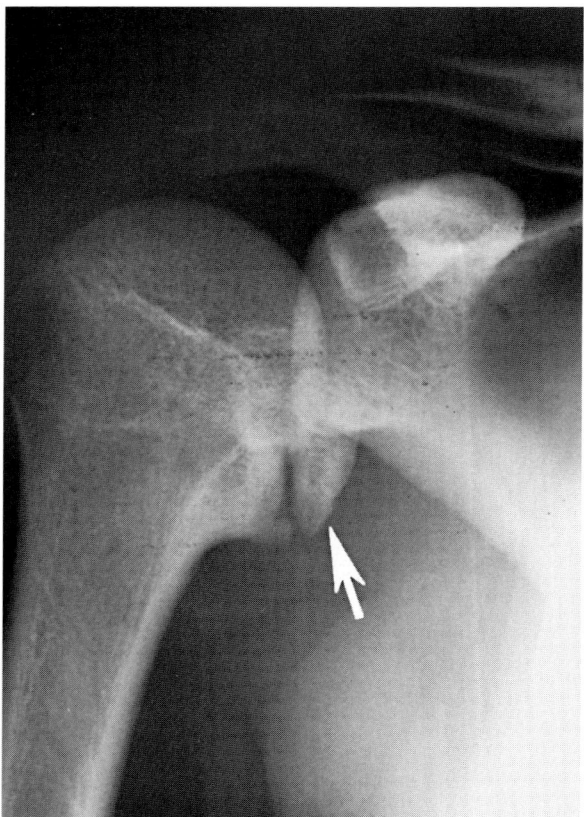

Figure 5-17 ■ Anteroposterior radiograph of the shoulder demonstrating exuberant new bone formation following an avulsion fracture of the lesser tuberosity. The subscapularis muscle inserts on the lesser tuberosity and may be pulled off *(arrow)* following a posterior dislocation of the shoulder.

usually prevents overdiagnosis, these lesions are occasionally biopsied.

Histologically, the distal femoral cortical irregularity syndrome shows a wide range of reactive tissues. Some lesions are densely fibrous, with bland fibroblasts in a highly collagenized matrix. Other lesions contain very cellular fibrous tissue (Fig. 5–19) and abundant osteoid. The osteoid seams are lined by typical osteoblasts. In addition, cartilage is occasionally present.

Although normal mitotic figures may be present in the fibrous tissue, cellular pleomorphism and atypical mitoses, necessary for the diagnosis of osteosarcoma, are not present in the distal femoral cortical irregularity syndrome.

PATHOLOGIC FRACTURES

Although normal bone has a great resistance to fracture, abnormal bone fractures with minimal trauma. In fact, severely weakened bone may fracture without trauma. Fractures may occur through large bony defects caused by neoplasms, or they may occur through bone that is structurally weak due to congenital or metabolic disease.

Fractures Through Neoplasms

Malignant bone tumors are the most common cause of pathologic fractures. In adults, metastatic bone disease, multiple myeloma, and lymphoma are the most common causes

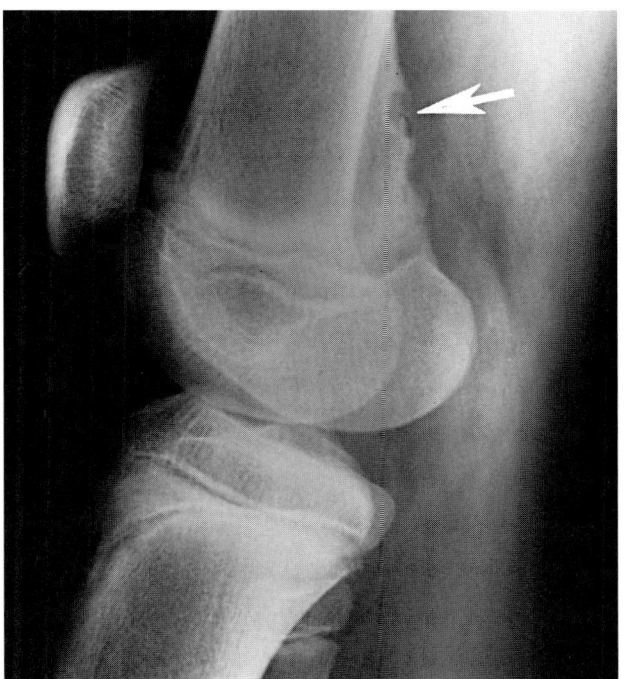

Figure 5–18 ■ Oblique radiograph of the distal femur demonstrating a lucent area in the cortex with periosteal new bone formation *(arrow)*. This is the typical location and appearance of the distal femoral cortical irregularity syndrome. (From McCarthy, E. F.: *Differential Diagnosis in Pathology. Bone and Joint Disorders.* New York and Tokyo, Igaku-Shoin, 1996. With permission from Williams & Wilkins.)

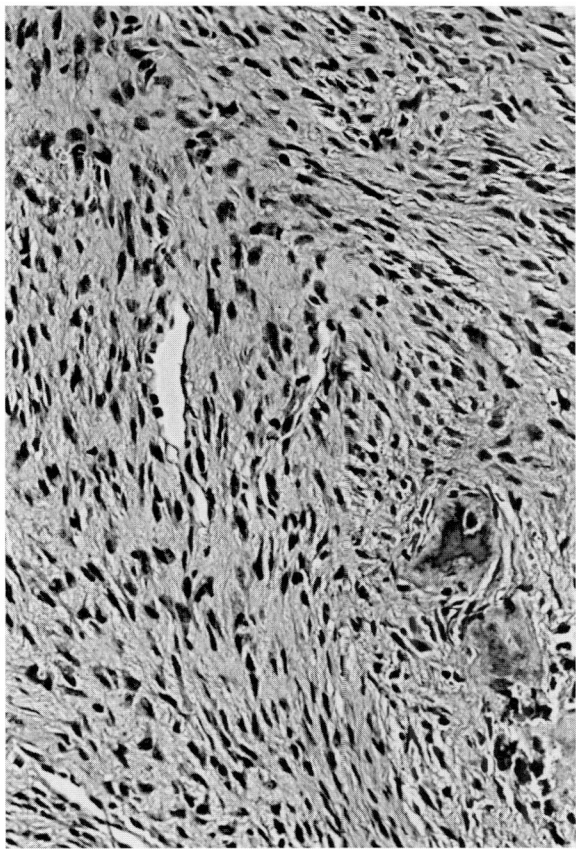

Figure 5–19 ■ Photomicrograph of distal femoral cortical irregularity syndrome. Cellular fibrous tissue contains a few spicules of woven bone.

of pathologic fractures. The tumor process activates the osteoclasts, and bone is resorbed. When more than 50% of the cortical bone has been destroyed, the risk of fracture is significant (Fig. 5–20). Lesions that are purely blastic, such as occur in metastatic breast and prostate carcinomas, seldom fracture. By contrast, purely lytic lesions are very prone to fracture.

In children, about 5 to 10% of osteosarcomas and Ewing sarcomas cause pathologic fractures. Usually the children describe antecedent pain in the extremity over the involved bone. Unicameral bone cysts, however, are the most common lesions that fracture in children. When these fractures occur in the proximal humerus, lesions may be injected with steroids when the fracture is healed. When the fracture occurs through a cyst in the proximal femur, the treatment is more difficult, and surgery with internal fixation may be necessary.

Fractures in Bone Weakened by Congenital or Metabolic Disease

Fractures are the most common presentation of patients with metabolic bone disease. Osteoporosis and osteomalacia are two metabolic bone diseases that commonly develop in pathologic fractures. By the time these diseases are apparent with plain radiographs, bones have lost as much as 50% of

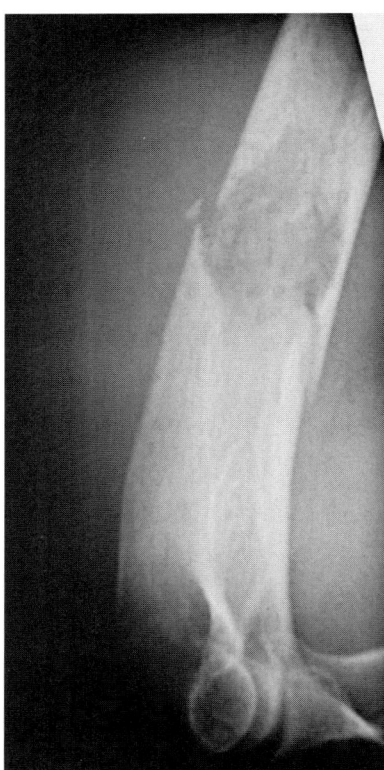

Figure 5-20 ■ Pathologic fracture through a focus of metastatic carcinoma in the humerus.

their strength (see Chapter 4). Therefore, in metabolic bone disease, fractures may occur through apparently normal bone. An important aspect of the evaluation of any fracture is to learn the exact mechanism of the fracture and the force that the patient sustained. Fractures with minimal or no trauma should raise the suspicion of an underlying bone disease.

Bone weakening can be due to many factors. In osteoporosis, both the matrix and mineral are reduced. In addition, osteoporotic bone is architecturally abnormal, and the collagen fibers are weak. In osteomalacia, the bones are poorly mineralized. In osteogenesis imperfecta, bone collagen is abnormal.

Bones do not have to be osteopenic to be weak. Dense bones can also be brittle if architectural distortion has occurred. For example, in Paget's disease and osteopetrosis, diseases characterized by radiodensity, bones fracture easily. This is because the hollow tube of the long bones is converted into a solid cylinder, a much weaker structure. Pathologic fractures through architecturally distorted bones are often transverse, a so-called "banana" or "chalk-stick" pattern of fracture.

REFERENCES

1. Ostrum, R. F., Chao, E. Y., Bassett, C. A., et al.: Bone injury, regeneration, and repair. Simon, S. R., Ed. *Orthopaedic Basic Science.* American Academy of Orthopaedic Surgeons, 1994, pp. 277–323.
2. Harkess, J. W., Ramsey, W. C., and Ahmadi, B.: Principles of fractures and dislocations. Rockwood, C. A., and Green, D. P., Eds. *Fractures in Adults,* 2nd ed. New York, Raven Press, 1984, pp. 1–9.
3. Chao, E. Y. S., and Aro, H. T.: Biomechanics of fracture fixation. Mow, V. C., and Hayes, W. C., Eds. *Basic Orthopaedic Biomechanics.* New York, Raven Press, 1991, pp. 293–328.
4. Gustillo, R. B., and Anderson, J. T.: Prevention of infection in the treatment of one thousand and twenty-five open fractures of long bones. *J Bone Joint Surg* 58A:453–458, 1976.
5. Perren, S. M.: Physical and biological aspects of fracture healing with special reference to internal fixation. *Clin Orthop* 138:175–196, 1979.
6. Perren, S. M., and Cordey, J.: Mechanics of interfragmentary compression by plates and screws. Uhthoff, H. K., Ed. *Current Concepts of Internal Fixation of Fractures.* Berlin, Springer-Verlag, pp. 184–191.
7. Bassett, C. A.: The development and application of pulsed electromagnetic fields (PEMFs) for ununited fractures and arthrodeses. *Orthop Clin North Am* 15:61–87, 1984.
8. Cruess, R. L.: Healing of bone, tendon, and ligament. Rockwood, C. A., and Green, D. P., Eds. *Fractures in Adults,* 2nd ed. New York, Raven Press, 1984, pp. 147–167.
9. Friedenberg, Z. B., and Brighton, C. T.: Bioelectric potentials in bone. *J Bone Joint Surg* 48A:915–923, 1966.
10. McBryde, A. M.: Stress fractures in athletes. *J Sports Med* 3:212–217, 1975.
11. Resnick, D., Goergen, T. G., and Niwayama, G.: Physical injury: Concepts and terminology. Resnick, D., Ed. *Diagnosis of Bone and Joint Disorders,* 3rd ed. Philadelphia, W. B. Saunders, 1995, pp. 2561–2692.
12. Sweet, D. E., and Allman, R. M.: Stress fracture. RPC of the month from the AFIP. *Radiology* 99:687–693, 1971.
13. Johnson, L. C.: Morphologic analysis in pathology. Frost, H. H., Ed. *Bone Biodynamics. Henry Ford Hospital International Symposium.* Boston, Little, Brown & Co., 1964, p. 607.
14. Burr, D. B., Milgrom, C., Boyd, R. D., et al.: Experimental stress fractures of the tibia. Biological and mechanical aetiology in rabbits. *J Bone Joint Surg* 72B:370, 1990.
15. Mori, S., and Burr, D. B.: Increased cortical remodeling following fatigue damage. *Bone* 14:103–109, 1993.
16. Barnes, G. R. Jr., and Gwinn, J. L.: Distal irregularities of the femur simulating malignancy. *Am J Roentgenol* 122:180, 1974.
17. Brower, A. C., Culver, J. E. Jr., and Keats, T. E.: Histologic nature of the cortical irregularity of the medial posterior distal femoral metaphysis in children. *Radiology* 99:389–392, 1971.
18. Bufkin, W. J.: The avulsive cortical irregularity. *Am J Roentgenol* 112:487–492, 1971.
19. Dunham, W. K., Marcus, N. W., Enneking, W. R., and Haun, C.: Developmental defects of the distal femoral metaphysis. *J Bone Joint Surg* 62A:801–806, 1980.
20. Johnson, L. C., Genner, B. A. III, Engh, C. A., and Brown, R. H.: Cortical desmoids. *J Bone Joint Surg* 50A:828, 1968.
21. Kimmetstiel, P., and Rapp, I. H.: Cortical defect due to periosteal desmoids. *Bull Hosp Joint Dis* 12:286, 1951.
22. Kreis, W. R., and Hensinger, R. N.: Irregularity of the distal femoral metaphysis simulating malignancy. Case report. *J Bone Joint Surg* 59A:838, 1977.
23. Sontag, L. W., and Pyle, S. I.: The appearance and nature of cyst-like areas in the distal femoral metaphyses of children. *Am J Roentgenol* 46:185, 1941.
24. Resnick, D., and Greenway, G.: Distal femoral cortical defects, irregularities, and excavations. A critical review of the literature with the addition of histologic and paleopathologic data. *Radiology* 143:345–354, 1982.

CHAPTER 6
Skeletal Manifestations of Systemic Disease

Over 100 systemic diseases cause secondary changes in bone. In this chapter, we discuss the most common of these disorders and those that produce the most striking osseous lesions. The skeletal manifestations of these systemic diseases may be severe and present very difficult problems in patient management. For example, as discussed in Chapter 2, all patients with chronic renal disease develop osseous abnormalities, and in some, the changes are a source of significant morbidity. By contrast, bone involvement in other systemic diseases—sarcoidosis, for example—is only an occasional and clinically insignificant finding.

The systemic diseases that most commonly affect the skeleton fall into two major categories: proliferative disorders of the hematopoietic system and proliferative disorders of the reticuloendothelial system. Bone changes occur in these disease categories because the affected cells of each reside in the bone marrow. Important hematopoietic proliferations include systemic mastocytosis, leukemia, sickle cell anemia, thalassemia, and myelofibrosis. The skeletal changes in these disorders tend to be diffuse and symmetric.

In the second category, proliferations of the reticuloendothelial system, diseases tend to be multifocal and asymmetric. Among these disorders are Langerhans' cell granulomatosis, sarcoidosis, sinus histiocytosis with massive lymphadenopathy, Erdheim-Chester disease, and multicentric reticulohistiocytosis.

In addition to hematologic or reticuloendothelial proliferations, bone changes occur in diseases of other organ systems. Of these we only discuss pulmonary hypertrophic osteoarthropathy, a skeletal complication of various disorders of the lung.

In almost all the systemic diseases that secondarily involve bone, the primary disease has been diagnosed before osseous changes are noted. Bone involvement is incidental and poses no diagnostic problems. However, in one disorder, Langerhans' cell granulomatosis, bone lesions are often the presenting complaint. In this disorder, the bone lesion often must be diagnosed without systemic clues.

RETICULOENDOTHELIAL DISEASES

Langerhans' Cell Granulomatosis

Langerhans' cell granulomatosis encompasses a group of disorders that have no known etiology and variable clinical outcomes.[1,2] Lichtenstein first popularized the term *histiocytosis X* for these disorders because the proliferating cells resembled histiocytes.[3-5] He felt that histiocytosis X represented a spectrum that encompassed three disorders: eosinophilic granuloma of bone, Hand-Schüller Christian disease, and Letterer-Siwe disease. Today, the terminology has changed. The term *histiocytosis X* is no longer used because the proliferating cells are not true histiocytes—they lack phagocytic capability. Also, the eponyms are no longer used for the systemic manifestations of the disease because of overlapping clinical features.

The hallmark of this disorder is the Langerhans' cell, a cell that is part of the widespread system of dendritic cells.[6] These cells arise from CD34+ progenitors and become specialized to present antigens for T-cell–mediated immunity.[6] They are normally present in the skin, lymph nodes, thymus, and other organs. These cells were first noticed in 1865 by a medical student, Paul Langerhans. He described them after applying Cohnheim's gold chloride to a section of epidermis, and, later, they came to bear his name.[7] In the past, the Langerhans' cells were thought to be histiocytes and part of the monocyte-macrophage system. Hence, proliferations of this cell were called histiocytosis or Langerhans' cell histiocytosis. Eosinophils are often found intermingled with the Langerhans' cells in these disorders, but they are not necessary for the diagnosis.

This disorder is now called Langerhans' cell granulomatosis, emphasizing the nonhistiocytic nature of the proliferating cell. Although most investigators feel that the disease is a reactive cellular proliferation, the recent finding of clonality in lesions suggests that it may be neoplastic.[8]

Langerhans' cell granulomatosis may be unifocal or

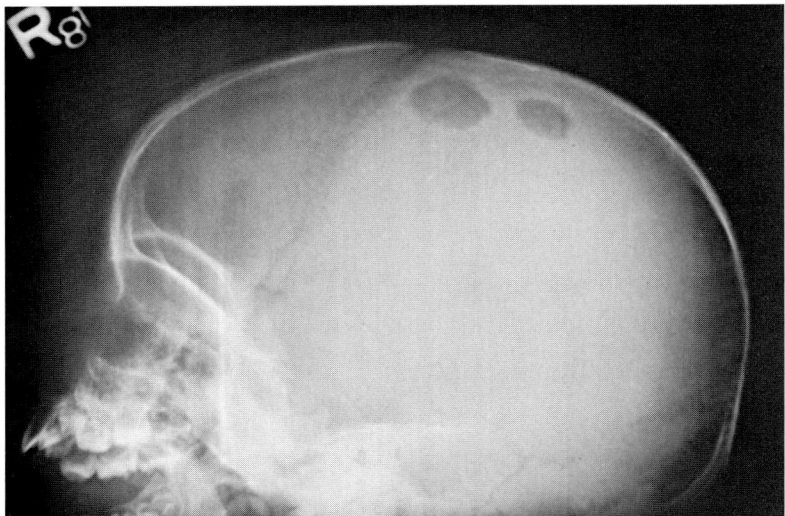

Figure 6-1 ▪ Eosinophilic granuloma of the skull. Two sharply defined lytic lesions are present.

multifocal, and lesions can involve bone, skin, soft tissue, and parenchymal organs. Destructive bone lesions are a constant feature of the disease, whereas visceral organ involvement is a variable feature. Localized lesions of Langerhans' cell granulomatosis are known as *eosinophilic granuloma*.

Unifocal Langerhans' Cell Granulomatosis (Eosinophilic Granuloma of Bone)

Eosinophilic granuloma is the localized form of the disease that occurs at single skeletal sites. Children are most commonly affected, and 90% are between ages 5 and 15 years.[9] However, a lesion may occasionally be found in patients as old as 60 years. Children generally present with symptoms related to the destructive lesion. Most present with a limp or well-localized pain in an extremity or the back. However, about 10% of lesions are asymptomatic and may be found incidentally when radiographs are taken for other reasons.

The most common locations of eosinophilic granuloma are the skull, femur, pelvis, ribs, and spine. Less common locations include the jaw, humerus, and clavicle. In the spine, the vertebral bodies are usually involved, and the posterior elements are spared.

The radiographs show a variable pattern of bone destruction. A well-circumscribed punched-out lesion with no periosteal reaction is the most common appearance (Fig. 6–1). Occasionally, lesions show a so-called "hole in a hole" pattern because of the different rates of bone destruction of the inner and outer cortical surfaces (Fig. 6–2). In contrast to the more common well-circumscribed lesions, the bone destruction may also have a permeative or moth-eaten pattern with periosteal reaction (Fig. 6–3). This aggressive appearance may be confused with osteomyelitis, Ewing sarcoma, or hematologic malignancies such as leukemia or lymphoma. Periosteal new bone formation is common once the lesion has destroyed the cortical bone, and occasionally an adjacent soft tissue mass is present.

Vertebral lesions have a characteristic appearance following fracture and collapse. The body flattens, losing about 75% of its height. It also gains a similar amount in width. This pattern is known as *vertebra plana* (Fig. 6–4). Clinicians must carefully evaluate children with a collapsed vertebral body because Ewing sarcoma and osteomyelitis can have a similar appearance.

Histologic features of all manifestations of Langerhans'

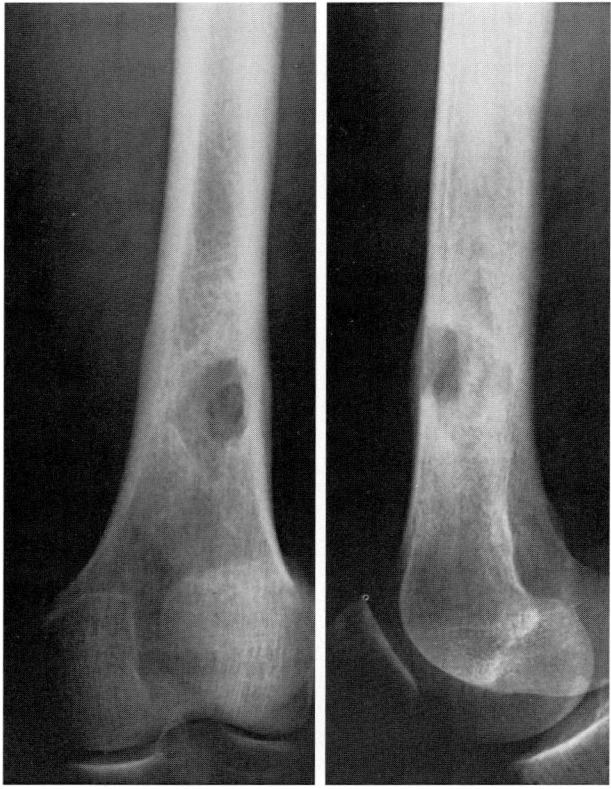

Figure 6-2 ▪ Anteroposterior *(left)* and lateral radiographs of eosinophilic granuloma of the femur. This lesion shows the characteristic "hole within a hole" pattern.

cell granulomatosis are similar. Lesions consist of heterogeneous inflammatory infiltrate. However, the diagnostic cell is the Langerhans' cell. This distinctive cell is characterized by abundant cytoplasm with a bean-shaped nucleus, often with a nuclear groove (Fig. 6–5). Occasionally, these cells fuse to form multinucleated giant cells. Unlike true histiocytes, the Langerhans' cell is positive with immunohistochemical stains for S-100 protein. Electron microscopy of these cells demonstrates cytoplasmic granules, known as Birbeck granules, which are invaginations of the cell membrane.[10–12]

The Langerhans' cells are usually grouped in loose clusters simulating granuloma (Fig. 6–6). However, discrete granulomas characteristic of fungal or tuberculous infections are not present.

In addition to Langerhans' cells, lesions contain other inflammatory cells, including true histiocytes, lymphocytes, plasma cells, and large numbers of eosinophils, although in rare lesions, eosinophils may be absent. In older lesions of Langerhans' cell granulomatosis, the Langerhans' cells may be obscured by dense fibrosis. In addition, these cells in older lesions stain much less strongly for S-100 protein.

Several treatment options are available for eosinophilic granuloma after a biopsy has established the diagnosis, including (1) observation only after biopsy, (2) curettage with or without bone grafting, (3) corticosteroid injection, (4)

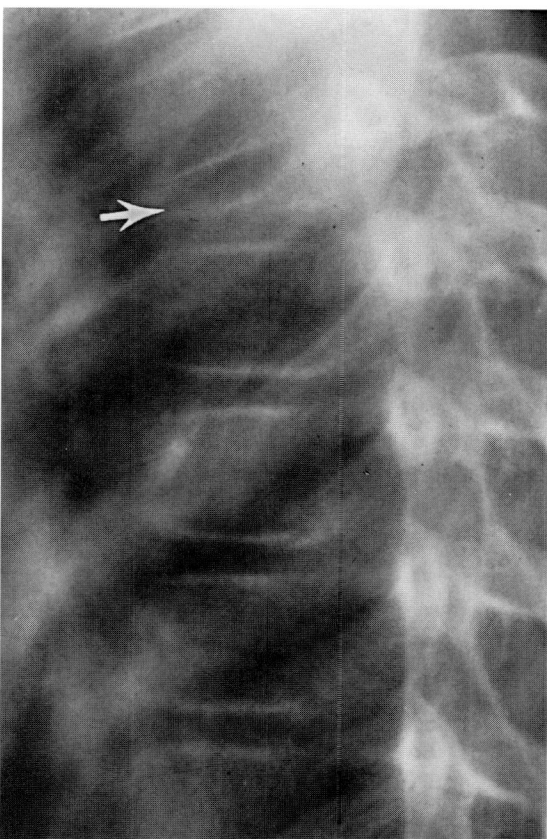

Figure 6-4 ■ Vertebra plana of a thoracic vertebra *(arrow)*.

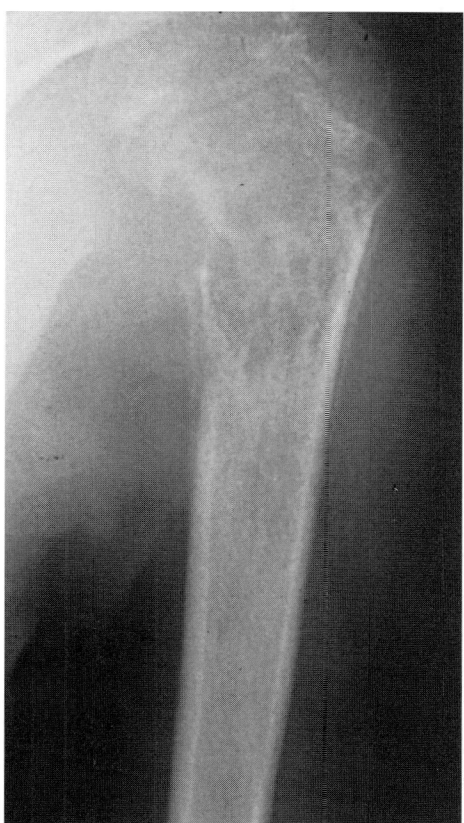

Figure 6-3 ■ Eosinophilic granuloma of the proximal humerus. The lesion is highly destructive and has a periosteal reaction. This pattern may be mistaken for a malignant neoplasm.

low-dose radiotherapy, and (5) chemotherapy with either systemic steroids or antimitotic medications. Observation alone is suitable for lesions that are asymptomatic and do not threaten skeletal structural stability. In one series, only 3 of 10 patients who were observed without treatment eventually required surgical intervention. Curettage with or without bone grafting is necessary for larger symptomatic lesions that have not destroyed the cortex. Alternatively, good results have been achieved by intralesional corticosteroid injection.[13,14]

Low-dose external beam irradiation can be used for inaccessible lesions or lesions that would require extensive reconstructive surgical procedures. Low doses of 600 to 1200 cGy in two to four fractions are effective. These low doses carry almost no risk for the development of a postradiation sarcoma. Chemotherapy can be used for multiple or recurrent lesions; however, this modality is seldom required.

The prognosis is excellent for patients with localized disease. In one large series, 21 of 30 patients were successfully treated without recurrence. Of the nine children with recurrent lesions, a second curettage was curative in all patients.

Disseminated Langerhans' Cell Granulomatosis

In contrast to the indolent, often self-limited course of unifocal Langerhans' cell granulomatosis, disseminated disease may be aggressive. Multifocal disease can involve a wide variety of sites and produce multiple signs and symptoms. For example, multifocal disease may be confined to several osseous locations, a presentation accounting for 62% of disseminated cases. A combination of bone and soft tissue sites accounts for 23% of cases, and soft tissue only sites account for only 15%.

The prognosis of multifocal disease depends on the age of the patient and the number of extraosseous sites involved. Generally, the younger the child at the time of diagnosis, the worse the prognosis. For example, children less than 6 months of age have a mortality rate as high as 80% compared with children older than age 3 years.[15] Although the prognosis of multifocal disease confined to bone is excellent, it worsens relative to the number of extraosseous sites. These sites include skin, liver, spleen, lung, central nervous system, lymph nodes, and bone marrow.

Disseminated disease results in many characteristic features.[9] For example, involvement of the face and skull may result in diabetes insipidus, exophthalmos, otitis media, or loose teeth. Hepatosplenomegaly may be prominent, and many patients have a skin rash. Involvement of the bone marrow results in anemia. Lung infiltrates can cause dyspnea and cyanosis, and liver involvement can lead to hepatic dysfunction.

Although many authors have described fatal cases of

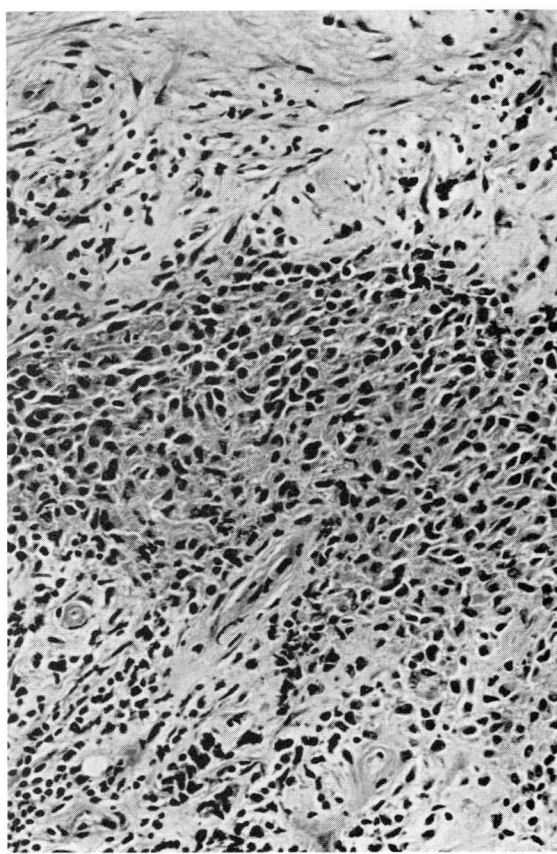

Figure 6-6 ■ Photomicrograph of eosinophilic granuloma. The Langerhans' cells are in a cluster that vaguely resembles a granuloma.

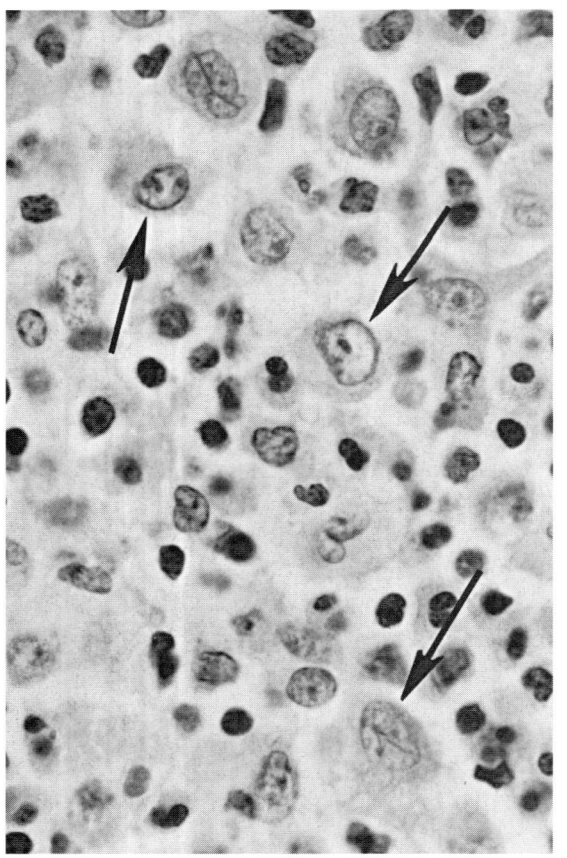

Figure 6-5 ■ Photomicrograph of a focus of Langerhans' cell granulomatosis. Numerous round Langerhans' cells are present (arrows).

multifocal form of the disease, Lieberman and colleagues,[6] in a series of 238 patients, reported no deaths that could be directly attributed to the Langerhans' cell granulomatosis. It is likely that even multifocal disease runs a benign, self-limited course that resolves within 5 to 7 years of diagnosis. Eight of 153 patients with unifocal disease and 12 of 85 with multifocal disease died during the period of this study. Although several patients died of chemotherapy complications, none died of a cause directly attributable to the Langerhans' cell granulomatosis.

Historically, numerous treatment regimens have been employed for disseminated disease. These have included pituitary extract, low-cholesterol diet, parathyroid extract, insulin, cod liver oil, arsenic, irradiated foods, and many others. The modern treatment of patients with systemic disease is corticosteroids (prednisolone), chemotherapy (vinblastine or 6-mercaptopurine), or a combination of the two. In one series, 5 of 10 patients had a complete response to medical treatment without evidence of recurrence. In the same series, three patients had no response to treatment, and two of these patients died from organ failure. Sessa and others[1] have outlined a treatment strategy based on the location, activity, and morbidity associated with each treatment (Table 6-1). Late sequelae following treatment include persistent diabetes insipidus, growth retardation, and chronic obstructive pulmonary disease.

Table 6-1 ■ **MANAGEMENT OF PATIENTS WHO HAVE LANGERHANS' CELL HISTIOCYTOSIS**

Type of Disease	Symptoms	Management Techniques
Localized disease		
Osseous lesion	Asymptomatic	Biopsy, observation, or curettage
Osseous lesion	Pain	Biopsy and
		Currettage or
		Low-dose radiation or
		Steroid injection or
		Observation
Inaccessible osseous lesion	Pain	Biopsy and
		Low-dose radiation or
		Steroid injection
Vertebral lesion	With or without neurologic signs and symptoms	Cast immobilization and
		Low-dose radiation or
		Steroid injection
Aggressive skeletal lesion: impending fracture	Pain	Biopsy, curettage, and bone grafting and/or internal fixation
Systemic disease without organ dysfunction		
Skin, osseous lesion	Asymptomatic	Biopsy, observation
Osseous lesion with organ dysfunction	Pain	Low-dose radiotherapy
Liver, lung, hematopoietic system	Organ dysfunction	Chemotherapy and/or corticotherapy

Modified from Sessa, S., Sommelet, D., Lascombes, P., and Prevot, J.: Treatment of Langerhans'-cell histiocytosis in children. *J Bone Joint Surg* 76A:1513–1525, 1994.

Sarcoidosis of Bone

Sarcoidosis is a chronic multisystem disorder of unknown etiology that primarily affects the lymph nodes, lungs, and skin. The disease is characterized by the accumulation of noncaseating epithelioid granulomas that distort the normal architecture of the involved organ. The disease probably results from an exaggerated cellular immune response (acquired, inherited, or both) to a limited class of antigens or self-antigens.

Sarcoidosis usually develops in young adults between ages 20 and 40, and women are more commonly affected than men. African-Americans are affected 10 times as often as whites.

Histologically, lesions of sarcoidosis are characterized by granulomatous inflammation. The granulomas are tight, compact aggregates of histiocytes with admixed multinucleated giant cells. Occasionally, focal necrosis is present within the granulomas. The histiocytes are usually surrounded by a rim of helper-inducer T lymphocytes and, to a lesser extent, B lymphocytes.[16]

Because the disease can affect many organs, the clinical symptoms are highly variable. They may reflect involvement of the lungs, lymph nodes, skin, eye, nasal mucosa, liver, kidney, nervous system, or musculoskeletal system. A typical presentation is a young adult with constitutional complaints, erythema nodosum, blurred vision, and respiratory symptoms such as shortness of breath and cough.[16] A chest radiograph typically shows hilar adenopathy. Although sarcoidosis is a chronic disease, patients may present with acute symptoms. In the acute setting, the combination of hilar adenopathy, erythema nodosum, fever, and articular manifestations is known as Lofgren's syndrome.[17,18]

Sarcoidosis may involve the joints or the bones. Approximately 25% of sarcoidosis patients have joint involvement. They have either an acute or a chronic polyarthritis.[19] In the acute form, patients usually present with pain in the ankles, knees, elbows, wrists, and hands.[19] These joint symptoms usually occur in association with extraskeletal manifestations, such as erythema nodosum, hilar lymph node enlargement, fever, and uveitis.

The chronic form of polyarthritis occurs in patients with long-standing sarcoidosis. Patients have a long history of joint pain, especially in the ankles, knees, shoulders, wrists, and small joints of the hands. These symptoms may wax and wane. Most patients have concurrent skin and pulmonary involvement. Synovial biopsy shows the typical noncaseating granulomas in both the acute and chronic forms (Fig. 6–7).

From 5 to 10% of sarcoidosis patients have bone lesions.[19,20] Patients with osseous sarcoidosis usually have skin lesions as well, and from 80 to 90% have radiographic evidence of pulmonary disease. Therefore, because most patients have documented sarcoidosis, the osseous lesions present few diagnostic problems. Although any bone can be involved, the hand is the most common location, and lesions occur most commonly in the phalanges (Fig. 6–8). The lesions are almost always lytic and show several patterns of bone destruction. For example, diffuse resorption may result in a honeycomb pattern. Alternatively, lesions may be well-defined lytic areas with sclerotic rims.

In addition to focal lytic lesions, osseous sarcoidosis may present as diffuse osteopenia or as focal areas of osteosclerosis. This latter pattern, sometimes seen in the distal phalanges, is known as acroosteosclerosis.

Sinus Histiocytosis with Massive Lymphadenopathy

Langerhans' cell granulomatosis and sarcoidosis are relatively common proliferative disorders of the reticuloendothe-

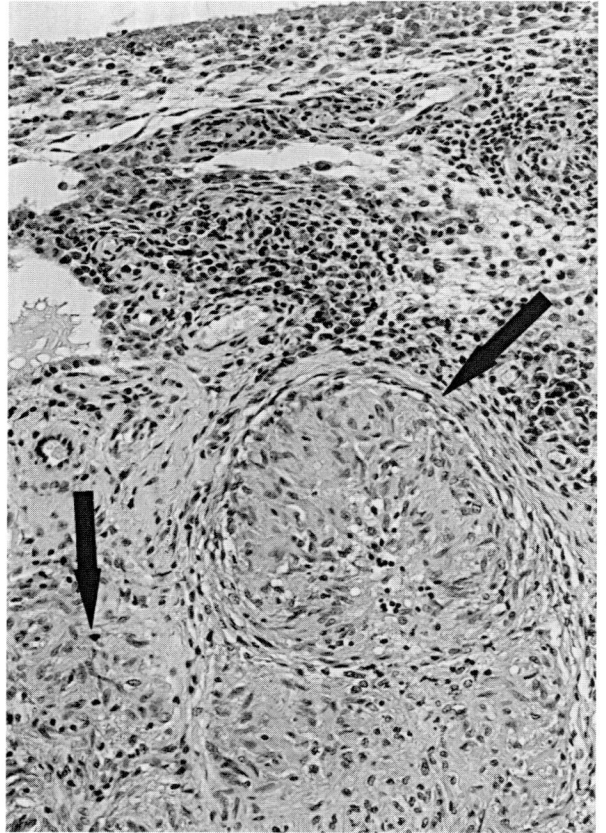

Figure 6–7 ■ Photomicrograph of a synovial membrane from a patient with sarcoidosis. The synovial membrane contains foci of granulomatous inflammation (arrows).

lial system that can involve bone. By contrast, several rare systemic diseases characterized by histiocyte proliferations may also affect the skeleton. One such disease is sinus histiocytosis with massive lymphadenopathy. This disorder, also known as Rosai-Dorfman disease, is an idiopathic proliferation of histiocytes that presents with lymphadenopathy. Typically, lymphadenopathy occurs in the neck, and patients also have fever, leukocytosis, an elevated erythrocyte sedimentation rate, and a polyclonal hyperglobulinemia. The histiocytes, which are probably recruited from the blood, fill the lymph sinuses until the nodes are massively enlarged and architecturally distorted.

Although sinus histiocytosis with massive lymphadenopathy primarily affects lymph nodes, about 40% of patients also have extranodal disease. Sites include the eye, upper respiratory tract, skin, central nervous system, and bone. Although most patients with extranodal disease also have lymphadenopathy, on rare occasions, extranodal involvement may be the presenting manifestation.

Bone involvement by sinus histiocytosis with massive lymphadenopathy is well documented.[21–23] Any bone can be involved in both the appendicular and axial skeleton (Fig. 6–9). However, the radius, ulna, and skull are most commonly affected. The bone lesions are well-defined lytic areas that are radiographically similar to the lesions of eosinophilic granuloma. Usually, osseous involvement is multifocal.

Histologically, the histiocytes have large vesicular nuclei and abundant foamy cytoplasm. These cells are positive with the S-100 stain, a feature that occasionally makes this disorder difficult to distinguish from Langerhans' cell granulomatosis. A characteristic feature of the histiocyte in this disorder is emperipolesis, the presence of intracytoplasmic intact lymphocytes (Fig. 6–10). This feature is most prominent in the involved lymph nodes and is less commonly seen in extranodal sites. In addition to the histiocytes, a lymphoplasmacytic histiocytic reaction is almost always present. Fibrosis is also common, particularly in extranodal locations.

The osseous lesions of sinus histiocytosis with massive lymphadenopathy can be mistaken histologically for eosinophilic granuloma or osteomyelitis. However, negative cultures and S-100–positive histiocytes distinguish these changes from infection. The histiocytes, although S-100 positive, differ from those in eosinophilic granuloma. Their cytoplasm is foamy, a feature not present in the Langerhans' cell. In addition, lymphadenopathy is usually present, and if not, it subsequently appears and confirms the diagnosis of sinus histiocytosis with massive lymphadenopathy.

Sinus histiocytosis with massive lymphadenopathy is usually a self-limited disease. In many cases, the disease undergoes rapid and complete resolution. In other cases, especially those with extensive extranodal disease, the disease follows an indolent course that may last for decades. A few patients with severe disease have responded to chemotherapy.

Erdheim-Chester Disease

Erdheim-Chester disease, also known as lipid granulomatosis, is another rare disorder characterized by the proliferation of histiocytes in bone and in extraosseous locations. In this disorder, thought perhaps to be a lipid storage disease, foamy lipid-laden histiocytes accumulate in the bone marrow. In addition, extravasated lipid results in cholesterol granulomas and a fibroinflammatory reaction. Parenchymal organs, such as lung, heart, and kidney, may also develop the xanthogranulomatous inflammation.

Adults in their 40s to 60s are affected by Erdheim-Chester disease. Although some patients are asymptomatic or some have mild constitutional symptoms from extraosseous involvement, most have bone pain and tenderness. Radiographic changes are invariably present in the long bones, particularly the femur and tibia. A patchy or diffuse osteosclerosis involves the medullary canal, a feature most prominent in the diaphysis and metaphysis. The cortices are also thickened because of periosteal new bone deposition. In this disease, the skeletal involvement is multifocal and is usually symmetric.[24] Histologically, the marrow is extensively replaced by foamy histiocytes and xanthogranulomatous inflammatory tissue. This tissue is associated with reactive trabecular thickening, a feature correlating with the radiodensity.[25]

The cause of Erdheim-Chester disease is unknown. Although this disorder bears some conceptual resemblance to Langerhans' granulomatosis, the histiocytes lack the ultrastructural features of Langerhans' cells.

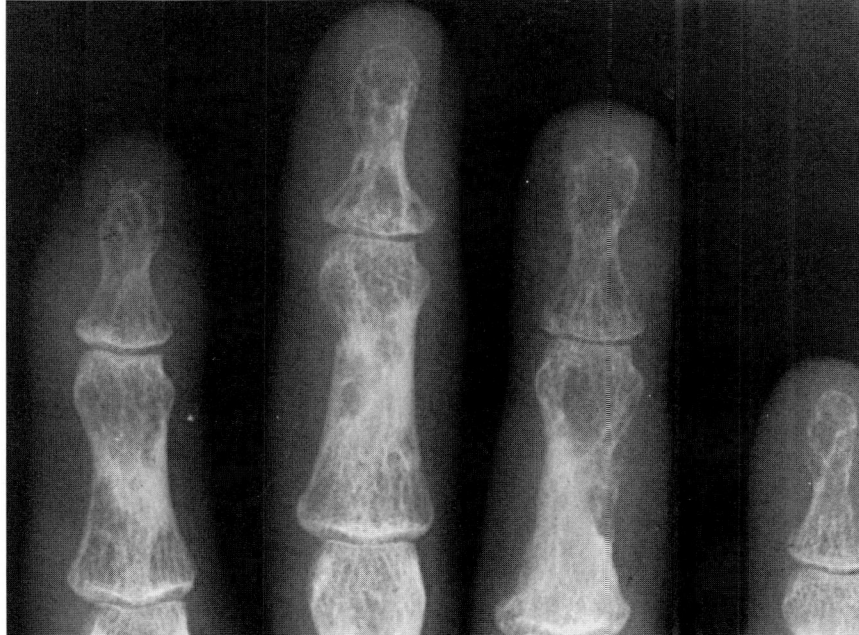

Figure 6-8 ■ Radiograph of hand in a patient with sarcoidosis. Numerous lytic lesions are present in the phalanges.

Multicentric Reticulohistiocytosis

Multicentric reticulohistiocytosis is a systemic disease of unknown etiology in which nodules of histiocytes proliferate in the skin and synovial membrane. The skin lesions are numerous and are firm nodules that develop most commonly in the face, scalp, forearms, and hands. Involvement of the synovial membrane produces a symmetric erosive arthritis that often affects the interphalangeal joints of the hands and feet, although other joints can be affected. The pattern of erosion resembles rheumatoid arthritis. However, unlike rheumatoid arthritis, periarticular osteoporosis is not present in multicentric reticulohistiocytosis. From 60 to 70% of patients develop these arthritic changes before skin lesions appear. Other areas of the body, such as eyelids, mucosal surfaces, tendons, and lymph nodes, may also be involved.[26]

Histologically, involved tissues contain sheets of histiocytes with large, eosinophilic glassy cytoplasms. Admixed with these cells are numerous multinucleated giant cells and variable amounts of lymphocytes and plasma cells. This histologic pattern is also characteristic of an isolated skin lesion known as reticulohistiocytoma. The synovial tissues in multicentric reticulohistiocytosis show villous hyperplasia secondary to the histiocytic proliferation. Bone erosions show similar infiltrates.[27]

Patients with multicentric reticulohistiocytosis are usually middle-aged adults, although any age group may be affected. They often develop other systemic diseases such as diabetes or Sjögren's syndrome. In addition, some develop neoplasms, including carcinomas of the colon, breast, or lung.

HEMATOLOGIC DISORDERS

Mastocytosis

Mastocytosis is a generic term referring to a spectrum of rare disorders characterized by the proliferation of mast cells in tissues. The most frequent presentation, known as *urticaria pigmentosa*, is localized mast cell proliferations in

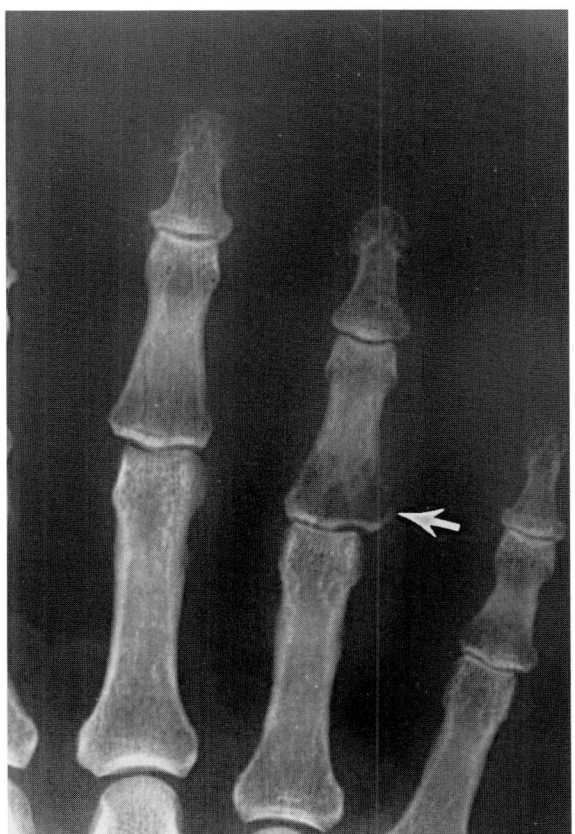

Figure 6-9 ■ Radiograph of a hand showing a lesion of sinus histiocytosis with massive lymphadenopathy. Multiple erosions are present at the base of the second phalanx *(arrow)*.

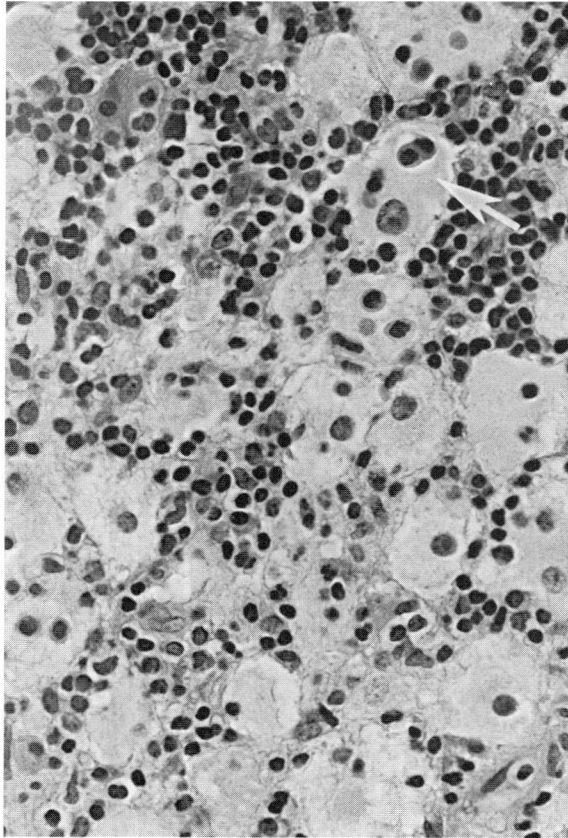

Figure 6-10 ■ Photomicrograph of the lesion in Figure 6-9. Numerous foamy histiocytes are present, some of which contain intact lymphocytes, a phenomenon known as emperipolesis *(arrow)*.

the skin of children. Only 10% of patients with mastocytosis have systemic disease in addition to skin lesions. Systemic mastocytosis usually affects adults, and mast cells accumulate in the bone marrow and sometimes in many other organs.

Mast cells are normally widely distributed throughout the body. These cells are sensitive sentinels for the immune system. They detect foreign proteins and initiate a local inflammatory response. This function is made possible by numerous chemical mediators contained in their cytoplasmic granules, among which are histamine, serotonin, and heparin. Many of the local or systemic signs of mastocytosis are caused by the release of these substances. These include urticaria, flushing, nausea, and diarrhea.[28]

Urticaria pigmentosa is usually a self-limited disease. Children present in infancy or early childhood with one or more macular lesions. They also have pruritus and dermatographia. These skin lesions disappear by late childhood. Systemic mastocytosis, however, is a more extensive disease, and usually adults in their 40s through 70s are affected.[29] Many of these patients have only osseous disease in addition to skin lesions. However, a small percentage of patients with osseous disease lack cutaneous involvement. In even more severe forms of this disease, mast cells infiltrate the parenchymal organs such as liver, spleen, and lymph nodes.[30] In addition to symptoms caused by mast cell degranulation, these patients present with weight loss, weakness, and hematologic abnormalities due to replacement of the bone marrow.

Osseous changes are the most constant abnormality in systemic mastocytosis.[31] In most cases, the bone lesions are asymptomatic, but about 28% of patients have bone pain. Lesions involve both the axial and appendicular skeleton, and they may be diffuse or focal. Both radiolytic and radiodense lesions occur. Radiographic change may include diffuse osteopenia, a pattern that mimics osteoporosis. Focal lytic lesions also may occur (Fig. 6-11). The diffuse pattern of radiolucency may be caused partly by the release of heparin, a potent bone-resorbing agent, from the mast cells. Bone from these osteopenic patients shows increased remodeling, a finding that suggests that mild mastocytosis may be responsible for many cases of so-called "idiopathic" osteoporosis.[32,33]

In contrast to radiolytic bone lesions, osteosclerotic lesions also develop in many patients. These lesions are poorly defined radiodensities and, when multiple, may mimic osteoblastic metastases from breast or prostate carcinoma. Occasionally, patients present with a diffuse increase in bone density.

Histologically, the bone marrow in mastocytosis is focally or diffusely infiltrated by mast cells. These cells may be admixed with other marrow elements, or they may be in

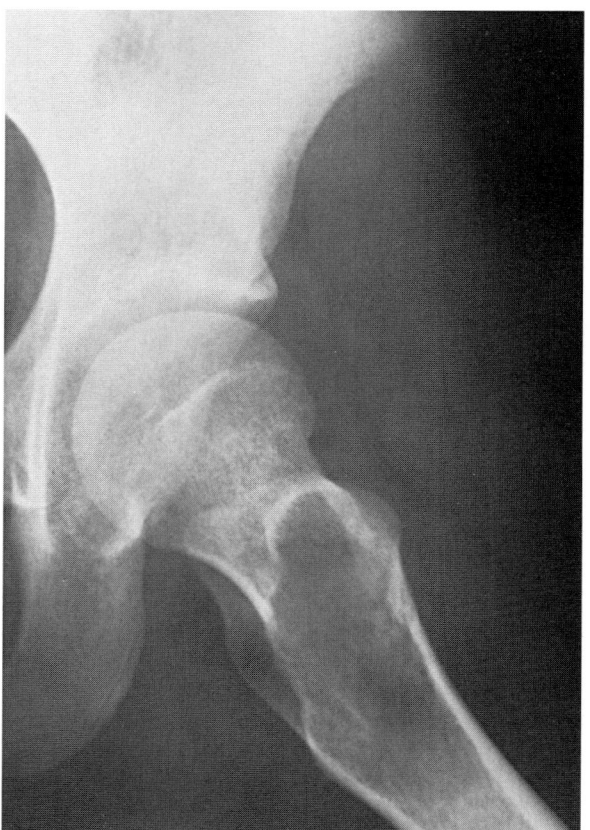

Figure 6-11 ■ A lytic lesion of mastocytosis in the proximal femur.

solid sheets.[34] Focal lesions, when admixed with other cellular elements, often contain numerous eosinophils and fibroblasts. When found in bone marrow biopsy specimens, these lesions have been called "eosinophilic fibrohistiocytic lesions."[35]

Mast cells have characteristic cytologic features. They have uniform round to vesicular nuclei (Fig. 6–12). These nuclei are centrally placed in a clear or pale cytoplasm with a crisp cytoplasmic membrane. In some areas, the mast cells assume a spindle shape. A frequent feature, which often obscures the typical mast cell morphology, is marrow fibrosis. This process occurs adjacent to bone trabeculae and is usually associated with appositional bone formation. This histologic feature corresponds to the increased bone density seen on plain radiographs of some lesions. Although mast cells can be recognized on routine hematoxylin and eosin stains, their positive identification requires demonstration of the characteristic granules with a Giemsa or toluidine blue stain. An immunohistochemical stain for mast cell tryptase also identifies these cells.[36] In contrast to typical morphology, mast cells may on rare occasions be large and anaplastic and have bizarre and hyperchromatic nuclei.

The prognosis of mastocytosis correlates with the extent of organ involvement. Patients with "bone-only" disease follow an indolent course. Patients die from unrelated causes. Those with significant parenchymal disease also pursue a long clinical course, but some die of complications of organ involvement. Treatment is supportive and is geared toward reducing systemic symptoms. On rare occasions, patients develop a mast cell leukemia.

Leukemias

The leukemias are a group of malignant proliferations of hematopoietic stem cells. The proliferations take place primarily in the bone marrow, and normal hematopoietic cells are replaced by sheets of neoplastic cells. In most cases, the neoplastic cells spill over into the peripheral blood where they cause a pronounced leukocytosis, a characteristic feature of these diseases. Because the neoplastic cells grow in the marrow, bone changes occur in almost all the leukemias, although radiographic abnormalities are not always present.

Leukemias are classified by cell type and the degree of maturity of the leukemic cells. The cell type may be either lymphocytic or myelocytic, and the cells may be immature or mature. Proliferations of immature white cells are the acute leukemias, whereas those of mature cells are the chronic leukemias.

Bone changes are most prominent in the acute leukemias of childhood, and *acute lymphoblastic leukemia* accounts for 80% of these cases. Approximately 2500 new childhood cases of this disease are diagnosed each year in the United States, and skeletal radiographic changes are present in 50 to 70% of cases.

Children with acute lymphoblastic leukemias present with symptoms of bone marrow replacement and the infiltration of parenchymal organs. They have anemia, fever, and bleeding tendencies. In addition, bone pain is common. Parenchymal involvement causes hepatosplenomegaly and lymphadenopathy. Central nervous system involvement also occurs.

Bone and joint symptoms are common presenting complaints in children with acute leukemia. These include bone tenderness and swelling, as well as arthralgias. In fact, children with leukemia are occasionally misdiagnosed as having osteomyelitis or juvenile rheumatoid arthritis.[37] The arthralgias, which symmetrically involve multiple joints, are caused by leukemic infiltration of synovial membrane.

The osseous lesions of acute leukemia are the result of replacement of bone marrow by malignant cells.[38] Four patterns of radiographic change exist: diffuse osteopenia, localized areas of bone destruction, periostitis, and, on rare occasions, osteosclerosis. Diffuse, symmetric osteopenia is the most common radiographic finding. The medullary canal is widened, and the cortices are thin (Fig. 6–13). Vertebral compression fractures also occur.[39] Focal radiolytic lesions occur in about 40% of patients. These areas show a permeative pattern of skeletal destruction, and, if solitary, can mimic a primary malignant bone tumor, such as Ewing sarcoma, or osteomyelitis. Periostitis, the third radiographic change, is caused by penetration of the leukemia cells through the cortex into the subperiosteal space. This change

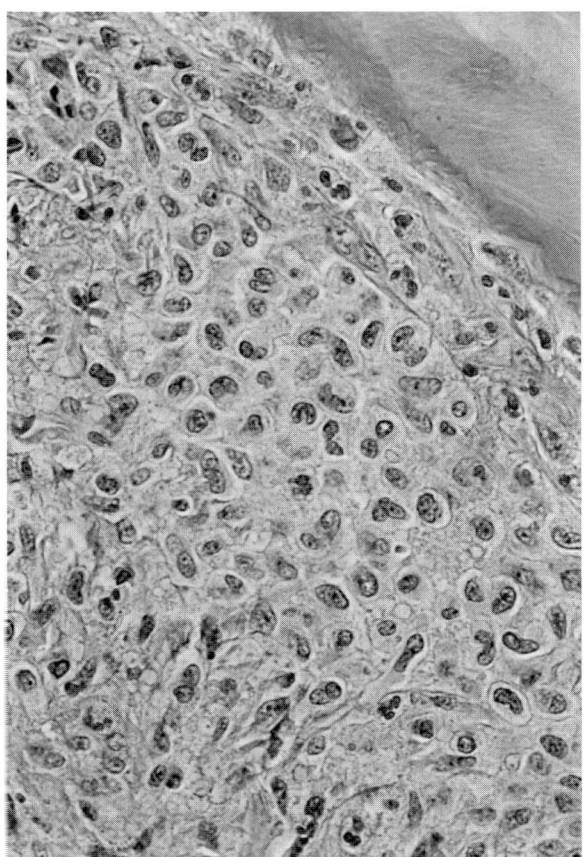

Figure 6-12 ▪ A bone marrow biopsy from a lesion of mastocytosis. The marrow is replaced by sheets of mast cells.

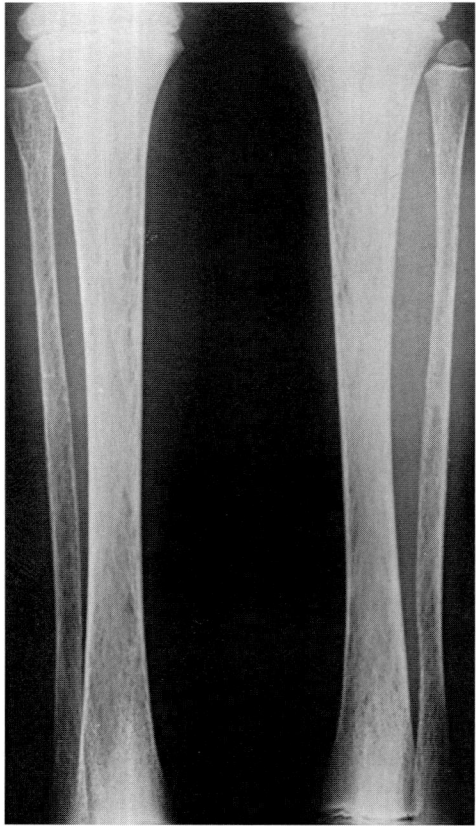

Figure 6–13 ■ Radiograph of a child with leukemia. There is diffuse lucency throughout the lower extremities.

is particularly prominent in the long bones. The final radiographic pattern, osteosclerosis, is uncommon. Increased bone density occurs in the long bone metaphyses and is the result of both reactive new bone deposition and osteonecrosis.

Another radiographic change commonly seen in acute lymphoblastic leukemia is not directly caused by leukemic infiltration. This change is the development of symmetric radiolucent metaphyseal bands.[40] This thin zone of radiolucency is not occupied by neoplastic cells. Instead, it is probably produced by defective osteogenesis due to a nutritional defect. Fractures through these radiolucent bands may occur.

Modern chemotherapy regimens have considerably improved the prognosis of acute lymphoblastic leukemia. More than 90% of children have a complete remission, and two thirds may be considered cured. Osseous lesions resolve, although many children with leukemia experience growth retardation.

Thalassemia

A wide variety of bone changes occur in patients with anemia, and, like with leukemia, changes are caused by expansion of marrow space. However, unlike the leukemias in which the marrow is infiltrated by neoplastic hematopoietic cells, the bone marrow in the anemias is expanded by normal but hyperplastic marrow elements. This hyperplasia, mainly of erythrocyte precursors, is an attempt to compensate for the diminished numbers of peripheral red cells. The marrow hyperplasia and resulting skeletal changes are most pronounced in the hemolytic anemias, diseases characterized by a shortened erythrocyte life span. Thalassemia and sickle cell anemia cause the most striking osseous lesions.

Thalassemia refers to a group of mendelian disorders characterized by the lack or decreased synthesis of either the alpha or beta globulin chain of hemoglobin A. As a result, the hemoglobin concentration in red cells is lower, and abnormal hemoglobin aggregates damage the red cell membranes. As a result of this latter defect, erythrocyte precursors are destroyed in the marrow, and secondary marrow hyperplasia occurs.

The thalassemias exhibit a wide range of clinical severity, depending on the dose of the abnormal gene. The most severe disease is β-thalassemia major, a disorder that occurs when patients are homozygous for the β-thalassemia gene. In this disease, anemia is very severe and first presents 6 to 9 months after birth. Regular blood transfusions are required to keep affected children alive.

All thalassemia patients, but particularly those with β-thalassemia major, have osseous abnormalities due to marrow expansion.[41] All bones are affected, but the most severe changes occur in the axial skeleton. Changes are striking in the skull. Widening of the diploic space and thinning of the outer table occur. Radial spicules of reactive bone lead to a hair-on-end appearance[42] (Fig. 6–14). As affected patients grow older, the entire calvarium thickens. Osseous expansion also occurs in the face and causes striking facial abnormalities.

Marrow space expansion is also evident in the spine. The number of trabeculae in the vertebral bodies is reduced, and the subchondral plates are thinned. Vertebral body deformities are common. In the appendicular skeleton, the tubular bones are symmetrically rarefied. The marrow cavity is wide, and the cortices are thin. In addition, the cancellous bone shows a trabeculated pattern due to coarsening and reduction in the number of trabeculae (Fig. 6–15).

Secondary osseous changes occur as a result of the generalized bone rarefaction. For example, fractures are common in thalassemia.[43] They usually occur in the long bones or in the vertebrae. Many of these fractures result in skeletal deformities. Another secondary change, developing in 10 to 15% of patients, is premature epiphyseal plate closure. This change is most often caused by epiphyseal injury secondary to the weakened cortices.

Sickle Cell Anemia

Sickle cell anemia is another red cell disorder that causes significant osseous abnormalities. Like thalassemia and the other hemolytic anemias, sickle cell disease is characterized by marrow hyperplasia and expansion of the medullary bone space. However, additional bone changes are caused by the

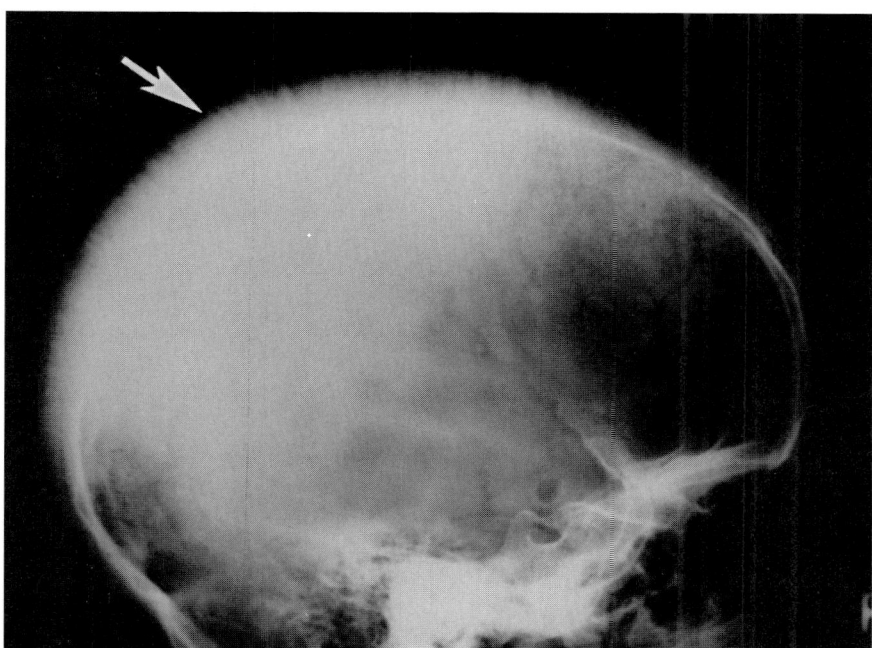

Figure 6-14 ■ Radiograph of a skull from a patient with thalassemia. The calvarium shows the characteristic "hair on end" appearance *(arrow)*.

principal feature of this disease—microvascular occlusion due to sickling of the erythrocytes. As a result, various presentations of osteonecrosis are common.

Sickle cell anemia is the result of a genetic defect that leads to a substitution of a valine for a glutamic acid in the sixth position of the beta globulin chain of the hemoglobin molecule. The abnormal hemoglobin molecule, known as hemoglobin S, has physiochemical properties that, in low-oxygen states, result in polymerization, and the red cells become sickled.

Sickle cell anemia occurs in people of African origin and, less commonly, in dark-skinned people in the Middle East. People who are heterozygous for the abnormal gene, a condition known as sickle cell trait, have only minimal symptoms. However, patients with sickle cell disease, the homozygous state, have lifelong complications of anemia and intermittent crises caused by episodic microvascular occlusion. In the United States, 7% of African-Americans have sickle cell trait, and about 1% have the disease.

The osseous changes due to marrow hyperplasia are similar to those in thalassemia. Widening of the medullary cavities and thinning of the cortices occur. Also, the trabeculae are fewer and coarser than normal. These changes are most pronounced in the axial skeleton. For example, the skull shows expansion of the diploic space, and the vertebrae are osteoporotic.

In addition to marrow expansion, a wide variety of osteonecrotic lesions occur. In the hands, particularly in young children, osteonecrosis occurs in the short tubular bones of the hands. Extensive infarction of marrow and trabecular bone occurs, and a periosteal reaction is often present. This presentation of osteonecrosis is extremely painful and is known as sickle cell dactylitis[44] (Fig. 6–16). Other manifestations of bone infarction occur in any bone in patients of any age. Medullary infarction of long bones is common and results in lesions with a smoke-ring pattern of radiodensity (see Chapter 7). In these lesions, the cortex may also be infarcted. A resulting periosteal reaction encases the native cortex, and when consolidated, this reaction leads to the

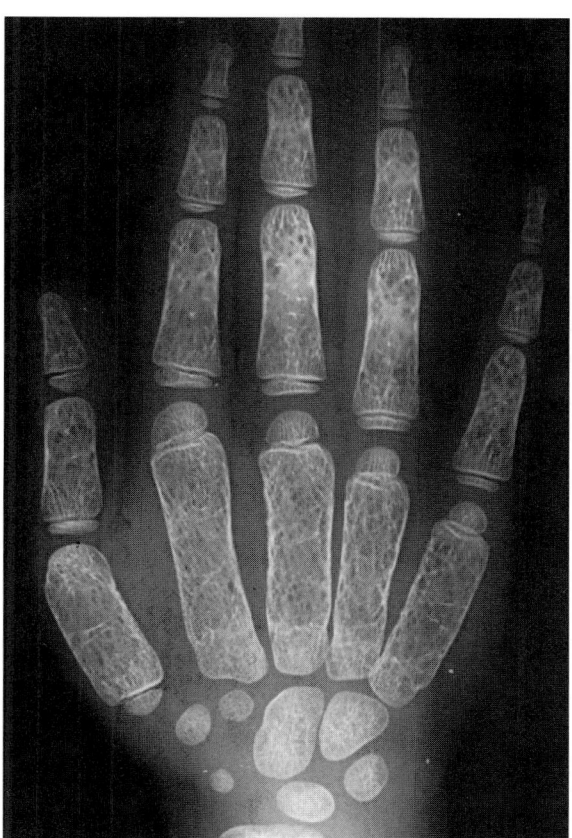

Figure 6-15 ■ Radiograph of a hand in a child with thalassemia. Extensive expansion of the marrow with thinning of the cortices and coarsening of the trabeculae is seen.

130 SKELETAL MANIFESTATIONS OF SYSTEMIC DISEASE

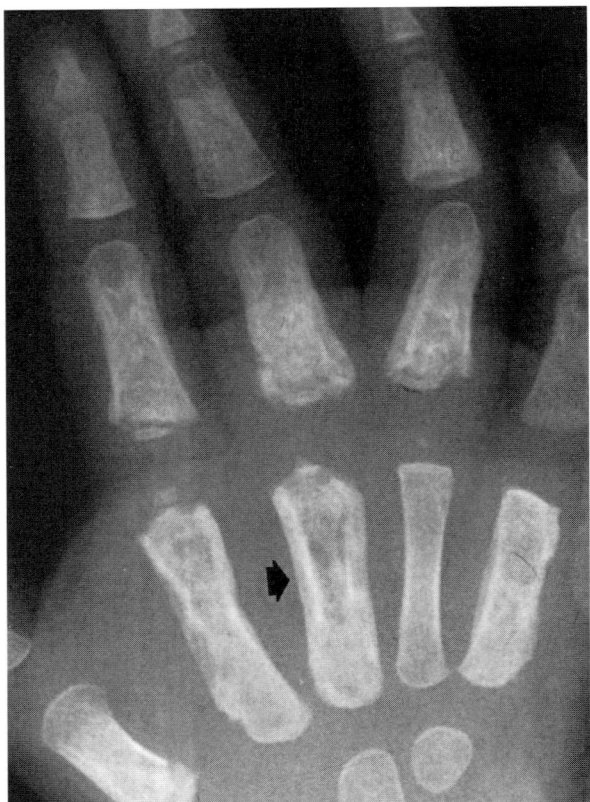

Figure 6-16 ■ Radiograph of a child with sickle cell anemia. The hand shows sickle cell dactylitis. A characteristic "bone within a bone" pattern is seen *(arrow)*.

so-called "bone within a bone" pattern.[45] Medullary bone infarction is often disseminated throughout the skeleton and can mimic osteoblastic metastases. In addition to medullary bone infarcts, osteonecrosis also occurs in epiphyseal locations and leads to arthritic symptoms similar to osteonecrosis caused by steroid therapy or alcohol abuse.

Another osseous complication of sickle cell anemia is osteomyelitis. Although *Staphylococcus aureus* is the most common etiologic organism, many cases are caused by *Salmonella* organisms. Bone infections caused by this organism occur almost exclusively in sickle cell anemia. The osteomyelitis in sickle cell disease is further discussed in Chapter 8.

Myelofibrosis

Myelofibrosis is another hematopoietic disorder that causes osseous lesions. However, unlike the anemias, which expand the marrow and produce bone rarefaction, myelofibrosis causes osteosclerosis. This disorder is one of the myeloproliferative disorders that are characterized by clonal neoplastic proliferations of multipotential myeloid stem cells. Other diseases in this group are chronic myeloid leukemia, polycythemia vera, and essential thrombocytemia.

In myelofibrosis, the neoplastic stem cell proliferation begins in the marrow and is manifested by a trilineage proliferation of cells, including normoblasts, granulocyte precursors, and megakaryocytes. Megakaryocytes are particularly numerous. As the disease progresses, the marrow gradually becomes fibrotic, and the myeloid proliferation shifts to the spleen and liver. In the end stage, the marrow is completely fibrotic.

The marrow fibrosis is accompanied by thickening of intraosseous trabeculae by appositional new bone deposition. Both the fibrosis and osteoblastic activity are stimulated by the same process—the inappropriate release of growth factors from the neoplastic megakaryocytes. Both platelet-derived growth factor and transforming growth factor β are synthesized by megakaryocytes and leak into the marrow

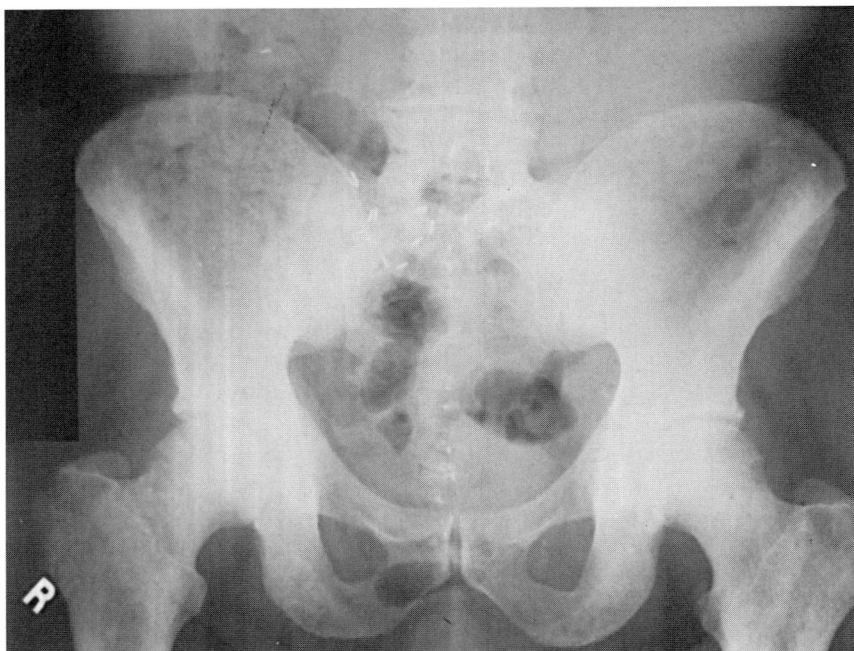

Figure 6-17 ■ Radiograph of the pelvis from a patient with myelofibrosis. Diffuse osteosclerosis is present.

space. There they stimulate fibrosis by increasing the number and synthetic activity of fibroblasts.[46]

Myelofibrosis affects older adults, and most present with anemia and hepatosplenomegaly. Many have bone pain, and from 40 to 50% of affected patients develop varying degrees of diffuse osteosclerosis (Fig. 6–17). This change is most prominent in the axial skeleton, particularly the pelvis and spine. This change is the result of thickening of both the cortex and trabecular bone.

The histologic changes of myelofibrosis are usually observed on bone marrow biopsies to evaluate the anemia that accompanies this disorder. In the early stages, the marrow is hypercellular and many megakaryocytes are present (Fig. 6–18). The fibrosis, usually mild at this point, is paratrabecular. In the late stages, the marrow is completely fibrotic, with only an occasional entrapped megakaryocyte. The bone trabeculae demonstrate successive layers of new bone deposition.

HYPERTROPHIC OSTEOARTHROPATHY

Hypertrophic osteoarthropathy is a syndrome that consists of clubbing of the digits of the hands and feet, enlargement of the extremities secondary to periosteal bone deposition, and painful, swollen joints.[47-50] This syndrome most com-

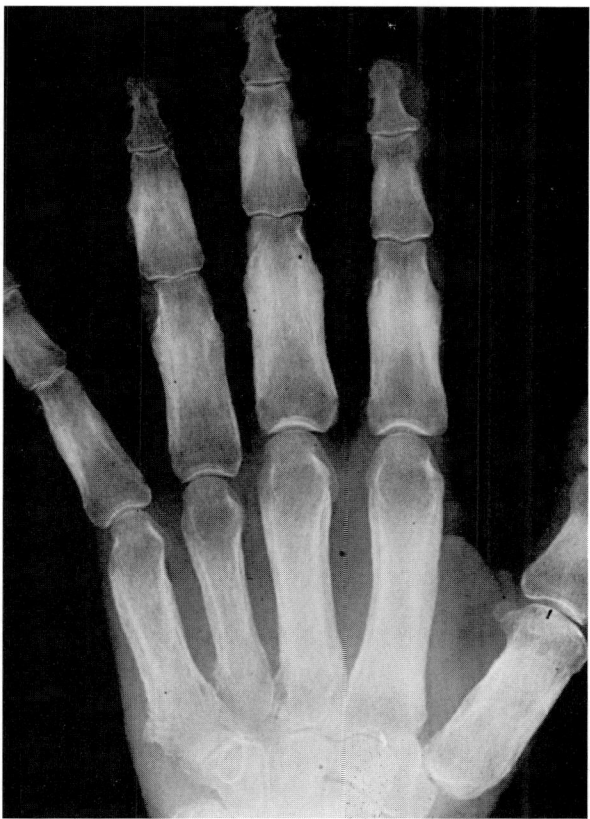

Figure 6-19 ■ Radiograph of the hand in hypertrophic osteoarthropathy. The bones are thickened owing to symmetric periosteal new bone deposition.

monly occurs in patients with chronic lung diseases, in whom it is known as secondary hypertrophic osteoarthropathy. It also may occur without an identifiable underlying disease, a condition known as primary hypertrophic osteoarthropathy.

Primary hypertrophic osteoarthropathy (pachydermoperiostosis) is a rare disorder that most commonly affects men and has a predilection for African-Americans. The disorder usually begins in adolescence with enlargement of the hands and feet, clubbing of the distal ends of the digits of the hands and feet, and convexity of the nails. Bones become progressively larger because of periosteal bone deposition. The tubular bones of the extremity, particularly the metacarpals, metatarsals, and phalanges, are most commonly affected (Fig. 6–19).

Secondary hypertrophic osteoarthropathy occurs most commonly in primary pulmonary disorders such as bronchogenic carcinoma, but it may also occur in other disorders as well (Table 6–2). The syndrome occurs in about 5 to 10% of patients with bronchogenic carcinoma. Interestingly, the incidence is highest in those tumors that are peripherally located and show squamous differentiation.[51-53] Clubbing of the fingers and toes also occurs.[54] The cause of the clubbing is not known, but the mechanism involves neovascularization of the bone surface and overlying soft tissues. Initially, thickening of the fibroelastic tissue occurs at the base of

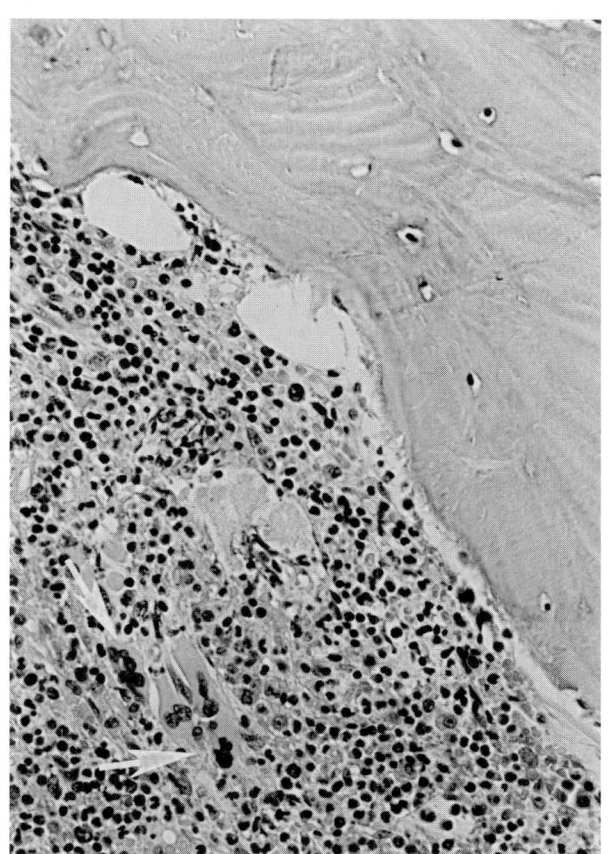

Figure 6-18 ■ Photomicrograph of a bone marrow biopsy specimen from a patient with myelofibrosis. The trabeculae are thickened, and numerous megakaryocytes are present in the marrow (arrows).

Table 6–2 ■ DISORDERS THAT MAY CAUSE SECONDARY HYPERTROPHIC OSTEOARTHROPATHY

Pulmonary	Bronchogenic carcinoma
	Abscess
	Bronchiectasis
	Emphysema
	Hodgkin's disease
	Metastasis
	Cystic fibrosis
Pleural, diaphragmatic	Mesothelioma
Cardiac	Congenital heart disease
Abdominal	Portal or biliary cirrhosis
	Ulcerative colitis
	Crohn's disease
	Dysentery
	Gastrointestinal polyposis
	Neoplasms
	Biliary atresia
Miscellaneous	Nasopharyngeal carcinoma
	Esophageal carcinoma
	Infected aortic or axillary artery grafts

the nail, followed by prominence, striations, shininess, and increased curvature of the nail. Large joints such as the knees, ankles, wrists, elbows, and ankles are often involved.[55,56] Patients present with pain, swelling, and limited range of motion.

The radiographs invariably show periosteal new bone formation.[57] The periostitis is usually found on the long bone diaphyses, particularly the tibias, fibulas, radii, ulnas, and, less commonly, the femurs, humeri, metacarpals, metatarsals, and phalanges (Fig. 6–20). The periosteal new bone formation increases with time. With chronic and long-standing disease, multiple periosteal layers may be seen. Various patterns of periosteal bone deposition occur. Simple elevation of the periosteum may occur, or it may have a laminated, "onion skin" appearance. It also may show cortical thickening. Technetium bone scans show a characteristic appearance—tracer accumulates diffusely on the bone surface. When viewed from the anteroposterior projection, increased activity can be seen on the medial and lateral cortices, giving the appearance of a "double stripe" or "parallel track."

The clinical manifestations often abate if the primary problem can be corrected. However, the radiographic alterations may persist.

REFERENCES

1. Sessa, S., Sommelet, D., Lascombes, P., and Prevot, J.: Treatment of Langerhans'-cell histiocytosis in children. *J Bone Joint Surg* 76A:1513–1525, 1994.
2. Nesbit, M. E.: Current concepts and treatment of histiocytosis X (Langerhans' cell histiocytosis). Voute, P. A., Bassett, A., Bloom, H. J. G., et al., Eds. *Cancer in Children. Clinical Management,* 2nd ed. New York, Springer, 1986, pp. 176–184.
3. Lichtenstein, L., and Jaffe, H. L.: Eosinophilic granuloma of bone, with report of a case. *Am J Pathol* 16:595, 1940.
4. Lichtenstein, L.: Histiocytosis X: Integration of eosinophilic granuloma of bone, "Letter-Siwe" and "Schüller-Christian disease" as related manifestations of a single nosologic disease entity. *Arch Pathol* 56:84–102, 1953.
5. Lichtenstein, L.: Histiocytosis X (eosinophilic granuloma of bone, Letter-Siwe disease, and Schüller-Christian disease). Further observations of pathological and clinical importance. *J Bone Joint Surg* 46A:76–90, 1964.
6. Lieberman, P. H., Jones, C. R., Steinman, R. M., Erlandson, R. A., Smith, J., Gee, T., Huvos, A., Garin-Chesa, P., Filippa, D. A., Urmacher, C., Gangi, M. D., and Sperber, M.: Langerhans' cell (eosinophilic) granulomatosis: A clinicopathologic study encompassing 50 years. *Am J Surg Pathol* 20:519–552, 1996.
7. Langerhans, P.: Ueber die Nerven der menschlichen Haut. *Virchows Arch (Pathol Anat)* 44:325–327, 1868.
8. Willman, C. L., Busque, L., Griffith, B. B., et al.: Langerhans' cell histiocytosis (histiocytosis X): A clonal proliferative disease. *N Engl J Med* 331:154–160, 1994.
9. Mirra, J. M.: Eosinophilic granuloma. *Bone Tumors: Clinical, Radiologic, and Pathologic Correlations.* London, Lea & Febiger, 1989, pp. 1023–1060.
10. Friedman, B., and Hanaoka, H.: Langerhans' cell granules in eosinophilic granuloma of bone. *J Bone Joint Surg* 51A:367–374, 1969.
11. Birbeck, M. S., Breathnach, A., and Everall, J. D.: An electron microscope study of basal melanocytes and high level clear cells (Langerhans' cells) in vitiligo. *J Invest Dermatol* 37:51–64, 1961.
12. Shamoto, M.: Langerhans' cell granule in Letterer-Siwe disease. An electron microscopic study. *Cancer* 26:1102–1108, 1970.
13. Cohen, M., Zornaza, J., Cangir, A., et al.: Direct injection of methylprednisolone sodium succinate in the treatment of solitary eosinophilic granuloma of bone—a report of nine cases. *Radiology* 136:289, 1980.
14. Capanna, R., Springfield, D. S., Ruggieri, P., et al.: Direct cortisone injection in eosinophilic granuloma of bone: A preliminary report on 11 patients. *J Pediatr Orthop* 5:339, 1985.
15. Lahey, M. E.: Prognosis in reticuloendotheliosis in children. *J Pediatr* 60:664–671, 1962.
16. Fanburg, B. L.: Sarcoidosis. Wyngaarden, J. B., Smith, L. H., and Bennett, J. C., Eds. *Cecil Textbook of Medicine,* 19th ed. Vol. I. Philadelphia, W. B. Saunders, 1992, pp. 430–435.

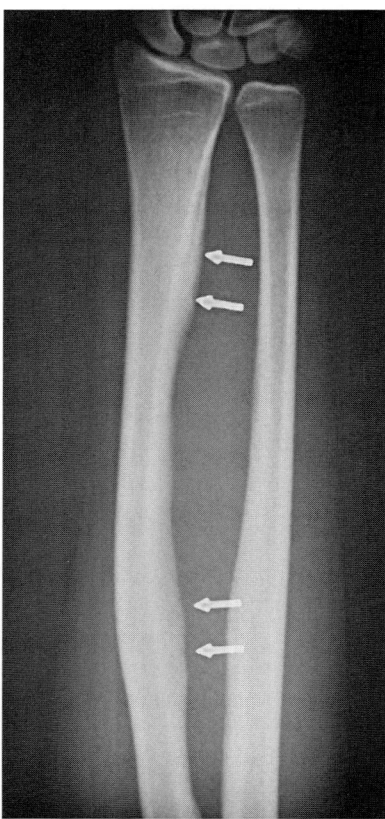

Figure 6–20 ■ Radiograph of a forearm in a patient with secondary hypertrophic osteoarthropathy. Extensive periosteal bone is present along the shaft of the radius *(arrows).*

17. Schumacher, H. R. Jr: Sarcoidosis. McCarty, D. J., Ed. *Arthritis and Allied Conditions: A Textbook of Rheumatology.* Lea & Febiger, 1989.
18. Lofgren, S.: Primary pulmonary sarcoidosis. I. Early signs and symptoms. *Acta Med Scand* 145:424–431, 1953.
19. Resnick, D., and Niwayama, G.: Sarcoidosis. *Diagnosis of Bone and Joint Disorders,* 2nd ed. Philadelphia, W. B. Saunders, pp. 4012–4032, 1988.
20. James, D. G., Neville, E., and Carstairs, L. S.: Bone and joint sarcoidosis. *Semin Arthritis Rheum* 6:53–81, 1976.
21. Lin, J., Lazarus, M., and Wilbur, A.: Sinus histiocytosis with massive lymphadenopathy: MRI findings of osseous lesions. *Skeletal Radiol* 25:279–282, 1996.
22. Unni, K. K.: Case report 457. *Skeletal Radiol* 17:129–132, 1988.
23. Foucar, E., Rosai, J., and Dorfman, R.: Sinus histiocytosis with massive lymphadenopathy (Rosai-Dorfman disease): Review of the entity. *Semin Diagn Pathol* 7:19–73, 1990.
24. Resnick, D., Greenway, G., Genant, H., Brower, A., Haghighi, P., and Emmett, M.: Erdheim-Chester disease. *Radiology* 142:289–295, 1982.
25. Lantz, B., Lange, T. A., Heiner, J., and Herring, G. F.: Erdheim-Chester disease. A report of 3 cases. *J Bone Joint Surg* 71A:456–464, 1989.
26. Melton, J. W., and Irby R.: Multicentric reticulohistiocytosis. *Arthritis Rheum* 15:221–226, 1972.
27. Nakajima, Y., Sato, K., Morita, S., Hidano, A., Nishioka, K., and Kashiwazaki, S.: Severe progressive erosive arthritis in multicentric reticulohistiocytosis: Possible involvement of cytokines in synovial proliferation. *J Rheumatol* 19:1643–1646, 1992.
28. Galli, S. J.: New concepts about the mast cell. *Semin Med Beth Israel Hosp Boston* 328:257–265, 1993.
29. Webb, T. A., Li, C.-Y., and Yam, L. T.: Systemic mast cell disease: A clinical and hematopathologic study of 26 cases. *Cancer* 49:927–938, 1982.
30. Brunning, R. D., McKenna, R. W., Rosai, J., Parkin, J. L., and Risdall, R.: Systemic mastocytosis. Extracutaneous manifestations. *Am J Surg Pathol* 7:425–238, 1983.
31. Travis, W. D., Li, C. Y., Bergstrahl, E. J., Yam, L. T., and Swee, R. G.: Systemic mast cell disease. Analysis of 58 cases and literature review. *Medicine (Baltimore)* 67:345–368, 1988.
32. Cundy, T., Beneton, M. N., Darby, A. J., Marshall, W. J., and Kanis, J. A.: Osteopenia in systemic mastocytosis: Natural history and responses to treatment with inhibitors of bone resorption. *Bone* 8:149–155, 1987.
33. Fallon, M. D., Whyte, M. P., and Teitelbaum, S. L.: Systemic mastocytosis associated with generalized osteopenia. Histopathological characterization of the skeletal lesion using undecalcified bone from two patients. *Human Pathol* 12:813–820, 1981.
34. Horny, H. P., Parwaresch, M. R., and Lennert, K.: Bone marrow findings in systemic mastocytosis. *Hum Pathol* 16:808–814, 1985.
35. teVelde, J., Vismans, F. J., Leenheers-Binnendijk, L., Vos, C. J., Smeenk, D., and Bijvoet, O. L.: The eosinophilic fibrohistiocytic lesion of the bone marrow. A mastocellular lesion in bone disease. *Virchows Arch (A)* 377:277–285, 1978.
36. Horney, H. P., Reimann, O., and Kaiserling, E. Immunoreactivity of normal and neoplastic human tissue mast cells. *Am J Clin Pathol* 89:335–340, 1988.
37. Silverstein, M. N., and Kelly, P. J.: Leukemia with osteoarticular symptoms and signs. *Ann Intern Med* 59:637–645, 1963.
38. Simmons, C. R., Harle, T. S., and Singleton, E. B.: The osseous manifestations of leukemia in children. *Radiol Clin North Am* 6:115–130, 1968.
39. Ribeiro, R. C., Pui, C. H., and Schell, M. J.: Vertebral compression fracture as a presenting feature of acute lymphoblastic leukemia in children. *Cancer* 61:589–592, 1988.
40. Willson, J. K. V.: The bone lesions of childhood leukemia. *Radiology* 72:672–681, 1959.
41. Caffey, J.: Cooley's anemia: A review of the roentgenographic findings in the skeleton. *Am J Roentgenol* 78:381, 1957.
42. Ponec, D. J., and Resnick, D.: On the etiology and pathogenesis of porotic hyperostosis of the skull. *Invest Radiol* 19:313–317, 1984.
43. Exarchou, E., Politu, C., Vretou, E., et al.: Fractures and epiphyseal deformities in beta-thalassemia. *Clin Orthop* 189:229–233, 1984.
44. Watson, R. J., Burko, H., and Megas, H.: Hand-foot syndrome in sickle cell disease in young children. *Pediatrics* 31:975–982, 1963.
45. Jaffe, H. L.: *Metabolic, Degenerative, and Inflammatory Disorders of Bones and Joints.* Philadelphia, Lea & Febiger, 1972, pp. 693–720.
46. Groopman, J. E.: The pathogenesis of myelofibrosis in myeloproliferative disorders. *Ann Intern Med* 92:857–858, 1980.
47. Vogel, A., and Goldfischer, S.: Pachydermoperiostosis. Primary or idiopathic hypertrophic osteoarthropathy. *Am J Med* 33:166–187, 1962.
48. Ursing, B.: Pachydermoperiostosis. *Acta Med Scand* 188:157, 1970.
49. Herman, M. A., Massaro, D., Katz, S., and Sachs, M.: Pachydermoperiostosis. Clinical spectrum. *Arch Intern Med* 116:918–923, 1965.
50. Lazarus, J. H., and Galloway, J. K.: Pachydermoperiostosis. An unusual cause of finger clubbing. *Am J Roentgenol* 118:308–313, 1973.
51. Aufses, A. H.: Primary carcinoma of the lung. 14 year survey. *J Mt Sinai Hosp* 20:212, 1953.
52. Hansen, J. L.: Bronchial carcinoma presenting as arthralgia. *Acta Med Scand* 266:467–472, 1952.
53. Wierman, W. H., Clagett, O. T., and McDonald, J. R.: Articular manifestations in pulmonary diseases. An analysis of their occurrence in 1024 cases in which pulmonary resection was performed. *J Am Med Assoc* 155:1459–1463, 1954.
54. Mendolowitz, M.: Clubbing and hypertrophic osteoarthropathy. *Medicine* 21:269–306, 1942.
55. Calabro, J. J.: Cancer and arthritis. *Arthritis Rheum* 10:553–567, 1967.
56. Segal, A. M., and McKenzie, A. H.: Hypertrophic osteoarthropathy: A ten year retrospective analysis. *Semin Arthritis Rheum* 12:220–232, 1982.
57. Greenfeld, G. B., Schorsch, H. A., and Shkolnik, A.: The various roentgen appearances of pulmonary hypertrophic osteoarthropathy. *Am J Roentgenol* 101:927–931, 1967.

CHAPTER 7 Osteonecrosis

When deprived of a blood supply, bone dies just like any other tissue. As with other tissues, the blood supply to bone may be interrupted by various mechanisms—primary vascular occlusion, infiltrative processes, or trauma. The first of these, bone death due to vascular occlusion, is the main subject of this chapter. Secondary subjects are radiation necrosis and a group of related syndromes known as the osteochondroses. However, before turning to these, a brief description of bone death due to infiltrative processes and trauma is in order.

Infiltrative processes, such as infections or neoplasms, commonly isolate portions of trabecular bone or cortex. The blood vessels supplying these portions of bone are either destroyed or compressed by the infiltrating tissue; the bone then dies and becomes necrotic. In infection, the isolated portion of necrotic bone is called a sequestrum (see Chapter 8).

Trauma may also interrupt the blood supply to bone and cause osteonecrosis. Two important clinical situations exemplify this manner of bone death. First, necrosis of the femoral head commonly follows intracapsular femoral neck fracture. Second, severe joint trauma may shear off a portion of articular cartilage and bone, a condition known as *osteochondritis dissecans*. In the first situation, femoral neck fracture, necrosis is caused by peculiarities of blood supply. For example, the femoral head in adults is primarily supplied by the lateral epiphyseal vessels, which are branches of the profunda femoris artery. These vessels, running in close association with the femoral neck, may become lacerated or occluded following displaced femoral neck fractures. As many as 75% of these fractures are complicated by focal osteonecrosis of the femoral head.[1] The amount of necrosis varies, depending on the degree of displacement and the time interval to reduction. Occasionally, the entire femoral head dies. The osteonecrosis often leads to nonunion of the femoral neck fracture, and after about a year, the femoral head collapses. In addition to the femoral head, other bones prone to developing focal necrosis following fracture are the talus and the carpal navicular.

The second form of traumatic bone death, osteochondritis dissecans, affects adolescents. In this disorder, joint trauma shears from the joint surface a portion of articular cartilage and underlying bone, together known as an *osteochondral fragment*.[2] The trauma, probably an excessive rotary force, usually detaches the osteochondral fragment from the bone, and it becomes a loose body in the joint cavity. Occasionally, however, the fragment remains attached. The lateral portion of the medial femoral condyle is the most common site of osteochondritis dissecans; the dome of the talus is also a frequent site. Osteochondritis dissecans of the distal femur usually affects patients between the ages of 15 and 20, and, in about one fourth of the cases, the lesion is bilateral.

The radiographic features of osteochondritis dissecans are diagnostic.[3] A cup-shaped radiolucent defect, usually with a sclerotic rim, is adjacent to the articular surface (Fig. 7–1). If the osteochondral fragment remains attached, a radiodensity may be present in this lytic zone. In addition, the radiolucent defect may enlarge owing to cystic change in the adjacent viable trabecular bone. Histologically, the osteochondral fragment consists of viable articular cartilage and a portion of underlying necrotic bone. The bone is dead because it has been detached from its blood supply, but the articular cartilage, receiving nutrients from the synovial fluid, remains alive. The osteochondral fragment shows only scant evidence of a reparative reaction. However, a fibrous nonunion is usually present on the osseous side of the fragment.

OSTEONECROSIS DUE TO INTRAVASCULAR OCCLUSION

In addition to infiltrating processes and trauma, primary vascular occlusion also causes segmental bone death. The resulting changes are known as *osteonecrosis* or *bone in-*

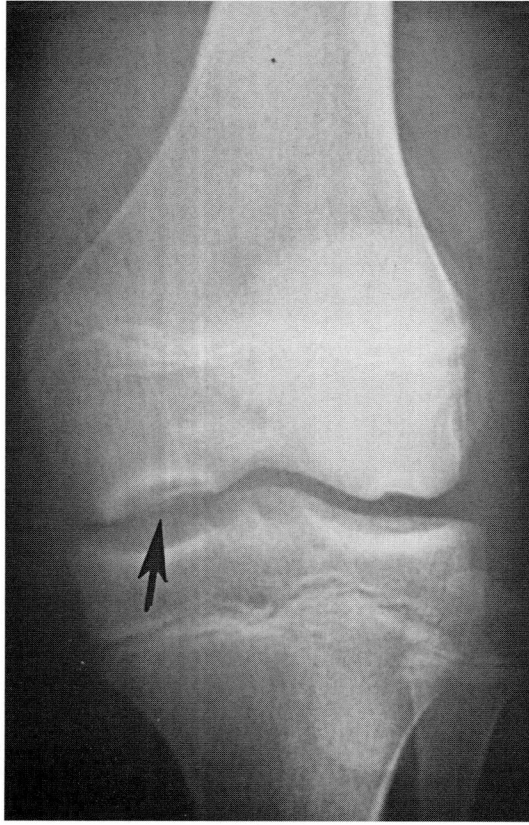

Figure 7-1 ■ Osteochondritis dissecans of the medial femoral condyle. A radiolucent defect in the articular surface is surrounded by a sclerotic rim *(arrow)*.

farction. Until a few years ago, this disorder was called aseptic necrosis or avascular necrosis. However, these terms are now outdated. Osteonecrosis of bone is a process similar to infarction in other organs, such as the heart or brain. Unlike infarcts in other organs, however, which are usually caused by atherosclerotic occlusion of arteries, bone infarction results from intravascular coagulation in small arterioles or venules. It is a common disorder and often leads to significant disability.

History

Osteonecrosis is a very ancient process. Evidence of this disease has been found in the humeral heads of fossilized mosasaurs, deep-diving marine reptiles from the Cretaceous period, 64 to 100 million years ago.[4] Fossils of other prehistoric deep-diving turtles also show evidence of osteonecrosis, presumably a manifestation of decompression sickness.[5] This disease occurred in comparatively recent antiquity as well. Radiologic evidence of osteonecrosis has been found in Egyptian mummies dating from the fourth century BC to the first century AD.[6]

The first clinical description of what was most probably osteonecrosis of the hip was by the German surgeon Franz Konig in 1888.[7] Although he called the lesion osteochondri-

tis dissecans, his description of the femoral head and joint space suggest osteonecrosis to the modern reader. In 1907, George Axhausen, a German pathologist, was the first to use the term *aseptic necrosis.*[8] Axhausen was an early student of bone grafts. By noting the evolution of changes in these grafts, he learned to recognize the histologic features of dead bone and its repair. Bone necrosis involving the hip was first recognized in 1924 by Schmorl.[9] Then in 1935, Fremont Chandler recognized the similarity of femoral head infarcts to coronary infarcts, and he postulated that the process was the result of vascular occlusion.[10] Because of Chandler's interest, osteonecrosis of the hip is occasionally called Chandler's disease.

Pathogenesis

Osteonecrosis can occur anywhere in any bone. However, the subchondral areas of bone are targeted because these regions have little or no collateral circulation. The most common site is the femoral head, but the distal femur, proximal humerus, talus, and scaphoid are also frequently involved. In addition to subchondral regions, the medullary canal in the shafts of long bones, particularly the femur and tibia, may also become infarcted.

Osteonecrosis rarely occurs in a healthy patient; usually an underlying medical problem is present. These problems include previous steroid therapy, alcoholism, sickle cell disease, dysbarism (decompression sickness), and Gaucher's disease. Bone infarction not associated with an underlying disease was formerly called "idiopathic" avascular necrosis. However, the idiopathic category is shrinking because close investigation of affected patients often reveals preexisting but not clinically obvious abnormalities. For example, many patients with so-called idiopathic necrosis have been found to have hypercoagulable blood.

The initial pathophysiologic events leading to osteonecrosis depend on the underlying disease state. However, the various underlying diseases all lead to a final common pathway: *focal intravascular coagulation,* either in terminal arterioles or postsinusoidal venules. Two observations support this theory that intravascular coagulation is a final common pathway. First, fibrin thrombi can be found adjacent to infarcts that have occurred in a wide variety of clinical settings. Second, bone infarcts often occur in patients who survive disseminated intravascular coagulation (DIC).[11] For example, children with DIC due to meningococcemia develop bone infarcts.[12] Also, bone infarcts occur in patients with anaphylactic shock, a condition often complicated by DIC.[13]

Many predisposing factors lead to the final common pathway of intravascular thrombosis (Table 7–1). These factors include vascular stasis, fat embolism, and hypercoagulability of blood. In addition, increased intraosseous pressure due to fat swelling or marrow edema also compromises blood flow.

The first factor, *vascular stasis,* contributes to the development of most bone infarcts. The microanatomy of the blood

Table 7-1 ■ **PATHOGENETIC FACTORS IN OSTEONECROSIS**

> Intravascular coagulation
> Vascular stasis
> Fat embolization and hyperlipidemia
> Increased intraosseous pressure
> Hypercoagulability of blood

supply to the ends of long bones predisposes to vascular stasis. For example, the subchondral bone of the femoral head, the most common site of osteonecrosis, is supplied by endarterioles. Because the ends of long bones are encased by articular cartilage, almost no collateral circulation flows to these areas. In the femoral head, the endarterioles blend into vascular arcades that make 180° turns beneath the subchondral plate. This microanatomy favors vascular stasis and predisposes to fibrin thrombosis.

The next predisposing factor, *fat embolism and hyperlipidemia,* plays a major etiologic role in many cases of osteonecrosis. In these cases, fat emboli to subchondral bone may be the initial event that triggers intravascular coagulation. The fat emboli may originate by several mechanisms—disrupted marrow fat, mobilization of fat from a fatty liver, or coalescence of serum lipids. Whatever their origin, the fat emboli are trapped in the endarterioles of subchondral bone where they damage the endothelium and initiate the clotting cascade. The fat embolism theory was first postulated by Jones in 1965[14] and received experimental support the following year.[15] This theory is supported by the observation that most of the systemic conditions that predispose to osteonecrosis are characterized by disturbed lipid metabolism.[16] Indeed, the two most common associated conditions, alcoholism and steroid therapy, are often complicated by fatty livers. In addition, fat emboli have been demonstrated near bone infarcts in patients on corticosteroids[17] and in alcoholics. Jones and colleagues[18] also have suggested that fat emboli released from the marrow are the cause of dysbaric related infarcts. Other hyperlipidemic syndromes associated with osteonecrosis are pancreatitis[19] and pregnancy.[20]

The fat embolism theory is controversial. Some investigators have not been able to demonstrate fat emboli near bone infarcts.[21,22] In addition, several observations contradict the theory. First, osteonecrosis does not occur following multiple fractures or following the bone reaming necessary for internal fixation, yet both conditions are known to be complicated by major fat embolization. In addition, bone necrosis is not a complication of lipiodol lymphangiograms. To explain the absence of bone necrosis in these settings, Jones has postulated that multiple embolic showers over a period of time are required to produce infarction.[18]

Increased intraosseous pressure, well documented in osteonecrosis of the hip[23,24] is another important contributing factor to bone infarction. When caused by bone marrow edema or hemorrhage, increased intraosseous pressure probably occurs secondarily in all cases of osteonecrosis and further compromises blood supply. However, in certain circumstances, such as fat cell swelling secondary to steroid therapy, the increased intraosseous pressure may be the primary cause of bone death. Just as steroids cause fat swelling in the face and trunk (so-called "cushingoid" features), they also cause swelling of bone marrow fat cells.[25] However, fat swelling in the rigid, nonexpansile compartment of bone increases the intraosseous pressure and compresses the microvasculature. The local bone architecture may exaggerate this effect. For example, trabecular bone is most concentrated in weight-bearing, subchondral areas. Therefore, these areas are the most rigid and are the most susceptible to damage by increased intraosseous pressure. Indeed, osteonecrosis is most common in these weight-bearing areas; e.g., the anterolateral portion of the femoral head.

A final systemic factor that may predispose to bone infarction is *hypercoagulability of blood,* a finding in many patients who develop osteonecrosis. Altered hemostasis and capillary sludging was first described in patients with osteonecrosis in 1970.[26] More recently, specific syndromes of congenital and acquired hypercoagulability have been documented.[21,27] Among these syndromes are protein C and protein S deficiency. Reduction of these proteins, which are inhibitors of the clotting cascade, causes hypercoagulability and a tendency for thrombosis to occur. These conditions are not uncommon. For example, protein C deficiency, an autosomal dominant disorder, may be present in as many as 1 in 60 adults.[28] Blood hypercoagulability may also be caused by hypofibrinolysis, a condition that may be either congenital or acquired. Congenital hypofibrinolysis, a familial disorder, is due to high levels of plasminogen activator inhibitor. Acquired hypofibrinolysis occurs in several conditions, such as pregnancy or certain malignancies. Various hypofibrinolytic syndromes have, in fact, been documented in patients with osteonecrosis.[29]

Associated Conditions

Alcohol Abuse

A wide variety of associated diseases or behaviors predispose patients to osteonecrosis (Table 7–2). Of these, alcoholism and steroid therapy account for 90% of the reported associated conditions.[30] Alcoholism may even account for some of the remaining 10% of cases because some patients give an inaccurate drinking history. Most drinkers downplay the amount of alcohol they consume, and alcoholics rarely

Table 7-2 ■ **ASSOCIATED BEHAVIORS AND DISEASES**

> Alcoholism
> Steroid therapy
> Decompression sickness
> Sickle cell anemia
> Gaucher's disease (see Chapter 3)
> Pancreatitis
> Gout

admit they are alcoholic. However, not much alcohol is needed. As little as 400 ml/wk of pure alcohol (about three beers per day) raises the risk of developing osteonecrosis. Chronic alcohol intake predisposes to bone infarction by interference with lipid metabolism. Drinkers may have a fatty liver, or they may be hyperlipidemic; both of these conditions can lead to fat embolism. Hypofibrinolysis is another complication of heavy drinking that predisposes to bone infarction. In alcoholics, the femoral head is the most common site of osteonecrosis. The proximal humerus and distal femur may also be involved. Almost 75% of patients with alcohol-related bone necrosis have synchronous or metachronous bilateral disease.[30]

Steroid Therapy

Patients receiving steroids are also at risk of developing osteonecrosis. As with alcoholism, many of these patients are predisposed to fat embolism secondary to fatty liver or hyperlipemia, both known complications of steroid therapy. The risk of bone necrosis correlates with the amount of steroids. However, a critical dose level that correlates with an increased risk of necrosis is difficult to establish. This is because susceptibility of steroid-induced bone infarction varies from patient to patient. The shortest reported steroid course associated with bone necrosis was 24 mg of oral dexamethasone for 7 days. The smallest reported dose was 16 mg of prednisone for 30 days.[31] One suggested guideline for all steroid-treated patients is that a total dose of 2800 mg of oral prednisone within 4 months significantly increases the risk of bone infarction.[32] Because high doses of oral steroids are commonly used for lupus erythematosus and immunosuppression following renal transplantation, patients in these situations are the most susceptible. As many as 40% of these patients develop bone infarcts,[33] and magnetic resonance imaging (MRI) studies indicate that they occur from 3 to 4 months after treatment is started.[34] Lupus patients with Raynaud's phenomenon or cushingoid features are even more likely to develop this complication of steroid therapy. Interestingly, lupus patients not treated with steroids also have a higher incidence of osteonecrosis. This is because many have antiphospholipid antibodies, another condition associated with hypercoagulability and bone necrosis.[35] Osteonecrosis complicates steroid therapy for other diseases. These include asthma, multiple sclerosis, rheumatoid arthritis, inflammatory bowel disease, and polymyalgia rheumatica. Steroid-treated patients develop infarcts in many locations. The femoral head, distal femur, and proximal humerus are common sites. Also, the medullary shafts of the femur and tibia are frequently affected. Sensitive imaging tools such as MRI demonstrate that as many as 90% of patients with osteonecrosis have multiple sites of involvement.[36]

Dysbaric Osteonecrosis

Persons who work in environments of compressed air, such as divers and caisson workers, are also predisposed to bone infarction. (Caissons are chambers which, when filled with compressed air, allow underwater work on bridges.) Rapid return to normal atmospheric pressure results in dysbarism and, occasionally, bone infarcts. The association between bone infarcts and high-pressure environments was first noted in 1911 by Borstein and Plate.[37] These authors studied late joint changes in caisson workers and published the first radiographs of osteonecrosis. Tunnel workers also are exposed to compressed air. In these professions, bone infarction occurs in as many as 20% of workers.[38] Some divers are also liable to develop osteonecrosis. Because bone infarction is rare unless significant exposure to pressures greater than 17 psi (the equivalent of 60 ft of water) occurs, sport scuba divers are almost never affected. However, 4 to 6% of navy divers, even following rigid decompression schedules, develop bone lesions.[39] A greater incidence of bone infarcts is present among the diving fishermen of Japan and Hawaii. Because these divers pay little attention to decompression tables, over 50% suffer osteonecrosis.[40] Dysbaric-related bone infarcts occur in subarticular zones and in the medullary cavity with equal frequency. For unknown reasons, lesions in compressed air workers are most common in the humeral head. In other associated conditions, the femoral head is the most common site.

Osteonecrosis in compressed air workers is initiated by the formation of nitrogen bubbles in tissue. Rapid decompression allows nitrogen, which has been dissolved in the tissues, to come out of solution and form bubbles. Bubbles that form in the marrow cavity disrupt fat cells and lead to fat embolism.[18]

Osteonecrosis in Sickle Cell Disease

Bone necrosis has also been reported in many of the common variants of the sickle cell disorder. The sickled erythrocytes cause capillary sludging and vascular thrombosis. Infarcts are most common in SC disease, occurring in 20 to 68% of patients.[41] A lower incidence is reported with SS disease, presumably because patients with this disease have a decreased life expectancy. In patients with sickle cell anemia, acute infarcts may be very difficult to distinguish from osteomyelitis, another complication of this disorder. However, bone infarction is at least 50 times more common in these patients than bacterial osteomyelitis.[42] Patients with sickle cell disease develop both subarticular and medullary bone infarcts. Infarcts also occur in unusual locations, such as the vertebral bodies and phalanges.

A wide variety of other diseases predispose to osteonecrosis. These include Gaucher's disease, pancreatitis, and gout.

Histopathology

The histologic features of necrotic bone are uniformly empty osteocyte lacunae and fat necrosis of the marrow. However, depending on the cell type, these features of necrosis take varying periods to evolve after bone death. First, the hematopoietic cells begin to show necrotic features 2 to 3

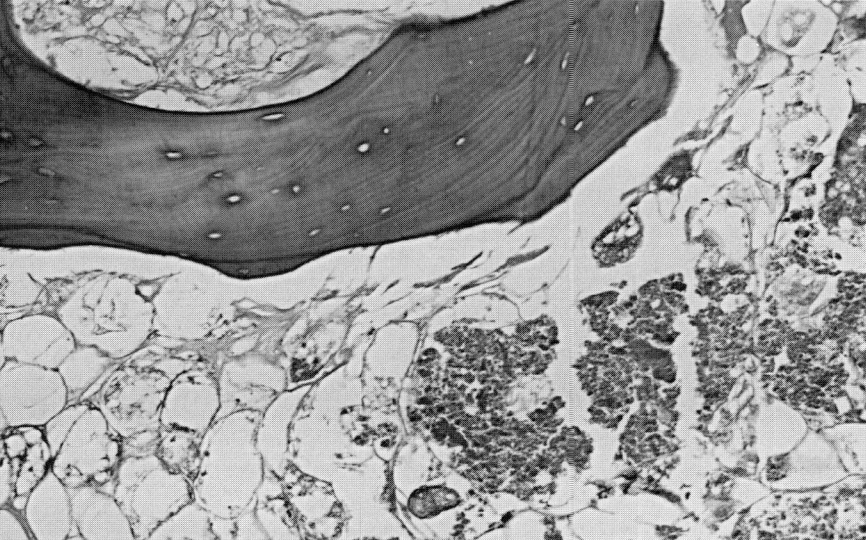

Figure 7-2 ■ Photomicrograph showing necrotic bone. The lacunae in the bone are empty, and the marrow is necrotic.

days after death. Second, osteocyte dropout takes anywhere from 2 days to 4 weeks. Finally, the marrow fat begins to show necrosis about 5 days after death. Therefore, bone may not be recognizably dead until 5 days or more after the irreversible cessation of cellular metabolism.

Further complicating the histologic interpretation of vascular compromise, the various cell types have different sensitivities to anoxia, and this may result in death of some cellular elements and not others. For example, the hematopoietic cells are the most sensitive, requiring only about 6 hours of anoxia to die. The bone cells, however, may survive anoxia for 6 hours to 2 days. The marrow fat is the most resistant tissue; it may survive 2 to 5 days of anoxia. Therefore, because of this variation in sensitivity, an anoxic event may produce death of only the hematopoietic cells, the other cells remaining viable.

As previously stated, both empty osteocyte lacunae and marrow fat alterations are necessary for the diagnosis of osteonecrosis (Fig. 7–2). All the lacunae in a zonal area of trabecular bone must be empty, a feature that remains constant. However, histologic changes evolve in the marrow. For the first few weeks after an infarct, the marrow shows only fat necrosis. The nuclei of the lipocytes are absent, and their cellular membranes are indistinct. In addition, foam cells, multinucleated giant cells, and a few lipid-filled cysts are present. Eventually, the marrow space is filled with amorphous acellular debris, and small particles of dead bone are surrounded by foreign body giant cells. Sometimes, focal dystrophic calcification occurs in the necrotic fat of the marrow space (Fig. 7–3).

The viable bone at the margin of the infarct shows reactive changes and is the source of repair of the infarct. First,

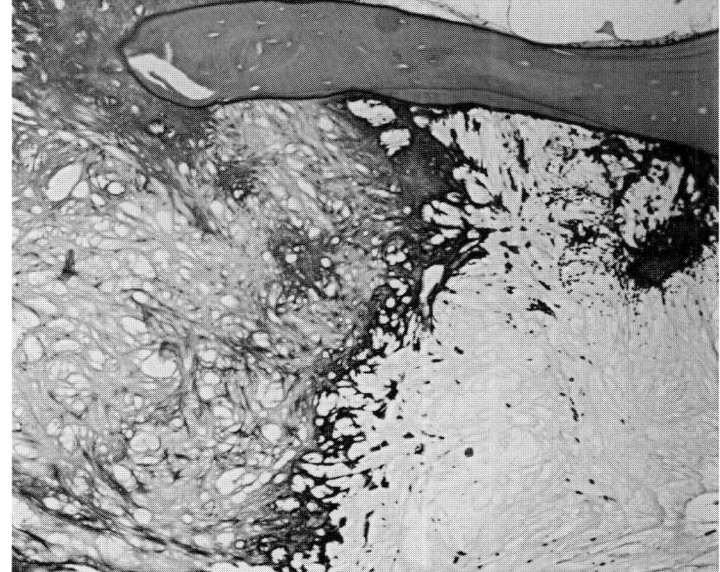

Figure 7-3 ■ Photomicrograph of necrotic bone. Calcification of the necrotic marrow is present.

these marginal areas show bone marrow edema. Faintly eosinophilic edema fluid is present between the marrow fat cells, and small blood vessels are dilated and congested. The trabeculae in this region show mild osteoclastic resorption.

After several weeks, a reparative reaction begins. First, a zone of granulation tissue develops at the interface between viable and dead bone. This tissue often contains scattered mononuclear inflammatory cells. Then, gradual encroachment of reparative tissue into the necrotic zone replaces dead fat with a highly collagenized fibrous tissue. Osteoblasts, having differentiated from the granulation tissue, deposit seams of appositional bone on the dead trabecular bone (Fig. 7–4). The new bone, containing viable osteocytes, is sharply demarcated from the necrotic bone, which shows only empty lacunae. New viable bone also forms in resorption cavities within the dead bone, a process known as *creeping substitution* (Fig. 7–5). Weakened by osteoclastic resorption at the margin of the infarct, the dead trabeculae eventually fracture beneath the subchondral plate. This process, leading to collapse of the articular surface, correlates with the crescent sign seen radiographically.

Clinical Syndromes

Medullary Infarcts

Medullary infarcts occur in the metaphyseal and diaphyseal regions of a bone. This manifestation of osteonecrosis

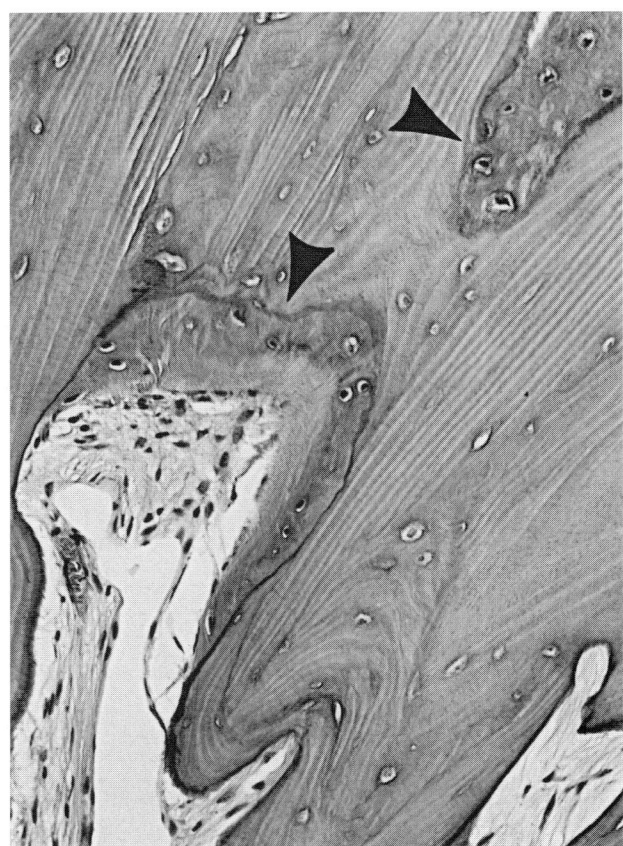

Figure 7-5 ■ Photomicrograph of creeping substitution. Necrotic bone is being replaced by viable new bone *(arrowheads)*.

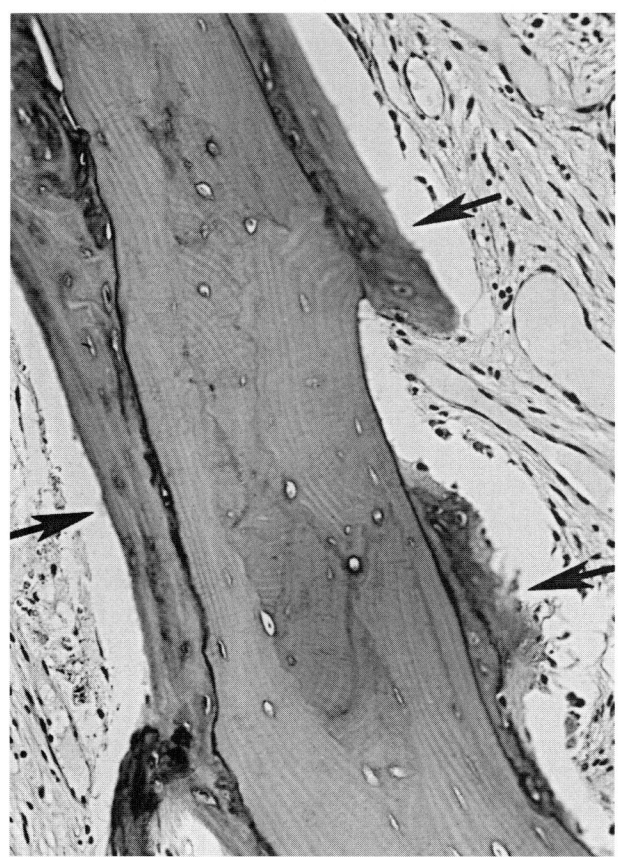

Figure 7-4 ■ Photomicrograph of necrotic bone with repair. A central necrotic trabecula, evidenced by empty lacunae, is surrounded by seams of viable reparative bone *(arrows)*.

frequently occurs in patients with sickle cell disease or patients treated with steroids, and usually the femur or tibia is involved. During the early phases of medullary infarction, bone pain may be present, and the process may be misdiagnosed as infection or neoplasm.[43] Most medullary infarcts, however, are asymptomatic and are discovered incidentally during imaging procedures for other areas of bone or joint pain.

The radiologic features of an old medullary infarct are characteristic. A well-defined, mottled radiodensity involves a 2- to 10-cm segment of the medullary canal. The radiodensities, due to calcification of dead marrow and reparative new bone, assume a "smoke-ring" shape (Fig. 7–6). Very old infarcts may show partial or complete cystic change.

Recent medullary infarcts may also be diagnosed radiographically. Plain radiographs are usually normal, although a small periosteal reaction may be present. A bone scan characteristically shows decreased uptake in the area of infarction. After a few weeks, the bone scan shows tracer uptake when revascularization and repair begin at the margins of the lesion. The MRI, however, is the most sensitive tool to diagnose early bone infarction. Signal abnormalities may appear as early as a few days after infarction. Typically, an inhomogeneous signal change is present in a well-demarcated zone with serpiginous borders (Fig. 7–7). Infarcts usually show low signal intensity on T_1-weighted images and an intermediate or high signal intensity on T_2-weighted images. The T_2-weighted images often show the "double-line sign," a pattern highly characteristic of necrosis. This double line is thought to represent a zone of hypervascular granulation tissue at the interface between viable and necrotic bone.

Osteonecrosis of the Femoral Head

Osteonecrosis of the femoral head (ONFH), a common disease that often leads to significant disability, is the most important clinical syndrome of bone infarction. In the United States, approximately 10,000 to 20,000 new cases occur each year. Unlike medullary infarcts, which are usually asymptomatic, the subchondral location of an infarct in the femoral head causes hip pain. Osteonecrosis of the femoral head most commonly affects patients between the ages of 20 and 40. Usually, the disease leads to structural failure of the femoral head, and a total hip arthroplasty is required. However, hip arthroplasty for osteonecrosis is problematic. Results of total hip surgery in these patients are less satisfactory than in patients with primary osteoarthritis. One reason for this is that patients with osteonecrosis require hip arthroplasty earlier, the average age being only 38.[30] It is, therefore, unlikely that a total hip prosthesis will last the remainder of the person's life. Another reason is that hip arthroplasties fail earlier in these patients. This early failure

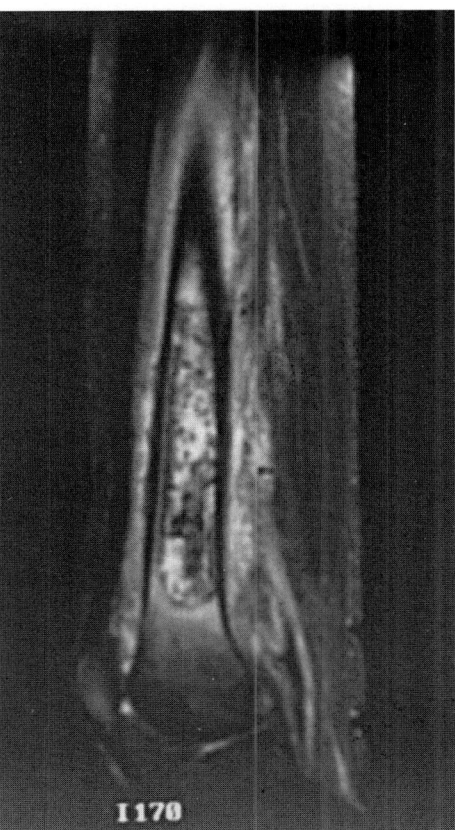

Figure 7-7 ▪ A T_2-weighted MRI of an acute medullary infarct. There is a well-defined area of irregular signal. This area is bounded by a crisp zone of low signal.

may be the result of the systemic disease that led to the necrosis or an increased activity level of this younger age group. The failure rate of total hip arthroplasty for osteonecrosis may be as high as 25%, significantly higher than the 5% failure rate of this procedure for primary osteoarthritis (Hungerford, D., Personal communication, 1996).

Staging. The clinical, radiographic, and pathologic evolution of osteonecrosis of the hip may be divided into various stages. Many staging systems exist, most of which are modifications of the very practical system proposed by Ficat and Arlet in 1980[44] (Table 7-3). This four-stage system is based on the observation that dead bone appears normal on plain radiographs. Radiographic changes appear as secondary repair and degenerative changes develop. In *stage I,* patients

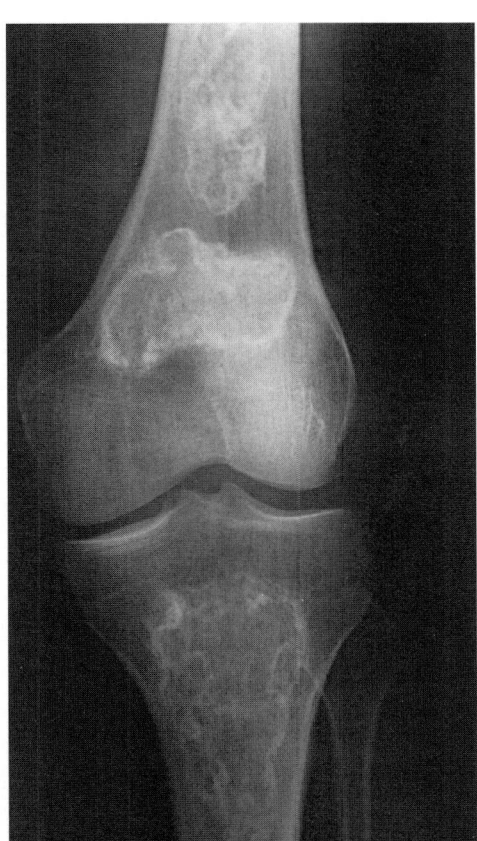

Figure 7-6 ▪ Medullary infarcts of the femur and tibia. Calcification of necrotic fat results in this smoke-ring pattern of radiodensity.

Table 7-3 ▪ **STAGES OF OSTEONECROSIS OF THE FEMORAL HEAD**

Stage	Symptoms	Results of Plain Radiographs	Results of Magnetic Resonance Imaging
0	None	No change	Positive change
I	Pain	No change	Positive change
II	Pain	Mottled sclerosis	Positive change
III	Pain	Crescent sign	Positive change
IV	Pain	Osteoarthritis	Positive change

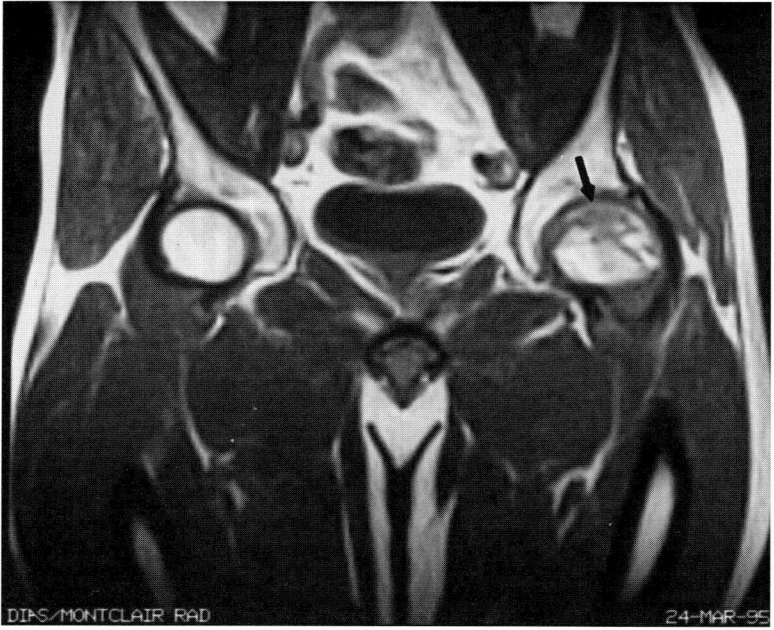

Figure 7–8 ■ Stage 1 of osteonecrosis of the femoral head. A distinct margin of low signal is apparent on this T_1-weighted image *(arrow)*. (From McCarthy, E. F. Jr.: *Differential Diagnosis in Pathology. Bone and Joint Disorders.* New York and Tokyo, Igaku-Shoin, 1996. With permission from Williams & Wilkins.)

have hip pain and normal plain radiographs. In this stage, a segment of the femoral head is dead, but reparative changes have not yet occurred. Although plain radiographs are normal, the bone scan is positive at the margins of the infarct, indicating early repair. The MRI is the most sensitive imaging modality and shows changes very early in stage I.[45] Dead marrow fat, not visible on plain radiographs, appears as a well-demarcated zone of signal change in the anterosuperior portion of the femoral head. This is best seen as a linear dark band on T_1-weighted images (Fig. 7–8).

Evidence of the bone's reaction to the necrotic segment is visible on plain radiographs in *stage II*. Mottled radiodensity appears in the femoral head, but the articular contour is unaltered (Fig. 7–9). These radiodensities correspond to calcification of the dead marrow and the ingrowth of reparative new bone. Moreover, the radiodensities may be enhanced by relative disuse osteopenia of the adjacent viable bone.

Stage III is characterized by structural failure of the femoral head. A radiolucent crescent, the so-called "crescent sign," appears beneath the subchondral plate (Fig. 7–10). The crescent is secondary to microfractures through dead bone trabeculae that have been weakened by partial resorption (Fig. 7–11). Ultimately, these microfractures lead to collapse or flattening of the articular surface (Fig. 7–12).

Changes of secondary osteoarthritis indicate *stage IV*. The joint space may be narrowed, and osteophytes and subchondral cysts may be present (Fig. 7–13). Occasionally, extensive fragmentation of the necrotic segment leads to rapid deterioration of a large segment of the femoral head. In this event, an intense synovitis results from embedded detritic bone.

Other more complicated staging systems of osteonecrosis of the femoral head are based on that of Ficat and Arlet. Some of these systems include size of the necrotic segment or its location in the femoral head. Whether these additional parameters significantly correlate with prognosis has not been determined.

Evolution of an Infarct. The time required for a necrotic lesion to evolve through the four stages is not known. Most patients do not seek medical attention until stage III, when pain develops due to collapse of the articular surface. In most patients, the early stages are asymptomatic or minimally symptomatic. Therefore, the duration of each stage cannot be calculated. However, experience with dysbaric osteonecrosis

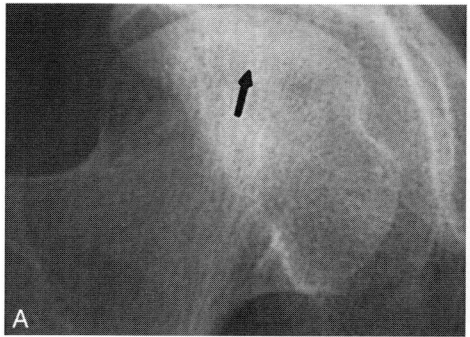
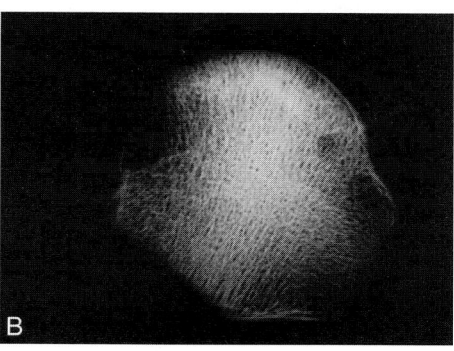

Figure 7–9 ■ Radiographs of stage II osteonecrosis of the femoral head. **A,** Plain radiograph showing increased density beneath the articular surface *(arrow)*. **B,** This zone is better seen on a slab section of the femoral head.

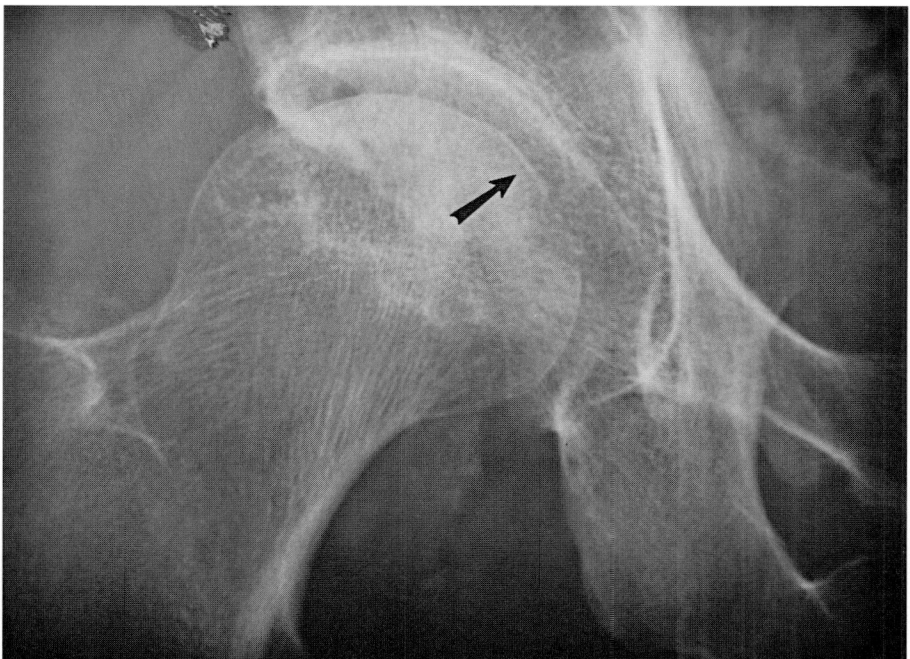

Figure 7-10 ■ Stage III of osteonecrosis of the femoral head. Mottled radiolucency and density are present. A linear lucent zone (the crescent sign) is present beneath the articular surface *(arrow)*.

provides a clue. An exposure to compressed air marks a starting point in the evolution of a necrotic lesion. Plain radiographic features do not become evident until 4 to 5 months after a hyperbaric exposure.[21] Articular collapse, marking the onset of stage III, occurs from 15 months to a few years after such an event. These observations suggest that a long window of time—more than a year—exists to salvage the integrity of the articular surface.

Dysbaric-related osteonecrosis provides another clue to the evolution of bone infarcts. Scintigraphic studies of compressed air workers show that some bone infarcts may never become visible on plain radiographs. In these workers, asymptomatic and radiographically normal hot spots persist as long as 10 years following compressed air exposure.[46]

Because at least 50% of patients with osteonecrosis of the femoral head eventually have bilateral disease, close study of the contralateral, "silent" hip provides clues to the evolution of a lesion. The most important observation is that, in many instances, an MRI demonstrates an infarct long before the hip becomes symptomatic. This setting, MRI changes in

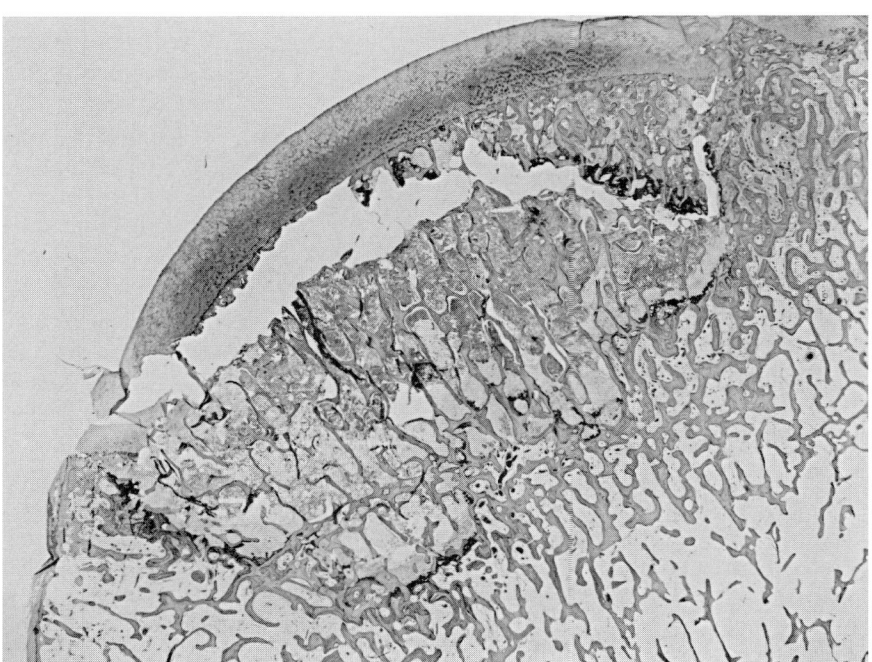

Figure 7-11 ■ Osteonecrosis of the femoral head, stage III. This macrophotomicrograph shows a fracture beneath the subchondral bone, which corresponds to the crescent sign.

an asymptomatic patient, has been called stage 0 by Hungerford and Lennox.[47] Treatment in this stage affords the best prognosis.

Treatment of Osteonecrosis of the Femoral Head. Because of the suboptimal results of total hip surgery in patients with osteonecrosis of the femoral head, this procedure should be delayed as long as possible. Therefore, efforts should be directed at preserving the integrity of the articular surface before stage III occurs. Excellent results have been achieved in early cases with a decompression core biopsy. This procedure relieves the increased intraosseous pressure and provides a path for the ingrowth of reparative tissue.[48] Insertion of a vascularized fibular bone graft is also effective in preserving the integrity of the articular cartilage. A stage III or IV lesion, however, usually requires total hip surgery.

Spontaneous Osteonecrosis of the Knee

Bone infarction also occurs in the subchondral regions of the knee, particularly in the distal femur. Risk factors, such as alcoholism or steroid therapy, are identifiable in many patients with infarcts in these regions. Presumably, the pathogenesis of infarction in these patients—fat embolism and intravascular coagulation—is similar to that of infarcts elsewhere. However, unlike patients with osteonecrosis of the hip, a large group of patients with osteonecrosis of the knee, usually women older than 60 years, have no identifiable risk factors.[49,50] This syndrome in patients without risk factors

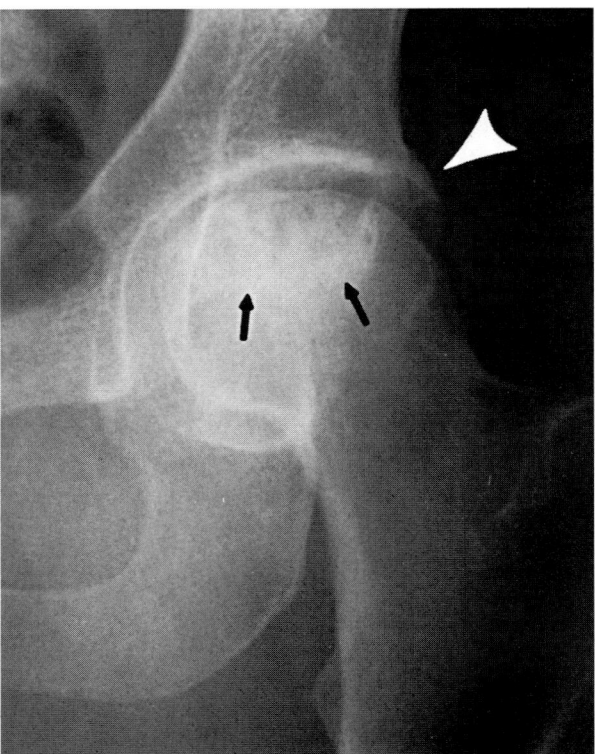

Figure 7-13 ■ Osteonecrosis of the femoral head, stage IV. Collapse of the articular surface has occurred within the margins of the infarct *(bounded by arrows)*. An osteophyte in the acetabulum indicates early osteoarthritis *(arrowhead)*.

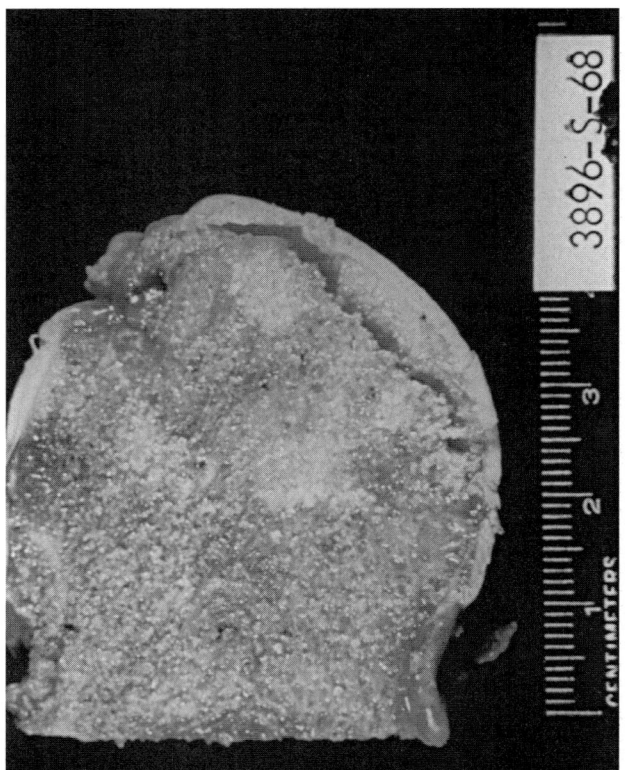

Figure 7-12 ■ Gross specimen of osteonecrosis of the femoral head showing the subchondral fracture.

has been called *spontaneous osteonecrosis of the knee* or osteonecrosis-like syndrome of the knee. The pathogenesis of infarction in these patients may be trauma rather than intravascular coagulation, a theory supported by the observation that a meniscal injury is often present. Possibly, microfractures through osteoporotic subchondral bone cause marrow hemorrhage and edema, a process that may lead to necrosis. In fact, some of these lesions may not be examples of necrosis but rather syndromes of bone marrow edema, similar to focal osteoporosis of the hip (see Chapter 4).

The location of the infarct in the knee depends on the clinical setting. The lateral condyle is more commonly affected in patients with risk factors, such as steroid therapy or sickle cell disease. In these patients, both knees are involved in 50% of cases. In addition, infarcts are often present in other locations, such as the hip or proximal humerus. In contrast to patients with risk factors, the medial femoral condyle is usually affected in elderly patients without risk factors.

Spontaneous osteonecrosis of the knee presents with acute pain, which is typically worse at night. Patients often have localized tenderness, stiffness, and an effusion. Plain radiographs are initially normal, although a bone scan shows intense uptake. After weeks to months, plain radiographic changes become evident. Flattening and sclerosis of the femoral condyle occur (Fig. 7-14), and a demarcated zone of radiolucency appears, a change presumably caused by

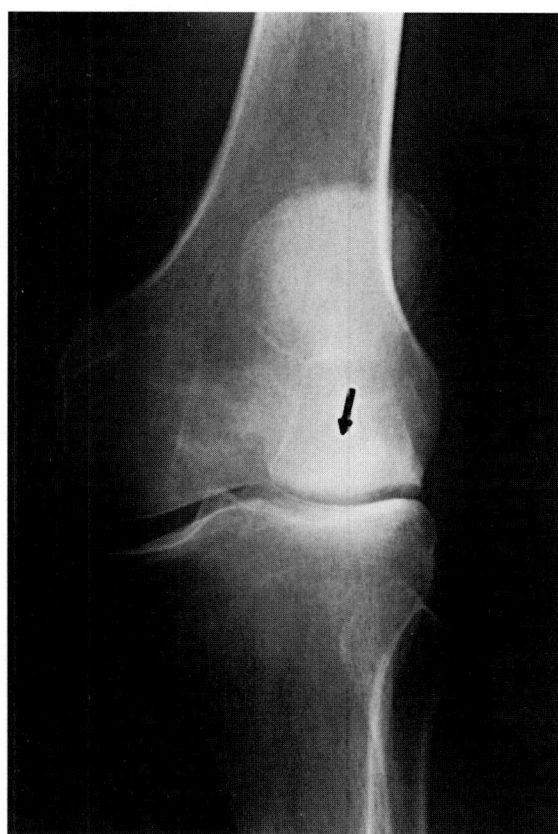

Figure 7-14 ■ Spontaneous osteonecrosis of the knee. The lateral femoral chondyle is collapsed, and the bone is radiodense *(arrow)*.

compression and fragmentation of subchondral necrotic bone. As in osteonecrosis of the hip, the MRI is a very sensitive diagnostic tool, and imaging features are similar.[51] A well-defined zone of low signal intensity is present in T_1-weighted images, and a surrounding zone of high signal is visible on T_2-weighted images.

THE OSTEOCHONDROSES

The osteochondroses are a heterogeneous group of epiphyseal or apophyseal disorders that affect children and adolescents. At least 30 other eponymic syndromes in this group of diseases correspond to lesions at particular sites. Radiographically, they are characterized by bone fragmentation and sclerosis. Frequently, reparative new bone is present. Previously, all the osteochondroses were believed to be manifestations of osteonecrosis. However, it is now known that osteonecrosis is not present in all these lesions. Moreover, in those lesions characterized by osteonecrosis, the bone death is probably secondary to trauma rather than intravascular coagulation. In fact, trauma to the vulnerable growing skeleton is the likely cause of most of these disorders whether or not necrosis is present. Only the most common of these disorders is discussed in this chapter (Table 7-4). Of these, four syndromes are characterized by osteonecrosis: Legg-Calvé-Perthes disease, Freiberg's disease, Köhler's disease, and Kienböck's disease. Two other disorders, Osgood-Schlatter disease and Scheuermann's disease, although not characterized by necrotic bone, also are discussed.

Legg-Calvé-Perthes Disease

Legg-Calvé-Perthes disease is osteonecrosis of the capital femoral epiphysis in children who are usually between ages 5 and 7. This disorder is the childhood counterpart of osteonecrosis of the femoral head in adults. Boys are affected five times as often as girls. Usually only one hip is involved, although minimal asymptomatic radiographic features are often present in the contralateral hip.

Pathogenesis

The cause of the osteonecrosis in Legg-Calvé-Perthes disease is unknown, although various hypotheses exist. One theory postulates that the disease is initiated by trauma, a history of which is present in 25% of cases. Trauma may cause an acute transient synovitis, which compresses the retinacular vessels and causes ischemia of the epiphysis.[52] Another hypothesis suggests that the disease is a manifestation of a transient generalized disorder of the epiphyseal cartilage.[53] Studies supporting this theory have demonstrated a thickened and disorganized growth plate in affected patients, an abnormality that possibly interferes with the epiphyseal blood supply. Further evidence of a growth plate disorder is that patients with Legg-Calvé-Perthes disease are shorter than normal and have other signs of delayed skeletal maturation, such as small feet. A final etiologic theory, similar to that proposed for adult osteonecrosis, is that affected patients have hypercoagulable blood and are predisposed to venous thrombosis. Indeed, 75% of affected children have identifiable syndromes of hypercoagulability, including protein C or S deficiency, hypofibrinolysis, or increased lipoprotein (a).[54]

Unlike osteonecrosis of the hip, which almost always leads to an end-stage joint, Legg-Calvé-Perthes disease has a variable evolution, depending on the age of onset and the extent of epiphyseal involvement. Various classification systems, reviewed by Wenger and colleagues,[55] have been developed to predict the outcome. In general, patients younger than age 6 or with involvement of less than 50% of the capital femoral epiphysis do well. Presumably, collateral

Table 7-4 ■ **OSTEOCHONDROSES**

Disease	Site
Legg-Calvé-Perthes disease	Capital femoral epiphysis
Freiberg's disease	Second metatarsal head
Kienböck's disease	Carpal lunate
Köhler's disease	Tarsal navicular
Osgood-Schlatter disease	Tibial tubercle
Scheuermann's disease	Vertebral endplates

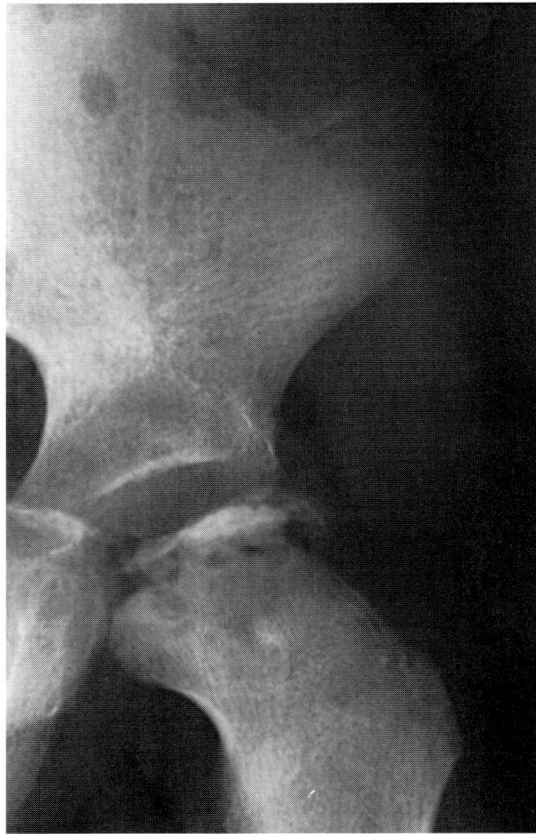

Figure 7-15 ■ Legg-Calvé-Perthes disease. The femoral capital epiphysis is collapsed, and the bone is sclerotic.

blood supply to the growing epiphyses, absent in the adult, enables many of these patients to reconstitute an almost normally shaped femoral head.

Clinical and Radiographic Presentation

Legg-Calvé-Perthes disease is not uncommon; a pediatric orthopedist in a university medical center sees as many as 25 new cases per year. The diagnosis is made by clinical and plain radiographic features. Children present with hip pain, a limp, and decreased range of motion. Several radiographic features may be present. In the early stages, the femoral epiphyseal ossification nucleus is sometimes displaced laterally in the acetabulum and is smaller than that of the contralateral hip. Later in the course of the disease, the ossific nucleus fractures, and it may become flattened and sclerotic (Fig. 7–15). Another late manifestation is the appearance of radiolucent defects on the metaphyseal side of the physis. These defects correspond to islands of uncalcified cartilage displaced into the metaphysis from a distorted epiphyseal plate. End-stage radiographic features of a severely affected child are a flattened femoral head with a wide, short femoral neck.

Pathology

The pathologist has only rare opportunities to study tissue from an active lesion of Legg-Calvé-Perthes disease. Tissue is occasionally obtained from core biopsies and, rarely, at autopsy. Osteonecrosis is a constant histopathologic feature, and fracture and collapse of necrotic bone trabeculae often are seen. As in osteonecrosis in the adult femoral head, evidence of repair is present. Granulation tissue grows into the necrotic zone, with new bone deposition on dead trabeculae. Unlike femoral head necrosis in the adult, however, complete repair of the necrotic area usually occurs, although in some cases the femoral head is severely distorted.

Freiberg's Disease

Freiberg's disease, also known as Freiberg's infarction, is osteonecrosis of the metatarsal head. Typically, the second metatarsal head is involved, but the third or fourth metatarsal may, although rarely, be affected. This disorder usually affects girls between the ages of 13 and 18.[56] They present with pain, tenderness, and swelling over the affected metatarsal head. Radiographically, the metatarsal head is flattened and sclerotic (Fig. 7–16). In the late stages, loose osteochondral fragments are visible in the joint space. The histopathologic features seen in excised metatarsal heads show osteonecrosis with varying degrees of repair. Repeated trauma to the second metatarsal head is a likely cause of this disorder.[57] This metatarsal, being longer and more firmly fixed to the tarsus than the others, is more vulnerable to

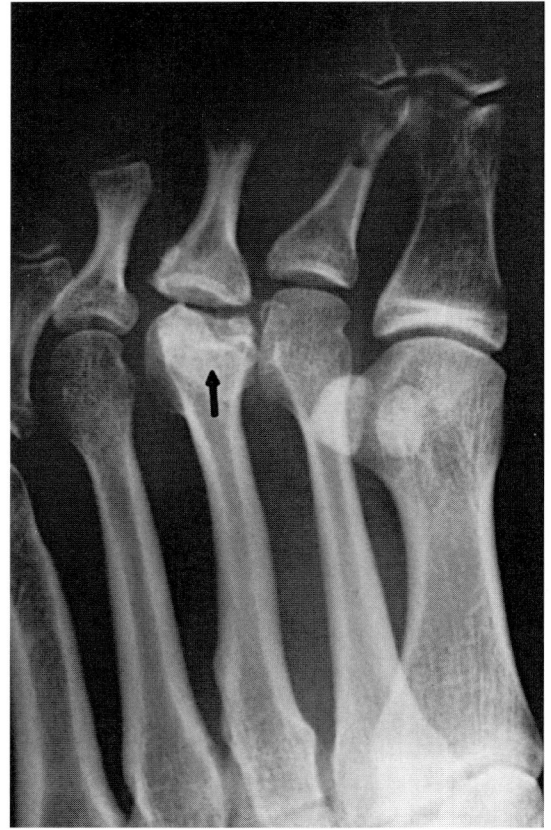

Figure 7-16 ■ Freiberg's disease of the third metatarsal head (arrow).

trauma. Its higher incidence in female patients is possibly related to their wearing high-heeled shoes.

Kienböck's Disease

Kienböck's disease is osteonecrosis of the carpal lunate, a disorder that targets patients in their 20s and 30s. They present with pain and stiffness of the wrist. Radiologic changes in the lunate include sclerosis, fracture, and collapse (Fig. 7–17). As in Freiberg's disease, the pathologic changes show necrosis and repair. This disease often follows severe or repeated injury to the wrist, suggesting, like in Freiberg's disease, that trauma is a likely cause. In addition, many patients have a slightly shortened ulna (an ulnar minus variance), which possibly exposes the lunate to more stress.[58]

Köhler's Disease

Köhler's disease affects the tarsal navicular bone. Patients, usually boys between ages 3 and 7, present with pain, swelling, and decreased ankle motion. Radiographs reveal increased density, flattening, and fragmentation of the ossific nucleus of the tarsal navicular. MRI studies, however, reveal that the cartilage anlage is not compressed, suggesting that this disease is a manifestation of abnormal endochondral

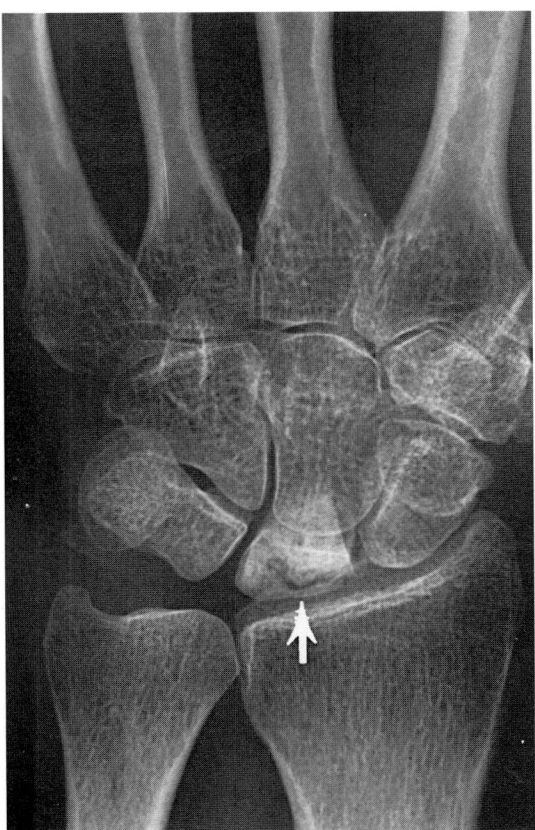

Figure 7–17 ■ Kienböck's disease of the carpal lunate. The lunate is fractured and focally radiodense (arrows).

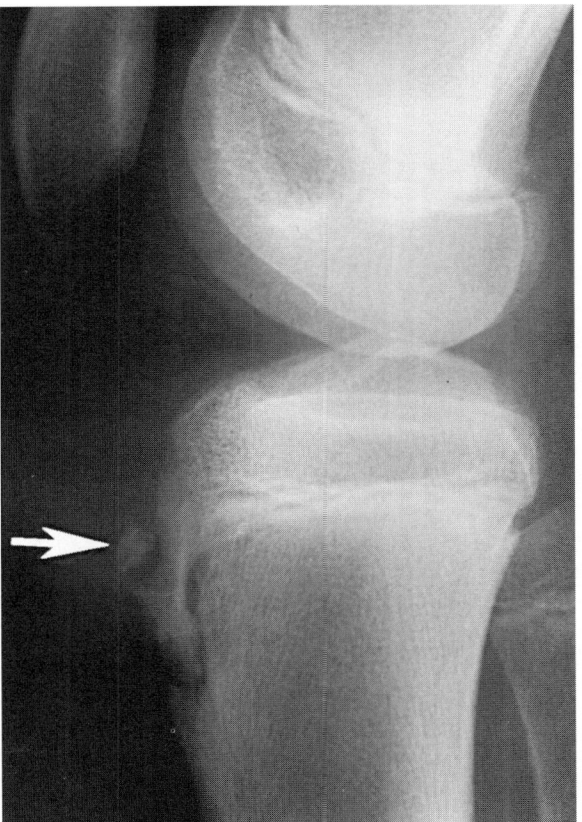

Figure 7–18 ■ Osgood-Schlatter disease. A portion of the tibial tubercle is detached (arrow).

bone formation rather than osteonecrosis.[59] However, osteonecrosis has been demonstrated in the bony nucleus. Köhler's disease is probably caused by stresses on the ankle at a vulnerable point in skeletal development.[60]

Osgood-Schlatter Disease

Osgood-Schlatter disease is an avulsion of a portion of the patellar tendon from the tibial tuberosity resulting in inflammatory and reparative changes.[61] This common disorder occurs in adolescents, usually boys between the ages of 11 and 15 years. Patients often have a history of a recent growth spurt or vigorous participation in sports. They present with pain, swelling, and a very tender tibial tuberosity. Radiographically, Osgood-Schlatter disease is characterized by displaced fragments of bone in the region of the tibial tuberosity (Fig. 7–18). Cartilage is also avulsed; therefore, the detached fragments enlarge by endochondral ossification as the patient gets older. Symptoms of Osgood-Schlatter disease may persist for several years until the tuberosity is fused to the tibia. Although symptoms almost always disappear, a rare patient may develop a nonunion of the tibial tuberosity.

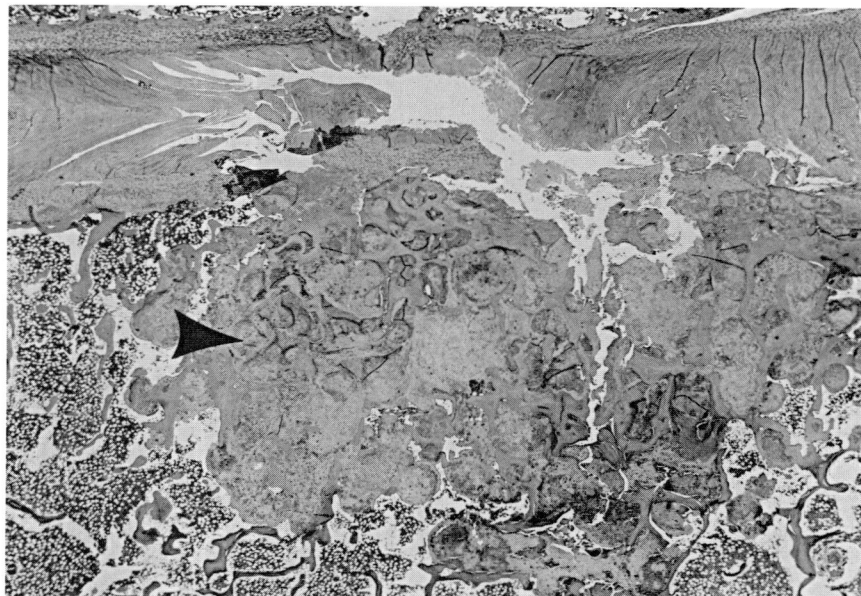

Figure 7-19 ▪ Low-power photomicrograph showing a Schmorl's node. A portion of a vertebral disc is present in the vertebral body (arrowhead).

Scheuermann's Disease

Scheuermann's disease is a disorder of the vertebral endplates, which results in varying degrees of thoracic kyphosis. Formerly felt to be a result of osteonecrosis of the vertebral apophyseal rings, this disorder is now recognized to be caused by herniation of intervertebral disc material into the vertebral body (Fig. 7–19). Isolated herniations of vertebral disc material and cartilage into the vertebral body, known as *Schmorl's nodes,* are common in elderly patients, especially those with osteoporosis. However, unlike isolated Schmorl's nodes, which occur in older patients, Scheuermann's disease affects adolescents, usually between the ages of 13 and 17, and the process is multifocal.[62] The cause of this process is unknown, although congenital defects in the vertebral endplates or endplate fracture at a vulnerable point in skeletal maturation has been suggested.[63] A family history of this disorder is present in 25% of cases, suggesting a heritable weakness of the vertebral endplates in these patients.[64]

Radiographically, Scheuermann's disease is characterized by irregular or disrupted vertebral endplates with adjacent lytic lesions in the vertebral bodies. Eventually, the vertebral body becomes wedged and the disc space is narrowed, usually more so in the anterior zone (Fig. 7–20). This results in varying degrees of a kyphosis, which often becomes fixed as the patient ages. Occasionally, bony fusion of affected vertebral bodies occurs. A spectrum of severity exists in this disease. Minimal endplate irregularity is not uncommon in the general population. However, involvement of at least three contiguous vertebrae, each with wedging of 5° or more, is required to establish the diagnosis.[65]

RADIATION OSTEODYSPLASIA

Clinical Features

Radiation osteodysplasia, an uncommon disease, is now seen almost exclusively after external beam radiation therapy for malignant neoplasms. Clinical evidence of bone damage occurs in 1 to 7% of patients treated with this modality. The affected bone may have been the target of the radiation, or it may have been normal bone included in the radiation field for treatment of a visceral or soft tissue neoplasm.

The degree of bone damage is a function of the type

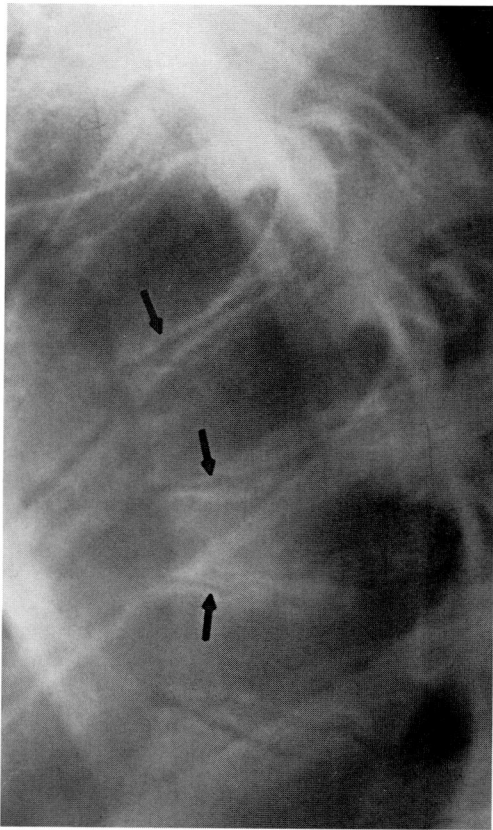

Figure 7-20 ▪ Scheuermann's disease. Erosion of the vertebral endplates (arrows) and anterior wedging of the vertebral bodies are present.

of irradiation, the dose, and the method of administration. Osteodysplasia usually does not occur below 3000 rads. Some changes occur between 3000 and 5000 rads, and doses above 5000 rads cause permanent bone damage. Osteodysplasia does not usually manifest until 5 to 10 years after radiotherapy. Therefore, patients who develop bone disease are long-term survivors of their malignancies. Some patients present with pathologic fracture. Others present with collapse of joint surfaces secondary to osteonecrosis, an important feature of this disease.

Although any bone in an irradiation field can be affected, certain sites are common. Mandibular involvement follows irradiation for oral cancers. The ribs, clavicle, and proximal humerus are involved after treatment for breast, lung, or mediastinal malignancies. The pelvis and proximal femurs are affected after irradiation for rectal, prostate, or gynecologic cancers. Finally, long bones adjacent to irradiated soft tissue sarcomas may be severely affected. Children irradiated for childhood malignancies may also develop radiation damage to bone. In children, the growth plates are also damaged and result in such skeletal deformities as severe scoliosis or limb length discrepancy. These growth deformities manifest sooner than osteodysplasia.

Radiology

Although radiation produces immediate damage to bone, the radiographic features of osteodysplasia evolve slowly. The first radiographic change is osteopenia, which develops 5 months to 1 year after therapy. A pathologic fracture, particularly in the femoral neck, often accompanies the osteopenia. Other radiographic features develop even more slowly, usually over 5 to 10 years following therapy.[66] A fully developed lesion shows patchy areas of radiodensity in the medullary canal and coarsening of the trabeculae (Fig. 7–21). In addition to the radiodense areas, irregular areas of longitudinally oriented radiolucencies are present. The pattern of mixed radiolysis and radiodensity simulates a permeative neoplasm. However, unlike most permeative neoplasms, a periosteal reaction (in unfractured lesions) and a soft tissue mass are absent. Also, the bone scan in radiation osteodysplasia usually shows no increased uptake of radioisotope.

Histology

Fully developed radiation osteodysplasia is characterized by patchy osteonecrosis and evidence of increased bone resorption.[67,68] These changes are produced by a combination of microvascular injury and direct cell damage, and they take years to evolve following the initial radiation damage. Irradiation immediately damages most of the marrow elements and some bone cells. These elements are only partially restored. Normal bone remodeling is shifted in favor of osteoclastic resorption and results in osteopenia, the initial change seen on plain radiographs. The damaged marrow is

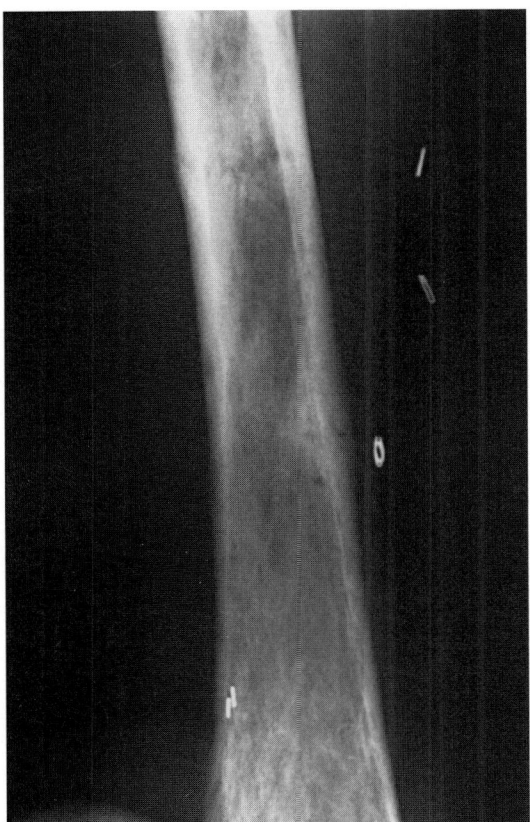

Figure 7–21 ■ Radiation osteodysplasia. A moth-eaten pattern of bone destruction can be seen throughout the entire length of the femur.

replaced by poorly vascular scar tissue, which results in chronic ischemia and, eventually, necrosis.

Histologic changes are evident in both the bone and in the marrow. The bone is focally necrotic; osteocytes are absent from trabeculae and segments of cortex. Cortical haversian canals are dilated, a result of increased osteoclastic activity, and many of these dilated haversian canals fuse to form intracortical cavities. Some haversian canals and osteocyte lacunae are filled with amorphous calcified debris. In addition to changes in the bone, the marrow shows features of prior damage and abortive repair. The marrow space is filled with sparsely cellular fibrous tissue (Fig. 7–22). A few of the spindle cells show bizarre and hyperchromatic nuclei. These cells may be mistaken for recurrent or metastatic neoplasm. However, keratin stains are negative. In addition, the fibrous areas show calcification and deposits of deeply basophilic woven bone (Fig. 7–23). A distinctive histologic feature of severe radiation osteodysplasia is an absent or minimal reparative reaction in the damaged areas. The limited repair is presumably caused by failure of precursor cells to differentiate into osteoblasts secondary to the damaged microvascular system. However, resorption continues, although at a lower rate. Less severe osteodysplasia shows seams of appositional bone deposited on dead trabeculae. Vascular occlusive changes seen in other irradiated organs are not usually present in osteodysplasia.

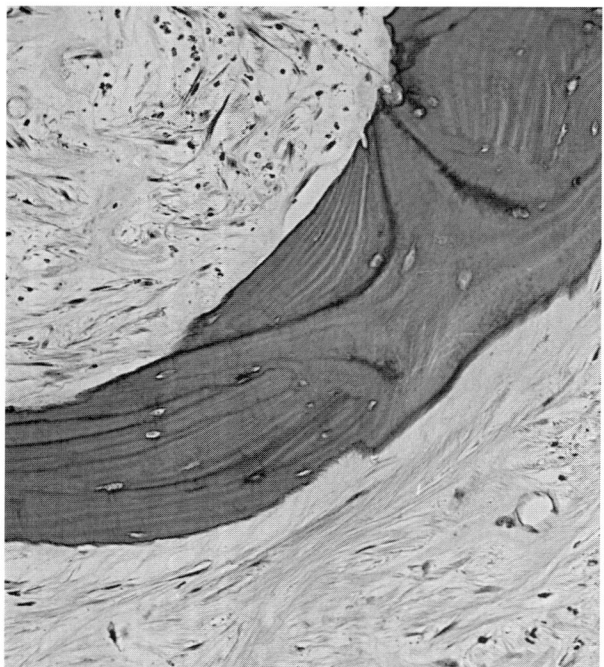

Figure 7-22 ■ Photomicrograph of radiation osteodysplasia. Necrotic trabeculae are surrounded by fibrotic marrow.

Management

The pathologic fractures resulting from radiation osteodysplasia heal slowly and often require internal fixation. Collapsed, necrotic femoral heads are best treated by total joint arthroplasty. The most devastating complication of radiation osteodysplasia is the development of postradiation sarcoma in the area of bone previously irradiated. The incidence of this complication is about 0.2% in patients who have received up to 7000 rads. The average latent period following therapy is 14.3 years, although on rare occasions, a sarcoma may develop 2 years after therapy. The malignancy is usually an osteosarcoma or a malignant fibrous histiocytoma.

REFERENCES

1. Catto, M.: A histological study of avascular necrosis of the femoral head after transcervical fracture. *J Bone Joint Surg* 47B:749–776, 1965.
2. Petrie, P. W. R.: Aetiology of osteochondritis dissecans. Failure to establish a familial background. *J Bone Joint Surg* 59B:366–367, 1977.
3. Milgram, J. W.: Radiological and pathological manifestations of osteochondritis dissecans of the distal femur. A study of 50 cases. *Radiology* 126:305–311, 1978.
4. Rothschild, B. M.: Decompression syndrome in fossil marine turtles. *Ann Carnegie Museum* 56:253–258, 1987.
5. Rothschild, B. M.: Stratophenetic analysis of avascular necrosis in turtles: Affirmation of the decompression syndrome hypothesis. *Comp Biochem Physiol* 100A:529–535, 1991.
6. Gray, P. H. K.: Bone infarction in antiquity. *Clin Radiol* 19:436–437, 1968.
7. Konig, F.: Über freie Korper in den Gelenken. *Dtsch Z Chir* 27:90, 1888.
8. Axhausen, G.: Kritisches und Experimentelles zur Genese der Arthritis deformans, insbesondere über die Bedeutung der aseptischen Knochen und Knorpelnechrose. *Arch Klin Chir* 94:331, 1911.
9. Schmorl, G.: Anaemische Nekrose in Schenkelkopf. *Zentralbl Allg Pathol* 35:261, 1924.
10. Chandler, F.: Aseptic necrosis of the head of the femur. *Wis Med J* 35:609, 1936.
11. Harigaya, K., Watanabe, S., Watanabe, Y., et al.: Multiple bone marrow necrosis and disseminated intravascular coagulation. *Arch Pathol Lab Med* 101:652–654, 1977.
12. Duncan, J. S., and Ramsay, L. E.: Widespread bone infarction complicating meningococcal septicaemia and disseminated intravascular coagulation. *Br Med J* 288:111–112, 1984.
13. Jones, J. P.: Fat embolism, intravascular coagulation, and osteonecrosis. *Clin Orthop* 292:294–308, 1993.
14. Jones, J. P., Engleman, E. P., Steinbach, H. L., et al.: Fat embolization as a possible mechanism producing avascular necrosis. *Arthritis Rheum* 8:449, 1965.
15. Jones, J. P. Jr., and Sakovich, L.: Fat embolism of bone. A roentgenographic and histological investigation, with use of intra-arterial lipiodol, in rabbits. *J Bone Joint Surg* 48A:149–164, 1966.
16. Jacobs, B.: Epidemiology of traumatic and nontraumatic osteonecrosis. *Clin Orthop* 130:51–67, 1978.
17. Jones, J. P. Jr.: Alcoholism, hypercortisolism, fat embolism and osseous avascular necrosis. Zinn, W. M., Ed. *Idiopathic Ischemic Necrosis of the Femoral Head in Adults*. Stuttgart, Georg Thieme, 1971, pp. 112–132.
18. Jones, J. P., Ramirez, S., and Doty, S. B.: The pathophysiologic role of fat in dysbaric osteonecrosis. *Clin Orthop* 296:256–264, 1993.
19. Lee, P. C., and Howard, J. M.: Fat necrosis. *Surg Gynecol Obstet* 148:785–789, 1979.
20. Zolla-Pazner, S., Pazner, S. S., Lanyi, V., et al.: Osteonecrosis of the femoral head during pregnancy. *JAMA* 244:689–690, 1980.
21. Catto, M.: Pathology of aseptic bone necrosis. Davidson, J. K., Ed. *Aseptic Necrosis of Bone*. New York, American Elsevier, 1976, pp. 3–100.
22. Solomon, L.: Mechanisms of idiopathic osteonecrosis. *Orthop Clin North Am* 16:655–667, 1985.
23. Hungerford, D. S.: Bone marrow pressure, venography, and core decompression in ischemic necrosis of the femoral head. *The Hip: Proceedings of the Seventh Open Scientific Meeting of The Hip Society*. St. Louis, C. V. Mosby, 1979, pp. 218–237.
24. Hungerford, D. S.: Pathogenetic considerations in ischemic necrosis of bone. *Can J Surg* 24:583–587, 590, 1981.
25. Wang, G., Sweet, D. E., Reger, S. I., and Thompson, R. C.: Fat-cell changes as a mechanism of avascular necrosis of the femoral head in cortisone-treated rabbits. *J Bone Joint Surg* 59A:729–735, 1977.

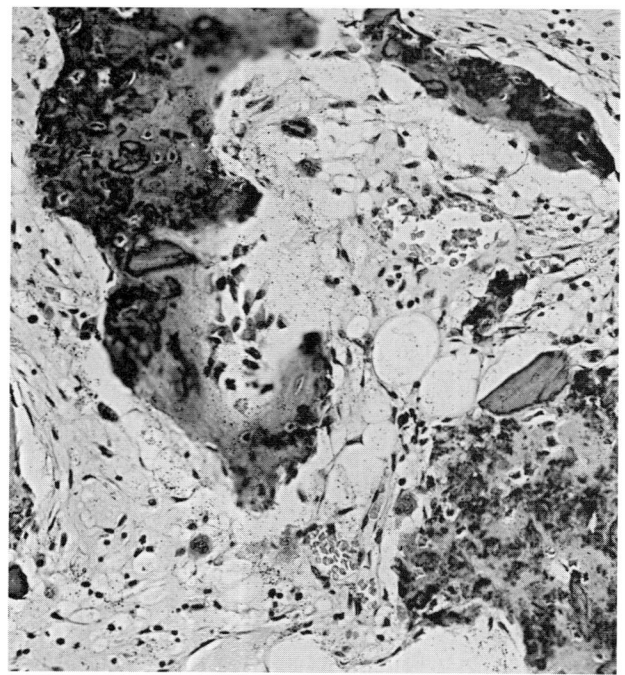

Figure 7-23 ■ Photomicrograph of radiation osteodysplasia. Deeply basophilic woven bone is present in a fibroinflammatory background.

26. Boettcher, W. G., Bonfiglio, M., Hamilton, H. E., et al.: Non-traumatic necrosis of the femoral head: Part I, Relation of altered hemostasis to etiology. *J Bone Joint Surg* 52A:312–329, 1970.
27. Jones, J. P. Jr.: Avascular necrosis of bone. McCarty, D. J., and Koopman, W. J., Eds. *Arthritis and Allied Conditions. A Textbook of Rheumatology.* Philadelphia, Lea & Febiger, 1993, pp. 1677–1696.
28. Jones, J. P.: Concepts of etiology and early pathogenesis of osteonecrosis. Instructional Course Lectures. *Am Acad Orthop Surg* 43:499–512, 1994.
29. Glueck, C. J., Freiberg, R., Glueck, H. I., Henderson, C., Welch, M., Tracy, T., Stroop, D., Hamer, T., Sosa, F., and Levy, M.: Hypofibrinolysis: A common, major cause of osteonecrosis. *Am J Hematol* 45:156–166, 1994.
30. Mont, M. A., and Hungerford, D. S.: Current concepts review: Nontraumatic avascular necrosis of the femoral head. *J Bone Joint Surg* 77A:459–474, 1995.
31. Anderton, J. M., and Helm, R.: Multiple joint osteonecrosis following short-term steroid therapy. *J Bone Joint Surg* 64A:139, 1982.
32. Shpall, E. J., Efremidis, A. P., Kasambalides, E., Sedlin, E., and Hermann, G.: Case report 352. *Skeletal Radiol* 15:170–174, 1986.
33. Zizic, T. M., and Hungerford, D. S.: Avascular necrosis of bone. Kelley, W. N., Harris, E. D., Ruddy, S., Sledge, C. B., Eds. *Textbook of Rheumatology.* Philadelphia, W. B. Saunders, 1985, pp. 1689–1710.
34. Sakamoto, M., Shimizu, K., Iida, S., Akita, T., Moriya, H., and Nawata, Y.: Osteonecrosis of the femoral head. A prospective study with MRI. *J Bone Joint Surg* 79B:213–219, 1997.
35. Nagasawa, K., Ishii, Y., and Mayumi, T.: Avascular necrosis of bone in systemic lupus erythematosus: Possible role of haemostatic abnormalities. *Ann Rheum Dis* 48:672–676, 1989.
36. Koo, K., Kim, R., Cho, S. H., Song, H. R., Lee, G., and Ko, G. H.: Angiography, scintigraphy, intraosseous pressure, and histologic findings in high-risk osteonecrotic femoral heads with negative magnetic resonance images. *Clin Orthop* 308:127–138, 1994.
37. Borstein, A., and Plate, E.: Über chronische Gelenkveränderungen, entstanden durch Presslufterkrankung. *Fortschr Geb Roentgenstr* 18:197, 1911.
38. McCallum, R., Stanger, J., Walder, D., Barnes, R., Catto, M., Davidson, J., Fryer, D., Golding, F., and Paton, W.: Bone lesions in compressed-air workers with special reference to men who worked on the Clyde Tunnels 1958 to 1963. Report of decompression sickness. Panel Medical Research Council. *J Bone Joint Surg* 48B:207–235, 1966.
39. Elliott, D., and Harrison, J.: Bone necrosis—an occupational hazard of diving. *J Med Serv* 56:140–161, 1970.
40. Ota, Y., and Matsunaga, H.: Bone lesions in divers. *J Joint Surg* 56B:3–16, 1974.
41. Moran, M.: Osteonecrosis of the hip in sickle cell hemoglobinopathy. *Am J Orthop* 24:18–24, 1995.
42. Keeley, K., and Buchanan, G.: Acute infarction of long bones in children with sickle-cell anemia. *J Pediatr* 101:170–175, 1982.
43. Rajah, R., Young, J., and Conway, W.: Acute hemorrhagic infarct with edema. *Skeletal Radiol* 24:158–159, 1995.
44. Ficat, R., and Arlet, J.: Functional investigation of bone under normal conditions. Hungerford, D. S., Ed. *Ischemia and Necrosis of Bone.* Baltimore, Williams & Wilkins, 1980, pp. 29–52.
45. Thickman, D., Axel, L., Kressel, H., Steinberg, M., Chen, H., Velchick, M., Fallon, M., and Dalinka, M.: Magnetic resonance imaging of avascular necrosis of the femoral head. *Skeletal Radiol* 15:133–140, 1986.
46. Gregg, P., and Walder, D.: A study of old lesions of caisson disease of bone by radiography and bone scintigraphy. *J Bone Joint Surg* 63B:132–137, 1981.
47. Hungerford, D., and Lennox, D.: Diagnosis and treatment of ischemic necrosis of the femoral head. Evarts, C. M., Ed. *Surgery in the Musculoskeletal System.* New York, Churchill-Livingstone, 1990, pp. 2757–2794.
48. Smith, S., Fehring, T., Griffin, W., and Beaver, W.: Core decompression of the osteonecrotic femoral head. *J Bone Joint Surg* 77A:674–680, 1995.
49. Ahuja, S., and Bullough, P.: Osteonecrosis of the knee. A clinicopathological study in twenty-eight patients. *J Bone Joint Surg* 60A:191–198, 1978.
50. Rozing, P., Insall, J., and Bohne, W.: Spontaneous osteonecrosis of the knee. *J Bone Joint Surg* 62A:2–7, 1980.
51. Pollack, M., Dalinka, M., Kressel, H., Lotke, P., and Spritzer, C.: Magnetic resonance imaging in the evaluation of suspected osteonecrosis of the knee. *Skeletal Radiol* 16:121–127, 1987.
52. Landin, L., Danielsson, L., and Wattsgaerd, C.: Transient synovitis of the hip. Its incidence, epidemiology and relation to Perthes' disease. *J Bone Joint Surg* 69B:238–242, 1987.
53. Ponseti, I., Maynard, J., Weinstein, S., et al.: Legg-Calvé-Perthes disease. Histochemical and ultrastructural observations of the epiphyseal cartilage and physis. *J Bone Joint Surg* 65A:797–807, 1983.
54. Glueck, C., Crawford, A., Roy, D, Freiberg, R., Glueck, H., and Stroop, D.: Association of antithrombotic factor deficiencies and hypofibrinolysis with Legg-Perthes disease. *J Bone Joint Surg* 78A:3–13, 1996.
55. Wenger, D., Ward, W., and Herring, J.: Current concepts review Legg-Calvé-Perthes disease. *J Bone Joint Surg* 73A:778–786, 1991.
56. Hoskinson, J.: Freiberg's disease: A review of the long-term results. *Proc R Soc Med* 67:106–107, 1974.
57. Smillie, I.: Freiberg's infraction (Koehler's second disease). *J Bone Joint Surg* 39B:580, 1957.
58. Gelberman, R., Salamon, P., and Jurist, J.: Ulnar variance in Kienbock's disease. *J Bone Joint Surg* 57A:674–676, 1975.
59. Resnick, D.: *Diagnosis of Bone and Joint Disorders,* 3rd ed. Philadelphia, W. B. Saunders, 1995, pp. 3559–3610.
60. Scaglietti, O., Stringa, G., and Mizzau, M.: Plus-variant of the astragalus and subnormal scaphoid space, two important findings in Koehler's scaphoid necrosis. *Acta Orthop Scand* 32:499–508, 1962.
61. La Zerte, G., and Rapp, I.: Pathogenesis of Osgood-Schlatter's disease. *Am J Pathol* 34:803–813, 1958.
62. Aufdermaur, M.: Juvenile kyphosis (Scheuermann's disease): Radiography, histology, and pathogenesis. *Clin Orthop* 154:166–174, 1981.
63. Alexander, C.: Scheuermann's disease. A traumatic spondylodystrophy. *Skeletal Radiol* 1:209–221, 1977.
64. Bradford, D., Moe, J., Montalvo, F., and Winter, R. B.: Scheuermann's kyphosis and roundback deformity. Results of Milwaukee brace treatment. *J Bone Joint Surg* 56A:740–758, 1974.
65. Sorensen, K.: *Scheuermann's Juvenile Kyphosis.* Copenhagen, Munksgaard, 1964.
66. Paling, M., and Herdt, J.: Radiation osteitis: A problem of recognition. *Radiology* 137:339–342, 1980.
67. Sugimoto, M., Takahashi, S., Toguchida, J., Kotoura, Y., Shibamoto, Y., and Yamamuro, T.: Changes in bone after high-dose irradiation. Biomechanics and histomorphology. *J Bone Joint Surg* 73B:492–497, 1991.
68. Maeda, M., Bryant, M., Yamagata, M., Li, G., Earle, J., and Chao, E.: Effects of irradiation on cortical bone and their time-related changes. *J Bone Joint Surg* 70A:392–399, 1988.

CHAPTER 8
Infections of Bones and Joints

Infection of bone, known as *osteomyelitis,* has two serious consequences for the patient. First, the infection destroys bone, which may threaten the structural stability of the skeleton. Second, the reactive bone response insulates the microorganisms and makes their eradication extremely difficult. Therefore, immediate diagnosis and therapy is imperative to prevent possible lifetime disability.

Microorganisms find their way into bone by two mechanisms: via the bloodstream or via direct invasion. When bone is infected via the bloodstream, a syndrome known as *hematogenous osteomyelitis,* organisms originate elsewhere in the body. In direct invasion, often referred to as *secondary osteomyelitis,* organisms are inoculated directly into bone from an adjacent soft tissue infection or, as in some open fractures, from a source outside the patient.

Bone infections are usually caused by bacteria, although they may result from any kind of microorganism. The clinical syndrome associated with the initial invasion of microorganisms is known as *acute osteomyelitis.* If the infection is not completely eradicated, a continuous interaction of microbial growth and reactive bone formation results in *chronic osteomyelitis.* On occasion, an episode of acute osteomyelitis is subclinical. A patient's defenses confine the infection to a localized zone of the bone. This presentation is called *subacute osteomyelitis.*

Microorganisms may also infect joint cavities without producing osteomyelitis, a condition known as *septic arthritis.* The modes of entry into joints are similar to those into bone—via the bloodstream or via direct inoculation. Because the inflammatory exudate in septic arthritis is rapidly destructive to articular cartilage, these infections must also be promptly recognized and treated to prevent irreversible joint damage.

HISTORY

Archaeological evidence suggests that osteomyelitis has affected humans for thousands of years.[1] For example, a tibia specimen from a Neolithic grave in Switzerland shows radiographic and histologic features highly suggestive of subacute osteomyelitis.[2] The earliest medical reference to chronic draining osteomyelitis is found in the aphorisms of Hippocrates: "When ulcers continue open for a year or upward there must necessarily be exfoliation of bone, and the cicatrices are hollow." Later, Roman and medieval medical treatises, such as those by Celsus[3] and Albucasis,[4] described how to probe the draining sinuses of osteomyelitis.

In the preantibiotic era, most documented cases of osteomyelitis resulted from open fractures. However, by the end of the 18th century, the syndrome of acute hematogenous osteomyelitis had also been described by Alexander Mackenzie (1762)[5] and William Bromfeild (1773)[6]. Since most preantibiotic cases resulted in devitalization of bone, osteomyelitis was often called "necrosis." The most extensive early description of necrosis was by Nathan Smith in 1827,[7] who recognized that this disease occurred almost exclusively in adolescents and children. Further contributions were made by Benjamin Brodie, who in 1845 described chronic abscesses of the tibia, a syndrome that still bears his name.[8] Brodie was able to successfully treat these lesions by trephination and drainage. The term *osteomyelitis* was first used for this condition in 1852 by the French surgeon E. Chassaignac.[9]

Although surgeons were familiar with the course of osteomyelitis, its etiology was not established until the last part of the 19th century. In 1863, Pasteur found bacteria associated with pus, and in 1878, Robert Koch suggested that these bacteria were the causal agents of infections. Also in 1878, the bacterial cause of osteomyelitis was confirmed by Rosenbach,[10] who produced the disease experimentally by injecting pus into the marrow of various animals. Further experiments led him to conclude that spontaneous osteomyelitis resulted from organisms carried to the bone via the bloodstream. Thus, the etiology of osteomyelitis had been firmly established. However, until the advent of penicillin in

1946, its treatment was limited to surgical drainage, dressings, and support of the bone.

HEMATOGENOUS BACTERIAL OSTEOMYELITIS

Hematogenous osteomyelitis is usually caused by *Staphylococcus aureus* and almost always begins in the metaphyseal region of long bones. Patients are usually children younger than 15 years. The infection is a result of a bacteremia that has its origin elsewhere in the body, such as impetigo, otitis media, or tonsillitis. However, half of affected patients have no clinical evidence of a distant site of infection, making them apparently part of that 30% of the general population who are asymptomatic carriers of *S. aureus*. They carry the organisms in their anterior nose, and septicemia may result from a breakdown of normal mucocutaneous defense mechanisms.

Although *S. aureus* is the most common etiologic organism for all cases of hematogenous osteomyelitis, *Hemophilus influenzae* occurs frequently in children younger than 3 years and is the most common agent in children younger than 2 years. In the neonate, in addition to *S. aureus*, Group B *Streptococcus* and the coliform bacteria are major etiologic agents.

Pathogenesis

As a result of the bacteremia, organisms seed the metaphysis of bone adjacent to the physis. This region contains fenestrated capillaries,[11] which permit bacteria to pass from the blood to the marrow. Once bacteria leave the blood, they bind to the bone surface. This is possible because certain bacteria, especially *S. aureus*, have receptors to bone surface proteins, such as sialoproteins and collagens.[12] Perhaps trauma makes these bone-protein binding sites more accessible to bacterial receptors. This is suggested by clinical and experimental studies, which have shown that blunt trauma is an important cofactor in the establishment of hematogenous osteomyelitis.[13]

After initial binding, bacteria, stimulated by the solidity of bone, secrete a thick coat of mucopolysaccharide, which causes even tighter adhesion to the bone surface. This coat, called a glycocalyx, favors bacterial survival by inhibiting both penetration of antibiotics and phagocytosis by host immune cells.

Following adhesion to the bone surface, the bacteria stimulate an acute purulent inflammatory reaction, which percolates through the trabecular bone to the cortex. There, the inflammatory reaction seeps through Volkmann's canals and forms a subperiosteal abscess. If the cortical penetration of the abscess occurs at a site inside a joint capsule, a septic arthritis also results. Usually the epiphyseal plate is a barrier to the inflammatory reaction. However, in infants, because they have transphyseal blood vessels, the epiphysis may become secondarily infected. On rare occasions, the epiphysis may be the site of the primary abscess.[14]

The next phase in the pathogenesis of osteomyelitis is bone destruction. Cytokines, released from the inflammatory cells, activate osteoclasts to resorb bone. These cytokines include tumor necrosis factor, interleukin-1, prostaglandin E_2, and others. Although osteoclasts are responsible for resorption of viable bone in all physiologic and pathologic states, some evidence has been found that inflammatory cells may be able to resorb necrotic bone.[15]

In addition to osteoclast-mediated bone destruction, the integrity of the bone is further compromised by the growing subperiosteal abscess. The elevated periosteum over the abscess disrupts blood vessels, and this causes segmental cortical necrosis. These necrotic segments are known as a *sequestra*. In contrast, the periosteum, which has an external blood supply, remains viable and produces reactive new bone. This reactive bone, known as an *involucrum*, encases the abscess and the sequestra.

Clinical Features

Hematogenous osteomyelitis has distinctive clinical features. In the usual presentation, a child younger than 15 years presents with fever, pain, and loss of function around a joint. Severe local bone tenderness is a cardinal sign of osteomyelitis.[16] A septic or a sterile reactive effusion in the joint adjacent to the site of tenderness also may be present. Laboratory studies usually show a marked leukocytosis, and the erythrocyte sedimentation rate is elevated in 90% of patients.[17]

Radiographic Features

Imaging studies are critical in the diagnosis of bone infections. The most sensitive indicator of acute osteomyelitis is the bone scan,[18] an imaging modality that is positive within 48 to 72 hours after the onset of symptoms. The bone scan, however, is nonspecific. Other processes, such as neoplasms, can cause similar changes.

The plain radiograph is more specific, but the changes are not apparent until 10 to 14 days after the onset of symptoms. The first change is usually the appearance of a poorly defined lytic area in the metaphysis adjacent to the physis. Usually, the amount of lucency seen on the plain radiograph does not reflect the total amount of bone tissue involved by the inflammatory process. A sequestrum, if present, appears as a radiodensity within the area of bone destruction.

Appearing about the same time as the lytic area, a thin line of periosteal new bone forms on the adjacent cortex (Fig. 8–1). Generally, the amount of periosteal new bone parallels the amount of medullary bone destruction. This characteristic radiographic pattern of acute osteomyelitis helps distinguish it from other permeative processes in which the amount of bone destruction and periosteal reaction are not equivalent.[16]

INFECTIONS OF BONES AND JOINTS

The computed tomography (CT) scan is also useful. A very well defined lytic area is present in the center of the metaphysis. This area is surrounded by a thin rim of sclerotic bone (Fig. 8–4).

SECONDARY OSTEOMYELITIS

Direct inoculation of microorganisms into bone may also cause osteomyelitis, a syndrome known as *secondary osteomyelitis*. Secondary osteomyelitis may be caused by an adjacent soft tissue infection, a contaminated open fracture, or a puncture wound or may be a complication of bone surgery. Any bone may be invaded by microorganisms in this manner. Secondary osteomyelitis presents diagnostic problems because many patients have only vague constitutional symptoms. In addition, radiographic changes may be misleading. For example, bone destruction due to infection may be impossible to distinguish from disuse osteopenia. Therefore, it is especially difficult to diagnose bone infection at the base of a decubitus ulcer or in an ulcerated, infected foot of a diabetic patient. Often, a bone biopsy with a microbiologic culture is the only way to confirm the diagnosis of osteomyelitis.

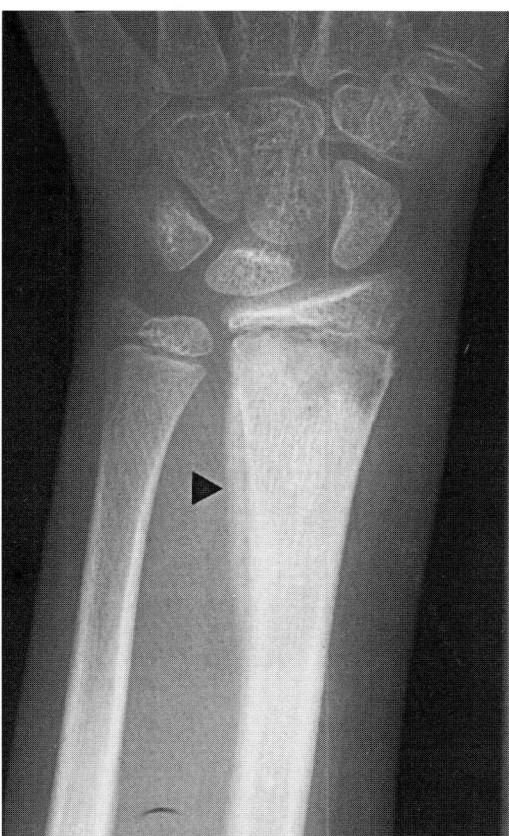

Figure 8-1 ■ Acute osteomyelitis of the distal radius. An area of medullary bone destruction and a periosteal reaction *(arrow)* is present.

On occasion, adults develop hematogenous osteomyelitis in long bones. In these patients, the primary abscess is often intracortical, usually in the diaphysis. Plain radiographs show a streak of intracortical lucency, which may have minimal or no associated periosteal reaction (Fig. 8–2).

SUBACUTE OSTEOMYELITIS

Occasionally, the body's defense mechanisms are able to contain but not eradicate the initial infection of hematogenous osteomyelitis. In this event, patients may be asymptomatic. Usually, however, mild symptoms, such as vague pain and low-grade fever, are present for months. This syndrome is known as subacute osteomyelitis or a *Brodie's abscess*. Plain radiographs show a well-defined metaphyseal lytic area surrounded by a rim of reactive bone. It is most commonly seen in the tibia, but the femur and tarsal bones are also favored sites (Fig. 8–3).

Although the magnetic resonance imaging (MRI) scan is nonspecific in most presentations of bone infection, subacute osteomyelitis shows distinctive changes with this imaging modality. A well-defined focus of high marrow signal intensity, representing the active disease, is surrounded by a crisp rim of low signal activity. This zone is known as the "rim sign" and is dark on all sequences.

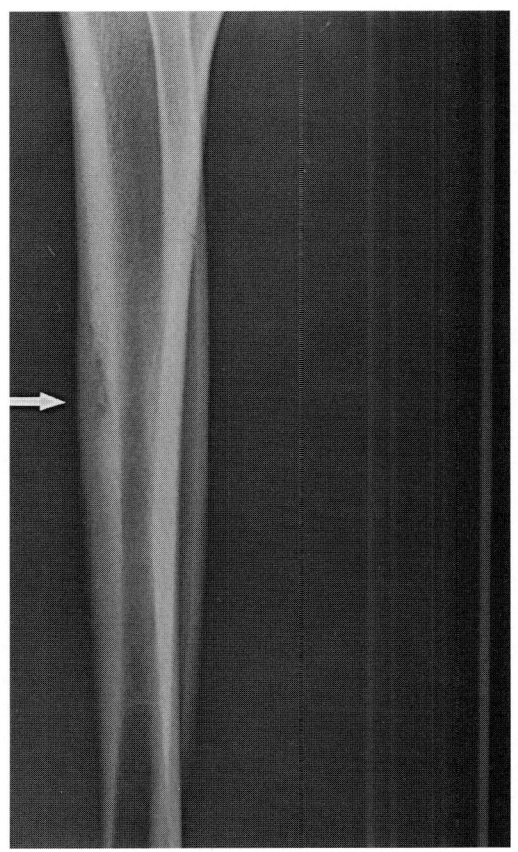

Figure 8-2 ■ Acute osteomyelitis in an adult. A linear intracortical abscess is present in the tibia *(arrow)*. A periosteal reaction is not present.

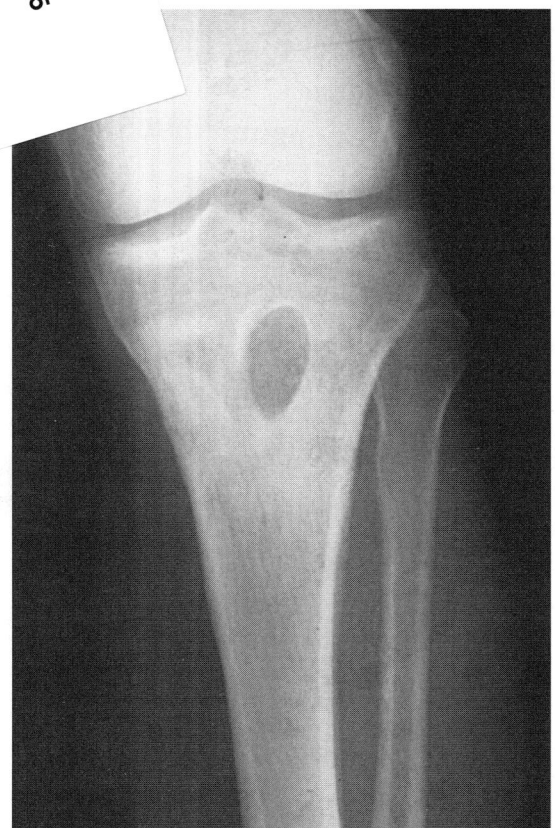

Figure 8-3 ■ A Brodie's abscess of the proximal tibia. A well-defined lytic defect and mottled sclerosis of the adjacent metaphysis is present.

CHRONIC OSTEOMYELITIS

Chronic osteomyelitis is the symptomatic, long-term infection of bone due to failure to eradicate hematogenous or secondary osteomyelitis. This condition is associated with marked disability and is always difficult, sometimes impossible, to eradicate. Most cases of chronic osteomyelitis result from open fracture–related secondary osteomyelitis. In fact, 5% of open fractures result in this syndrome. In addition, 5% of cases of acute hematogenous osteomyelitis also become chronic bone infections (Fig. 8-5). The progression usually becomes clinically evident within 1 year of the primary infection, although an 80-year interval has been reported.[19]

The characteristic feature of chronic osteomyelitis is the tenacious persistence of microorganisms. These organisms cause continuous, smoldering bone destruction and sequestration. The dead bone fragments harbor the microorganisms and insulate them from both host defense mechanisms and antibiotics. In addition, continuous reactive bone formation makes surgical débridement difficult. As a result, infection persists for many years, and sometimes it lasts for the remainder of a patient's life.

Clinically, patients have intermittent episodes of pain and constitutional symptoms that are separated by months or years. These episodes may be accompanied by the extrusion of sequestra and pus through sinus tracts from the bone to the skin. Sinus tracts that drain for 20 years or more may, on rare occasions, develop a squamous cell carcinoma. This complication is rare, affecting only 1% of chronic osteomyelitis cases.

Plain radiographs show evidence of continuous bone destruction and repair, processes that alter the shape of the bone. Multiple ill-defined radiolucent areas alternate with radiodense reactive bone. Also, extensive periosteal new bone formation occurs, which increases the diameter of the bone (Fig. 8-6). This periosteal bone reaction may be extensive and markedly distort the bone contour (Fig. 8-7). Small radiodense areas, representing sequestra, may be present within the radiolucent areas. A CT scan is often necessary to localize these sequestra.

THE PATHOLOGY OF OSTEOMYELITIS

Osteomyelitis is characterized by bone destruction, the replacement of bone marrow by inflammatory tissue, and reparative new bone formation. The pathologist must be aware of two diagnostic principles: (1) the diagnosis of osteomyelitis should only be made in the proper clinical and radiographic setting, and (2) the various syndromes of osteomyelitis—acute, subacute, and chronic—cannot usually be distinguished histologically.

The first principle is based on the fact that in the bone marrow, inflammation is not synonymous with infection. Marrow fibrosis with an inflammatory cell infiltrate is a nonspecific reactive change that occurs focally or diffusely in many other clinical settings. For example, inflammation of the marrow is present in healing fractures, osteoarthritis, inflammatory arthritis, and bone adjacent to neoplasms or infarcts. Therefore, the unequivocal diagnosis of osteomyelitis should only be made in a clinical and radiographic setting consistent with the disease. In ambiguous cases, the pathologist should suggest that an unexplained inflammatory reaction in bone be correlated with the radiographs, clinical history, or microbiologic cultures.

The second principle in the diagnosis of osteomyelitis is that the various syndromes—acute, subacute, and chronic osteomyelitis—are clinicoradiologic entities. Because the microscopic features of inflammatory reactions in these syndromes overlap, they cannot be distinguished histologically. For example, tissue from an active focus of chronic osteomyelitis may contain an acute purulent exudate, a feature commonly seen in acute osteomyelitis. The pathologist should only render a diagnosis of osteomyelitis.

Despite overlapping histologic features, certain patterns of inflammation are suggestive of each syndrome, although they should never be used to render diagnoses of specific syndromes. In acute osteomyelitis, for example, suppuration in the marrow is common, and extensive osteoclastic bone resorption is present (Fig. 8-8). In subacute osteomyelitis, acute purulent inflammation is less prominent. The marrow is replaced by edematous granulation tissue containing, in addition to neutrophils, a mixture of lymphocytes and plasma

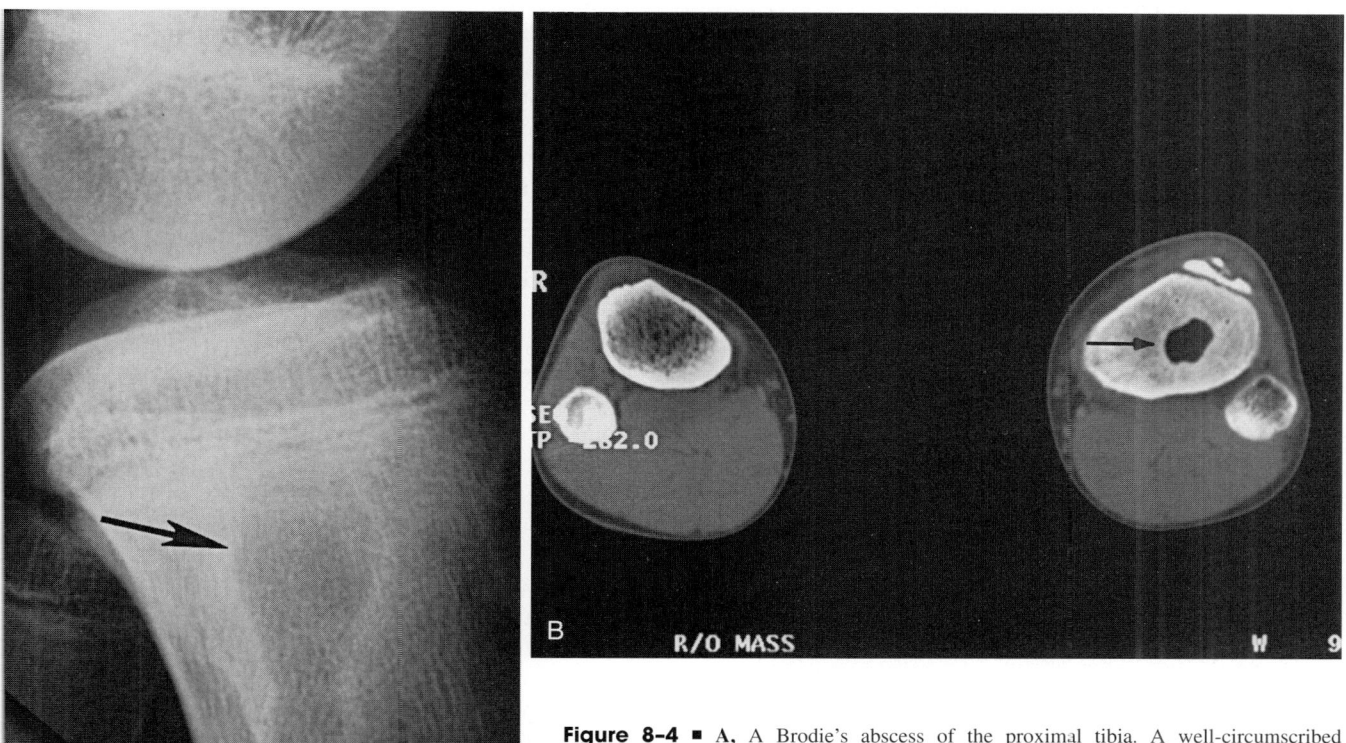

Figure 8-4 ■ **A,** A Brodie's abscess of the proximal tibia. A well-circumscribed metaphyseal lytic lesion is surrounded by a sclerotic rim *(arrow).* **B,** The central well-defined lucency apparent on the CT scan is surrounded by a rim of sclerotic bone *(arrow).*

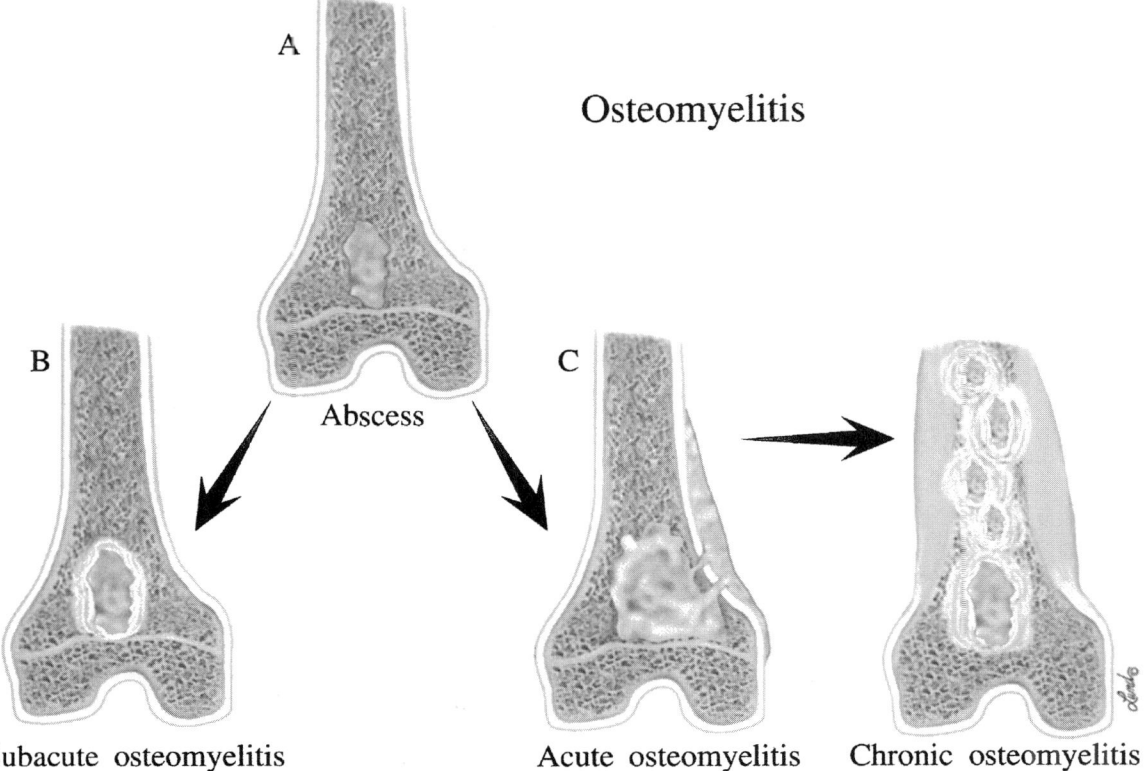

Figure 8-5 ■ The various stages of osteomyelitis. A metaphyseal abscess *(panel A)* can progress to either an acute osteomyelitis *(panel C)* or a subacute osteomyelitis *(panel B).* Some cases of acute osteomyelitis progress to chronic osteomyelitis *(see panel C).*

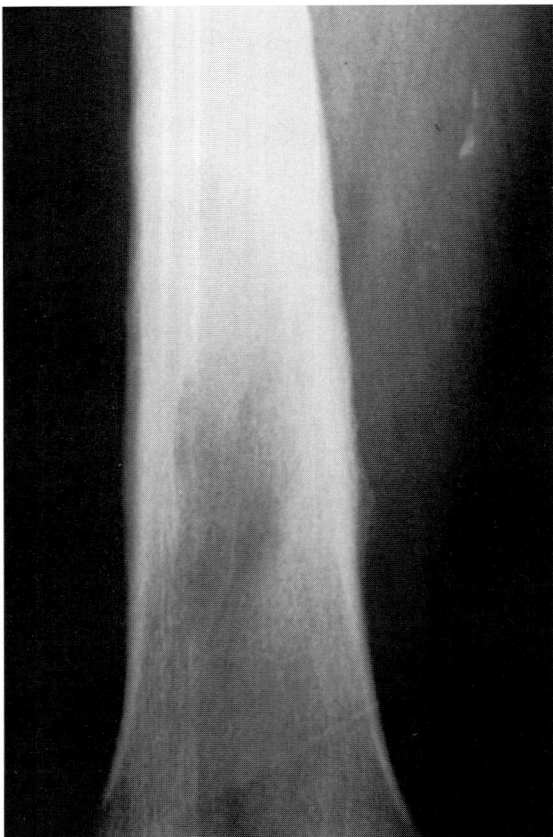

Figure 8-6 ■ Chronic osteomyelitis of the femur. A poorly defined lytic area is surrounded by dense reactive bone.

The main clinical feature is back pain and tenderness. However, because 50% of patients with this condition are afebrile, and two thirds lack leukocytosis, the back pain of osteomyelitis may be difficult to distinguish from back pain of other causes.[20] The erythrocyte sedimentation rate, almost always elevated in infection, is therefore a critical laboratory test.

The most distinctive radiographic feature of vertebral osteomyelitis is narrowing of a disc space and destruction of the adjacent vertebral endplates (Fig. 8–11). In addition, the vertebrae often show partial collapse. In the presence of vertebral destruction, loss of the disc space is highly suggestive of osteomyelitis. This feature helps distinguish vertebral osteomyelitis from a neoplasm or an osteoporotic compression fracture. Although neoplasms may cause vertebral destruction, they usually leave the disc intact. Similarly, the disc space is preserved in compression fractures secondary to osteoporosis.

In vertebral osteomyelitis, plain radiographic changes may be very subtle or not present at all in the early stages of the disease. Therefore, ancillary imaging modalities such as CT and MRI are frequently necessary to study patients with suspected spondylitis. CT scanning often shows early bony changes before they are visible on plain radiographs.[21,22] Small endplate erosion and paravertebral abscesses are visible with this modality. Later in the course of the disease,

cells (Fig. 8–9). In chronic osteomyelitis, marrow fibrosis with varying numbers of chronic inflammatory cells usually is present (Fig. 8–10). Often, native trabecular bone is encased by layers of appositional reactive bone, a feature leading to radiodensity. Although focal bone necrosis is present in all syndromes of osteomyelitis, necrotic bone is especially prominent in chronic osteomyelitis.

VERTEBRAL OSTEOMYELITIS

Unlike hematogenous osteomyelitis of childhood, which typically affects the metaphysis of long bones, hematogenous osteomyelitis in adults usually involves the spine, a disease sometimes called *spondylitis*. Organisms reach the vertebral bodies via arterial blood or via backflow through the perivertebral venus plexus of Batson. Infection begins in the vertebral body near the endplate and then erodes into the disc space and the adjacent vertebral body.

As with osteomyelitis in children, *S. aureus* is the most common etiologic agent. However, in adults with special risk factors, gram-negative organisms are often the causative organism. Risk factors include a history of genitourinary tract surgery or infection, diabetes, or intravenous drug abuse.

Vertebral osteomyelitis presents diagnostic difficulties.

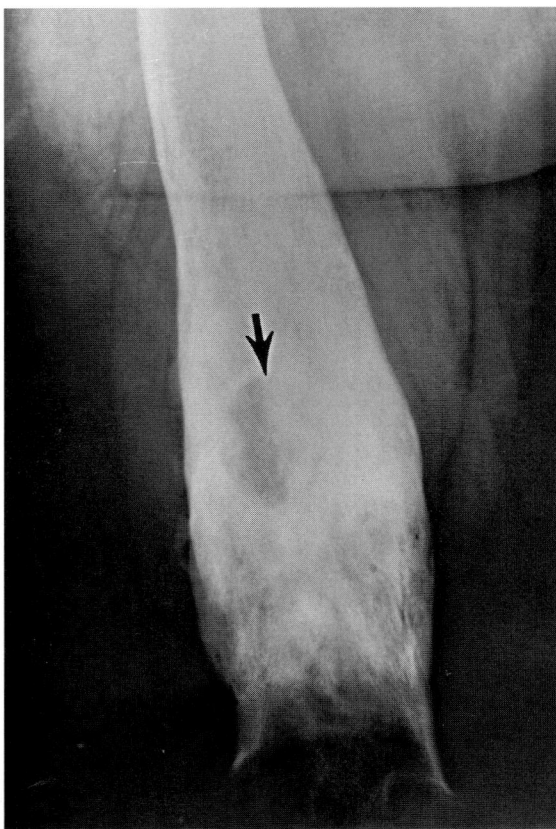

Figure 8-7 ■ Long-standing chronic osteomyelitis of the femur. A central lytic zone *(arrow)* is encased by extensive reactive bone, which alters the contour of the entire femoral shaft.

CT helps define the degree of spinal cord compression. MRI is also very sensitive in detecting vertebral infections.[23,24] Osteomyelitis is associated with bone marrow edema and is therefore seen as a bright signal on T_2-weighted images and a low signal on T_1-weighted images.

Children also develop a syndrome of spinal osteomyelitis. In this condition, known as *discitis,* the inflammatory process begins in the intervertebral disc space and secondarily involves bone.[25] Because organisms are not always isolated in the discitis of children, some clinicians feel that many cases are noninfectious inflammatory or traumatic disorders. Cultures are negative in 50 to 90% of cases, but when positive, *S. aureus* is the most common organism.

Discitis usually presents in a child between ages 3 and 6, although the age range is 1 to 16 years. Often, the child has had a recent infection, such as an upper respiratory tract or middle ear infection. The child usually has a low-grade fever and an elevated erythrocyte sedimentation rate. A leukocytosis is also common. Characteristically, the child has back pain and tenderness. Usually the lumbar spine is affected, and radiographs show disc space narrowing and faint subchondral bone erosion and sclerosis. Histologically, disc material removed from these children shows inflamed granulation tissue. The adjacent bone shows reactive fibrosis and paratrabecular new bone deposition.

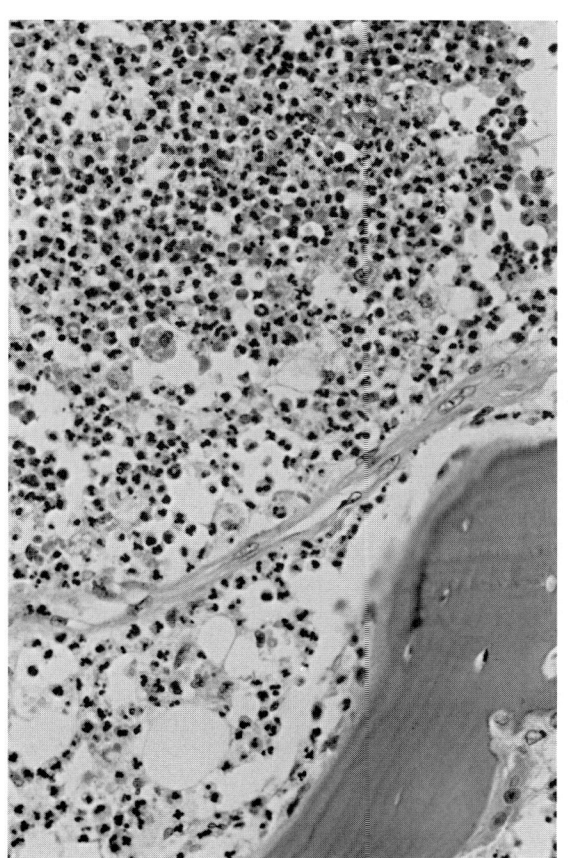

Figure 8-8 ■ Acute osteomyelitis. A suppurative inflammatory reaction is present in the marrow.

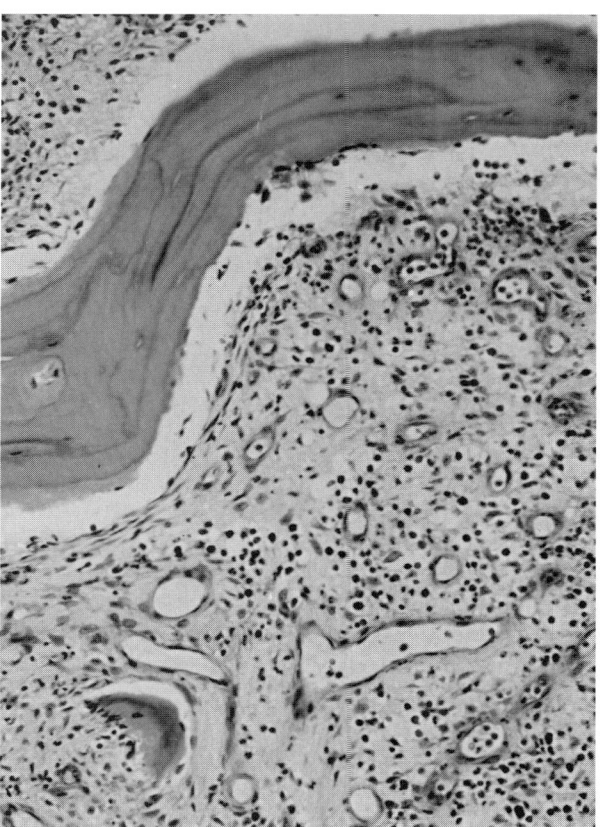

Figure 8-9 ■ Subacute osteomyelitis. The marrow is replaced by edematous granulation tissue.

OSTEOMYELITIS IN PATIENTS AT RISK

Certain groups of patients are at a greater risk of developing osteomyelitis. In these patients, the disease often has distinctive features. Patients at risk include those with human immunodeficiency virus (HIV) infection and sickle cell anemia. Also at risk are intravenous drug abusers and patients on hemodialysis.

Patients with Human Immunodeficiency Virus

Patients with acquired immunodeficiency syndrome (AIDS) are at risk for developing both osteomyelitis and septic arthritis.[26] Although *S. aureus* is a common pathogen, AIDS patients also develop infection with a wide range of other organisms, including various fungal and mycobacterial species. These infections usually occur in the end stage of the disease and pursue a fulminant course. AIDS patients may also develop *bacillary angiomatosis of bone,* an exuberant, highly vascular granulation tissue secondary to the cat-scratch bacillus. This disease usually occurs in the skin but when in bone produces a highly destructive lesion that may be confused radiographically and histologically with an aggressive malignant neoplasm.[27]

Patients on Hemodialysis

Patients on long-term hemodialysis also have an increased incidence of osteomyelitis, presumably due to bacteremia originating in infected catheter sites. The ribs and the thoracic spine are the most common bones affected.[28] Patients present with bone pain, which unfortunately may be attributed to the bone pain of renal osteodystrophy, also a common complication of end-stage renal disease.

Patients with Sickle Cell Anemia

Patients with sickle cell anemia are at risk of developing osteomyelitis because they have repeated episodes of sepsis. Although *S. aureus* is the most common causative organism, many cases of osteomyelitis in sickle cell anemia are caused by *Salmonella* organisms. In these cases, microinfarction of the gut, common in sickle cell anemia, leads to breakdown of mucosal barriers, and organisms enter the blood. Also, impaired macrophage function may render these patients susceptible to infection.[29] In sickle cell anemia, osteomyelitis may be extremely difficult to distinguish from bone infarction, a complication of this disease that is 50 times more common.[30] Clinical, laboratory, and imaging features are almost identical. A positive blood culture favors a diagnosis

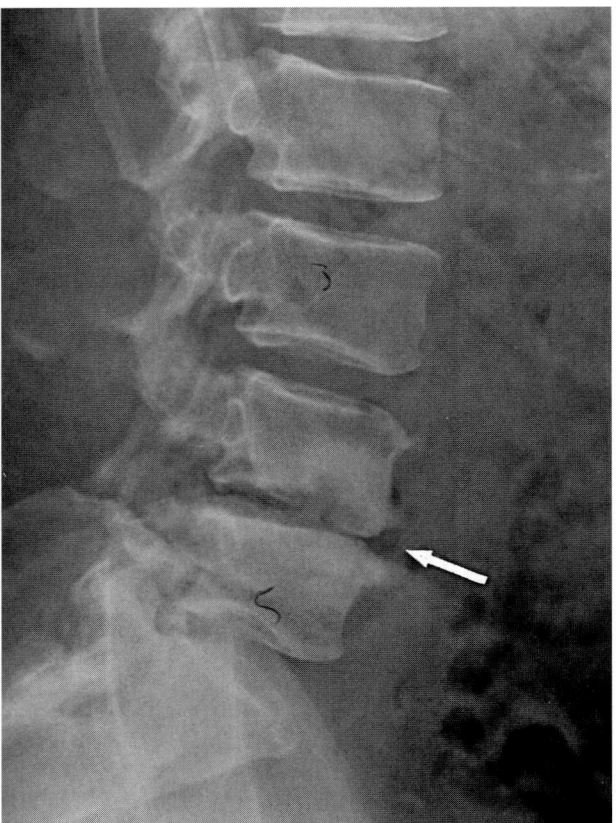

Figure 8-11 ■ Radiograph of spine showing spondylitis. Narrowing of the disc space and destruction of the vertebral endplates are present *(arrow)*.

of osteomyelitis as does the image of a subperiosteal abscess on ultrasound.

Drug Abusers

The pattern of osteomyelitis in intravenous drug abusers, the final risk group, is also distinctive. In these patients, *Pseudomonas aeruginosa* is the most common infecting organism, and the sites of infection are often unusual locations. For example, fibrocartilaginous joints, such as the symphysis pubis and the sternocostal or sternoclavicular joints, are frequently involved. Infection of the symphysis pubis, known as *osteitis pubis,* occurs in heroin addicts who inject into the groin. Osteitis pubis may also occur in patients who have had prior pelvic surgery or pelvic instrumentation (Fig. 8–12). In many of these patients, organisms cannot be isolated.

TREATMENT OF OSTEOMYELITIS

The treatment of acute osteomyelitis requires vigorous antibiotic therapy and, in most cases, surgical drainage of pus.[31] Although most cases of acute osteomyelitis are caused by *S. aureus*, attempts should be made to isolate an organism to obtain sensitivity studies. A needle aspiration at the site of maximum bone tenderness often provides material for

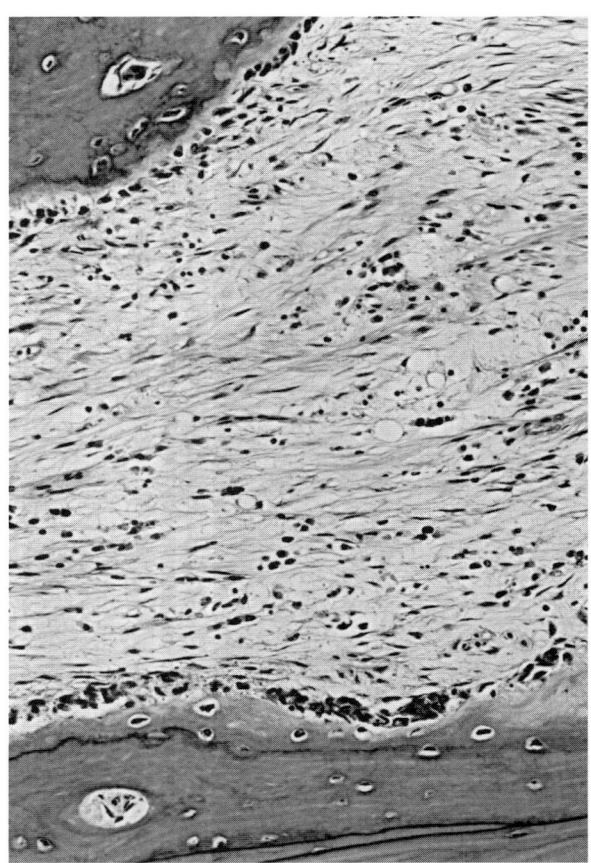

Figure 8-10 ■ Chronic osteomyelitis with marrow fibrosis. Appositional new bone deposition on native trabeculae also can be seen.

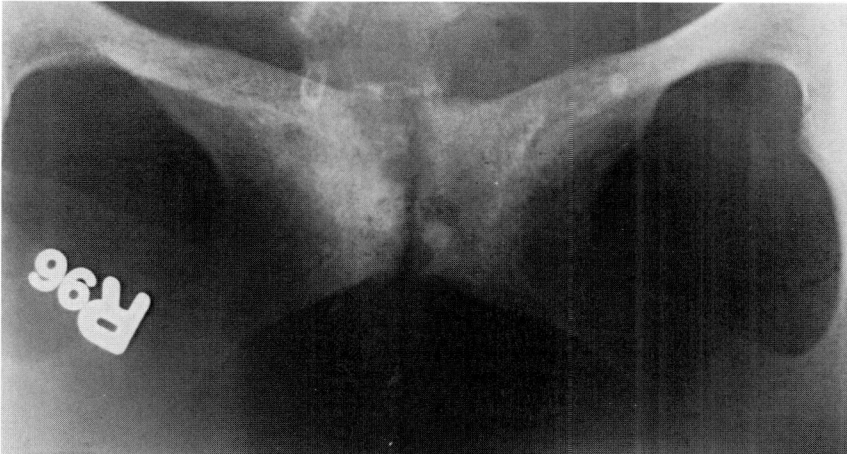

Figure 8-12 ■ Osteitis pubis. Destruction of the margins of the symphysis pubis has occurred.

microbiologic studies. Parenteral administration of the appropriate antibiotics for at least 4 to 6 weeks is usually necessary to achieve an acceptable rate of cure. This is followed by several weeks of oral antibiotic therapy.

The need for surgical drainage in acute osteomyelitis is controversial. Although some patients can be cured with antibiotics alone, surgery is often necessary because the diagnosis is sometimes delayed and a significant subperiosteal abscess has developed. The surgical procedure must include drainage of subperiosteal and intramedullary pus and débridement of necrotic tissue.

Whereas the role of surgery in acute osteomyelitis remains controversial, chronic osteomyelitis always requires aggressive surgical management. Two aspects of surgery exist—removal of all infected tissue and reconstruction of resulting tissue defects. Cure can be obtained only after complete débridement of all dead bone and soft tissue. Traditionally, tissue is removed until briskly bleeding soft tissue is reached. This often creates large defects in bone, soft tissue, and skin—defects that must be reconstructed. Skin grafts are frequently necessary to cover wound sites, and local muscle pedicle flaps or myocutaneous flaps fill the space created by surgery. These flaps, in addition to filling defects, also revascularize the débrided area. Large bone defects may be filled with cancellous bone grafts or vascularized fibular grafts.

Vertebral osteomyelitis also requires intensive antibiotic therapy, and often surgery is required. Although blood cultures may identify an organism that can be presumed to cause the spinal infection, tissue from the infection site is a better source of organisms for culture and sensitivity studies. Tissue may be obtained by CT-guided Craig needle biopsies, but an open biopsy is usually required. Two indications for surgery in vertebral osteomyelitis exist: (1) to drain a paravertebral abscess, and (2) to stabilize a spine that has been weakened by vertebral destruction. The latter is best achieved by anterior interbody fusion.

SEPTIC ARTHRITIS

Sometimes bacteremia results in infection of the synovial membrane and joint cavity without infecting bone. Alternatively, organisms may enter a joint from an intracapsular focus of osteomyelitis or from a puncture wound. This condition, known as *acute septic arthritis,* is less common than hematogenous osteomyelitis. It is, however, an important clinical problem that demands immediate diagnosis and treatment because the inflammation is rapidly destructive to articular cartilage and can lead to permanent joint damage.

Pathogenesis

As with hematogenous osteomyelitis, septic arthritis is most commonly caused by *S. aureus.* In infants and young children, *H. influenzae* and *Streptococcus* species are also important pathogens. These organisms first seed the synovial membrane and cause an acute purulent synovitis. Then, pus flows into the joint cavity from the synovial membrane and distends the joint capsule, a condition known as *pyarthrosis.* If treatment is delayed, the infected synovial membrane becomes an aggressive pannus, which, by means of proteolytic enzymes, destroys the articular cartilage. Also, bacteria participate directly in the destruction of articular cartilage by stimulating chondrocytes to produce endogenous proteinases.

Infants and Children

Like osteomyelitis, septic arthritis is usually a disease of children.[32,33] Patients present with fever, leukocytosis, and a swollen painful joint, most frequently the knee. Infants and young adults have special manifestations of this disease. The hip is the most common site of pyogenic arthritis in infants.[34] This syndrome often presents diagnostic problems because clinical signs do not localize to the hip. The infants present with only nonspecific signs of irritability and fever. Failure to move the affected extremity may be the only clue to the pyarthrosis.

Adults

In adults younger than 30 years, *Neisseria gonorrhoeae* is the most common cause of septic arthritis. The joint infection results from disseminated gonococcal infection originating in the genital mucosa.[35] About 2% of patients with gonorrhea develop disseminated infection, and about 25% of these patients develop a septic joint. Therefore, 1 of 200 patients with gonorrhea develops septic arthritis. Usually, the knee, wrist, or ankle is involved. On occasion, a migratory polyarticular pattern of joint involvement is associated with a pustular dermatitis. In this setting, the arthritis is usually sterile and is presumably caused by a reactive synovitis secondary to an immune reaction to gonococcal antigens. This presentation, known as *reactive arthritis,* occurs most frequently in patients who are human leukocyte antigen–B27 positive (see Chapter 16).

TUBERCULOSIS AND FUNGAL INFECTION OF BONE

A gradual decline in the incidence of tuberculosis followed the introduction of chemotherapy in the 1940s. However, in recent years, this trend has been reversed. The incidence of tuberculosis is increasing because of three factors: the growing population of immunocompromised patients, the influx of immigrants with active tuberculosis, and the emergence of antibiotic-resistant strains of the tubercle bacillus.

Approximately 5% of patients with tuberculosis have bone or joint involvement.[36] Osteoarticular tuberculosis results from dissemination of microorganisms from the primary lesion, which in only half of these patients is in the lungs.[37] Three main presentations of osteoarticular tuberculosis occur. First, accounting for half of all cases of bone and joint tuberculosis, is involvement of the spine, a disorder known as tuberculous spondylitis. The second presentation is tuberculous arthritis, a condition that affects primarily the hip and knee. The third common presentation is involvement of the bones or the tenosynovium of the hands and feet.

Whereas hematogenous spread of organisms occurs in tuberculosis, spinal involvement is most likely caused by spread of organisms from the lungs to the vertebrae via lymphatics.[38] Skip lesions, uncommon in patients with nontuberculous spondylitis, occur in two thirds of patients with spinal tuberculosis. In addition, patients with tuberculous spondylitis commonly develop paravertebral abscesses, a result of collapse of the vertebral bodies, disc involvement, and spread of organisms into the soft tissue. Two thirds of patients with vertebral collapse develop kyphosis, and when it is severe or associated with a paravertebral abscess, it may result in paraplegia. This syndrome—kyphosis with paraplegia—is known as *Pott's disease.*

Involvement of joints, accounting for 30% of osteoarticular tuberculosis, results from a hematogenous spread of microorganisms to the synovial membrane. Radiographically, tuberculous arthritis is characterized by extensive destruction of the bone ends with little reactive bone. An adjacent soft tissue mass is usually present. An important feature of healed cases of articular tuberculosis is that disease can be reactivated by total joint replacement.[39]

In addition to the spine and large joints, *M. tuberculosis* may infect bone without involving nearby joints. This most commonly occurs in the small bones of the hands and feet. In addition to bone and joint infection, any bursa or tendon sheath may be involved. Often, the tendon sheaths of the wrist are infected, a syndrome described in 1923 by Kanavel.[40]

The histologic features of *M. tuberculosis* infection of bone are similar to tuberculous infection in other tissues. An acute inflammatory and granulomatous reaction is associated with varying amounts of caseating necrosis. Stains for acid-fast organisms are seldom positive in osteoarticular tuberculosis caused by *M. tuberculosis.*

Atypical mycobacterial species also cause bone and joint infection, particularly in immunocompromised patients. In these infections, caused by organisms such as *Mycobacterium kansasii* and *Mycobacterium avium intracellulare,* the histologic features are somewhat different. Granulomas are usually not present, and only a nonspecific inflammatory reaction with numerous macrophages may be present.[41] In these cases, acid-fast stains are usually positive.

Fungal organisms can also cause bone and joint infection, especially in immunocompromised patients or those receiving long-term corticosteroid therapy. In these patients, infection results from hematogenous dissemination of opportunistic organisms such as *Candida,*[42] *Cryptococcus,*[43] and *Aspergillus* species.[44] Like tuberculosis, the spine is the most common site of fungal infections, although any bone may be involved. Radiologically, fungal infections produce nonspecific osteolytic defects. Therefore, fungal infection should be suspected as a cause of any osteolytic defect in an immunocompromised host, and appropriate diagnostic measures should be taken. For example, bone lesions should be cultured for all types of microorganisms, and tissue should be routinely stained with methenamine silver. Unlike the acid-fast stain for tuberculosis, fungal stains usually demonstrate the offending organism.

Some fungal organisms, such as *Histoplasma capsulatum,*[45] *Coccidioides* species,[46] and *Blastomyces* species[47] can cause osteomyelitis in apparently healthy individuals. These infections probably result from hematogenous spread from a primary lung lesion. Like with infection with *M. tuberculosis* or the opportunistic fungi, the spine is the most commonly involved site. A distinctive pattern of spine infection is seen in patients with coccidioidomycosis—involvement of the posterior elements of the vertebral body and preservation of the disc space.

SYPHILITIC BONE INFECTION

Like tuberculosis, the incidence of syphilis is also increasing. However, syphilitic infection of bone is still rare. In the secondary or tertiary stages, three syndromes of bone infection can occur: synovitis, periostitis, and osteomyelitis.[48] Synovitis, which may involve multiple joints, is a result of hematogenous spread of the organisms. Periostitis, which occurs in 20% of patients in the secondary phase, is the most distinctive manifestation of syphilitic bone disease because of its unusual radiographic presentation: The bones are expanded with layers of periosteal new bone, which, when involving the tibia, produce the characteristic "saber shin" deformity. The third manifestation of osteoarticular syphilis, osteomyelitis, occurs in the tertiary phase. This form of bone infection produces an osteolytic defect with abundant reactive bone. Histologically, lesions show the typical gumma—a central necrotic area surrounded by chronic inflammatory cell infiltrate. Syphilitic lesions are also characterized by many plasma cells and vasculitis.

CHRONIC MULTIFOCAL OSTEOMYELITIS

An unusual syndrome of multiple metachronous inflammatory bone lesions in young patients, usually women, was described in 1972.[49] This syndrome, known as *chronic recurrent multifocal osteomyelitis*, is characterized by malaise, bone pain, and multiple bone lesions. The bone lesions, numbering as many as 5 to 10, appear and resolve spontaneously over a period of years. Radiologically, lesions are poorly defined zones of mixed lytic and sclerotic changes (Fig. 8–13). Histologically, lesions show inflammatory tissue similar to that seen in subacute or chronic bacterial osteomyelitis. Marrow fibrosis and necrotic bone trabeculae are particularly prominent, and plasma cells are usually numerous. Bacteria are rarely cultured from these lesions, and most resolve without antibiotics. An indolent organism, such as *Mycoplasma*, has been suggested as the cause,[50] although the definite etiology is not known.

Chronic multifocal osteomyelitis is often associated with other disorders, suggesting an autoimmune cause.[51] Some patients have pustulosis palmoplantaris, a psoriasiform rash on the soles and palms. Other patients may have chronic bowel disease or other skeletal lesions such as condensing osteitis of the clavicle or sternoclavicular hyperostosis. A full constellation of associated disorders is known as the *SAPHO (synovitis, acne, pustulosis, hyperostosis, and osteitis) syndrome*.[52]

Although each osteolytic bone lesion is self-limiting, the active disease may be present for many years. In addition, the radiographic changes often persist into adulthood, long after symptoms have abated.[53]

REFERENCES

1. Roney, J. G.: Palaeopathology of a California archeological site. *Bull Hist Med* 33:97–109, 1959.
2. Lagier, R., Baud, C., and Kramar, C.: Brodie's abscess in a tibia dating from the Neolithic period. *Virchows Arch (Pathol Anat)* 401:153–157, 1983.
3. Celsus, A. C.: *De Medicina*. Spencer, W. G. (Ed.). Cambridge, MA, Harvard University Press, 1935, pp. 307–309.
4. Abu al-Qasim, K., Spink, M. S., and Lewis, G. L. (Eds.): *Albucasis on Surgery and Instruments*. Berkeley, CA, University of California Press, 1973, pp. 347–348.
5. Mackenzie, A.: A remarkable separation of part of the thigh bone. *Medical Observations and Inquiries* 2:299–303, 1762.
6. Smith, D. A., and LaTorence, T.: *Notes on Mr. William Bromfeild's Chirurgical Observations and Cases*. London, T. Cadell, 1773, pp. 20–24.
7. Smith, N.: Observations on the pathology and treatment of necrosis. *Phil Month J Med* 1:11–19, 1827.
8. Brodie, B. C.: Lecture on abscess of the tibia. *London Medical Gazette* 1399–1403, 1845.
9. Chassaignac, E.: De l'osteo-myelite. *Bull Mem Soc Chir Paris* 3:431–436, 1852.
10. Rosenbach, J.: Beitrage zur Kenntniss der Osteomyelitis: Experimentell-Klinische Studie uber die Aetiologie der Osteomyelitis. *Dtsch Zeit Chir* 10:369–393, 1878.
11. Alderson, M., Speers, D., Emslie, K., and Nade, S. M. L.: Acute haematogenous osteomyelitis and septic arthritis—a single disease. *J Bone Joint Surg* 68B:268–274, 1986.
12. Ryden, C., Yacoub, A. I., Maxe, I., et al.: Specific binding of bone sialoprotein to *Staphylococcus aureus* isolated from patients with osteomyelitis. *Eur J Biochem* 184:331–336, 1989.
13. Whalen, J. L., Fitzgerald, R. H., and Morrissy, R. T.: A histological study of acute hematogenous osteomyelitis following physeal injuries in rabbits. *J Bone Joint Surg* 70A:1383–1392, 1988.
14. Sorensen, T. S., Hedeboe, J., and Christensen, E. R.: Primary epiphyseal osteomyelitis in children. *J Bone Joint Surg* 70B:818–820, 1988.
15. Athanasou, N. A., Quinn, J., and Bulstrode, C. J.: Resorption of bone by inflammatory cells derived from the joint capsule of hip arthroplasties. *J Bone Joint Surg* 74B:57–62, 1992.
16. Norden, C., Gillespie, W. J., and Nade, S.: *Infections in Bones and Joints*. Boston, Blackwell Scientific Publications, 1994, pp. 3–12.
17. Schulak, D. J., Rayhack, J. M., Lippert, F. G., and Convery, F. R.: The erythrocyte sedimentation rate in orthopaedic patients. *Clin Orthop* 167:197–202, 1982.
18. Merkel, K. D., Fitzgerald, R. H., and Brown, M. L.: Scintigraphic evaluation in muscolo-skeletal sepsis. *Orthop Clin North Am* 15:401–416, 1984.
19. Gallie, W. E.: First recurrence of osteomyelitis eighty years after infection. *J Bone Joint Surg* 33B:110–111, 1951.

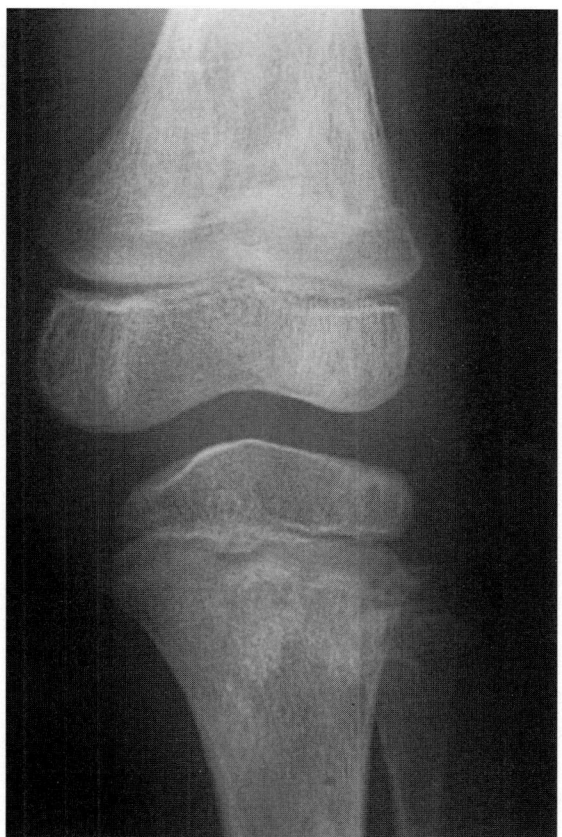

Figure 8-13 ▪ Chronic multifocal osteomyelitis. A mixed lytic and sclerotic lesion is present in the metaphysis of both the femur and the tibia.

20. Silverthorn, K. G., and Gillespie, W. J.: Pyogenic spinal osteomyelitis: Review of 61 cases. *N Z Med J* 99:62–65, 1986.
21. Abbey, D. M., and Hosea, S. W.: Diagnosis of vertebral osteomyelitis in a community hospital by using computed tomography. *Arch Intern Med* 149:2029–2035, 1989.
22. Burke, D. R., and Brant-Zawadzki, M.: CT of pyogenic spine infection. *Neuroradiology* 27:131–137, 1985.
23. Meyers, S., and Wiener, S.: Diagnosis of hematogenous pyogenic vertebral osteomyelitis by magnetic resonance imaging. *Arch Intern Med* 151:683–687, 1991.
24. Modic, M. T., Feiglin, D. H., Piraino, D. W., et al.: Vertebral osteomyelitis: Assessment using MR. *Radiology* 157:157–166, 1985.
25. Schmorl, G., and Junghanns, H.: *The Human Spine in Health and Disease*, 2nd ed. New York, Grune & Stratton, 1971, p. 325.
26. Hughes, R., Rowe, I., Shanson, D., and Keat, A.: Septic bone, joint and muscle lesions associated with human immunodeficiency virus infection. *Br J Rheumatol* 31:381–388, 1992.
27. Baron, A. L., Steinbach, L. S., LeBoit, P. E., Mills, C. M., Gee, J. H., and Berger, T. G.: Osteolytic lesions and bacillary angiomatosis in HIV infection: Radiologic differentiation from AIDS-related Kaposi sarcoma. *Radiology* 177:77–81, 1990.
28. Leonard, A., Comty, C. M., Shapiro, F. L., and Raij, L.: Osteomyelitis in hemodialysis patients. *Ann Intern Med* 78:651–658, 1973.
29. Hook, E. W., Kay, D., and Gill, F. A.: Factors influencing host resistance to *Salmonella* infection: The effects of hemolysis and erythrophagocytosis. *Trans Am Clin Climatol Assoc* 78:230–241, 1967.
30. Keeley, K., and Buchanan, G. R.: Acute infarction of long bones in children with sickle-cell anemia. *J Pediatr* 101:170–175, 1982.
31. Lew, D. P., and Waldvogel, F. A.: Current concepts. Osteomyelitis. *N Engl J Med* 336:999–1007, 1997.
32. Dan, M.: Septic arthritis in young infants: Clinical and microbiologic correlations and therapeutic implications. *Rev Infect Dis* 6:147–155, 1984.
33. Almquist, E. E.: The changing epidemiology of septic arthritis in children. *Clin Orthop* 68:96–99, 1970.
34. Hook, E. W.: Septic gonococcal arthritis is much more common in the USA than in the UK. *Br J Rheumatol* 29:283, 1990.
35. Hansfield, H. H.: *Neisseria gonorrhoeae*. Mandell, G. L., Douglas, R. G., and Bennett, J. E., Eds. *Principles and Practice of Infectious Diseases*. New York, Churchill-Livingstone, 1990, pp. 1613–1631.
36. Rieder, H. L., Snider, D. E., and Cauthen, G. M.: Extrapulmonary tuberculosis in the United States. *Am Rev Respir Dis* 141:347–351, 1990.
37. Davidson, P. T., and Horowitz, I.: Skeletal tuberculosis. A review with patient presentations and discussion. *Am J Med* 48:77–84, 1970.
38. Burke, H. E.: The pathogenesis of certain forms of extrapulmonary tuberculosis. *Am Rev Tuberc* 62:48–67, 1950.
39. Hecht, R. H., Meyers, M. H., Thornhill-Joynes, M., and Montgomerie, J. Z.: Reactivation of tuberculous infection following total joint replacement. *J Bone Joint Surg* 65A:1015–1016, 1983.
40. Kanavel, A. B.: Tuberculous tenosynovitis of the hand. *Surg Gynaecol Obstet* 37:635–647, 1923.
41. Klatt, E. C., Jensen, D. F., and Meyer, P. R.: Pathology of *Mycobacterium avium-intercellulare* infection in acquired immunodeficiency syndrome. *Hum Pathol* 18:709–714, 1987.
42. Gathe, J. C., Harris, R. L., Garland, B., Bradshaw, M. W., and Williams, T. W.: *Candida* osteomyelitis. Report of five cases and review of the literature. *Am J Med* 82:927–937, 1987.
43. Rolston, K. V. I.: Treatment of osseous cryptococcosis. Report of a case and review of the literature. *Orthopedics* 5:1610–1614, 1982.
44. Tack, K. J., Rhame, F. S., Brown, B., and Thompson, R. C.: *Aspergillus* osteomyelitis. Report of four cases and review of the literature. *Am J Med* 73:295–300, 1982.
45. Jones, R. C., and Goodwin, R. A.: Histoplasmosis of bone. *Am J Med* 70:864–866, 1981.
46. Drutz, D., and Catanzaro, A.: Coccidioidomycosis—part 1. *Am Rev Respir Dis* 117:559–585, 1978.
47. Wagner, D. K., Varkey, B., and Head, M. D.: Blastomycotic osteomyelitis of the mandible: Successful treatment with ketoconazole. *Oral Surg Oral Med Oral Pathol* 60:370–371, 1985.
48. Olle-Goig, J. E., Barrio, J. L., Gurgui, M., and Mildvan, D.: Bone invasion in secondary syphilis: Case reports. *Genitourin Med* 64:198–201, 1988.
49. Giedion, A., Holthusen, W., Masel, L. F., and Vischer, D.: Subacute and chronic "symmetrical" osteomyelitis. *Ann Radiol (Paris)* 15:329–342, 1972.
50. Hummell, D. S., Anderson, S. J., Wright, P. F., Cassell, G. H., and Waites, K. B.: Chronic recurrent multifocal osteomyelitis: Are mycoplasmas involved? *N Engl J Med* 317:510–511, 1987.
51. Pelkonen, P., Ryoppy, S., Jaaskalainen, J., Rapola, J., Repo, H., and Kaitila, I.: Chronic osteomyelitis-like disease with negative bacterial cultures. *Am J Dis Child* 142:1167–1173, 1988.
52. Reith, J. D., Bauer, T. W., and Schils, J. P.: Osseous manifestations of SAPHO (synovitis, acne, pustulosis, hyperostosis, osteitis) syndrome. *Am J Surg Pathol* 20:1368–1377, 1996.
53. Jurik, A. G., Moller, S. H., and Mosekilde, L.: Chronic sclerosing osteomyelitis of the iliac bone. *Skeletal Radiol* 17:114–118, 1988.

CHAPTER 9
Paget's Disease

Paget's disease of bone is a chronic condition characterized by exaggerated, nonphysiologic bone remodeling that affects one or multiple sites of the skeleton. The disease begins as a wave of bone resorption caused by an increased number of abnormally large osteoclasts. Next, a compensatory osteoblastic response leads to rapid and disorganized bone formation. Over the years, the affected bone becomes dense and architecturally distorted. As a result, the bone is brittle, and patients experience pain, deformity, and fractures.

HISTORY

In the late 19th century, Sir James Paget, the most famous surgeon in England, described numerous pathologic conditions that now bear his name. The two best known are Paget's disease of the breast, which is the intraepithelial spread of mammary carcinoma, and Paget's disease of bone. Paget originally called this latter disease *osteitis deformans*, believing it was an inflammatory process that led to skeletal deformity. Although two cases of this disorder had been described earlier by Wrany[1] and Wilks,[2] Paget's clear and extensive clinical description of five patients in 1877 has remained unsurpassed.[3]

By 1901, Packard and colleagues had tabulated 66 cases from the literature,[4] and numerous pathologists had attempted to understand the histologic process. However, these early attempts to understand Paget's disease were confused by von Recklinghausen's description of generalized *osteitis fibrosa cystica*. His description led most German pathologists to believe that *osteitis fibrosa* and *osteitis deformans* were the same disease at different ends of the spectrum.[5] This confusion was not resolved until 1926, when *osteitis fibrosa* was linked to parathyroid disease, finally distinguishing it from *osteitis deformans*.[6]

In 1926, Schmorl characterized the specific histologic features of *osteitis deformans*, and he defined it as a specific diagnostic entity, which he called Paget's disease.[7] Schmorl was also able to estimate the incidence of this disease based on meticulous examination of thousands of autopsy skeletons.

Although no evidence proves that Paget's disease exists in any other species,[8] it has affected humans for a long time. Unequivocal paleopathologic specimens have been found of Paget's disease from prehistoric Native American populations[9] and from an Anglo Saxon skeleton dating from 950 AD.[10] In addition, a highly probable example has been found in a Neolithic femur.[11]

EPIDEMIOLOGY

Three significant epidemiologic features characterize Paget's disease: (1) its predilection for older people, (2) its geographical variation in prevalence, and (3) its tendency to cluster in families. First, Paget's disease primarily affects the elderly. At least 3 to 4% of people older than 50 years have evidence of this disease, and the incidence increases with age. Ten to 15% of the population older than 80 years are affected. By contrast, Paget's disease is rarely diagnosed in patients younger than 40, although patients in their 20s have been reported. The youngest convincing case is that of an 18-year-old man.[12]

The second epidemiologic feature is that the prevalence of Paget's disease varies in different parts of the world. It is fairly common in England and other areas of Europe (excluding Scandinavia). It is also common in countries influenced by European migration, such as North America, Australia, Argentina, and South Africa. By contrast Paget's disease is rare in Asia and most of sub-Saharan Africa.

The third epidemiologic factor—clustering in families—suggests that Paget's disease has a genetic component.[13] Twenty-five percent of affected patients have one or more family members who also have the disease.[14] This figure rises to 40% if family members are studied with sensitive bone scans that identify subclinical disease.[15] Generally, the more severely affected a patient, the more likely a family member will also be affected.[15] Further evidence of a genetic component is suggested by the increased incidence of the human leukocyte antigen–DQW1 haplotype in affected patients.[14]

CLINICAL FEATURES

Paget's disease usually involves several bones (polyostotic), and on rare occasions, it may be so extensive that all the major bones of the skeleton are affected. By contrast, in 15% of patients, only one bone is involved (monostotic). During the course of the disease, the number of foci in a patient does not increase, but each focus slowly enlarges. The most common sites are in the axial skeleton: pelvis (involved in 80% of cases), spine, and skull. It is also common in the femurs and tibias. On the other hand, Paget's disease is uncommon in the ribs, the fibula, and the small tubular bones of the hands and feet.

Paget's disease usually presents with pain, a result of microfractures and periosteal tension produced by the enlarging bone. However, it is often asymptomatic and may be found incidentally on plain radiographs taken for other reasons. Because of this, calculations of the incidence of this disease, based on retrospective reviews of plain radiographs[16] and on autopsy studies,[17] are probably underestimated.

ETIOLOGY

The cause of Paget's disease has not been unequivocally established. Suggested causes include trauma, vascular occlusions, or endocrine abnormalities. However, the most widely accepted theory is that an infectious agent causes this disease—specifically, a slow virus like that causing kuru or subacute sclerosing panencephalitis. This viral theory originated in 1974, when investigators demonstrated with the electron microscope that the osteoclasts in pagetic bone contain intranuclear and intracytoplasmic inclusions. These inclusions are similar to those seen in cells infected by RNA paramyxoviruses, particularly measles virus, canine distemper virus, and the respiratory syncytial virus (RSV).[18] They are not seen in any other bone disease except in rare cases of giant cell tumor of bone.[19]

In addition to electron microscopic findings, other evidence supports a viral etiology. First, measles and RSV virus have been identified by immunohistochemistry in pagetic osteoclasts,[20] and measles antibodies have been detected in the serum of affected patients.[21] Second, in situ hybridization techniques to identify viral RNA have detected evidence of measles virus in pagetic osteoclasts.[22] Finally, measles virus nucleocapsid transcripts have been detected in osteoclast precursors from pagetic bone marrow,[23] as well as in peripheral blood cells derived from granulocyte-macrophage progenitors.[24]

The theory that a virus induces a generalized osteoclast disorder would suggest a systemic disease. Inconsistent with this interpretation, however, are two features of Paget's disease: its focality and the fact that once the disease is established, new foci do not appear. These inconsistencies can be explained away by findings of high concentrations of interleukin-6 in pagetic foci. This suggests that alterations in the microenvironment of bone may account for the distribution and progression of the disease.[25] Perhaps the increased levels of cytokines or other growth factors at sites of Paget's disease direct virally infected osteoclast precursors at those locations to become active osteoclasts.

Alteration in the microenvironment is supported by several observations. First, grafts of normal bone that are placed in pagetic lesions develop Paget's disease. Second, the disease process does not spread across a normal joint, but it does spread to an adjacent bone if the joint is fused.[26] Third, heterotopic ossification adjacent to a lesion of Paget's disease is often involved by the pagetic process.[27] Finally, the callus of a pagetic fracture frequently develops histologic features of active disease.

HISTOPATHOLOGY

Each focus of Paget's disease evolves in a sequence of changes that may be divided into three phases: (1) an initial phase of bone resorption (the hot phase), (2) a phase in

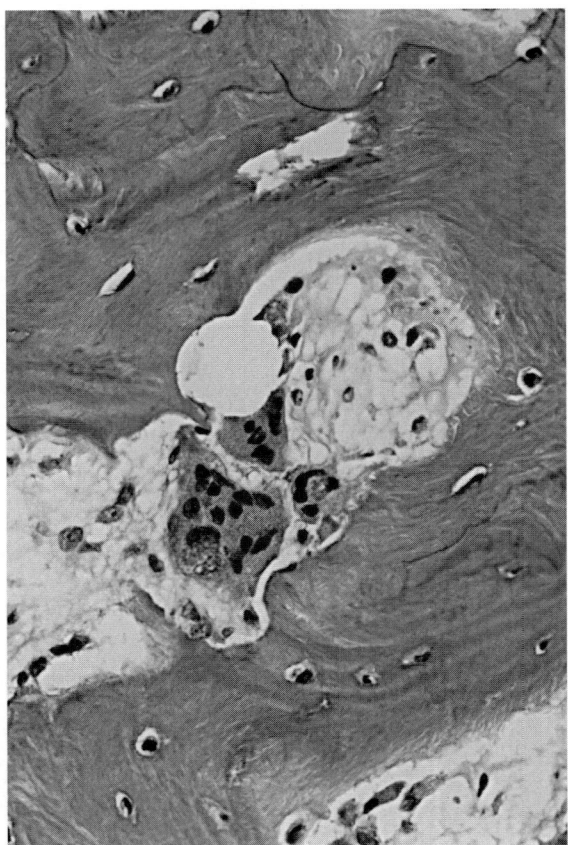

Figure 9-1 ■ Photomicrograph of Paget's disease showing osteoclastic resorption.

which rapid osteoblastic activity keeps pace with bone resorption (the intermediate phase), and (3) the final stage, in which resorption has almost ceased and continued bone formation results in dense bone (the cold phase). The histologic features of each phase correlate with radiographic changes. We discuss the histologic changes first.

The hot phase is marked by rapid bone resorption. The number of osteoclasts is increased, and they are much larger than normal, sometimes having as many as 100 nuclei. The osteoclasts are present in large, irregular resorption cavities (Fig. 9–1), and the marrow is replaced by a vascular fibrous tissue (Fig. 9–2). The histologic features of this phase resemble the osseous changes of secondary hyperparathyroidism. With the electron microscope, the characteristic intranuclear and cytoplasmic inclusions can be seen. The intranuclear inclusions are tight bundles of microfilaments, whereas the cytoplasmic inclusions are randomly distributed filaments.

In the intermediate phase, a compensatory increase in bone formation occurs. Many osteoblasts form irregular, thick seams of osteoid, which are mineralized at twice the normal rate. The functional trabecular arrangement is markedly altered, and marrow fibrosis with increased vascularity is present. Woven bone is prominent, especially beneath the periosteum.

In the late or cold phase of Paget's disease, the active remodeling is less prominent. However, evidence of prior

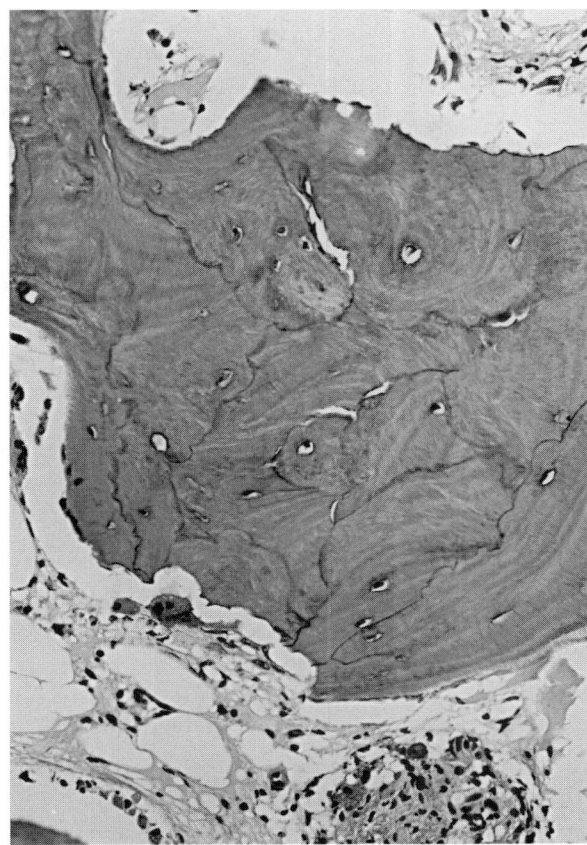

Figure 9-3 ■ Photomicrograph of late-stage Paget's disease. Many intersecting remodeling lines form a mosaic pattern.

chaotic remodeling is apparent—many intersecting cement lines form a "mosaic" pattern throughout the coarsely thickened trabeculae (Fig. 9–3). In addition, the woven bone deposited in the intermediate phase has been converted to lamellar bone. These changes obliterate distinction between the medullary bone and the highly porous cortex.

RADIOLOGIC FEATURES

The radiologic features parallel the histologic changes, and in many cases, the diagnosis can be made solely on the basis of plain radiographs. Paget's disease is usually encountered in its late (radiodense) phase. However, the earliest radiographic pattern, corresponding to the initial wave of osteoclastic resorption, is radiolucency. In the long bones, the first change is a wedge- or flame-shaped area of lucency in the metaphysis pointing toward the diaphysis (Fig. 9–4). At a rate of about 1 cm/y, the radiolucency extends like a wave into the diaphysis to involve the shaft of the bone (Fig. 9–5). Sometimes the entire shaft of the bone is involved (Fig. 9–6). Then, the compensatory osteoblastic response begins, and the lytic areas of the radiograph become radiodense in the older portions of the lesions (Fig. 9–7). In the late stages of the disease, the entire lesion is radiodense. It takes many years for the disease to travel

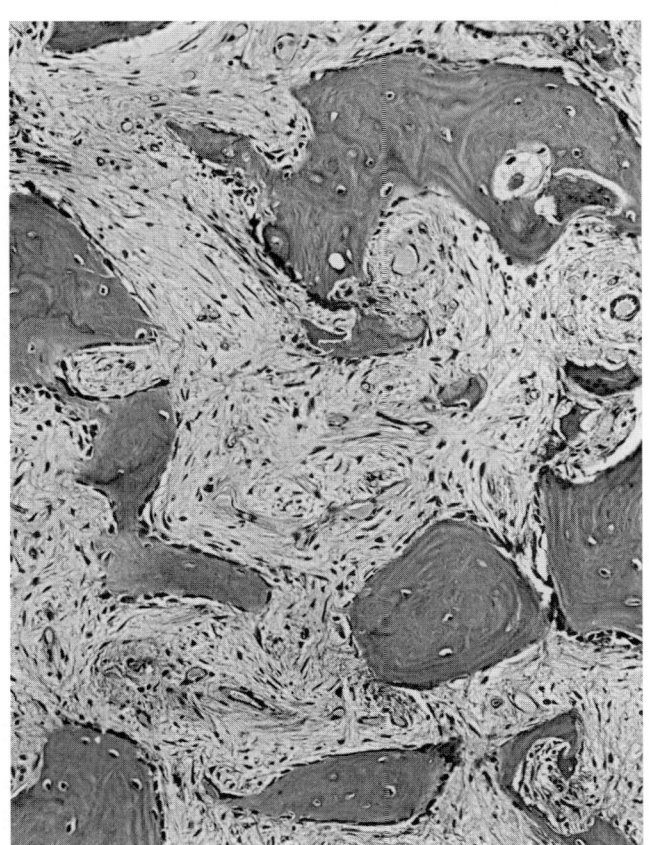

Figure 9-2 ■ Photomicrograph of hot phase Paget's disease. Osteoclastic resorption is present, and the marrow is fibrotic.

down the shaft of a long bone. For example, in the tibia, the process may take at least 12 years.[28] In polyostotic Paget's disease, each focus is in approximately the same stage of evolution, suggesting that the disease commenced everywhere at the same time. However, scintigraphic characteristics of various lesions may not all be synchronous.

Distinctive radiographic features of later stages of the disease include coarsening of trabeculae, blurring of the cortical-medullary junction, narrowing of the medullary canal, and thickening or enlargement of the bone (Fig. 9–8). This combination of features leads to radiodense bones (Fig. 9–9). In addition to radiodensity, bone enlargement is another highly suggestive feature of this disease. This feature is caused, in part, by periosteal new bone deposition.

Paget's disease in the spine, a very commonly involved site, produces distinctive radiographic and clinical features. In this location, the lumbar vertebrae are most commonly affected. In the early phases of vertebral involvement, compression fractures are common. In later stages, symmetric cortical thickening produces the so-called "picture frame" vertebra (Fig. 9–10). Symptoms result from enlargement of the vertebral body and involvement of the posterior elements. This often causes cord or nerve root compression, a problem best evaluated with a computed tomography scan.

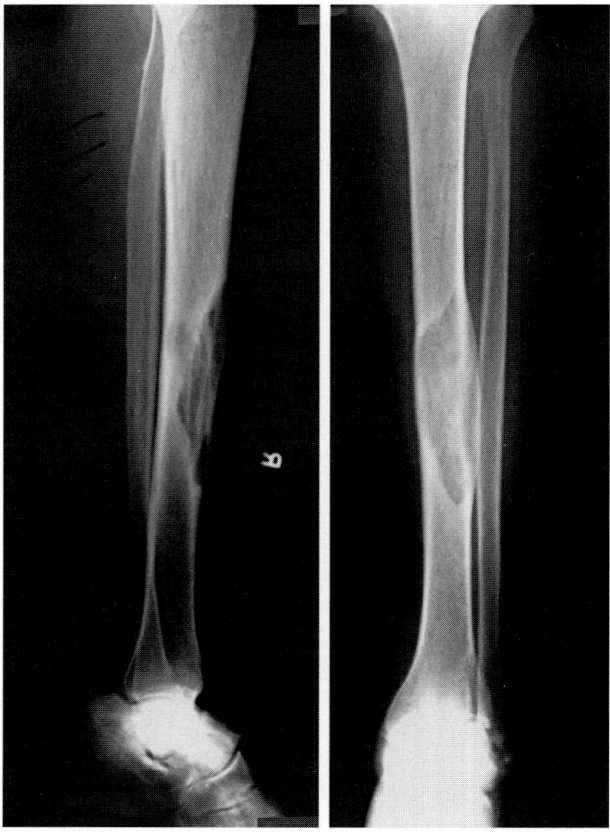

Figure 9–5 ■ Hot-phase Paget's disease. A well-defined radiolucent defect in the midshaft of the tibia. Both the proximal and the distal margins of this defect show the typical flame-shaped pattern.

The skull is also a common site of Paget's disease. In the hot phase of calvarial involvement, large areas of radiolucency are present in the frontal or occipital regions. These lytic areas, known as *osteoporosis circumscripta,* may progress to involve most of the skull. In the intermediate phase, an osteoblastic response causes a mixed osteolytic and osteoblastic pattern, the so-called "cotton wool" pattern. Involvement of the basilar portions of the skull occasionally causes platybasia and the neurologic symptoms of hydrocephalus. In addition, the mandible or maxilla may be involved and result in hypercementosis of the teeth.

Although plain radiographic features are usually diagnostic, the sensitive radionuclide bone scan is useful to quantify the extent of involvement. From 5 to 26% of lesions found on bone scan are not yet apparent with plain radiograph.[29] Characteristically, the radionuclide uptake is intense and involves long segments of cortex.

LABORATORY STUDIES

Laboratory tests are useful to confirm a radiographic suspicion of Paget's disease.[30] The most helpful test is the serum alkaline phosphatase, a measurement of osteoblastic activity. In Paget's disease, alkaline phosphatase is elevated, sometimes extremely, and levels are proportional to the ex-

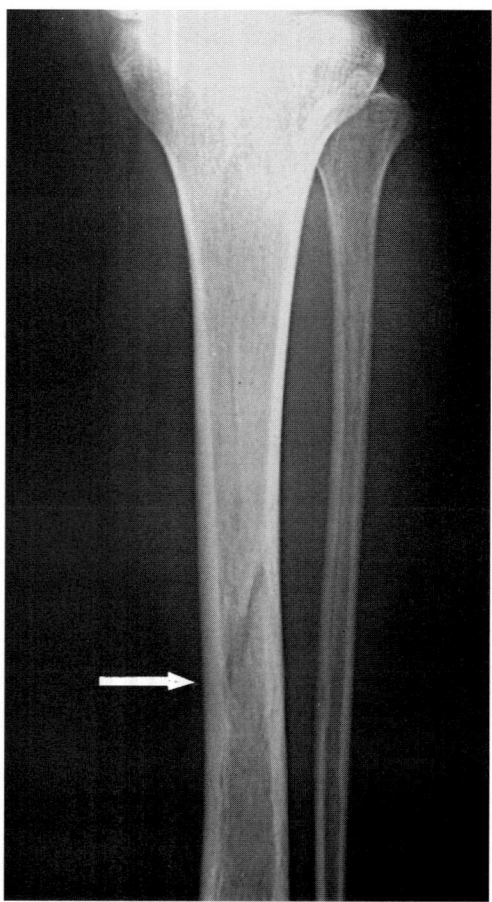

Figure 9–4 ■ Radiograph showing the earliest change of Paget's disease. A flame-shaped radiolucent area is present in the midshaft of the tibia *(arrow).*

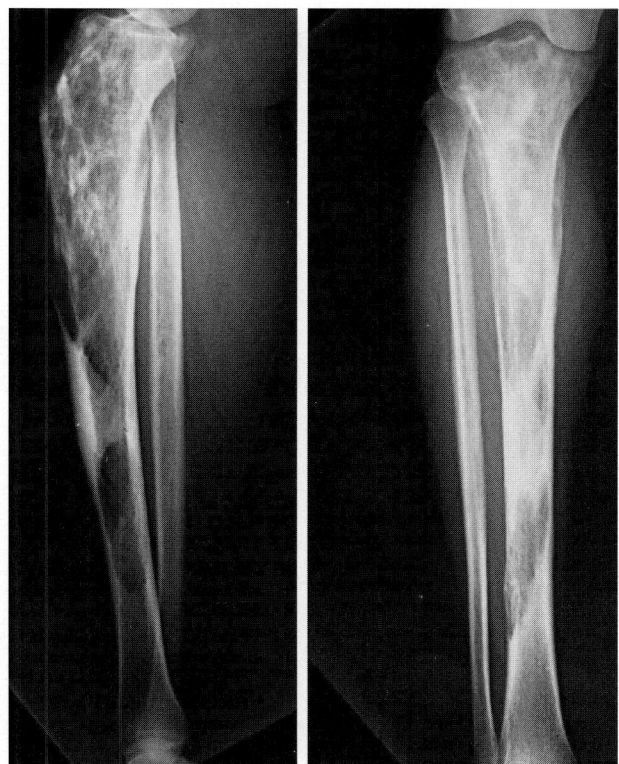

Figure 9-6 ■ Extensive hot-phase Paget's disease involving almost the entire shaft of the tibia.

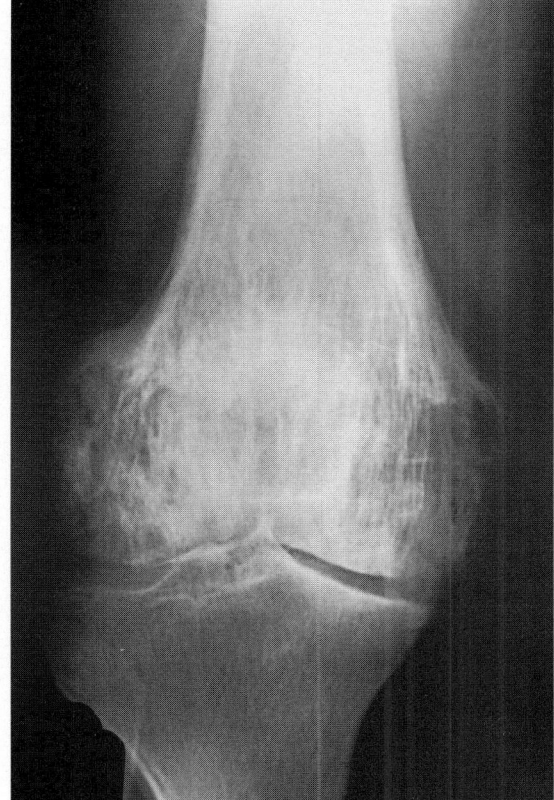

Figure 9-8 ■ Paget's disease of the distal femur. Compare the coarse trabeculae in the femur with the normal trabecular pattern in the tibia.

tent of skeletal involvement. Liver disease also elevates alkaline phosphatase, but if other liver enzymes are normal, elevations are probably caused by bone disease. Other indices of bone turnover are also elevated in Paget's disease. These include serum osteocalcin and the collagen breakdown products. The collagen of pagetic bone is normal, but four times the normal amount is synthesized. Therefore, levels of collagen breakdown products—urinary hydroxyproline and pyridinium cross-links—are elevated.

COMPLICATIONS

Osteoarticular Complications

Patients who have symptomatic Paget's disease suffer a wide variety of orthopedic complications.[31] Because pagetic bone is brittle, fractures are common. The strength of the long bones is due, in part, to the dense cortical tube. In Paget's disease, this tube is converted into a solid mass of porous bone, which does not bend with usual stress and therefore fractures easily. Fractures through this dense but structurally weak bone are transverse, producing the so-called "banana" or "chalk stick" pattern (Fig. 9–11). Unfortunately, complete fractures through pagetic bone often heal poorly.[32]

Stress fractures, common on the convex side of long bones, are also a result of bone brittleness (Fig. 9–12). The gradual accumulation of stress fractures causes the characteristic long bone deformity of Paget's disease. Deformity may

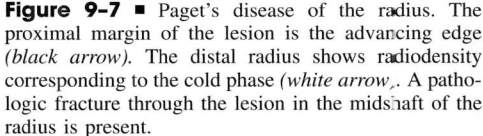

Figure 9-7 ■ Paget's disease of the radius. The proximal margin of the lesion is the advancing edge *(black arrow)*. The distal radius shows radiodensity corresponding to the cold phase *(white arrow)*. A pathologic fracture through the lesion in the midshaft of the radius is present.

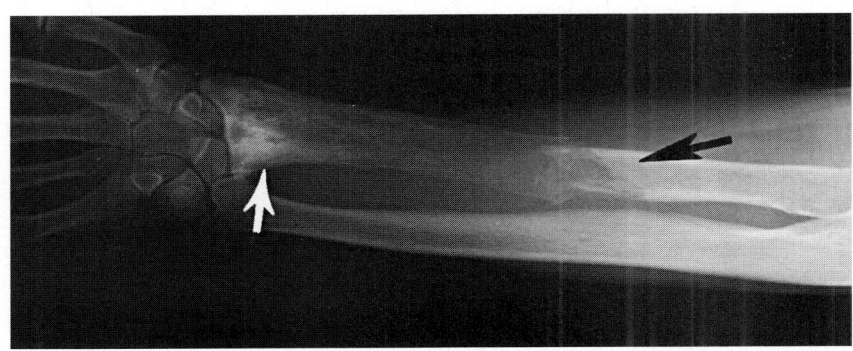

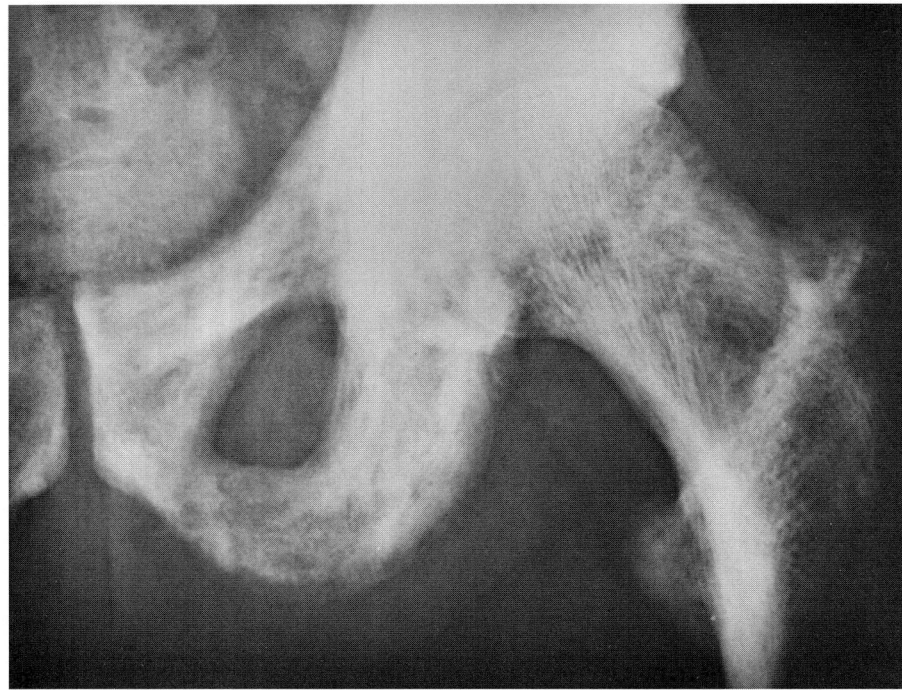

Figure 9-9 ■ Extensive Paget's disease of the pelvis and proximal femur. Blurring of the cortical medullary junction and expansion of the bone are present. The overall pattern is an increase in radiodensity.

also result from softening of the bone, which is present in the early phases of the disease.

Paget's disease adjacent to joints leads to another painful complication—the rapid development of osteoarthritis.[33] Because Paget's disease most frequently involves the pelvis, the hip joint is most often affected by this complication. Other commonly involved joints include the knee and the joints of the spine. Several mechanisms contribute to the development of osteoarthritis. First, enlarged pagetic bones alter joint biomechanics and cause uneven wear on the articular cartilage. In addition, deformed bones in the lower extremity cause an abnormal gait, resulting in increased stresses on the joints. Finally, pagetic bone is dense and noncompliant. As a result, the articular cartilage is subjected to more trauma than if it were supported by bone of normal density and compliance.

Cardiovascular Complications

Because pagetic bone is highly vascular and requires increased blood flow, demands are placed on the cardiovascular system. For example, cardiac enlargement often occurs if Paget's disease involves more than 35% of the skeleton.[34] On rare occasions, high-output cardiac failure results. Additionally, skin and soft tissue overlying involved bone have a higher blood flow. This causes local heat, a feature that led Paget to conclude that an inflammatory process was present.

Neurologic Complications

Neurologic symptoms are also a complication of Paget's disease. As pagetic bone enlarges, neural foramina are narrowed, and nerve impingement results. Peripheral nerve impingement syndromes may occur anywhere along the spine, and they are made worse by vertebral compression fractures.

Another neurologic complication may occur if the disease involves the cervical spine. This complication, known as the "spinal artery steal" syndrome, results from the increased blood flow to the vertebrae. In this syndrome, blood is shunted away from the spinal cord, which results in paraparesis.

When the skull is involved, various mechanisms of neurologic impairment occur. The thickened calvarium leads to brain compression and severe headache. Platybasia, basilar invagination of the posterior cranial fossa, may cause symptoms of hydrocephalus. Additionally, involvement of the base of the skull may lead to cranial nerve palsies, particularly of the optic and auditory nerves. It has been suggested that Beethoven's deafness was due to skull involvement by Paget's disease.[35] Although his temporal bones were not examined at autopsy, portrait images of his bust suggest skull thickening. However, this diagnosis is only conjectural; other possible causes include sarcoidosis[36] and neurosyphilis.[37]

Neoplastic Complications

Paget's disease is not life threatening except in the rare occurrence of one fatal complication—the development of a high-grade sarcoma in pagetic bone.[38] These sarcomas arise in the setting of the rapid bone turnover characteristic of the disease. This complication, known as Paget's sarcoma, occurs in about 1% of all patients with the disease and causes approximately 100 deaths per year in the United States.[8] The incidence rises to 20% in those patients who suffer with symptomatic polyostotic Paget's disease for 20 years or more. Patients with asymptomatic solitary lesions are the least likely to develop this complication.

The sarcomas develop in the same bones most frequently affected by Paget's disease—the bones of the axial skeleton. However, they also commonly occur in the humeri and femora. Sixteen percent of Paget's sarcomas are multifocal. Histologically, they are usually either osteosarcomas or malignant fibrous histiocytomas. The osteosarcomas are often the telangiectatic variant and are rich in multinucleated giant cells.[39] Therefore, these lesions are easily mistaken for giant cell tumors. Paget's sarcoma is almost always rapidly fatal, the average survival being only 9 months. This complication should be suspected if a patient with known Paget's disease has an increase in pain or develops an area of bone destruction associated with a soft tissue mass or fracture (Fig. 9–13). Magnetic resonance imaging is an important imaging modality in evaluating patients in whom Paget's sarcoma is suspected.

In addition to sarcomatous transformation, another neoplastic complication, although rare, is the development of a benign giant cell lesion.[40] This complication occurs almost exclusively in the face and skull. Early reports of this com-

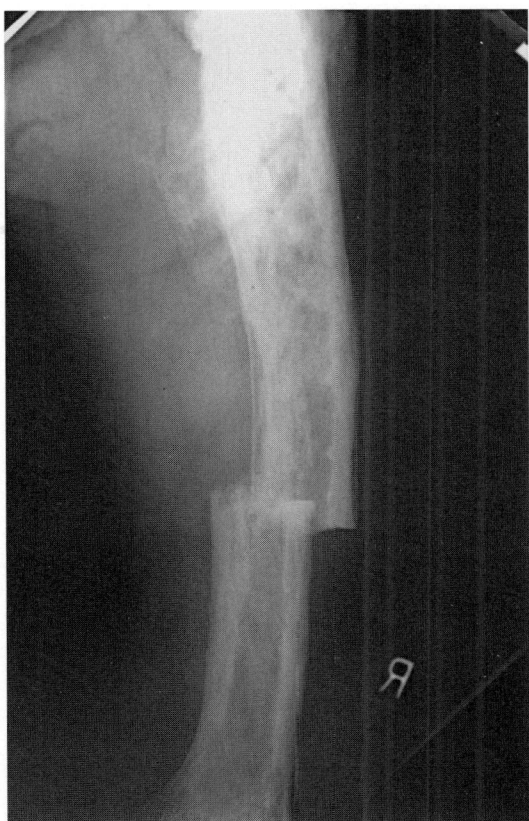

Figure 9–11 ■ Paget's disease of the entire length of the femur. A transverse fracture of the midshaft conforming to a so-called "banana fracture" pattern is present.

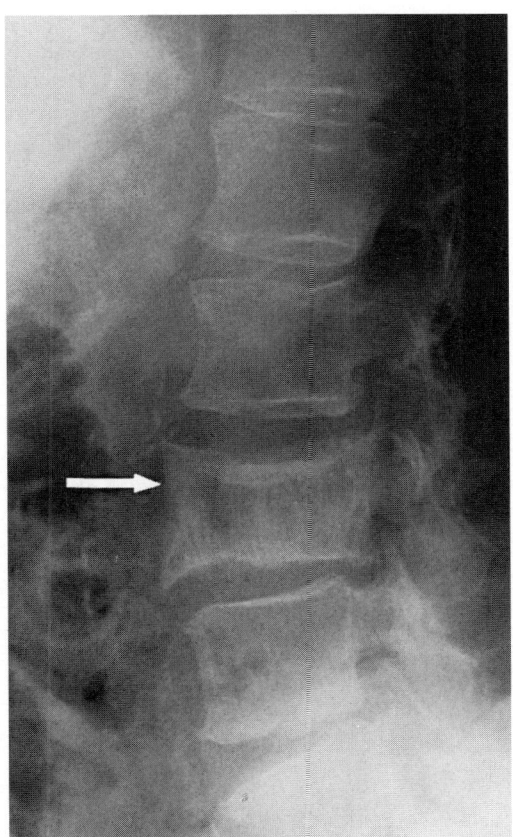

Figure 9–10 ■ Paget's disease of the vertebra. Enlargement of the vertebral body can be seen *(arrow)*. Sclerosis beneath the endplates and anteriorly is beginning to form the "picture frame" pattern.

plication regarded this lesion to be conventional giant cell tumor of bone. However, it is more likely that they are giant cell reparative granulomas.[41] Of interest, one such giant cell lesion contained intranuclear inclusions similar to those in the pagetic osteoclasts.[42]

Metastatic carcinomas also occur in pagetic bone because of the prominent vascularity of pagetic lesions.[43] Importantly, metastatic carcinoma may radiologically mimic Paget's sarcoma. Therefore, all destructive lesions associated with Paget's disease must be biopsied.

DIFFERENTIAL DIAGNOSIS

The radiologic features of trabecular coarsening and bone enlargement are diagnostic of Paget's disease. Similarly, a radiolytic focus with an advancing flame-shaped edge is highly suggestive of Paget's disease. When these features are not present, a biopsy is often necessary to rule out other radiodense or radiolytic lesions. One radiodense lesion often confused with Paget's disease is an osteoblastic focus of metastatic carcinoma. However, the radiodensity of a blastic metastasis is usually amorphous, similar to "wet cotton." This differs from the coarsened trabeculae of Paget's disease. If a biopsy is needed, keratin stains may be necessary to

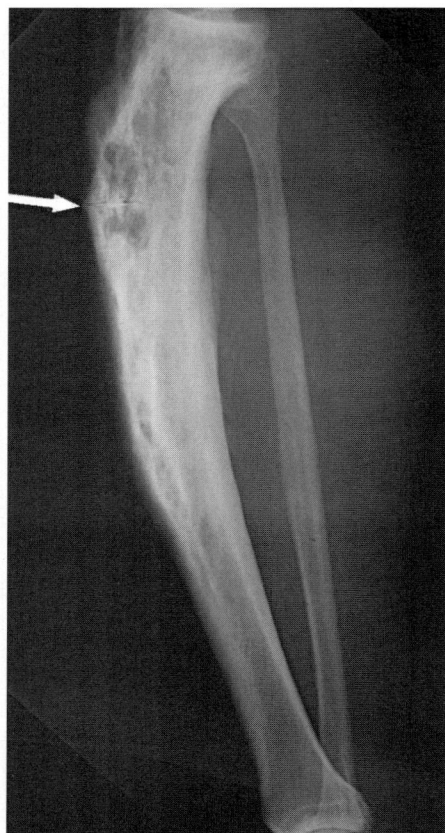

Figure 9-12 ■ Paget's disease of the tibia. Multiple stress fractures *(arrow)* result in anterior bowing deformities.

diagnose metastatic carcinoma. Other radiodense lesions may also be misdiagnosed as Paget's disease. For example, malignant lymphoma of bone may induce extensive reactive bone and produce long segments of radiodensity. Also, chronic osteomyelitis may mimic Paget's disease, especially if prominent periosteal bone enlargement is present. A biopsy usually distinguishes these lesions.

In the lytic phase, Paget's disease may be confused with other lesions microscopically. The extensive marrow fibrosis and woven bone production, characteristic of hot phase Paget's disease, may mimic fibrous dysplasia. If osteoblasts are numerous, osteoblastoma may be considered. Clinical and radiographic correlation is necessary to avoid these diagnostic pitfalls.

TREATMENT

The two aspects of therapy for Paget's disease are (1) the medical treatment of the primary disease process and (2) the surgical management of the complications. The high bone turnover of active Paget's disease is successfully quieted by many of the drugs that inhibit osteoclasts.[44] Among these, calcitonin has been used with some success. However, most endocrinologists currently use the bisphosphonates. Of these, oral alendronate or intravenous pamidronate is highly effective. These drugs reduce bone turnover by inhibiting osteoclast activity.[45] By binding to the apatite crystal, they render it less soluble. In addition, they inhibit the recruitment of osteoclasts and reduce their longevity. After bisphosphonate therapy, the indices of bone turnover decrease by as much as 50%. The decreased bone turnover, which lasts for many months after therapy, is reflected in a decreased uptake of radionuclide tracer on bone scans, decreased bone pain, and improvement of neurologic complications. The most frequent surgical procedures performed to ameliorate complications are total joint arthroplasty and nerve decompressions.

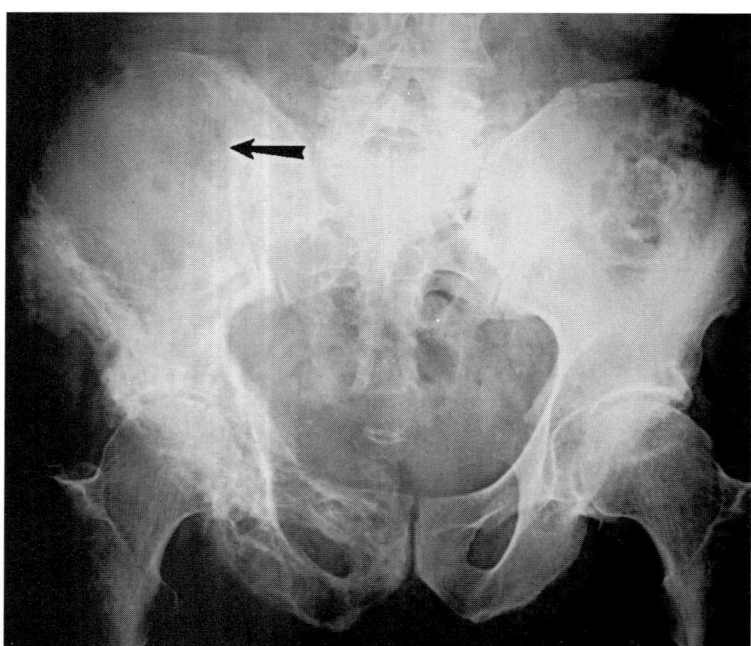

Figure 9-13 ■ Paget's disease of the pelvis. A huge lytic defect in the wing of the ilium *(arrow)* corresponds to a Paget's sarcoma.

REFERENCES

1. Wrany: Spongrose Hyperostose des Schadels, des Beckins und des linken Oberschenkels. *Vjsch Prakt Heilk* 93:79–95, 1877.
2. Wilks, S.: Case of osteoporosis, or spongy hypertrophy of the bones (calvaria, clavicle, or femoris and rib, exhibited at the Society). *Trans Pathol Soc Lond* 20:273, 1869.
3. Paget, J.: On a form of chronic inflammation of bones (osteitis deformans). *Med Chir Trans* 60:37–63, 1877.
4. Packard, F. A., Steele, J. D., and Kirkbride, T. S.: Osteitis deformans. *Am J Med Sci* 122:552–568, 1901.
5. Jaffe, H. L.: The classic. Paget's disease of bone. *Clin Orthop* 127:4–22, 1977.
6. Mandl, F: Klinisches und Experimentelles zur Frage der lokalisierten und generalisierten ostitis fibrosa. *Arch Klin Chir* 143:1, 245, 1926.
7. Schmorl, G.: *Verhandl d Deutsch Path Gesellsch* 21:71, 1926.
8. Altman, R. D.: Paget's disease of bone. Coe, F. L., and Favus, M. J. (Eds.): *Disorders of Bone and Mineral Metabolism*. New York, Raven Press, 1992, pp. 1027–1064.
9. Denninger, H.: Paleopathological evidence of Paget's disease. *Ann Med Hist* 5:73–81, 1933.
10. Wells, C. and Woodhouse, N.: Paget's disease in an Anglo-Saxon. *Med Hist* 19:396–400, 1975.
11. Pales, L.: Maladie de Paget prehistorique. *Anthrop* 39:263–270, 1929.
12. Wagner, M.: Report of a case of Paget's disease in an eighteen-year-old male with a review of the literature. *Wis Med J* 46:1098, 1947.
13. Siris, E. S.: Epidemiological aspects of Paget's disease: Family history and relationship to other medical conditions. *Semin Arthritis Rheum* 23:222–225, 1994.
14. Kaplan, F. S., and Singer, F. R.: Paget's disease of bone: Pathophysiology and diagnosis. *J Am Acad Orthop Surg* 3:336–344, 1995.
15. Morales-Piga, A. A., Rey-Rey, J. S., Corres-Gonzales, J., et al.: Frequency and characteristics of familial aggregation of Paget's disease of bone. *J Bone Miner Res* 10:663–670, 1995.
16. Rosenbaum, H. D., and Hanson, D. J.: Geographic variation in the prevalence of Paget's disease of bone. *Radiology* 92:959–963, 1969.
17. Schmorl, G.: Uber osteitis deformans Paget. *Virchow Arch Pathol Anat* 283:694–737, 1932.
18. Rebel, A., Malkani, K., Basle, M., Bregeon, C. H., et al.: Particularites ultrastructurales des osteoclastes de la maladie de Paget. *Rev Rheum* 41:767–771, 1974.
19. Welsh, R., and Meyer, A.: Nuclear fragmentations and associated fibrils in giant cell tumor of bone. *Lab Invest* 22:63–72, 1970.
20. Mills, B. G., Singer, F. R., Weiner, L. P., Suffin, S. C., Stabile, E., and Holst, P.: Evidence for both respiratory syncytial virus and measles virus antigens in the osteoclasts of patients with Paget's disease of bone. *Clin Orthop* 183:303–311, 1984.
21. Morgan-Capner, P., Robinson, P., Clewley, G., Darby, A., and Pettingale, K.: Measles antibody in Paget's disease. *Lancet* 1:733, 1981.
22. Basle, M. F., Fournier, J. G., Rozenblatt, S., et al.: Measles virus RNA detected in Paget's disease bone tissue by in situ hybridization. *J Gen Virol* 67:907–913, 1986.
23. Reddy, S. V., Singer, F. R., and Roodman, G. D.: Bone marrow mononuclear cells from patients with Paget's disease contain measles virus nucleocapsid messenger ribonucleic acid that has mutations in a specific region of the sequence. *J Clin Endocrinol Metab* 80:2108–2111, 1995.
24. Reddy, S. V., Singer, F. R., Mallette, L., and Roodman, G. D.: Detection of measles virus nucleocapsid transcripts in circulating blood cells from patients with Paget's disease. *J Bone Miner Res* 11:1602–1607, 1996.
25. Roodman, G. D., Kurihara, N., and Ohsaki, Y.: Interleukin-6: A potential autocrine/paracrine factor in Paget's disease of bone. *J Clin Invest* 89:46–52, 1992.
26. O'Driscoll, S., and Hastings, D. E.: Extension of monostotic Paget's disease from the femur to the tibia after arthrodesis of the knee. *J Bone Joint Surg* 71A:129–131, 1989.
27. Hadjipavlou, A., Lander, P., Boudreau, R., Srolovitz, H., and Palayew, M.: Pagetoid changes in a heterotopic center of ossification. *J Bone Joint Surg* 63A:1339–1341, 1981.
28. Zadek, R. E., and Milgram, J. W.: Progression of Paget's disease in the tibia. *J Bone Joint Surg* 58A:876–878, 1963.
29. Buchoff, H. S., and Altman, R. D.: Paget's disease: Correlation of pain, x-rays, and bone scans. *Arthritis Rheum* 24:572, 1981.
30. Russell, R. G. G., Colwell, A., Hannon, R. A., et al.: Biochemical measurements in Paget's disease of bone. *Semin Arthritis Rheum* 23:240–241, 1994.
31. Kaplan, F. S.: Paget's disease of bone: Orthopedic complications. *Semin Arthritis Rheum* 23:250–252, 1994.
32. Dove, J.: Complete fractures of the femur in Paget's disease of bone. *J Bone Joint Surg* 62B:12–17, 1980.
33. Altman, R. D.: Articular complications of Paget's disease of bone. *Semin Arthritis Rheum* 23:248–249, 1994.
34. Howarth, S.: Cardiac output in osteitis deformans. *Clin Sci* 12:271–275, 1953.
35. Naiken, V. S.: Paget's disease and Beethoven's deafness. *Clin Orthop* 89:103–105, 1972.
36. Palferman, T. G.: Beethoven: A medical biography. *J Med Biol* 1:35–45, 1993.
37. McCabe, B. F.: Beethoven's deafness. *Ann Otol* 67:192–205, 1958.
38. Wick, M. R., Siegal, G. P., Unni, K K., McLeod, R. A., and Greditzer, H. G.: Sarcomas of bone complicating osteitis deformans (Paget's disease). *Am J Surg Pathol* 5:47–59, 1981.
39. Schajowicz, F., Araujo, E. S., and Berenstein, M.: Sarcoma complicating Paget's disease of bone. *J Bone Joint Surg* 65-B:299–307, 1983.
40. Jacobs, T. P., Michelsen, J., Polay, J. S., D'Adamo, A. C., and Canfield, R. E.: Giant cell tumor in Paget's disease of bone: familial and geographic clustering. *Cancer* 44:742–747, 1979.
41. Upchurch, K. S., Simon, L. S., Schiller, A. L., Rosenthal, D. I., Campion, E. W., and Krane, S. M.: Giant cell reparative granuloma of Paget's disease of bone: A unique clinical entity. *Ann Intern Med* 98:35–40, 1983.
42. Mirra, J. M., Bauer, F. C. H., and Grant, T. T.: Giant cell tumor with viral-like intranuclear inclusions associated with Paget's disease. *Clin Orthop* 158:243–251, 1981.
43. Agha, F. P., Norman, A., Hirschl, S., and Klein, R.: Paget's disease: Coexistence with metastatic carcinoma. *N Y State J Med* 76:734, 1976.
44. Delmas, P. D., and Meunier, P. J.: The management of Paget's disease of bone. *N Engl J Med* 336:558–566, 1997.
45. Fleisch, H.: Bisphosphonates: Pharmacology. *Semin Arthritis Rheum* 23:261–262, 1994.

CHAPTER 10
Metastatic Carcinoma in Bone

Metastatic carcinoma is the most common cause of destructive bone lesions in adults. In fact, it occurs so frequently that physicians should assume that any destructive bone lesion in a patient older than 45 years is metastatic carcinoma. The diagnosis and treatment of metastatic carcinoma to bone composes the major part of the practice of an orthopedic oncologist.

Any malignant neoplasm can metastasize to bone, but most commonly, the primary lesion is a carcinoma, the main subject of this chapter. Sarcomas, on rare occasions, also metastasize to bone. Even primary bone tumors, such as malignant fibrous histiocytoma, Ewing sarcoma, and osteosarcoma, can spread to other osseous sites. In these cases, patients are usually children or young adults. Metastatic bone lesions may occur in young children, particularly in disseminated neuroblastoma.

INCIDENCE

Although carcinomas of any organ can spread to bone, the most common are carcinomas of the lung, breast, prostate, kidney, or thyroid. Primary carcinoma of these organs are the most common of all cancers, accounting for one half of the 1.3 million new cancer cases each year in the United States.[1]

Although the incidence of bone metastases in all patients dying of cancer is reported to be as high as 70%, it is probably more common.[2] This is because detection methods are limited. Radiographic studies are insensitive, and histologic examination is subject to sampling error. Therefore, because about 525,000 Americans die from cancer each year, the diagnosis and management of bone metastases is an enormous clinical burden.

In men, the most common metastatic tumors are from the lung and prostate. Formerly, before widespread screening with prostate-specific antigen, almost one third of patients already had bone metastasis when the diagnosis of prostate cancer was made.[3] This incidence will almost certainly be reduced. In patients with lung carcinoma, bone marrow involvement is present in 5 to 21% of patients at the time of initial presentation.[4] Small cell carcinoma is the most common to metastasize.

Breast carcinoma is the most common type of metastatic tumor in women. As many as 21% of patients have bone marrow metastases at the time of diagnosis,[5] and probably all of the 45,000 women who die of breast cancer each year in the United States have bone metastases.

CLINICAL SETTINGS

Metastatic tumors to bone occur in two clinical settings—in patients with known primary cancer and in patients with no history of prior disease. The first clinical setting is the more common. A patient with a history of carcinoma presents with one or more destructive bone lesions. In this setting, establishing the diagnosis of metastatic carcinoma often changes the stage of the disease and requires important therapeutic decisions. Although a destructive bone lesion in a patient with a history of carcinoma can be presumed to be a metastasis, we do not recommend treatment without histologic confirmation. This is especially true if the bone lesion is solitary or if the patient has had a long disease-free interval. Two reasons for this exist. First, other lesions, such as Paget's disease, large bone islands, and osteoporotic compression fractures, may radiographically mimic metastatic carcinoma. Second, the bone lesion may be from another, yet undiagnosed primary source, a situation that occurs in almost 10% of cases.

The second setting is the development of a destructive bone lesion in a patient without a prior history of a malignant neoplasm. In this clinical setting, the diagnostic challenges are greater. This situation requires a biopsy of the lesion, and a search for the primary tumor is necessary. Before computed tomographic (CT) scanning, the primary site could be discovered in only about 35% of cases.[6] With total body CT scanning, however, the primary tumor may be identified in as many as 85% of cases.[7] When the primary tumor can be found, it is usually in the lung. Those that cannot be found are usually adenocarcinomas. In 27% of these cases, classified as adenocarcinomas of unknown primary source, the primary tumor cannot be identified even at autopsy.[8]

PATHOPHYSIOLOGY

Bone, after lung and liver, is the third most common site of metastatic carcinoma. Although carcinomas frequently spread to other organs via lymphatics, bone metastases develop secondary to hematogenous spread of cancer cells (Fig. 10–1). The most common locations are the bones of the axial skeleton, particularly the spine. The pelvis and proximal femurs are also common sites (Fig. 10–2). In adults, these sites of predilection correspond to the distribution of hematopoietic marrow. The hematopoietic marrow has open vascular sinuses and easily allows embolic tumor cells to pass from blood to the marrow.

Routes of Cancer Cells to Bone

Malignant cells can reach bone via the arterial side of the body's circulatory system after passing through arterive-

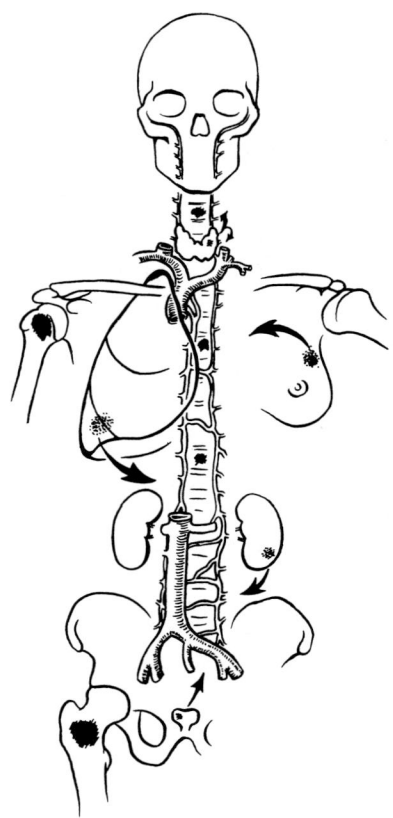

Figure 10-2 ■ Sites of metastasis. The spine, proximal femur, pelvis, and proximal humerus are the most common sites. The venus plexus of Batson allows retrograde blood flow around the spine.

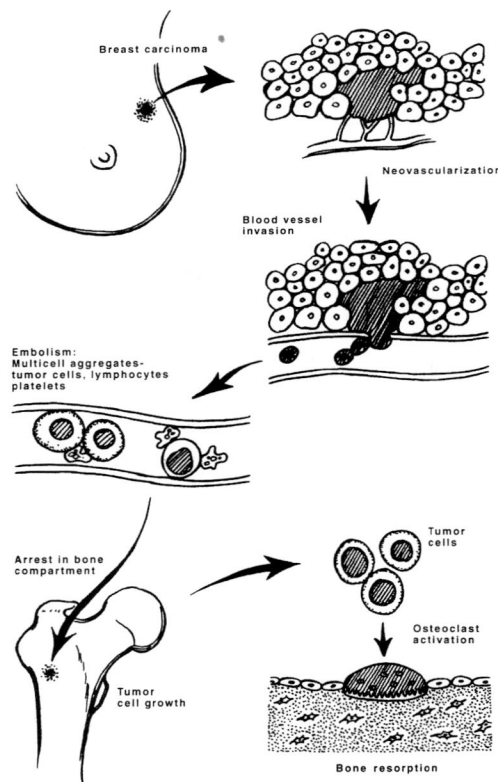

Figure 10-1 ■ The mechanism of bone metastasis. Cancer cells at the primary site invade arteries and veins. They pass via the bloodstream to the bone. Bone destruction is mediated by osteoclasts stimulated by the cancer cells.

nous anastomoses. Lung carcinoma cells, by direct invasion of pulmonary veins, take a more direct route to the arterial circulation. Metastases may also reach bone through retrograde flow through the venous system. In 1940, Oscar Batson, after meticulous experiments on cadaver and animal spines, demonstrated a valveless plexus of veins around the spine.[9] This plexus, now known as *Batson's plexus,* extends from the sacrum to the dural venous sinuses of the skull. Because valves are absent, malignant cells can percolate in any direction through this plexus and enter the vertebral bodies at any level. Increased intraabdominal pressure, such as occurs in coughing or abdominal compression, enhances retrograde blood flow. Batson's plexus is a major factor in the development of spine metastases in carcinomas of the prostate, breast, and kidney. It accounts for the occasional observation of widespread spinal metastases without lesions in other bones.

On rare occasions, metastatic carcinomas occur in the distal extremities. For example, we have observed a focus of metastatic bile-secreting hepatoma in the distal phalanx of the thumb. The thumb was green! Most commonly, however, these distal metastasis, known as *acral metastases,* are from lung carcinoma.[10] In the small bones of the feet, metastatic prostate or colon carcinoma occasionally occurs. The mechanism for this is probably gravitational. Tumor cells, through communications with the iliofemoral venous system, descend to the feet through incompetent veins.[11]

Effects of Cancer Cells on Bone

Some oncologists distinguish between bone marrow metastasis and bone metastasis. *Bone marrow metastasis* refers to the presence of malignant cells in bone biopsies performed in areas where no scintigraphic or radiographic abnormalities are present. This implies that the malignant cells have not yet activated native bone cells. Although occasionally this phase may last for a few months or possibly even years, neoplastic cells in the bone marrow eventually cause a bone reaction.[12]

The bone changes in metastatic carcinoma are always a result of native bone cells. The most frequent change is osteolysis. Osteoclasts are activated by cytokines secreted by the malignant cells[13] (Fig. 10-3). These include various growth factors and prostaglandins. Interleukin 1, secreted by some squamous carcinomas, also stimulates osteoclasts.[14]

Malignant cells in the bone marrow also provoke a dense fibrous tissue response. Local osteoblasts can also be activated, and reactive new bone can be formed (Fig. 10-4). In metastatic prostate or breast cancer, new bone formation can

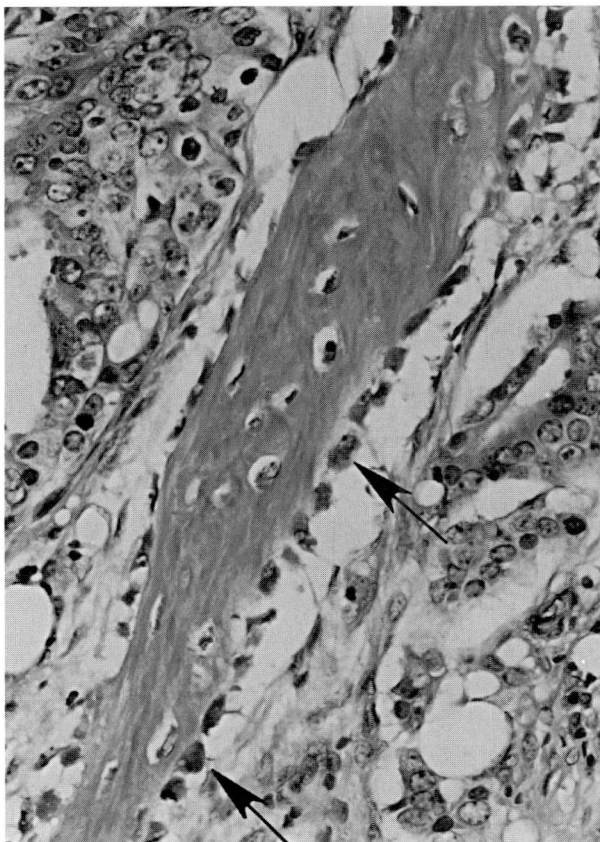

Figure 10-4 ■ Photomicrograph of reactive bone at a site of metastatic carcinoma. The bone is synthesized by native osteoblasts *(arrows)* stimulated by the neoplastic cells.

be extensive. In fact, prostate cancer cells have been shown to secrete an osteoblast-stimulating factor.[15]

CLINICAL FEATURES

Patients with metastatic carcinoma are usually in their 50s or 60s, ages at which cancer commonly occurs. A patient in this age group with a destructive bone lesion and no current cancer should be questioned carefully about previous illnesses. A remote history of cancer may be uncovered and provide a clue to the current problem. For example, one of our patients with a destructive lesion in the humerus denied a history of cancer. But when she was told that the tumor in her arm was a leiomyosarcoma, she replied, "Oh, I had one of those once in my uterus."

Carcinomas usually metastasize within 5 years, so a destructive bone lesion is easily connected to the primary cancer diagnosis. However, some cancers may not metastasize until years after the primary therapy. For example, a metastasis from a breast carcinoma may develop 20 years after a mastectomy.

Usually, a patient presents with more than one bone lesion. Although only one lesion may be symptomatic, a technetium bone scan demonstrates other sites of involvement in 90%

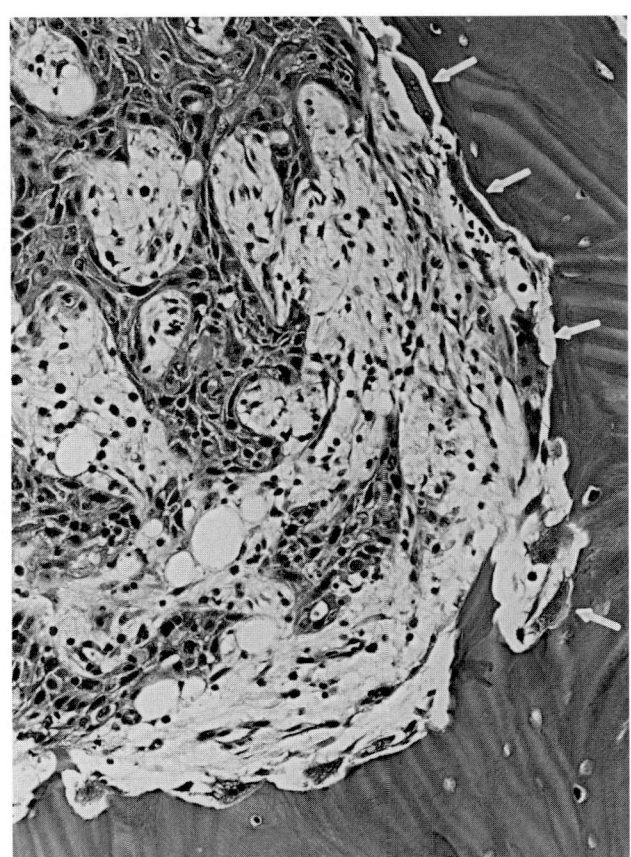

Figure 10-3 ■ Photomicrograph of organoid clusters of carcinoma cells. The local osteoclasts *(arrows)* are resorbing bone. These cells are stimulated by the neoplastic cells.

of cases. Occasionally, however, only a single metastatic focus is present. Renal cell carcinoma, for example, is well known for its serendipitous metastatic behavior. A single osseous metastasis may be the only manifestation of disseminated spread for many years. However, other metastases almost always appear eventually. Therefore, ablative surgical procedures for a single focus of metastatic renal cell carcinoma almost always fail to cure the patient.

Patients with metastatic carcinoma to bone present with pain. At first, the pain may be present only with activity, but it rapidly progresses to pain at rest. It is particularly severe at night. Abrupt severe pain is usually caused by a pathologic fracture, a presenting complaint of 25% of patients.[16] Pathologic fracture is related to the amount of cortical destruction. If more than 50% of the cortical circumference is destroyed, then the bone is at great risk of fracturing.

Patients with metastatic carcinomas to bone also have systemic complaints. Many have a normochromic normocytic anemia and are easily fatigable. Patients also have an abnormal serum alkaline or acid phosphatase,[17] a reflection of increased osteoblastic and osteoclastic activity. Some patients have elevated serum lactic dehydrogenase and elevated serum uric acid, both because of tumor necrosis.

A systemic complication of metastatic carcinoma that often requires therapy is hypercalcemia. Hypercalcemia complicates about 10 to 15% of all cancer cases.[18] In fact, cancer is one of the two most common causes of hypercalcemia. Unlike the hypercalcemia of hyperparathyroidism, the other common cause, the calcium levels in cancer rise rapidly and to very high, sometimes life-threatening, levels. However, the degree of hypercalcemia does not necessarily correlate with the number, or even presence, of bone metastases. Whereas in some cases, such as metastatic breast cancer, the hypercalcemia is the result of prostaglandin-mediated bone destruction, in other cases, the mechanism is humoral. The humoral mechanism is thought to be caused by the synthesis and secretion of parathyroid hormone–related protein by the tumor cells. For example, 10% of squamous carcinomas secrete this protein.[19] In these cases, the bone not involved by metastatic carcinoma shows features similar to hyperparathyroid bone disease.[20]

RADIOGRAPHIC FEATURES

The technetium bone scans are the most sensitive imaging modality to detect skeletal metastases.[21] In fact, with this technique, metastatic foci can be identified as long as 4 months before they become apparent by plain radiography.[22] Therefore, any adult patient with a destructive bone lesion should have a bone scan. The presence of other lesions raises the probability that bone metastases are present, and the extent of disease can be delineated. On occasion, widespread metastatic carcinoma can produce a false negative scan because tracer accumulates uniformly throughout the entire skeleton and is imaged as normal by the scanner's computer. This phenomenon is known as a *superscan*.

Metastatic carcinoma in bone is remarkable for its wide range of plain radiographic patterns. In contrast to most primary bone tumors, which have distinctive, often diagnostic, plain radiographic features, metastatic carcinoma can look like anything. Lesions may be radiolytic or radiodense; they may be permeative or well defined; or they may be periosteal, intracortical, or intramedullary. The only distinctive feature of metastatic carcinoma in bone is its predilection for the axial skeleton.

Certain metastatic carcinomas, however, produce consistent radiographic patterns. For example, metastatic prostate cancer usually produces radiodense lesions—so-called osteoblastic metastases (Fig. 10–5). Sometimes, the osteoblastic metastases of prostatic carcinoma are widely distributed throughout the entire skeleton (Fig. 10–6). The osteoblastic response imparts to the skeleton a consistency almost as hard as rock (Fig. 10–7). Cutting through these bones binds even the most powerful bandsaw. Breast carcinoma can also be osteoblastic, but lesions are often mixed osteolytic and osteoblastic.

Metastatic lung carcinoma, by contrast, almost always produces radiolytic lesions. Lesions can be permeative (Fig. 10–8) or well defined (Fig. 10–9), and cortical destruction often occurs. Characteristically, periosteal reactive bone is minimal. Often, lesions are associated with a large soft tissue mass. Metastatic renal cell and thyroid carcinomas produce a distinctive pattern of radiolysis. Radiographs show a huge,

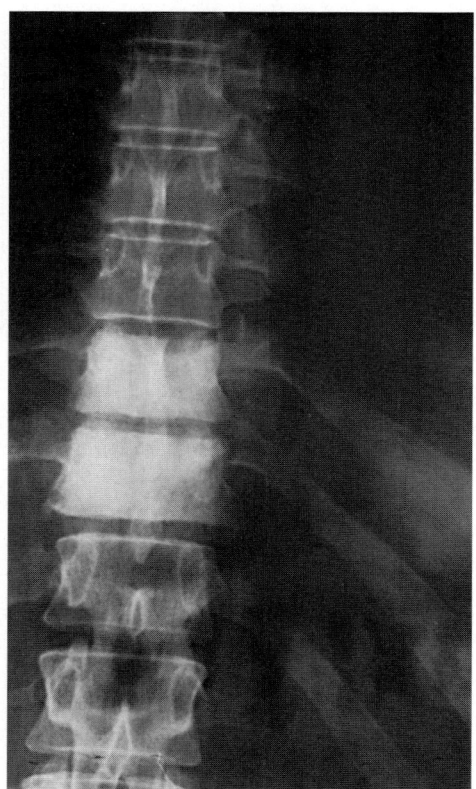

Figure 10–5 ■ Two vertebrae with metastatic prostate carcinoma. Prostate carcinoma typically produces osteoblastic lesions.

Figure 10-6 ■ Pelvis in disseminated prostate carcinoma. The entire skeleton shows increased radiodensity.

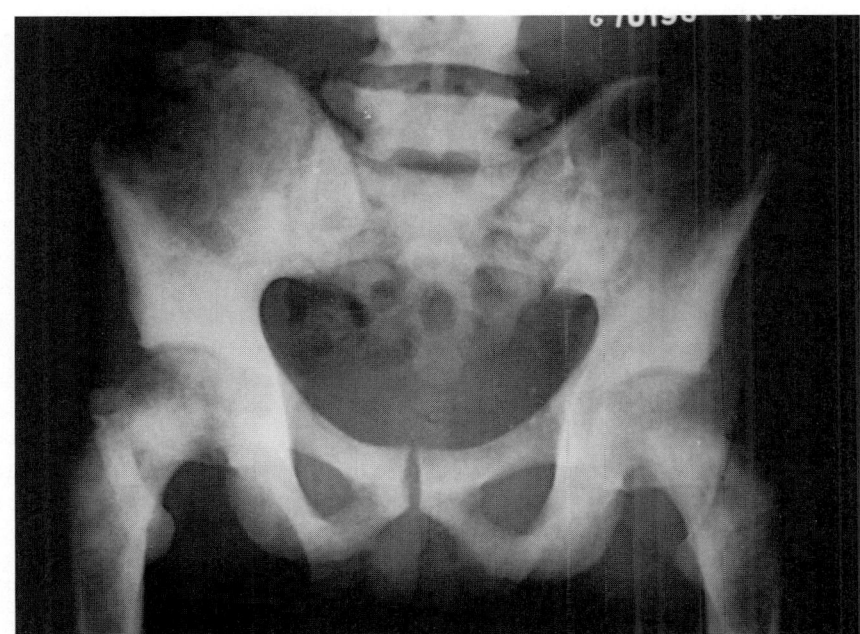

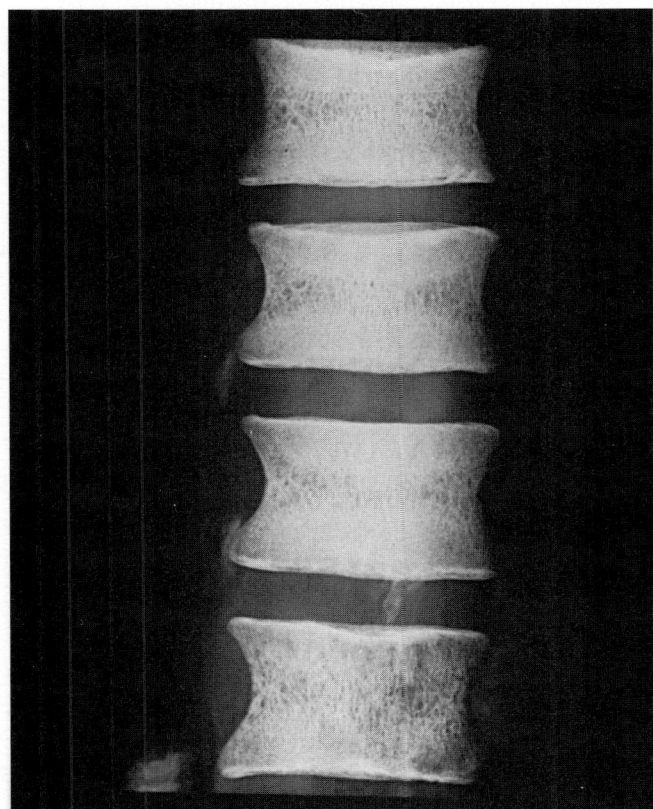

Figure 10-7 ■ Specimen radiograph of a portion of a spine with metastatic prostate cancer. The osteosclerosis is extreme.

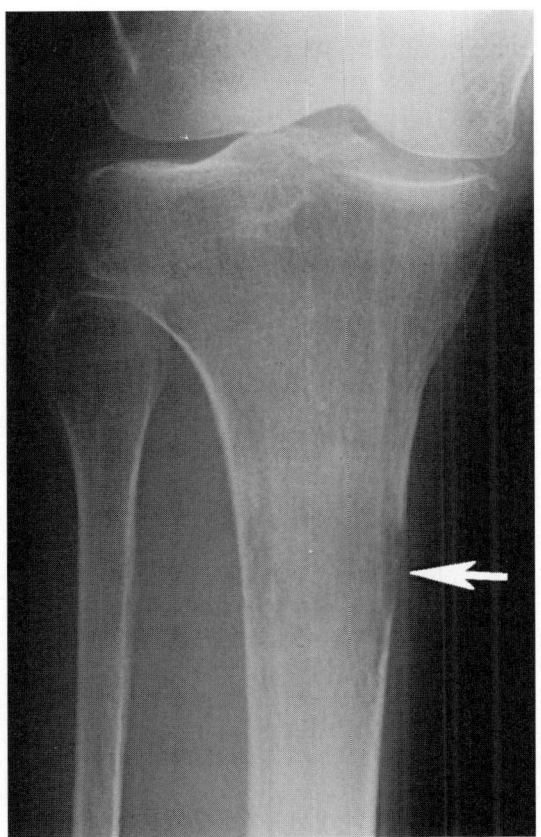

Figure 10-8 ■ Metastatic carcinoma from the lung to the tibia. A poorly defined, permeative pattern of radiolucency can be seen *(arrow)*.

bubbly, expansile pattern of bone destruction, a pattern that is highly suggestive of these primary sites (Fig. 10–10).

Although most metastatic carcinomas are centered in the medullary canal, some occur intracortically or subperiosteally on the bone surface.[23,24] Although some cortical scalloping may occur, the principal feature is exuberant reactive periosteal bone formation. This pattern is most commonly produced by metastatic lung or prostate carcinoma (Fig. 10–11).

In the spine, multiple vertebral bodies are often affected, but intervening uninvolved vertebrae are common. Characteristically, metastatic carcinoma to the spine spares the intervertebral disc. Considerable destruction of the vertebral body may occur, but the disc space is not narrowed. This feature helps distinguish metastatic carcinoma from vertebral osteomyelitis, a disease that almost always causes a reduction in the disc space.

Whereas the magnetic resonance imaging (MRI) and CT scans contribute little to the diagnosis of metastatic carcinoma to bone, they are extremely important in planning management. MRI effectively demonstrates the amount of soft tissue invasion and therefore accurately quantitates the tumor burden. The CT scan is the most effective modality in determining the amount of cortical destruction. The probability of pathologic fracture can be estimated, and the most effective stabilization procedures can be planned.

PATHOLOGIC FEATURES OF METASTATIC BONE TUMORS

The characteristic feature of metastatic carcinoma in bone is an organoid growth pattern of neoplastic cells. The cells are grouped in tight clusters or lines that are separated by a fibrous stroma. Often the clusters assume a glandular shape, a pattern suggestive of adenocarcinoma (Fig. 10–12). Also, keratinization, if present, suggests squamous differentiation. The keratinization may be intracellular or appear as extracellular pearls.

Prior to the use of immunohistochemical stains, pathologists could rarely identify the primary site of the metastasis by histologic features. Although certain lesions, such as renal cell carcinoma, thyroid carcinoma, and oat cell carcinoma could be recognized with a moderate degree of certainty, identifying the primary source was a clinical and radiologic problem. Today, immunohistochemical stains not only confirm the diagnosis of carcinoma but also, in some cases, make possible the positive identification of the primary site. First, cytokeratin immunostains, almost always positive in metastatic carcinoma, confirm the diagnosis and rule out sarcomas and lymphomas. Because some leiomyosarcomas and malignant fibrous histiocytomas contain occasional keratin-positive cells,[25,26] the diagnosis of carcinoma rests on uniform keratin staining throughout the neoplastic cells. Second, prostatic carcinoma in bone can almost always be identified by stains for prostate-specific antigen or prostatic acid phosphatase. Similarly, thyroid carcinoma can be identified with immunostains for thyroglobulin, and breast carcinoma is likely if an alpha lactalbumin stain is positive. However, despite these immunochemical stains, many cases occur in which the histologic features of the metastasis offer no clue to the location of the primary site.

Occasionally, the presence of metastatic carcinoma in bone is not obvious, usually because the bone's response obscures the malignant epithelial cells. One bone reaction is myelofibrosis. Almost always, the epithelial cells in the bone marrow produce a stromal reaction. However, sometimes the stromal reaction is a dense fibrosis, and the carcinoma cells are barely visible (Fig. 10–13). Serial sections and cytokeratin stains are sometimes necessary to identify them.

The second bony response is reactive bone formation, the histologic correlate of radiodense metastases (Fig. 10–14). Sometimes the reactive bone can be so extensive that the lesion mimics a bone-forming neoplasm (Fig. 10–15). Occasionally, osteoclast-like giant cells may also be present. However, cytokeratin stains can identify epithelial cells scattered throughout these reactive elements.

Another diagnostic pitfall in the diagnosis of metastatic carcinoma in bone is the presence of spindle cell differentiation of the epithelial cells. The problem is complicated if the osseous lesion is solitary, a setting that may mimic a malignant primary bone tumor. We have seen, on more than one occasion, a solitary metastasis from a sarcomatoid renal cell carcinoma mistakenly treated as a malignant fibrous histiocytoma of bone. Therefore, we routinely do cytokeratin stains on spindle cell intraosseous lesions in older patients.

TREATMENT OF METASTATIC CARCINOMA IN BONE

Bone metastasis always indicates an advanced stage of cancer. About 50% of patients die within 8 months, and the remainder generally do not live longer than 2 years.[6] Therefore, treatment is aimed at making the remaining months of a patient's life comfortable. Most importantly, pathologic fractures must be treated or prevented. Various intramedullary fixation devices, including plates, nails, or intramedullary rods, are available. Methyl methacrylate can be used to enhance the fixation of these devices and to fill large bone defects. Sometimes total joint prostheses are effective, particularly in metastases to the proximal femur or acetabulum where the joint integrity has been compromised[27] (Fig. 10–16). Surgery on metastatic renal cell carcinoma poses a difficult problem. Lesions are extremely vascular, and any surgical manipulation results in dangerous blood loss. Blood loss can be minimized with preoperative embolization.[28]

Radiotherapy is also useful to relieve pain and shrink the size of the lesion. Approximately 50% of patients have an excellent response, and another 35% have a partial response.[29] Chemotherapy is also effective in reducing the size of some metastatic lesions. In addition to conventional anticancer drugs, the bisphosphonates are useful in inhibiting the bone resorption induced by the malignant cells.[30] These drugs are also used in treating the hypercalcemia of malignancy.[31]

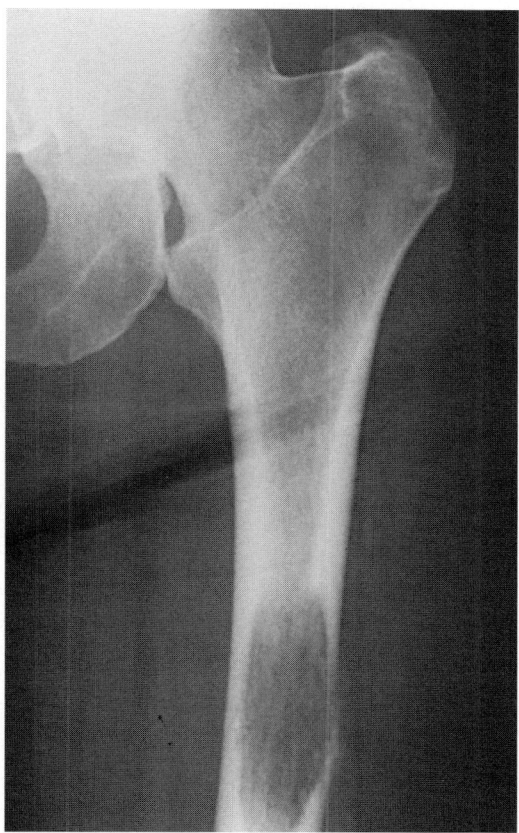

Figure 10-9 ■ Metastatic carcinoma from the lung to the femur. The lytic lesion is well defined, but one cortex is penetrated.

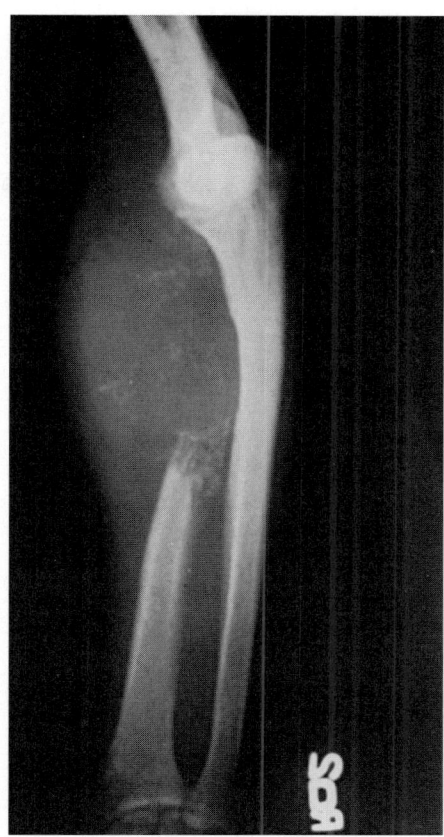

Figure 10-10 ■ Metastatic renal cell carcinoma to the radius. A large, expansile lytic area is common in renal cell carcinoma.

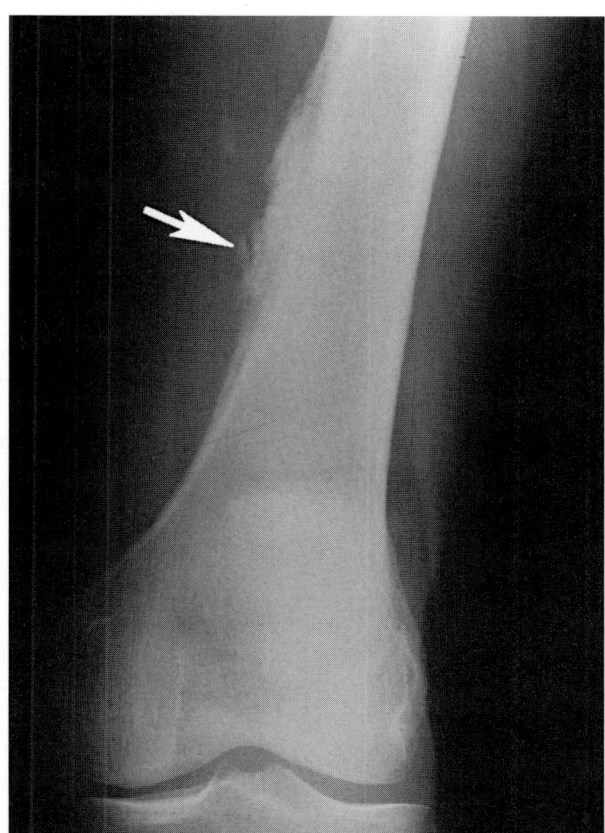

Figure 10-11 ■ Metastatic carcinoma to the femur. This periosteal location (*arrow*) suggests lung or prostate carcinoma.

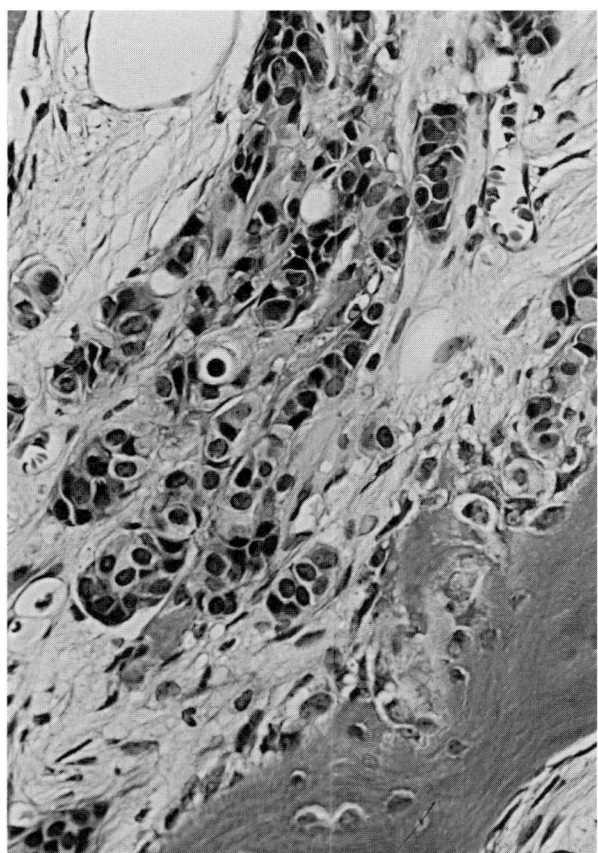

Figure 10-12 ■ Photomicrograph showing organoid pattern of epithelial cells.

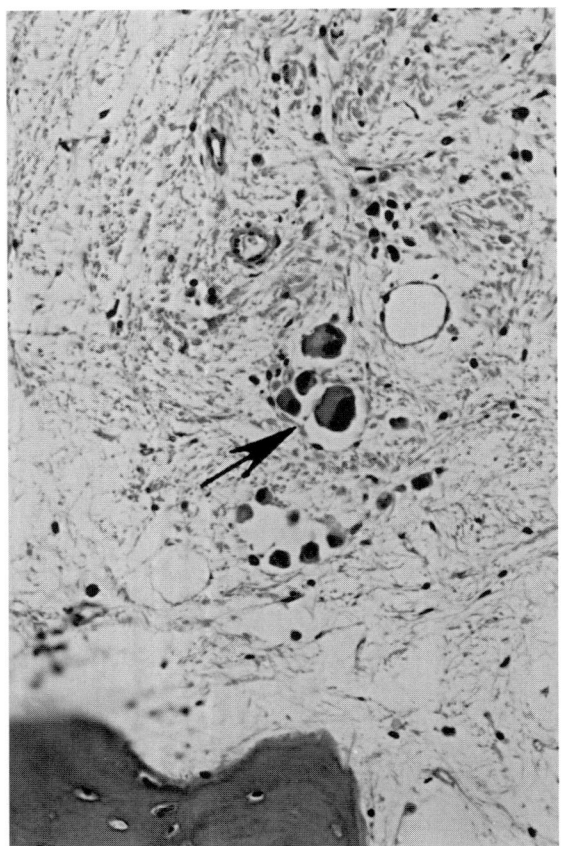

Figure 10-13 ▪ Dense stromal fibrosis. Only a few neoplastic cells *(arrow)* are recognizable.

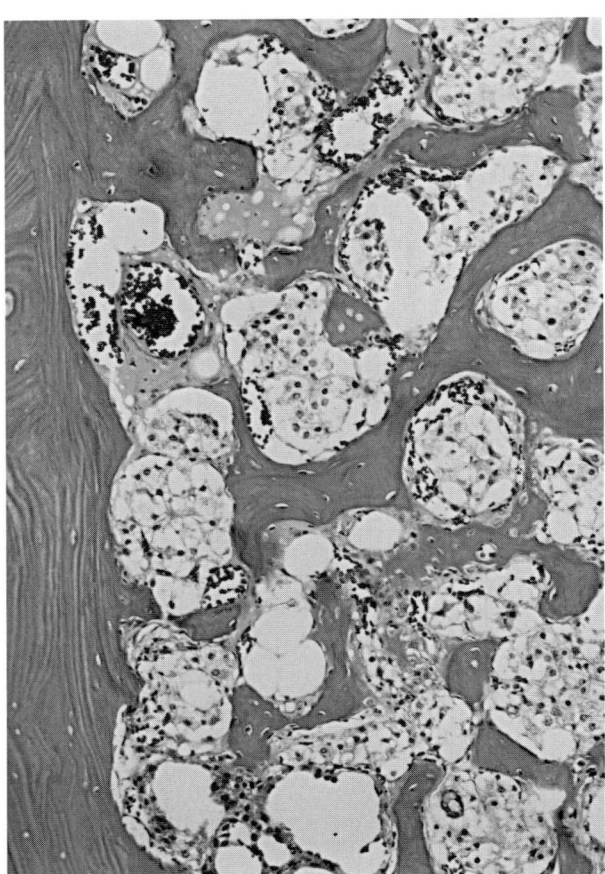

Figure 10-14 ▪ Photomicrograph of an osteoblastic metastasis. Extensive reactive bone is present.

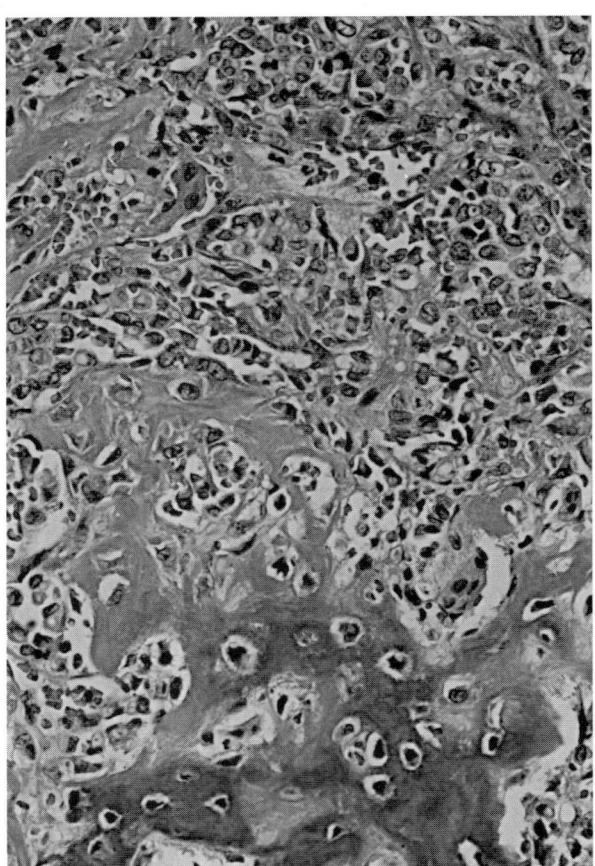

Figure 10-15 ▪ Reactive bone may be so extensive as to mimic a bone-forming neoplasm.

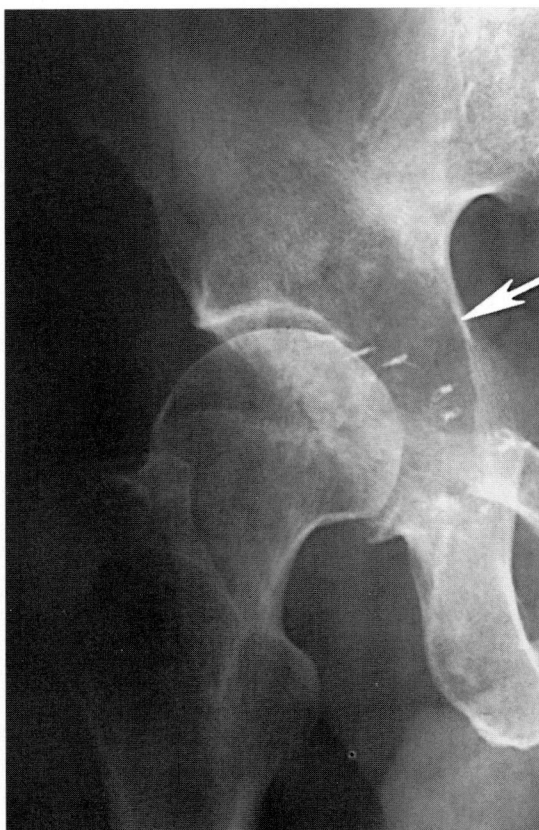

Figure 10-16 ▪ Metastatic lung carcinoma to the pelvis. The acetabulum is partially destroyed *(arrow)*. Reconstruction requires a total joint prosthesis.

REFERENCES

1. Boring, C. C., Squires, T. S., and Tong. T.: Cancer statistics. *C A Cancer J Clin* 43:7–26, 1993.
2. Jaffe, H. L.: *Tumors and Tumorous Conditions of the Bones and Joints.* Philadelphia, Lea & Febiger, 1958, p. 600.
3. Duchek, M., Lingardh, G., Saterborg, N. E., Winblad, B., and Angstrom, T.: Bone marrow examination as a diagnostic tool in carcinoma of the prostate. *Int Urol Nephrol* 7:59–64, 1975.
4. Anner, R. M., and Drewinko, B.: Frequency and significance of bone marrow involvement by metastatic solid tumors. *Cancer* 39:1337–1344, 1977.
5. Ingle, J. N., Tormey, D. C., and Tan, H. K.: The bone marrow examination in breast cancer: Diagnostic considerations and clinical usefulness. *Cancer* 41:670–674, 1978.
6. Simon, M. A., and Bartucci, E. J.: The search for the primary tumor in patients with skeletal metastases of unknown origin. *Cancer* 58:1088–1095, 1986.
7. Rougraff, B. T., Kneisl, J. S., and Simon, M. A.: Skeletal metastases of unknown origin: A prospective study of a diagnostic strategy. *J Bone Joint Surg* 75A:1276–1281, 1993.
8. Didolkar, M. S., Fanous, N., Elias, E. G., and Moore, R. H.: Metastatic carcinomas from occult primary tumors. *Ann Surg* 186(5):625–630, 1977.
9. Batson, O. V.: The function of the vertebral veins and their role in the spread of metastases. *Ann Surg* 112:138–149, 1940.
10. Healey, J. H., Turnbull, A. D. M., Miedema, B., and Lane, J. M.: Acrometastases. A study of twenty-nine patients with osseous involvement of hands and feet. *J Bone Joint Surg* 68A:743–746, 1986.
11. Libson, E., Bloom, R. A., Husband, J. E., and Stocker, D. J.: Metastatic tumors of the bones of the hand and foot. A comparative review and report of 43 additional cases. *Skeletal Radiol* 16:387–392, 1987.
12. Liotta, A.: Mechanisms of cancer invasion and metastasis. DeVita, V. T. Jr., Hellman, S., Rosenberg, S. A., Eds. *Important Advances in Oncology.* Philadelphia, J. B. Lippincott, 1985, pp. 28–41.
13. Mundy, G. R.: Hypercalcemia of malignancy revisited. *J Clin Invest* 82:1–6, 1988.
14. Sato, K., Mimura, H., Han, D. C., et al.: Production of bone resorbing activity and colony-stimulating activity in vivo and in vitro by a human squamous cell carcinoma associated with hypercalcemia and leukocytosis. *J Clin Invest* 78:145–154, 1986.
15. Jacobs, S. C., Pikna, D., and Lawson, R. K.: Prostatic osteoblastic factor. *Invest Urol* 17:195–198, 1979.
16. Koskinen, E. V., and Nieminen, R. A.: Surgical treatment of metastatic pathological fracture of major long bones. *Acta Orthop Scand* 44:539–549, 1973.
17. Tavassoli, M., Rizo, M., and Yam, L. T.: Elevation of serum acid phosphatase in cancers with bone metastasis. *Cancer* 45:2400–2403, 1980.
18. Mundy, G. R.: The hypercalcemia of malignancy. *Kidney Int* 31:142–155, 1987.
19. Dotts, J. T.: Diseases of the parathyroid gland and other hyper- and hypocalcemic disorders. Isselbacher, et al., Eds. *Harrison's Principles of Internal Medicine.* New York, McGraw-Hill, 1994, p. 2157.
20. Sharp, C. F., Rude, R. K., Terry, R., and Singer, F. R.: Abnormal bone and parathyroid histology in carcinoma patients with pseudohyperparathyroidism. *Cancer* 49:1449–1455, 1982.
21. Gold, R. H., and Bassett, L. W.: Radionuclide evaluation of skeletal metastases: Practical considerations. *Skeletal Radiol* 15:1–9, 1986.
22. Joo, K. G., Parthasarathy, K. L., Bakshi, S. P., and Rosner, D.: Bone scintigrams: Their clinical usefulness in patients with breast carcinoma. *Oncology* 36:94–98, 1979.
23. Deutsch, A., and Resnick, D.: Eccentric cortical metastases to the skeleton from bronchogenic carcinoma. *Radiology* 137:49–52, 1980.
24. Greenspan, A., and Norman, A.: Osteolytic cortical destruction: An unusual pattern of skeletal metastases. *Skeletal Radiol* 17:402–406, 1988.
25. Myers, J. L., Arocho, J., Bernreuter, W., Dunham, W., and Mazur, M. T.: Leiomyosarcoma of bone. A clinicopathologic, immunohistochemical, and ultrastructural study of five cases. *Cancer* 67:1051–1056, 1991.
26. Weiss, S. W., Bratthauer, G. L., and Morris, P. A.: Postirradiation malignant fibrous histiocytoma expressing cytokeratin: Implications for the immunodiagnosis of sarcomas. *Am J Surg Pathol* 12:554–558, 1988.
27. Harrington, K. D.: The management of acetabular insufficiency secondary to metastatic malignant disease. *J Bone Joint Surg* 63A:653–664, 1981.
28. Bowers, T. A., Murray, J. A., Charnsangavej, C., Soo, C.-S., Chuang, V. P., and Wallace, S.: Bone metastases from renal carcinoma. The preoperative use of transcatheter arterial occlusion. *J Bone Joint Surg* 64A:749–754, 1982.
29. Tong, D., Gillick, L., and Hendrickson, F. R.: The palliation of symptomatic osseous metastases: Final results of the study by the Radiation Therapy Oncology Group. *Cancer* 50:893–899, 1982.
30. Nemoto, R., Satou, S., Miyagawa, I., and Koiso, K.: Inhibition by a new bisphosphonate (AHBuBP) of bone resorption induced by the MBT-2 tumor of mice. *Cancer* 67:643–648, 1991.
31. Walls, J., Bundred, N., and Howell, A.: Hypercalcemia and bone resorption in malignancy. *Clin Orthop* 312:51–63, 1995.

CHAPTER 11
Plasma Cell Dyscrasia

The plasma cell dyscrasias encompass a spectrum of disorders characterized by the neoplastic proliferation of monoclonal plasma cells. This proliferation is most evident in the bone marrow, although other tissues are also affected. The plasma cells in these disorders preserve their function—they secrete immunoglobulins (Igs). Because these immunoglobulins are also monoclonal, these disorders can be recognized by a monoclonal immunoglobulin spike in an affected patient's serum. The monoclonal immunoglobulin, known as an M protein, can be any type of immunoglobulin. However, IgG is observed most frequently and accounts for 52% of cases. The next most common are IgA and IgM, which account for 21 and 12% of cases, respectively. In addition to a serum M protein, the light chains released from the breakdown of the immunoglobulins are excreted in the urine. These urinary light chains, known as Bence Jones proteins, can be identified by urinary immunoelectrophoresis. In one manifestation of plasma cell dyscrasia, multiple myeloma, they are present in the urine of 60 to 70% of patients.

Several well-defined syndromes exist on the spectrum of plasma cell dyscrasia. One syndrome, known as monoclonal gammopathy of undetermined significance, is an indolent disorder. More aggressive syndromes include multiple myeloma, solitary plasmacytoma, and amyloidosis. Other plasma cell dyscrasias also occur but are not discussed here. These include Waldenström's macroglobulinemia and heavy chain disease.

MONOCLONAL GAMMOPATHY OF UNDETERMINED SIGNIFICANCE

Monoclonal gammopathy of undetermined significance (MGUS) is a syndrome characterized only by low levels of serum M protein and very low levels of Bence Jones proteins. Patients are asymptomatic and have no bone lesions. The serum M protein indicates that a monoclonal population of plasma cells is present. However, bone marrow histology reveals only a minimal monoclonal plasma cell infiltrate (less than 10%), an amount insufficient to produce osseous changes.

Because symptoms and osseous lesions are not present, MGUS is usually diagnosed incidentally when patients are evaluated for other medical reasons. This syndrome is not uncommon—monoclonal proteins have been identified in 1% of the population older than 25 years and in 5% of all individuals older than 70.[1] The appearance of MGUS does not necessarily mean that a patient has a malignancy. However, as many as 11% of patients eventually are shown to develop multiple myeloma when followed up for 5 years.[2]

THE PATHOLOGY OF PLASMA CELL DYSCRASIAS

The plasma cell dyscrasias are characterized by monoclonal plasma cells in the bone marrow. Plasma cells are normally not residents of the marrow, although, on rare occasions, a few may be seen scattered around blood vessels. Many inflammatory diseases, however, are accompanied by a plasmacytosis. For example, plasmacytosis is especially prominent in rheumatoid arthritis and infection with human immunodeficiency virus. In these systemic inflammatory diseases, the plasma cells may account for as many as 25% of the marrow cells. However, the plasma cell population in these inflammatory disorders is polyclonal. Some contain kappa light chains and some contain lambda light chains. Kappa light chain–containing plasma cells are more abundant by a ratio of two or three to one.

In the plasma cell dyscrasias, however, the plasma cell population is monoclonal, and kappa light chain monoclonality is most common. Therefore, monoclonality of even a small number of plasma cells, even less than 10%, is consistent with MGUS if the patient has a serum M protein.[3]

Lytic bone lesions associated with sheets of plasma cells or a monoclonal plasmacytosis of more than 30% is diagnos-

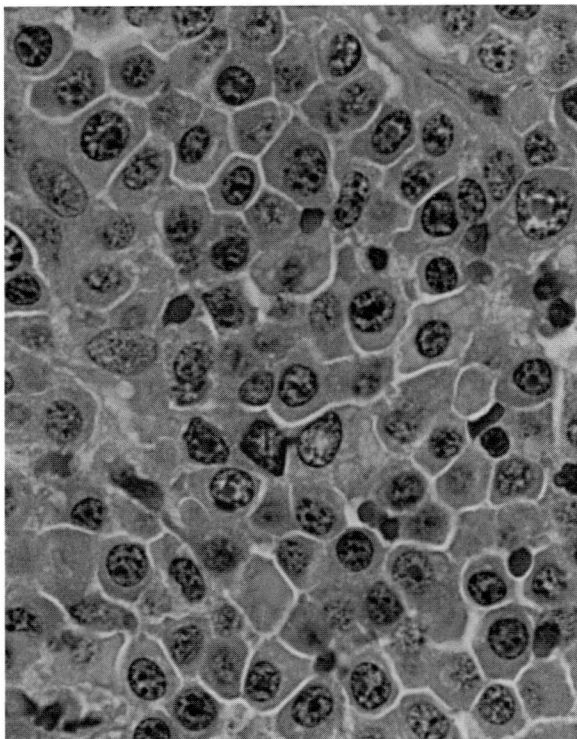

Figure 11–1 ■ Photomicrograph of a poorly differentiated plasma cell neoplasm. The nuclei are enlarged, and many have a prominent nucleolus. However, abundant cytoplasm is the clue to the plasma cell differentiation.

tic of multiple myeloma. The neoplastic plasma cells show a spectrum of differentiation that varies from patient to patient. In some patients, the neoplastic plasma cells are well differentiated and are almost indistinguishable from normal plasma cells. Other patients, however, have poorly differentiated lesions. The nuclei of the neoplastic cells are large and pleomorphic, often with a prominent nucleolus (Fig. 11–1). Unlike normal plasma cells, their cytoplasm may be scanty. However, within the small amount of cytoplasm, a paranuclear, amphophilic hof identifies their plasma cell differentiation.

Plasmacytoma Versus Chronic Osteomyelitis

Chronic osteomyelitis may, on rare occasions, be mistaken for a plasma cell neoplasm. This is because lesions of chronic osteomyelitis usually contain numerous plasma cells, and sometimes they are present in solid sheets. However, two features distinguish osteomyelitis from a plasmacytoma. First, chronic osteomyelitis almost always produces bone sclerosis, a reaction to the chronic infection. Plasmacytoma, by contrast, is a radiolytic lesion. Second, the plasma cells of chronic osteomyelitis are polyclonal—both kappa and lambda light chain–containing plasma cells are present. On the other hand, plasmacytomas are always monoclonal.

MULTIPLE MYELOMA

Multiple myeloma is a malignant manifestation of plasma cell dyscrasia that results in bone lesions.[4] Although plasma cells do not normally reside in the bone marrow, multiple myeloma is regarded as a primary bone tumor. Although multiple myeloma is not as common as MGUS, it is the most frequently observed malignant plasma cell dyscrasia (Table 11–1).[5–7] Other malignant plasma cell dyscrasias include solitary myeloma of bone, osteosclerotic myeloma, and amyloidosis of bone.

Incidence and Epidemiology

Multiple myeloma accounts for approximately 1% of all malignancies in the United States each year, with an annual incidence of about 13,000 cases.[8] This disease is twice as common in African-Americans and is more common in men than women (1.6:1.0).[9] It is second in incidence only to Hodgkin's disease among the nonleukemic hematologic malignancies. Multiple myeloma is a disease of older adults and is generally discovered between the ages of 50 and 80. Therefore, it should be considered in the differential diagnosis of all lytic bone lesions in patients in this age range. Less than 2% of cases occur in patients younger than 40. The etiology of myeloma is not known, although genetic, racial, occupational, and environmental factors have been implicated in some studies.[10–12] For example, multiple myeloma was found to occur with increased frequency in those exposed to the radiation of nuclear warheads in World War II after a 20-year latency.

Clinical Features

Among the primary malignant bone tumors, myeloma often has the most insidious and nonspecific presentation. Pain, present in two thirds of patients, is the most common symptom.[4] Back and chest pain (secondary to rib fractures) commonly occur. Unlike the pain of metastatic bone disease, which is worse at rest and at night, the pain of multiple myeloma is precipitated by movement. The pain is often

Table 11–1 ■ **MALIGNANT MONOCLONAL GAMMOPATHIES**

Multiple myeloma (IgG, IgA, IgD, IgE, and free light chains)
  Overt multiple myeloma
  Smoldering multiple myeloma
  Plasma cell leukemia
  Nonsecretory myeloma
  Osteosclerotic myeloma
Plasmacytoma
  Solitary plasmacytoma of bone
  Extramedullary plasmacytoma
Malignant lymphoproliferative diseases
  Waldenström's macroglobulinemia
  Malignant lymphoma

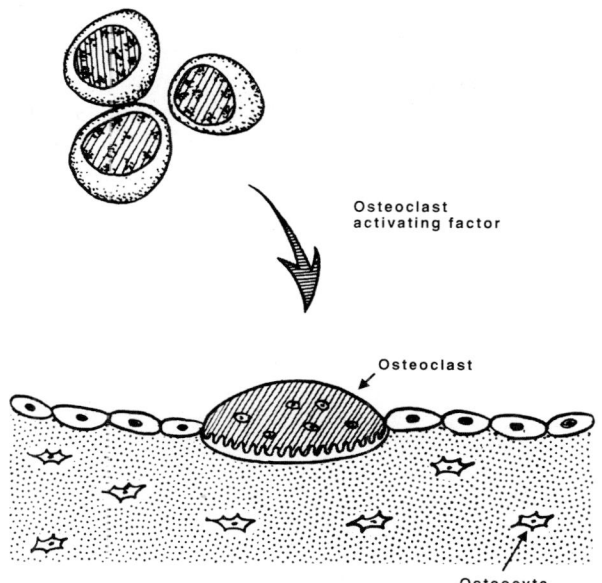

Figure 11-2 ■ The relationship of plasma cells to the process of bone resorption. Plasma cells secrete an osteoclast-stimulating factor that activates resorption.

sudden in onset, and many patients remember the exact date and time it began.

Other presenting symptoms in myeloma patients include bacterial infections (single or multiple), gross bleeding (most commonly epistaxis), and fever (only 1%).[4,13–16] Weakness and fatigue may occur secondary to anemia and may be found in as many as two thirds of patients.[4]

Patients may develop systemic complications from the myeloma protein. Renal insufficiency, hypercalcemia, and amyloid deposition often complicate the late stages of the disease.[7] Light chains are often deposited in tissue as amyloid and may cause congestive heart failure, hypercalcemia, nephrotic syndrome, orthostatic hypotension, peripheral neuropathy, or increased bleeding tendency.[17–19]

Pathophysiology

In multiple myeloma, bone marrow involvement is widespread throughout the skeleton. Bone marrow biopsy usually demonstrates a plasmacytosis of more than 30%. The bone destruction is caused by osteoclasts rather than the plasma cells.[20] The plasma cells secrete cytokines, which stimulate both replication and differentiation of osteoclast precursors. The osteoclasts then form resorption lacunae on the endosteal bone surface (Fig. 11-2). Although the exact cytokines are not known, lymphotoxin, interleukin-1, and interleukin-6 have been implicated as active agents.[21–24] In normal bone remodeling, osteoclastic resorption is coupled with osteoblastic new bone formation. However, in myeloma, bone resorption is uncoupled, and often no osteoblastic activity is present. This lack of new bone formation explains the low sensitivity of technetium bone scans in detecting myeloma bone lesions.

The pattern of bone destruction varies from patient to patient and in different bones of a single patient. In some patients, bone resorption is minimal, resulting in osteopenia. Other patients have small punched-out lesions, and still others have complete destruction of an involved bone.

Many patients develop nephropathy, which is known as myeloma kidney. Free light chain fragments of the myeloma protein (Bence Jones proteins) are filtered by the glomeruli, where they impair glomerular and tubular function.

Hypercalcemia is common in myeloma, but poor correlation exists between the hypercalcemia and the extent of the bone destruction.[25] The hypercalcemia may be more related to decreased renal function than to bone destruction. In contrast to other patients with malignancy and hypercalcemia, patients with myeloma often have an increased serum phosphorus level rather than a low level.[26]

Physical Examination

Often there are no diagnostic physical findings. Bone tenderness and pallor, secondary to anemia, may be detected by the careful examiner. Although extramedullary plasmacytomas are uncommon, they may, when present, produce large subcutaneous masses that have a purplish hue.[4] Purpura may also be present.

Laboratory Features

The most important laboratory studies in the diagnosis of multiple myeloma are the serum and urine immunoelectrophoresis. Almost 99% of patients have a serum immunoglobulin spike, Bence Jones proteinuria, or both. Because a small monoclonal immunoglobulin spike may be hidden under a polyclonal immunoglobulin curve, the much more sensitive *immune fixation electrophoresis* should be performed on any patient with suspected plasma cell dyscrasia.

Other laboratory tests may provide helpful clues (Table 11–2).[4] Anemia and an elevated erythrocyte sedimentation rate occur in 62% and 76% of patients, respectively. The anemia is usually normocytic and normochromic because the normal hematopoietic stem cells are displaced by the myeloma cells. Hypercalcemia and hyperuricemia are also common.

Table 11-2 ■ **INITIAL HEMATOLOGIC VALUES**

Laboratory Parameter	Frequency, %
Hemoglobin < 12 g/dl	62
Leukopenia < 4000/mm³	16
Thrombocytopenia < 100,000/mm³	13
Thrombocytosis > 300,000/mm³	11

Rate, mm/h	Erythrocyte Sedimentation Rate (Westergren) Frequency, %
< 10	6
10–20	4
21–50	14
51–100	38
> 100	38

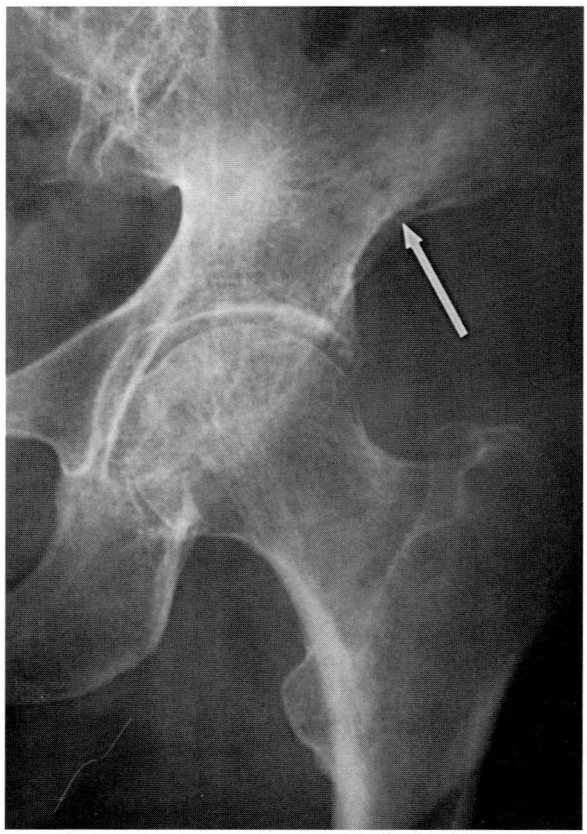

Figure 11-3 ■ Radiograph of pelvis showing faint moth-eaten radiolucencies. The most visible are those in the ilium *(arrow)*.

Radiographic Features

A wide range of radiographic changes characterize multiple myeloma. In keeping with the insidious evolution of this disorder, some patients present only with diffuse osteopenia. This change may mimic senile or postmenopausal osteoporosis, especially if a significant spinal involvement is present. As in osteoporosis, loss of height and biconcave deformities of the vertebrae may occur.[27] Single or multiple compression fractures may occur. As the disease progresses, very subtle moth-eaten radiolucencies appear (Fig. 11-3). A misdiagnosis of disuse osteoporosis is common in this radiographic presentation.

The most common radiographic change of myeloma, however, is multiple discrete punched-out lytic bone lesions. They are most commonly seen in the skull (Fig. 11-4), spine, pelvis, and proximal femurs or humeri. Lesions vary in size from 3 to 4 mm to 5 to 10 cm. They have well-defined borders and lack a sclerotic rim. In the long bones, a circular or elliptic lytic area may be seen on the endosteal bone surface[28] (Fig. 11-5). Larger lesions cause extensive cortical destruction (Fig. 11-6).

In other bone diseases, such as metastatic carcinoma, the technetium bone scan is useful to quantify the extent of skeletal involvement. However, in multiple myeloma, the bone scan often fails to identify all the lesions. This is because many lytic myeloma foci lack a secondary osteoblastic response and therefore do not concentrate radioactive tracer. However, because many myeloma lesions do accumulate tracer, a positive bone scan does not rule out this disease.

Diagnostic Criteria and Clinical Staging

Multiple myeloma is a common disease and should be included in the differential diagnosis of bone pain (pelvis, back, and chest wall) in an older person. The evaluation scheme should include serum hematologic and chemistry

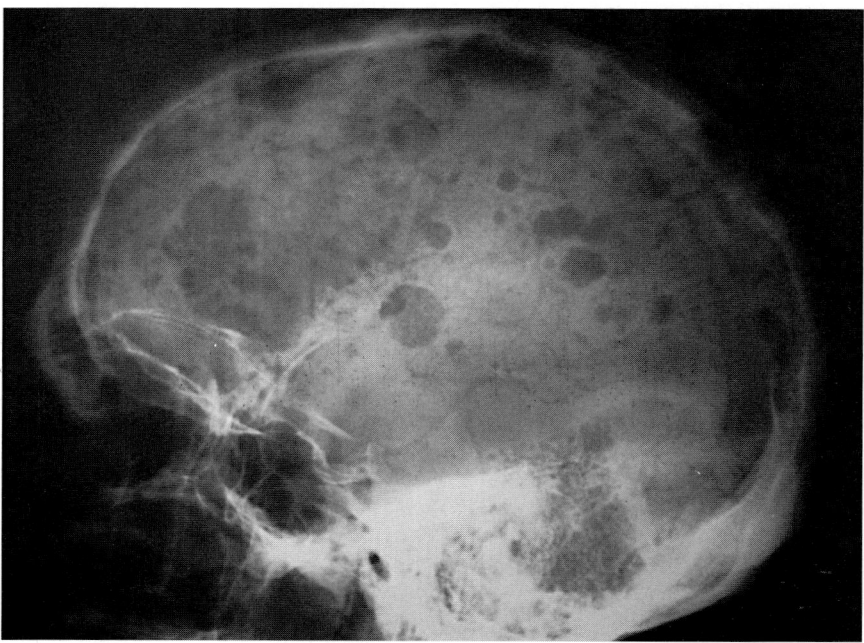

Figure 11-4 ■ Classic multiple myeloma involving the skull. Multiple well-defined, punched-out lesions are present.

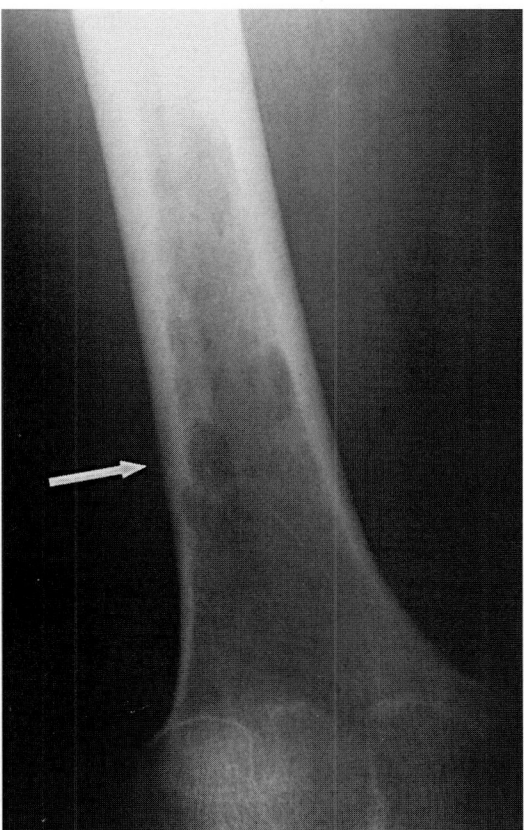

Figure 11-5 ■ A poorly defined radiolytic defect in the femur *(arrow)*.

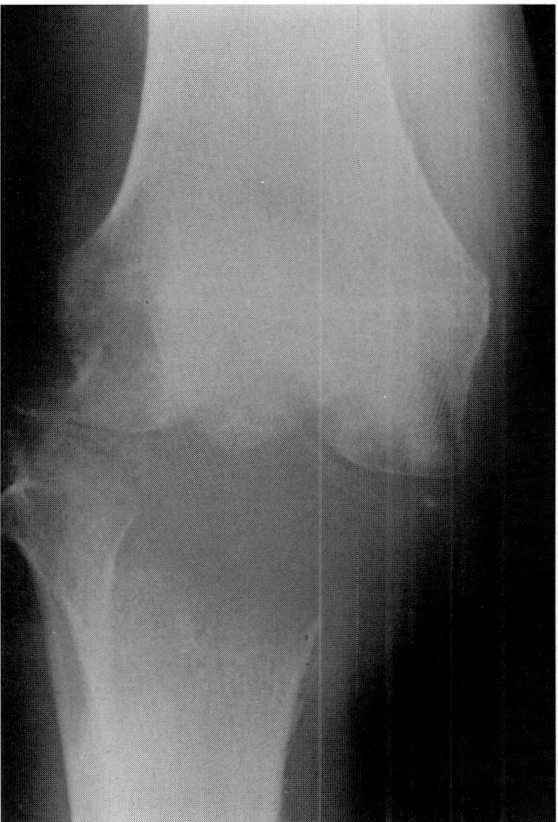

Figure 11-6 ■ A destructive lesion of multiple myeloma with penetration of the cortex.

studies and radiographs (Table 11–3). Bone marrow aspiration and biopsy should be performed when the serum and radiographic studies suggest myeloma.

Salmon and Cassady have developed a set of diagnostic criteria based on bone marrow biopsy, serum proteins, tissue biopsy, and radiographic findings for the more difficult cases (Table 11–4).[29] A staging system has also been developed that aids in predicting prognosis (Table 11–5).[30] Salmon and Cassady combined the results of eight series (1428 patients) and noted a median survival of over 60 months for stage I disease, 41 months for stage II disease, and 23 months for stage III disease.[29] Patients with abnormal renal function (subtype B) had a worse prognosis. Other authors have identified additional prognostic factors.[30–35]

Table 11-3 ■ EVALUATION STRATEGY FOR PATIENTS SUSPECTED OF HAVING MYELOMA

Serum hematologic studies
    Complete blood cell count, differential and platelets
    Serum protein electrophoresis
Serum chemistries
    Electrolytes
    Creatinine, calcium, uric acid
    Liver functions
Radiographs
    Skeletal survey
        Anteroposterior radiographs
            Humeri
            Radii/ulnae
            Femora
            Tibia/fibula
            Pelvis
        Anteroposterior/lateral radiographs
            Cervical spine
            Thoracic spine
            Lumbar spine

Table 11-4 ■ DIAGNOSTIC CRITERIA FOR MULTIPLE MYELOMA*

Major Criteria
  I. Plasmacytoma on tissue biopsy
  II. Bone marrow plasmacytosis with > 30% plasma cells
  III. Monoclonal immunoglobulin spike on serum electrophoresis exceeding 3.5 g/dl for G peaks or 2.0 g/dl for A peaks, 1.0 g/24 h of kappa or lambda light chain excretion on urine electrophoresis in the presence of amyloidosis
Minor Criteria
  a. Bone marrow plasmacytosis 10–30% plasma cells
  b. Monoclonal globulin spike present but less than the level defined above
  c. Lytic bone lesions
  d. Residual normal IgM < 50 mg/dl, IgA < 100 mg/dl, or IgG < 600 mg/dl
The diagnosis of myeloma requires a minimum of one major and one minor criteria or three minor criteria, which must include a and b.

*Adapted from DeVita, V. T., Hellman, S., and Rosenberg, S. A. (Eds.): *Cancer: Principles and Practice of Oncology*, 4th ed., Philadelphia, J. B. Lippincott, 1993, pp. 1984–2025.

Table 11-5 ■ MYELOMA STAGING SYSTEM*

Criteria	Measured Myeloma Cell Mass, cells $\times 10^{12}/m^2$

Stage I
All of the following
  Hemoglobin value > 10 g/dl
  Serum calcium value normal (< 12 mg/dl)
  On roentgenogram, normal bone structure or solitary plasmacytoma only
  Low M-complement production rates
    IgG value < 5 g/dl
    IgA value < 3 g/dl
    Urine light chain M-component on electrophoresis < 4 g/24 h
	< 0.6 (low)

Stage II Overall data not as minimally abnormal as shown for stage I and no single value as abnormal as defined for stage II	0.6–1.20 (intermediate)

Stage III
One or more of the following:
  Hemoglobin value < 8.5 g/dl
  Serum calcium value > 12 mg/dl
  Advanced lytic bone lesions
  High M-component production rates
    IgG value > 7 g/dl
    IgA value > 5 g/dl
    Urine light chain M-component on electrophoresis > 12 g/24 h
	> 1.20 (high)

Subclassification
  A = Relatively normal renal function (serum creatinine value < 2.0 mg/dl)
  B = Abnormal renal function (serum creatinine value 2.0 g/dl)	

*Adapted from DeVita, V. T., Hellman, S., and Rosenberg, S. A. (Eds.): *Cancer: Principles and Practice of Oncology*, 4th ed., Philadelphia, J. B. Lippincott, 1993, pp. 1984–2025.

SOLITARY MYELOMA OF BONE

About 5% of patients with malignant plasma cell dyscrasia present with only a solitary bone lesion. Because this lesion, known as *solitary myeloma* (or plasmacytoma) of bone, has a better prognosis than multiple myeloma, these two manifestations of plasma cell dyscrasia should be distinguished.[36–49] Three diagnostic criteria for solitary myeloma of bone exist: (1) a solitary lesion on skeletal survey, (2) histologic confirmation of a plasma cell neoplasm, and (3) a bone marrow biopsy at a noninvolved site showing less than 10% plasma cells. Patients with serum protein abnormalities and Bence Jones proteinuria of less than 1 g/24 h at presentation are not excluded if they meet the criteria given here.

Patients with solitary plasmacytoma are generally younger at presentation (median age, 56 years) than patients with multiple myeloma,[50] and men outnumber women by about two to one. Although any bone may be involved, the spine and the ribs are the most common sites.

Serum protein immunoglobulin spikes, Bence Jones proteinuria, or both are present in 50 to 77% of patients with solitary myeloma of bone, and the presence of these protein abnormalities is probably not an adverse prognostic factor. The protein abnormalities may persist following treatment.

The overall survival at 5 and 10 years for patients with solitary myeloma is about 75% and 50%, respectively.[50] Disease-free survival is lower, at about 45% and 25% at 5 and 10 years, respectively. By 10 years, over two thirds of patients will have progressed from solitary to multiple myeloma.

OSTEOSCLEROTIC MYELOMA

Although most cases of multiple myeloma are characterized by radiolytic bone lesions, a small number of patients (about 3%) have radiodense lesions.[51–56] This presentation, known as *osteosclerotic myeloma,* occurs in a slightly younger age group (median age, 56) and more often affects men.

In this presentation, the plasma cell infiltrate causes extensive reactive bone deposition in the marrow, resulting in numerous dense or mixed lytic and dense lesions throughout the skeleton. The vertebrae are the most commonly affected bones. Bone pain is uncommon in osteosclerotic myeloma.

Many patients with this presentation have disorders in other organ systems that are not caused by an infiltration of plasma cells or light chain deposition. The most common associated disorder, affecting 30 to 50% of patients with osteosclerotic myeloma, is polyneuropathy. However, numerous other organ systems may be involved and result in a disorder known as the POEM (polyneuropathy, organomegaly, endocrinopathy, and the presence of an M protein) syndrome.

The most important feature of this syndrome is a severe, progressive sensorimotor polyneuropathy. Hepatomegaly and lymphadenopathy occur in about two thirds of cases, and splenomegaly occurs in one third. Endocrine manifestations include amenorrhea in women and impotence in men. Gynecomastia, diabetes, and hirsutism also occur. In addition, the skin may be edematous and indurated. As in classical multiple myeloma, an M protein is present. However, the monoclonal protein usually contains lambda light chains rather than the typical kappa light chains. Also, affected patients rarely develop amyloidosis, and they usually lack Bence Jones protein. The cause of these nonosseous abnormalities is not known. However, an autoimmune pathogenesis is likely.

AMYLOIDOMA OF BONE

Amyloidosis is the pathologic deposition of protein in the extracellular space of various tissues and organs. This disorder occurs in a wide variety of clinical settings, and at least 15 biochemically distinct amyloid proteins have been identified. A common feature of all these proteins is their birefringence after histologic staining with the Congo red dye. In the United States, the most common form of amyloidosis occurs as a manifestation of plasma cell dyscrasia. The amyloid deposited is AL amyloid—the light chains of the immunoglobulin molecule.

Two presentations of this form of amyloidosis are possible. First, amyloidosis complicates 5 to 15% of established cases of multiple myeloma, and almost all these patients have Bence Jones proteinuria. In this setting, the amyloidosis is usually systemic, with deposits occurring in sites such as soft tissues, lung, skin, tongue, and gastrointestinal tract.

The second presentation is the development of amyloidosis without overt myeloma. However, the presence of a monoclonal gammopathy in almost all of these patients indicates that they have a plasma cell dyscrasia. Sometimes the amyloidosis presents as lytic bone lesions, and on rare occasions, a solitary lesion, known as *amyloidoma of bone*, is present. Thirty-seven cases of amyloidoma of bone have been well documented.[57] The average age of these patients is 57 years, and the most common locations are the skull and the spine. Radiologically, amyloidoma of bone is an expansile lytic lesion. However, stippled radiodensity reminiscent of cartilage calcification may be present (Fig. 11–7).

Histologically, waxy eosinophilic deposits, usually with a foreign body giant cell reaction, are present in the marrow space (Fig. 11–8). The eosinophilic material is identifiable as AL amyloid by permanganate-resistant Congo red birefringence. In addition, occasionally foci of amorphous calcification are present within the amyloid deposits, and metaplastic bone may occur at their periphery.[58] Another occasionally observed feature is the presence of a plas-

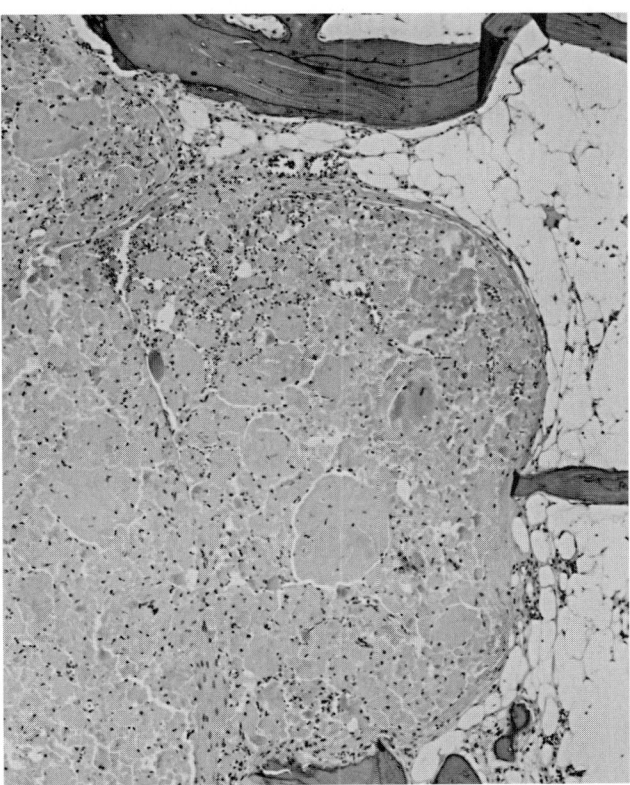

Figure 11-8 ■ Photomicrograph of amyloidosis in bone. Waxy eosinophilic material replaces the marrow fat.

macytosis in the cellular infiltrate surrounding the amyloid deposits. These plasma cells are monoclonal with kappa and lambda light chain immunostains, an observation suggesting that amyloidomas of bone represent plasmacytomas with massive amyloid deposition.

Solitary amyloidoma of bone almost always progresses to disseminated amyloidosis or multiple myeloma. Additional tumors develop after an interval of 3 months to 9 years. Most patients die within 3 years.

TREATMENT OF PLASMA CELL NEOPLASMS

Multiagent chemotherapy is the mainstay of treatment for patients with multiple myeloma. Unfortunately, few patients are cured. Bone marrow transplantation is under investigation as a potential modality. External beam irradiation is used to control pain or to stop progression of lesions that threaten skeletal integrity.[59–61]

Patients with solitary myeloma generally are treated with external beam irradiation to the affected site. Doses of 4500 to 5000 cGy are used, with excellent local control rates. Chemotherapy is necessary when patients progress to multiple myeloma. Osteosclerotic myeloma is difficult to treat. Chemotherapy, radiation, and plasmapheresis have all been utilized with variable results.

Surgery is utilized to prevent fractures and to rebuild the

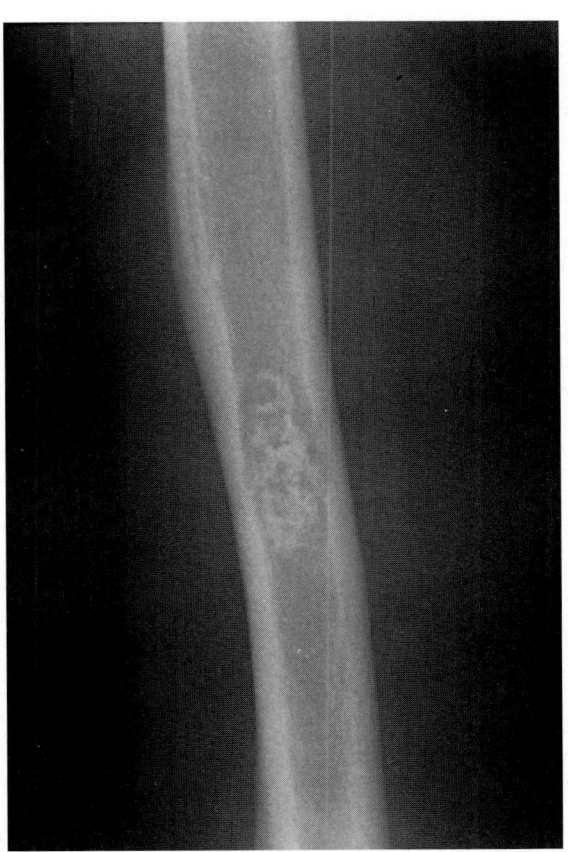

Figure 11-7 ■ Radiograph of an amyloidoma in bone. A lytic defect is present, and punctate densities correspond to calcification of the amyloid.

skeletal system once fracture has occurred. Internal fixation devices are very effective in strengthening the weakened bones, and they often afford full weight bearing and pain control. Prosthetic devices are utilized when rigid fixation is not feasible or the joint surfaces have been destroyed.

REFERENCES

1. Axelsson, U., Bachmann, R., and Hallen, J.: Frequency of pathologic proteins (M-components) in 6995 sera from an adult population. *Acta Med Scand* 179:235–247, 1966.
2. Longo, D. L.: Plasma cell disorders. Isselbacher, K. J., Braunwald, E., Wilson, J. D., Martin, J. B., Fauci, A. S., Kasper, D. L., Eds. *Harrison's Principles of Internal Medicine,* 13th ed. New York, McGraw-Hill, 1994, p. 1622.
3. Peterson, L. C., Brown, B. A., Crosson, J. T., and Mladenovic, J.: Application of the immunoperoxidase technique to bone marrow trephine biopsies in the classification of patients with monoclonal gammopathies. *Am J Clin Pathol* 85:688–693, 1986.
4. Kyle, R. A.: Multiple myeloma: Review of 869 cases. *Mayo Clin Proc* 50:29–40, 1975.
5. Kyle, R. A.: Monoclonal gammopathy of undetermined significance: Natural history in 241 cases. *Am J Med* 64:814–826, 1978.
6. Kyle, R. A., and Greipp, P. R.: Smoldering multiple myeloma. *N Engl J Med* 302:1347–1349, 1980.
7. Kyle, R. A.: Plasma cell proliferative disorders. Hoffmann, R., Ed. *Hematology: Basic Principles and Practice.* New York, Churchill-Livingstone, 1991, pp. 1021–1038.
8. Parker, S. L., Tong, T., Bolden, S., and Wingo, P. A.: Cancer statistics 1997. *CA Cancer J Clin* 47:5–27, 1997.
9. Linos A., Kyle, R. A., O'Fallon, M. W., and Kurland, L. T.: Incidence and secular trend of multiple myeloma in Olmstead County, Minnesota: 1965–77. *J Natl Cancer Inst* 66:17, 1981.
10. Maldonado, J. E., and Kyle, R. A.: Familial myeloma: Report of eight families and study of serum proteins in their relatives. *Am J Med* 57:875–884, 1974.
11. McPhedran, P., Heath, C. W. Jr., and Garcia, J.: Multiple myeloma incidence in metropolitan Atlanta, Georgia: Racial and seasonal variations. *Blood* 39:866–873, 1972.
12. Cuzick, J., and DeStavola, B.: Multiple myeloma: A case control study. *Br J Cancer* 57:516–520, 1988.
13. Meyers, B. R., Hirschman, S. Z., and Axelrod, J. A.: Current patterns of infection in multiple myeloma. *Am J Med* 52:87–92, 1972.
14. Norden, C. W.: Infections in patients with multiple myeloma [Editorial]. *Arch Intern Med* 140:1150–1151, 1980.
15. Twomey, J. J.: Infections complicating multiple myeloma and chronic lymphocytic leukemia. *Arch Intern Med* 132:562–565, 1973.
16. Wohlenberg, H.: Osteomyelitis and plasmacytoma. *N Engl J Med* 283:822–823, 1970.
17. Kyle, R. A., and Bayrd, E. D.: Amyloidosis: Review of 236 cases. *Medicine (Baltimore)* 54:271–299, 1975.
18. Fiedler, K., and Durie, B. G.: Primary amyloidosis associated with multiple myeloma: Predictors of successful therapy. *Am J Med* 80:413–419, 1986.
19. Glenner, G. G.: Amyloid deposits and amyloidosis: The beta-fibrilloses. *N Engl J Med* 302:1283–1292, 1980.
20. Mundy, G. R., and Bertolini, D. B.: Bone destruction and hypercalcemia in plasma cell myeloma. *Semin Oncol* 13:291–299, 1986.
21. Garrett, J. R., Durie, B. G. M., Nedwin, G. E., Gillespie, A., Bringman, T., Sabatini, M., Bertolini, D. R., and Mundy, G. R.: Production of lymphotoxin, a bone-resorbing cytokine by cultured human myeloma cells. *N Engl J Med* 317:526–532, 1987.
22. Bataille, R., Jourdan, M., Zhang, Z. G., et al.: Serum levels of interleukin-6, a potent myeloma cell growth factor, as a reflection of disease severity in plasma cell dyscrasias. *J Clin Invest* 84:2008–2011, 1989.
23. Cozzolini, F., Torcia, M., Aldinucci, D., Rubartelli, A., Miliani, A., Shaw, A. R., Lansdorp, P. M., and DiGugliemo, R.: Production of interleukin-1 by bone marrow myeloma cells. *Blood* 74:380–387, 1989.
24. Mundy, G. R., Raisz, L. G., Cooper, R. A., Schechter, G. P., and Salmon, S. E.: Evidence for the secretion of an osteoclast stimulating factor in myeloma. *N Engl J Med* 291:1041–1046, 1974.
25. Durie, B. G., Salmon, S. E., and Mundy, G. R.: Relation of osteoclast activating factor production to the extent of bone disease in multiple myeloma. *Br J Haematol* 47:21–30, 1981.
26. Mundy, G. R.: Hypercalcemia in hematologic malignancies and in solid tumors associated with extensive localized bone destruction. *Primer on the Metabolic Bone Disease and Disorders of Mineral Metabolism,* 3rd ed. Philadelphia, Lippincott-Raven, 1996, pp. 203–206.
27. Campanacci, M.: *Bone and Soft Tissue Tumors.* New York, Springer-Verlag, 1990, pp. 567–568.
28. Resnick, D.: Plasma cell dyscrasias and dysgammaglobulinemias. *Diagnosis of Bone and Joint Disorders.* Philadelphia, W. B. Saunders, 1988.
29. Salmon, S. E., and Cassady, J. R.: Plasma cell neoplasms. DeVita, V. T., Hellman, S. A., and Rosenberg, S. A., Eds. *Cancer: Principles and Practice of Oncology,* 4th ed. Philadelphia, J. B. Lippincott, 1993.
30. Durie, B. G. M., and Salmon, S. E.: A clinical staging system for multiple myeloma: Correlation of measured myeloma cell mass with presenting clinical features, response to treatment and survival. *Cancer* 36:842–852, 1975.
31. Alexanian, R., Balcerzak, S., Bonnet, J. D., Gehan, E. A., Hart, A., Hewlett, J. S., and Monto, R. W.: Prognostic factors in multiple myeloma. *Cancer* 36:1192–1201, 1975.
32. Bataille, R.: Localized plasmacytomas. *Clin Haematol* 11:113–121, 1982.
33. Feinleib, M., and MacMahon, B.: Duration of survival in multiple myeloma. *J Natl Cancer Inst* 24:1259–1269, 1960.
34. Merlini, G., Waldenstroem, J. C., and Jayakar, S. D.: A new improved clinical staging system for multiple myeloma based on analysis of 123 treated patients. *Blood* 55:1011–1019, 1980.
35. Woodruff, R. K., Wadworth, J., Malpas, J. S., and Tobias, J. S.: Clinical staging in multiple myeloma. *Br J Haematol* 42:199–205, 1979.
36. Bataille, R., and Sany, J.: Solitary myeloma: Clinical and prognostic features of a review of 114 cases. *Cancer* 48:845–851, 1981.
37. Chak, L. Y., Cox, R. S., Bostwick, D. G., and Hoppe, R. T.: Solitary plasmacytoma of bone: Treatment, progression, and survival. *J Clin Oncol* 5:1811–1815, 1987.
38. Corwin, J., and Lindberg, R. D.: Solitary plasmacytoma of bone versus extramedullary plasmacytoma and their relationship to multiple myeloma. *Cancer* 43:1007–1013, 1979.
39. Greenberg, P., Parker, R. G., Fu, Y. S., and Abemayor, E.: The treatment of solitary plasmacytoma of bone and extramedullary plasmacytoma. *Am J Clin Oncol (CCT)* 10:199–204, 1987.
40. Kvaloy, S., Abrahamsen, A. F., Landaas, T. O., Langholm, R., and Marton, P. F.: Solitary plasmacytoma of bone. *Scand J Haematol* 30(Suppl 39):23–29, 1983.
41. Loh, H. S.: A retrospective evaluation of 23 reported cases of solitary plasmacytoma of the mandible with an additional case report. *Br J Oral Maxillofac Surg* 22:216–224, 1984.
42. Mendenhall, C. M., Thar, T. L., and Million, R. R.: Solitary plasmacytoma of bone and soft tissue. *Int J Radiat Oncol Biol Phys* 6:1497–1501, 1980.
43. Meyer, J. E., and Schulz, M. D.: Solitary myeloma of bone. *Cancer* 34:438–440, 1974.
44. Ray, G., Fish, V., and Rabinowitz, L.: Solitary plasma cell tumors of bone and soft tissue: Natural history and response to radiotherapy. *Proc Am Soc Clin Oncol* 2:243, 1983.
45. Todd, I. D.: Treatment of solitary plasmacytoma. *Clin Radiol* 16:395–399, 1965.
46. Tong, D., Griffin, T. W., Laramore, G. E., Kurtz, J. M., Russell, A. H., Groudine, M. T., Herron, T., Blasko, J. C., and Tesh, D. W.: Solitary plasmacytoma of bone and soft tissues. *Radiology* 135:195–198, 1980.
47. Woodruff, R. K., Malpas, J. S., and White, F. E.: Solitary plasmacytoma II: Solitary plasmacytoma of bone. *Cancer* 43:2344–2347, 1979.
48. Wasserman, T. H. E., Trenker, D., Scharnhorst, K., and Holland, J.: Solitary plasmacytomas (SP): Response to radiation (XRT) and progression to multiple myeloma (MM). *Proc Am Soc Clin Oncol* 5:150, 1986.
49. Jacobson, R. J., Levy, J. I., Shulman, G., and DeMoor, N. G.: Solitary myeloma. *S Afr Med J* 49:1347–1351, 1975.
50. Frassica, D. A., Frassica, F. J., Schray, M. F., Sim, F. H., and Kyle, R. A.: Solitary plasmacytoma of bone: Mayo clinic experience. *Int J Radiat Oncol Biol Phys* 16:43–48, 1989.
51. Kelly, J. J. Jr., Kyle, R. A., Miles, J. M., and Dyck, P. J.: Osteosclerotic myeloma and peripheral neuropathy. *Neurology* 33:202–210, 1983.
52. Delauche, M. C., Clauvel, J. P., and Seligmann, M.: Peripheral neuropathy and plasma cell neoplasias: A report of 10 cases. *Br J Haematol* 48:384–392, 1981.
53. Driedger, H., and Pruzanski, W.: Plasma cell neoplasia with peripheral

polyneuropathy: A study of five cases and a review of the literature. *Medicine (Baltimore)* 59:301–310, 1980.
54. Osby, E., Noring, L., Hast, R., Kjellin, K. G., Knutsson, E., and Siden, A.: Benign monoclonal gammopathy and peripheral neuropathy. *Br J Haematol* 51:531–539, 1982.
55. Reitan, J. B., Pape, E., Fossa, S. D., Julsrud, D. J., Slettnes, D. N., and Solheim, O. P.: Osteosclerotic myeloma with polyneuropathy. *Acta Med Scand* 208:137–144, 1980.
56. Bardwick, P. A., Zvaifler, N. J., Gill, G. N., Newman, D., Greenway, G. D., and Resnick, D. L.: Plasma cell dyscrasia with polyneuropathy, organomegaly, endocrinopathy, M protein, and skin changes: The POEMS syndrome: Report on two cases and a review of the literature. *Medicine (Baltimore)* 59:311–322, 1980.
57. Pambuccian, S. E., Horyd, I. D., Cawte, T., and Huvos, A. G.: Amyloidoma of bone, a plasma cell/plasmacytoid neoplasm. *Am J Surg Pathol* 21(2):179–186, 1997.
58. Karasick, D., Schweitzer, M. E., Miettinen, M., and O'Hara, B. J.: Osseous metaplasia associated with amyloid-producing plasmacytoma of bone: A report of two cases. *Skeletal Radiol* 25:263–267, 1996.
59. Bosch, A., and Frias, Z.: Radiotherapy in the treatment of multiple myeloma. *Int J Radiat Oncol Biol Phys* 15:1363–1369, 1988.
60. Mill, W. B.: Radiation therapy in multiple myeloma. *Radiology* 115:175–178, 1975.
61. Mill, W. B., and Griffith, R.: The role of radiation therapy in the management of plasma cell tumors. *Cancer* 45:647–652, 1980.

CHAPTER 12
Primary Bone Tumors

Approximately 20 specific types of primary bone tumors exist, and many of these have well-defined variants. Each type and variant is recognized by not only its histologic features but also its growth pattern, as determined by the patient's radiographs. The radiographic images tell the physician what the lesion is doing to the patient. Whether a lesion is stationary, healing, growing slowly, or growing rapidly can be determined by radiographic patterns. These patterns then inform the pathologist how to interpret the histologic findings.

Bone tumors are partly defined by their location. For example, some bone tumors grow only on the bone surface, whereas others are confined to the medullary canal. In addition, some bone tumors predilect certain segments of bone. Some occur only in the metaphysis, and others involve the epiphysis. Studying the radiographs is the only way to locate a tumor's growth center.

Clinical information also supplies important clues to the correct diagnosis of a bone tumor. The age of the patient, the number of lesions present, and the presence or absence of pain must be considered when interpreting a biopsy.

Primary bone tumors usually affect adolescents and young adults. Although elderly patients do occasionally develop primary bone tumors, metastatic carcinoma and plasma cell myeloma are much more common in this age group. Presumably, adolescents and young adults are affected more often because their skeletons are more susceptible to neoplastic transformation. In fact, neoplasms occur more often in the bones that grow the most. Thus, the distal femur and proximal tibia are the most common sites for the development of almost all types of primary bone tumors.

Bone tumors may be benign or malignant. Malignant bone tumors are rare. Of the 1.3 million new cancer cases in the United States each year, only 2000 are primary malignant bone tumors. By contrast, benign lesions are fairly common. Some of the benign lesions are, in fact, not true neoplasms. For example, the most common lesions, osteochondromas and enchondromas, are hamartomas. The next most common lesion, nonossifying fibroma, is a developmental defect caused by disordered modeling during skeletal growth. Among malignant bone tumors, some, such as Ewing sarcoma, grow rapidly and metastasize early. Others, such as parosteal osteosarcoma, are slow growing and rarely metastasize.

Some bone tumors defy rigid classification as benign or malignant. For example, giant cell tumor and chondroblastoma are usually regarded as benign. Yet on very rare occasions, these "benign" lesions metastasize to the lungs. In these cases, the pulmonary lesions grow slowly, and the prognosis is good.

Two other general features of bone tumors are (1) the tendency of some to dedifferentiate and (2) their tendency to arise in damaged bone. Dedifferentiation is the sudden transformation of a benign or low-grade malignant neoplasm into a high-grade, rapidly fatal sarcoma. This transformation, although rare, occurs in cartilage lesions, giant cell tumors, low-grade osteosarcomas, and chordomas. Often the transformation is associated with incomplete removal of the original lesion. The second feature, the tendency to arise in damaged bone, is perhaps a reflection of a reparative reaction gone awry. Settings for this rare malignant transformation include bone infarcts, radiation osteitis, and Paget's disease.

Bone tumors are histologically classified according to what type of tissue the neoplastic cell is synthesizing. In general, tumors may be classified as benign or malignant osseous, cartilaginous, or fibrous lesions. Some neoplasms, such as giant cell tumor, Ewing sarcoma, and adamantinoma, are of uncertain differentiation and are usually considered specific entities.

Today, the classification, diagnosis, and therapy of bone tumors are extremely sophisticated. However, our current understanding of bone tumors would not be possible without the dedication of our predecessors. Important historical milestones are summarized in the following brief survey.

HISTORY

Humans have suffered from bone tumors for thousands of years. Paleopathologists have studied skeletal remains dating from the stone age. Using radiographic, histologic, and biochemical techniques, experts have identified in ancient bones many of the bone tumors we recognize today. For example, specimens containing osteochondromas, probable giant cell tumors, osteoid osteomas, and osteosarcomas have been found dating from Neolithic times through the Middle Ages.[1] One striking example of an osteosarcoma was unearthed from an Anglo-Saxon grave in Oxfordshire, England. An enormous osteosarcoma measuring approximately 25 cm × 27 cm was present at the knee of a young man. The specimen contained a pathologic fracture.

Although the awareness of cancer dates back to antiquity, the first attempts to study cancer scientifically did not occur until the beginning of the 19th century. The influence of one of the great anatomists of the previous century, John Hunter, led his pupil, John Abernethy, to formulate in 1804 the first classification of tumors based on pathologic anatomy.[2] The trend at that time was to classify all things according to the principles of Linnaeus (1707–1778); thus tumors were divided into various genera and species. Abernethy redefined the old term *sarcoma* to be a genus of tumors that had a "firm and fleshy feel." The various species of this genus were based on gross textural similarities to normal tissues; i.e., mammary sarcoma, pancreatic sarcoma, adipose sarcoma.

A year later, in 1805, Boyer defined the two species of bone tumors[3]: osteosarcoma, the conversion of bone to flesh, and *spina ventosa* (an ancient term meaning bag of wind), a cystic dilation of bone with a thin shell covering hemorrhagic tissue. Dupuytren[4] called the latter species of bone tumor *fungus hématode,* a name coined by Hey[5] and based on the idea that cancer had its origin in hematomas. Astley Cooper[6] in 1818 called this condition "fungus medullary exostosis." He documented the natural history, gave detailed anatomic descriptions, and provided some of the first gross pathologic drawings of this lesion, which would have included those tumors we would recognize today as giant cell tumors. Thus, for the first half of the 19th century until the application of the microscope, osteosarcoma and "spina ventosa" were the two recognized forms of bone tumors.

Although in 1665 Robert Hooke, with the aid of the microscope, described and named the cell, it was not until 1845 that the microscope began to find its way into medical practice.[7] This was facilitated by Lister's perfection in 1830 of the achromatic objective with which one could observe microscopic preparations with more resolution and less distortion than ever before.[8]

In 1838, the great German physiologist Johannes Müller published the first treatise on the microscopic appearance of tumors, *Üeber den feinern Bau und die Formen der Krankhaften Geschwülste*.[9] However, it was with great reluctance that surgeons and pathologists relied on the microscope for pathologic diagnosis or classification. This reluctance lasted to the end of the 19th century.

Lebert was the first to apply microscopic observations to the differentiation and classification of tumors. In his *Physiologie Pathologique* of 1845,[10] he stressed that tumors could not be understood without microscopic observation. All solid tumors that occurred in bone and that in the past were called osteosarcoma could now be subdivided on the basis of microscopic observations. When Lebert was just beginning to use the microscope to subclassify tumors in 1845, his observations were made on tissues that were unfixed, unembedded, unstained, and sectioned by hand with a sharp knife.[11]

An important milestone in the history of bone tumors was a classic paper published in 1879 by Samuel Gross (1837–1889).[12] Gross, who was working at Jefferson Medical College in Philadelphia, was one of the most prominent surgeons of the 19th century. This paper was the first attempt to classify a large series of bone tumors based on microscopic observations. He subdivided 165 tumors according to two parameters. One was location of the tumor—whether the tumor was central or periosteal. The other was cell type—giant cell, spindle cell, or round cell. For example, in his classification system, which influenced pathologists for many years, a central round cell sarcoma and a periosteal spindle cell sarcoma were described.

The next important milestone in the history of bone tumors was the establishment of the Registry of Bone Sarcoma in 1921 by Ernest Codman (1869–1940). The registry, sponsored by the American College of Surgeons, was the first tumor registry of any kind. Codman's vision was to collect cases of bone sarcoma from throughout the country and establish a nomenclature based on morphologic features and behavior. He invited two other experts in bone diseases, James Ewing and Joseph Bloodgood, to work with him. James Ewing (1866–1943) was a pathologist in New York, at that time working at Cornell University. He had already published his book *Neoplastic Diseases,*[13] and he had just described the entity diffuse endothelioma of bone, a malignant tumor that immediately (despite his protests) bore his name.[14] Joseph Bloodgood (1867–1935), a surgeon and director of surgical pathology at Johns Hopkins in Baltimore, also had an interest in bone tumors. He had already published his observations, based on his own cases and those he culled from the literature, that "giant cell sarcoma" behaved as a benign tumor.[15] Thus, the three physicians in charge of the Registry of Bone Sarcoma were the country's most respected experts on bone tumors.

The methods of the Registry were a model for methods used today. Only living patients could be registered. Surgeons sent the clinical history, details of the physical examination, radiographs, and histologic material (preferably wet tissue) to the Registry's headquarters at 227 Beacon Street in Boston.[16] The diagnosis and method of treatment were also submitted. The Registry sought yearly follow-up on each case and thus established the first national prospective study.

By 1925, the Registry had collected 560 cases. Tumors were grouped into eight categories:

Periosteal fibrosarcoma
Benign and malignant osteogenic tumors
Giant cell tumors
Angioma
Ewing sarcoma
Myeloma (what today are lymphomas and plasma cell myelomas)
Metastatic carcinoma
Tumor-like lesions

Interestingly, this system did not include chondrosarcoma. It was not until 1930 that Dallas Phemister suggested that this malignant tumor might be a distinct entity.

For over 15 years, the Registry of Bone Sarcoma had great prestige throughout the surgical world. Cases continued to be collected until about 1940, although in 1925 supervision was transferred to Dr. Dallas Phemister in Chicago. After World War II, the entire collection was transferred to the Armed Forces Institute of Pathology in Washington, D. C.

The many accomplishments of the Registry have had lasting influence. First, the classification system proposed by the Registry was the nucleus of all future classification systems. These systems are all based on the Registry's concept that bone tumors are defined by a combination of clinical, radiologic, and pathologic features. Second, the behavior of many of the entities was clarified. For example, the poor prognosis of osteosarcoma was firmly established. Third, epidemiologic data about bone tumors were gathered. Fourth, the concept of patient follow-up was established. Finally, the Registry provided a model for national cooperative clinical research. The Registry proved that, guided by a panel of experts, physicians across the country could communicate and use their collective experience to benefit future patients.

The achievements of the Registry of Bone Sarcoma were the starting point for the work of Henry Jaffe (1896–1979), the greatest bone pathologist of the 20th century. For 40 years, while working at the Hospital for Joint Diseases in New York City, Jaffe collected and studied cases of bone disease. With his astute eye and prodigious writing, he set the standards for the practice of bone pathology. That is, he correlated the gross specimens and histologic slides with the radiographs and clinical history. By carefully observing the behavior of each lesion, Jaffe named and characterized many of the entities discussed in this book. Working with colleagues, he established the nature of osteoblastoma (1932), osteoid osteoma (1935), giant cell tumor (1940), eosinophilic granuloma (1940), pigmented villonodular synovitis (1941), chondroblastoma (1942), nonossifying fibroma (1942), chondromyxoid fibroma (1948), and aneurysmal bone cyst (1952). In addition to these accomplishments, Henry Jaffe was a great teacher. He mentored or inspired many orthopedists, bone radiologists, and bone pathologists. His work culminated with the publication of two books, *Tumorous Conditions of Bones and Joints* in 1958 and *Metabolic, Degenerative, and Inflammatory Diseases of Bones and Joints* in 1972. Although many books on orthopedic pathology have since been published, they contain very little about bone disease that cannot be found in these works of Henry Jaffe.

GENERAL PRINCIPLES OF PRIMARY BONE TUMORS

Because of the rarity of bone tumors, most orthopedic surgeons have only limited experience in their management. Delays in diagnosis are common, and many patients receive improper therapy. Optimal treatment usually requires the guidance of an orthopedic oncologist, a specialist in these neoplasms, who, together with a team of radiologists, pathologists, and radiotherapists, provides the best therapeutic outcome for affected patients.

Presentation

Patients with rapidly growing, destructive bone tumors (high-grade malignancies and aggressive benign tumors) almost always present with pain. Initially, the pain may be associated only with activity. However, it quickly progresses to pain at rest. The most characteristic clinical feature of the pain of a growing bone tumor is its presence at night. Often, the patient is awakened several times from sleep. In contrast to the severe pain of malignant neoplasms, the pain of a slowly growing benign tumor is mild. If the bone lesion is not growing, pain may be absent.

Evaluation and Staging

The first step in the management of a patient with a bone tumor is the careful study of plain radiographs of the lesion. In fact, because each type of bone tumor has a characteristic radiographic pattern, many can be diagnosed with plain radiographs alone. Therefore, any patient presenting with a pain pattern suggesting a bony origin should have plain radiographs. Generally, the pain directs the radiologist to examine specific sites. However, in the pelvis and spine, the pain is difficult to localize, and the patient should have screening radiographs of both these areas. Similarly, patients with shoulder pain should have radiographs of the cervical spine, chest, and shoulder.

Sometimes a highly malignant bone tumor, such as a Ewing sarcoma, permeates the bone marrow so rapidly that plain radiographic changes are minimal or not present at all. Therefore, if a negative radiograph does not correlate with a patient's pain, the technetium bone scan should be used. This imaging modality identifies lesions before plain radiographic changes occur. Similarly, a magnetic resonance imaging (MRI) scan identifies bone lesions early, although, like with the bone scan, changes are nonspecific.

Once the presence of a bone tumor is identified, its speed and extent of growth should be determined. In addition to plain radiographs, this often requires cross-sectional imaging studies such as a computed tomography (CT) scan or an MRI. The process of judging the speed and extent of growth of a neoplasm is known as *staging*.

The staging system of the Musculoskeletal Tumor Society, known as the Enneking system, is the most useful (Table 12–1). Benign lesions are classified with Arabic numerals, and malignant ones, with Roman numerals. Stage 1 benign lesions are inactive processes and are usually asymptomatic. Observation is usually the only treatment required. Examples of stage 1 lesions include fibrous cortical defects, nonossifying fibromas, and enchondromas. Stage 2 benign lesions are active processes. Patients are generally symptomatic, and the radiographs show evidence of active growth, such as bone destruction, cortical thickening, or cortical erosion. Examples of active stage 2 lesions include chondroblastomas, osteoid osteomas, and periosteal chondromas. These lesions usually require removal. Stage 3 benign lesions are locally aggressive. These lesions cause significant bone destruction and often extend into the soft tissues. They may even destroy the articular surfaces or cause pathologic fractures. Examples of stage 3 aggressive lesions include some giant cell tumors, aneurysmal bone cysts, and desmoplastic fibromas.

Malignant lesions are classified according to whether the tumor is low or high grade and whether metastases are present. Stage I lesions are low grade, and staging studies show only localized disease. Stage I lesions have less than a 25% chance of metastasis. Stage II lesions are aggressive. They have a great risk for local recurrence and a greater than 25% chance of metastasis. Stage III lesions have already metastasized. The most common site of metastases for malignant bone tumors is to the lungs and other bones. Accordingly, a technetium bone scan and a CT scan of the lungs are necessary for accurate staging.

The treatment of bone tumors is based on their stage and histologic grade. Benign stage I lesions, such as bone islands and osteochondromas, often require no treatment. Active benign lesions are often treated with curettage and bone grafting. In contrast, aggressive lesions such as giant cell tumors often require extensive exteriorization, curettage, and adjuvant treatment, such as phenol cauterization. In some instances, the involved segment of bone must be removed and reconstructed.

Malignant tumors need to be removed completely with a tumor-free margin or they will recur locally. Characteristically, malignant lesions permeate soft tissues adjacent to the bone. These soft tissues must also be removed. Enneking has described the concept of a reactive zone that surrounds the tumor.[17] This zone consists of edema, inflammatory cells, fibrous tissue, and satellites of tumor cells. If the surgeon dissects through the reactive zone, a high risk of local recurrence exists. Careful preoperative planning is required to determine the plains of dissection needed to remove the tumor with a cuff of normal tissue. Postoperatively, the margins must be examined by the pathologist. The results of the evaluation place the margin in one of three categories (Table 12–2). First, an *intralesional* margin occurs when the surgeon cuts across the tumor. With an intralesional margin, the risk of local recurrence is high. Second, a *wide margin* is present if the surgeon has removed the entire tumor with a cuff of normal tissue. Third, a *radical margin* is achieved if the surgeon has removed an entire muscle compartment of bone (Fig. 12–1).

In the past, virtually all patients with malignant bone tumors were treated with amputation. Over the past 20 years, significant advances in imaging, preoperative chemotherapy regimens, and reconstructive techniques have been made. As a result of these advances, approximately 90% of patients are now treated with limb salvage surgery rather than amputation. Two major conditions are required for limb salvage surgery. First, the risk of local recurrence must be no greater than if an amputation were performed. Therefore, a complete removal with uninvolved margins must be possible. Second, the salvaged limb must be functional.

OSSEOUS LESIONS

Bone Island

A bone island, also known as an *enostosis*, is a focus of dense compact bone within the medullary cavity. This

Table 12–1 ■ **SURGICAL STAGING SYSTEM OF THE MUSCULOSKELETAL TUMOR SOCIETY (ENNEKING SYSTEM)**

Tumor Type and Stage*	Description
Benign	
Stage 1: Inactive, latent lesion	Usually asymptomatic
	No active growth on the radiograph
Stage 2: Active	Usually symptomatic
	Active destruction or remodeling seen on the radiograph
Stage 3: Aggressive	Always symptomatic
	Major bone or joint destruction; may be pathologic fracture
Malignant	
Stage I: Low grade	Primarily a local problem, and chance for systemic metastases is less than 25%
Stage II: High grade	High potential for local invasiveness, and the risk of systemic metastases exceeds 25%
Stage III: Metastases	May be pulmonary, bone, or other visceral organs

*Modifiers: The modifiers A or B are added to denote whether the lesion is intracompartmental (within the bone) or extracompartmental (outside the bone). Example: Stage IIB—high grade extracompartmental sarcoma.

Table 12–2 ■ **SURGICAL MARGINS (MUSCULOSKELETAL TUMOR SOCIETY)**

Intralesional	Plane of dissection goes through the tumor
Marginal	Plane of dissection goes through the zone of the tumor
Wide	The entire tumor with a cuff of normal tissue around it has been removed
Radical	The entire tumor and the compartment that it is within has been removed (e.g., a hip disarticulation is performed to remove an osteosarcoma of the distal femur)

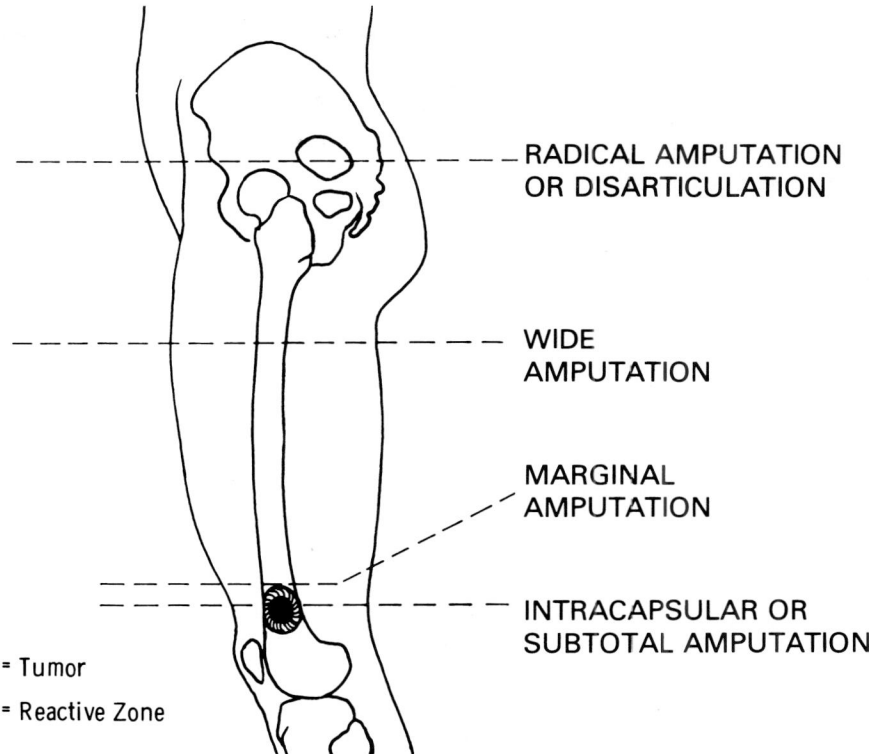

Figure 12-1 ■ Various types of amputations. An intracapsular amputation is through the neoplasm. A marginal amputation removes the reactive rim around the neoplasm. A wide amputation has a significant margin of uninvolved tissue. A radical amputation includes the joint proximal to the lesion. (From Enneking, W. F.: Musculoskeletal Tumor Surgery. Vol. I. New York, Churchill-Livingstone, 1983.)

nonneoplastic lesion most probably results from a remodeling error during skeletal growth. Although it is a developmental abnormality, a bone island may be mistaken radiographically for a neoplasm. Patients are asymptomatic. Therefore, a bone island is almost always discovered incidentally when a patient undergoes radiography for other reasons. A bone island can occur in any bone, and, occasionally, several bones may be involved. A hereditary syndrome, known as *osteopoikilosis*, results in hundreds of bone islands symmetrically distributed throughout the skeleton (see Chapter 3).

A bone island can usually be diagnosed with certainty by plain radiography. A well-defined round or oval radiodensity is present in the medullary canal, usually in the metaphysis (Fig. 12-2). The degree of radiodensity is comparable to the cortex. The size varies, but most are 1 mm to 2 cm in diameter. The margins of a bone island are usually sharply circumscribed. Occasionally, however, spicules of radiodensity radiate from the lesion and blend with the adjacent cancellous bone.[18] Often a bone island blends with the endosteal surface of the cortex.

Histologically, a bone island is a well-defined island of lamellar compact bone identical to the cortex. Also, mature haversian canals are usually present. Occasionally, a bone island has foci of spongy bone with a fibrovascular stroma and areas of remodeling.[19]

Three occasional features of bone islands may lead to its misdiagnosis as a neoplasm. First, bone islands may be very large; some reach 3 to 5 cm in greatest diameter.[20,21] Despite the large size, these giant bone islands exhibit the same radiographic features as their smaller counterparts. The second feature that may lead to misdiagnosis is the scintigraphic appearance of some lesions. Approximately one third of bone islands, irrespective of size, show mild positivity with a bone scan.[19,22] This feature is presumably due to remodeling activity present in some lesions. The final feature that may lead to misdiagnosis is growth of bone islands, observable in about one third of cases.[23] Growth is very slow, about 1 mm per year, and can be observed over several years. However, despite these occasional features—large size, positive bone scan, and minimal growth—the plain radiographic pattern may be relied on to differentiate a bone island from a neoplasm.

Osteoma

Osteomas are dense, slow-growing, bony projections that arise from the bone surfaces. Most commonly they arise in the craniofacial bones, where they project into the oral cavity or sinus, usually the frontal sinus. They vary in size from 1.5 to 3 cm[24] and can be discovered in 3% of patients requiring sinus radiographs.

On rare occasions, an osteoma may occur in the postcranial skeleton, where it is called a *parosteal osteoma*. The long bones are usually affected, but the pelvis or vertebrae may also be involved. Of the long bones, the tibia and femur are most commonly involved.[25] Parosteal osteomas tend to be larger than those in the craniofacial skeleton; some may reach a diameter of 6 to 8 cm.

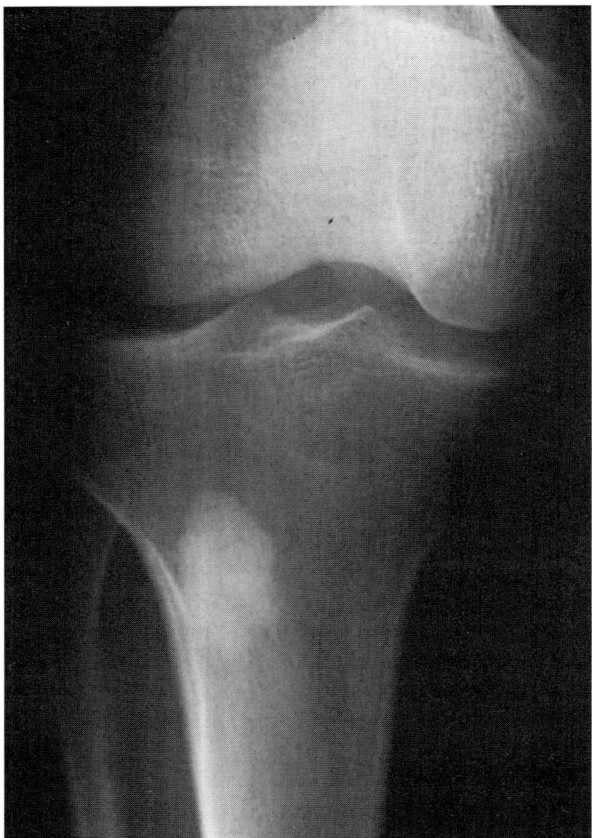

Figure 12–2 ▪ A bone island in the proximal tibial metaphysis. The lesion is a uniform radiodensity. The proximal margin is extremely well circumscribed, and the distal edge of the lesion shows radial streaks of radiodensity that blend in with normal trabeculae.

osteoma. Parosteal osteomas have very smooth contours and a uniform radiodensity, features that differ from the irregular borders and intralesional trabeculations usually seen in parosteal osteosarcomas. An osteoid osteoma can be distinguished from a parosteal osteoma by a CT scan. This study usually demonstrates the small radiolucent nidus of the osteoid osteoma in the center of the dense periosteal reactive bone.

Most osteomas of the cranial bones are asymptomatic, and excision is rarely indicated.[28] The treatment of parosteal osteomas is controversial. Complete surgical excision has been recommended.[29,30] However, we feel that parosteal osteomas should be treated conservatively without surgery. These lesions are self-limited and rarely cause significant symptoms. Furthermore, excision often requires extensive surgery with reconstruction. Conservative therapy, by contrast, eliminates the risk of surgical complications.

Osteoid Osteoma

Osteoid osteomas are benign osteoid-producing neoplasms with three important characteristics: a small size, self-limited growth, and a tendency to cause extensive reactive changes

Osteomas are not neoplasms. They result from the self-limited deposition of reactive periosteal new bone. Although the cause is unknown, a history of trauma is sometimes present.[26] Parosteal osteoma may be a limited form of melorheostosis, a disease characterized by longitudinal deposits of periosteal reactive bone in multiple sites, often in the same extremity (see Chapter 3).

Patients with parosteal osteomas are usually adults in their 30s and 40s, although an age range of 14 to 68 years has been reported.[25] A long history of swelling and sometimes dull aching pain are the presenting symptoms.

Radiographically, osteomas are smoothly contoured or lobulated radiodense lesions that are attached to the bone surface with a broad base (Fig. 12–3). The radiodensity is uniform and equal to that of the cortex. Histologically, osteomas consist of dense compact lamellar bone that shows evidence of remodeling (Fig. 12–4). Many mature haversian systems are present. Occasionally, osteomas of the craniofacial bones show some spongy bone with intervening loose fibrovascular tissue.[27]

Osteomas of the craniofacial bones are readily recognized radiographically. However, parosteal osteomas in the long bones may be confused radiographically with bone-forming neoplasms, particularly parosteal osteosarcoma and osteoid

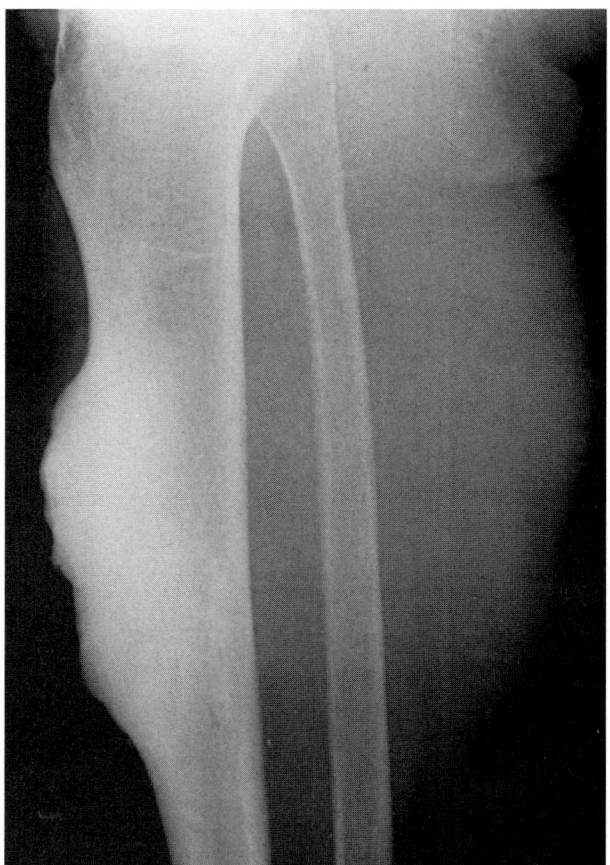

Figure 12–3 ▪ A parosteal osteoma of the proximal tibia. This is a smoothly contoured radiodense surface lesion. (From McCarthy, E. F.: *Differential Diagnosis in Pathology. Bone and Joint Disorders.* New York and Tokyo, Igaku-Shoin, 1996. With permission from Williams & Wilkins.)

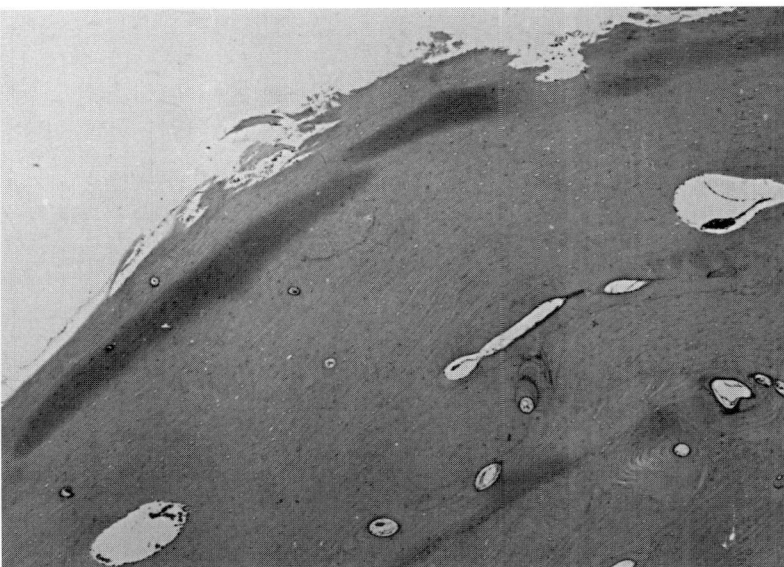

Figure 12-4 ■ Low-power photomicrograph of an osteoma. The lesion consists of dense compact bone with numerous haversian systems.

in adjacent tissues. The lesional tissue of an osteoid osteoma, known as a *nidus,* is almost always only 1 cm or less in diameter. Despite its small size, the lesional tissue causes intense pain and provokes an exuberant periosteal reaction, a reaction that often obscures the small nidus.[31,32]

Like most other primary bone tumors, osteoid osteomas affect children and young adults. Most cases present between the ages of 10 and 35, with the average being 19 years. Rarely, children younger than 5 years or adults older than 35 may be affected.[33] Patients invariably present with pain. Characteristically, the pain is worse at night and dramatically relieved by aspirin. This feature is present in more then 75% of cases and is an important diagnostic clue.[34]

In addition to causing pain, osteoid osteomas are highly irritative to adjacent tissues. These local effects may be caused by the prostaglandin synthesis demonstrated in some osteoid osteomas.[35] For example, a lesion in the spine can cause scoliosis,[36] and a lesion near a growth plate can stimulate lengthening of the extremity.[37] Also, an intraarticular lesion may cause an intense synovitis.[38] These intraarticular osteoid osteomas, particularly inside the hip or elbow capsule, may be difficult to diagnose. This is because the bone inside a joint capsule lacks a periosteum; therefore, lesions in these locations cannot stimulate the typical periosteal reaction. Another local effect of some osteoid osteomas is significant edema in the adjacent soft tissues.[39] This change, usually seen with MRI, should not be interpreted as evidence of a more aggressive infiltrative lesion. A final effect of some osteoid osteomas is muscular atrophy and osteopenia in the involved extremity.

Osteoid osteomas may occur in any bone, but lesions in the femur and tibia account for 50% of cases (Fig. 12–5). Other sites of predilection include the posterior elements of the spine (the vertebral body is a very rare location), the humerus, and the small bones of the hands and feet. A rare presentation of osteoid osteoma is multiple lesions occurring either synchronously or metachronously in one or several bones.[40,41]

Osteoid osteomas have a very characteristic radiographic appearance. A small radiolucent nidus is surrounded by dense reactive bone (Fig. 12–6). The nidus may be subperiosteal, intracortical, or subcortical. On rare occasions, the nidus is deep in the medullary canal. Occasionally, the reactive bone may be so dense that it obscures the nidus. In this

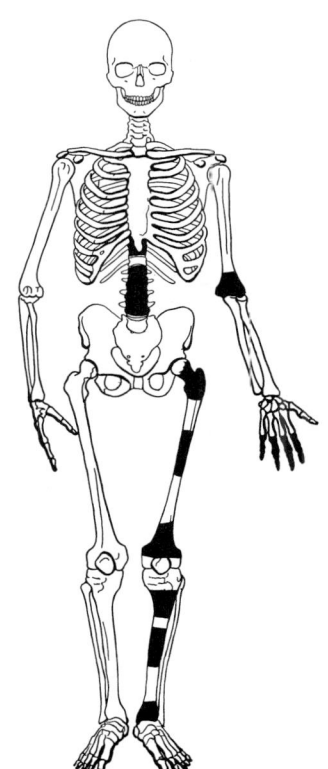

Figure 12-5 ■ Osteoid osteoma locations.

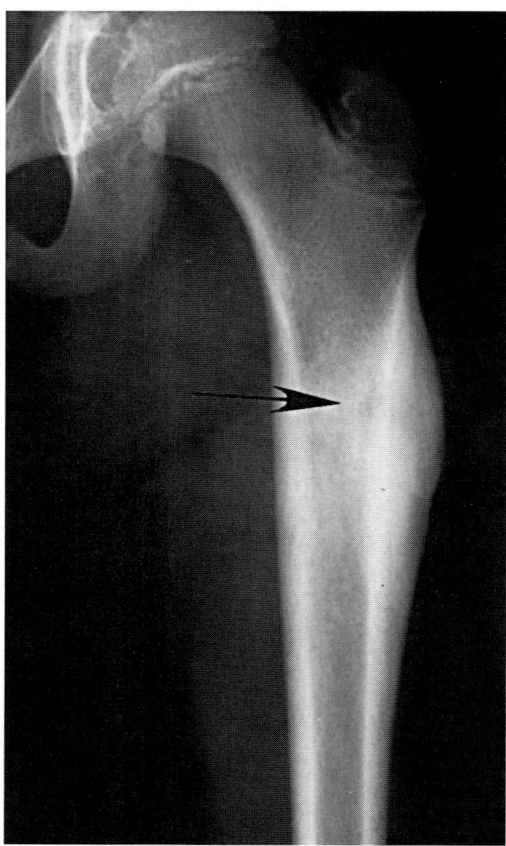

Figure 12-6 ■ Osteoid osteoma of the proximal femur. The lesion is a radiolucent nidus *(arrow)* surrounded by dense reactive periosteal bone.

situation, a CT or MRI scan usually identifies the small radiolucent focus in the center of the radiodense area (Fig. 12–7).

Histologically, osteoid osteomas are characterized by thin interconnecting seams of osteoid or woven bone lined by osteoblasts (Fig. 12–8). The osteoid seams are separated by a loose fibrous stroma with prominent vascularity. This lesional tissue is sharply demarcated from the dense surrounding bone (Fig. 12–9). Often, a few thick-walled blood vessels are present in the tissue between the surrounding reactive trabeculae.

The treatment of osteoid osteomas is surgical excision. This results in a dramatic relief of pain; patients often report that the night after surgery is the first good sleep they have had in many months.

Osteoid osteomas sometimes pose a surgical problem—the intraoperative localization of the lesion. The extensive periosteal reactive bone often hides the location of the nidus. Solving this problem requires cooperation of the surgeon, radiologist, and pathologist. Intraoperative radiographs are usually required. Ideally, the pathologist should find the nidus grossly before the operation is over. If the nidus is removed intact, it can be identified as a cherry red portion of trabecular bone about the size of a pea. Preoperative administration of tetracycline facilitates the intraoperative localization of the lesion. During surgery, Woods lamp illumination of the excised tissue identifies the brightly fluorescing nidus.[42] Alternatively, a small dose of technetium 99m may be administered a few hours preoperatively and the surgically removed specimens examined with a scintillation probe.[43] The nidus will have taken up more radioactivity. Occasionally, the nidus cannot be identified in surgically removed tissue despite these adjunctive procedures. For unknown reasons, symptoms are relieved in over three quarters of these patients.[44]

Two alternatives to en bloc surgery excision have been advocated for the treatment of osteoid osteoma. First, percutaneous CT-guided thermocoagulation (radiofrequency ablation) has proved an effective therapy. This minimally invasive procedure has few complications.[45] A second alternative therapy is the use of nonsteroidal antiinflammatory drugs.[46] Surgery has proved unnecessary in many patients treated with this regimen.

Osteoblastoma

Osteoblastomas are benign bone-forming neoplasms that share many histologic features with osteoid osteomas. However, these neoplasms differ in several important ways. First, osteoblastomas are rare neoplasms unlike osteoid osteomas, which are relatively common. Second, osteoblastomas are larger than osteoid osteomas. Third, unlike the self-limited growth of osteoid osteomas, osteoblastomas grow progressively. In fact, some grow very aggressively and may be mistaken for osteosarcomas. Fourth, osteoblastomas lack the highly irritative effect of osteoid osteomas.

Osteoblastomas may occur at any age; however, 80% occur between the ages of 10 and 25 years. Patients usually present with pain, and some have local swelling and tenderness. Any bone may be involved, including the calvarium and the small bones of the hands and feet. The spine, however, is the most common location, accounting for about a third of reported cases (Fig. 12–10). In this location, the vertebral posterior elements are the principal site of involvement, but occasionally the vertebral body may also be involved. Osteoblastomas almost never involve the vertebral body alone. All portions of the spine, including the sacrum, are equally affected. In the appendicular skeleton, the diaphysis or metaphysis of long bones, particularly the femur or tibia, are the most common locations. The mandible is also a common site. In addition to local symptoms, osteoblastomas have been associated with the oncogenic osteomalacia syndrome (see Chapter 4) and systemic toxicity syndromes.[47]

Radiographically, osteoblastomas are expansile, lytic lesions with variable amounts of fluffy mineralization (Fig. 12–11). Reported lesions have ranged from 1 to 11 cm. Most are well circumscribed, and occasionally they have a sclerotic rim. Many osteoblastomas expand the cortex and are bounded by a thin shell of reactive bone. About 25% of osteoblastomas show aggressive radiographic features with cortical destruction or penetration.[48]

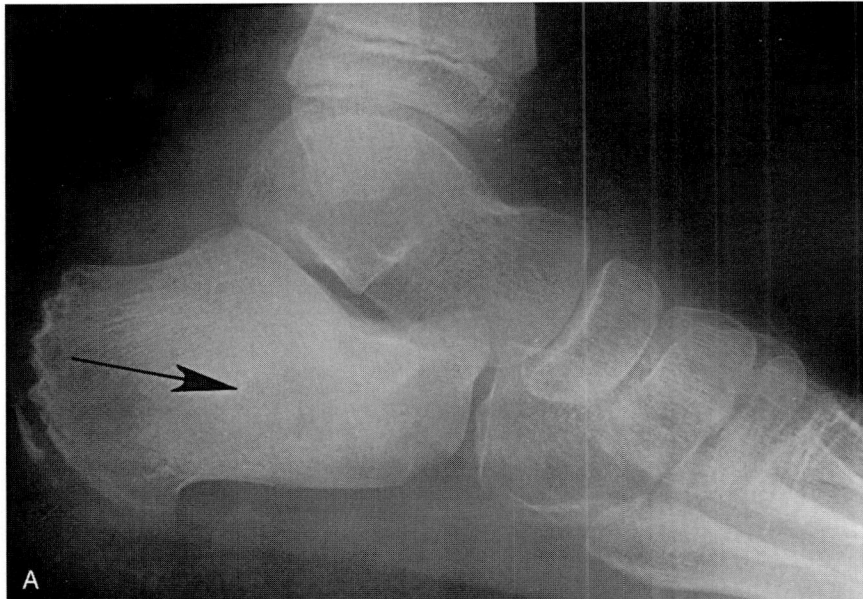
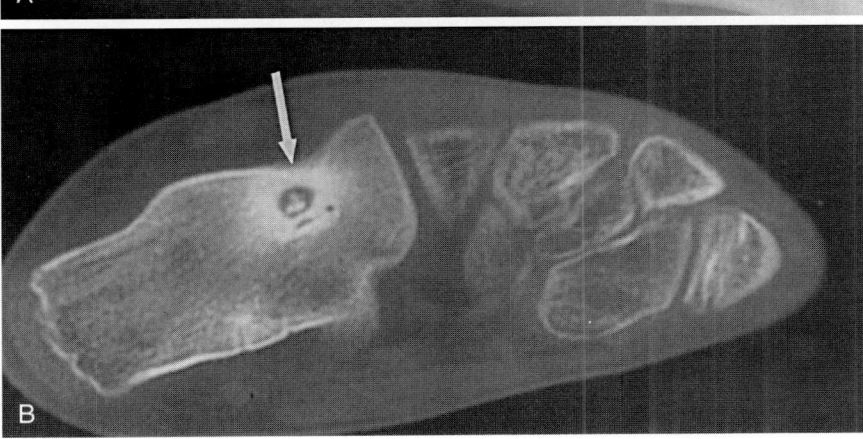

Figure 12-7 ■ Osteoid osteoma of the calcaneus. **A,** Lateral plain radiograph showing dense bone sclerosis with a faint radiolucent nidus *(arrow).* **B,** CT scan showing radiolucent nidus *(arrow)* surrounded by the rim of reactive bone. (From Frassica, F. J., Waltrip, R. L., Sponseller, P. D., Ma, L. D., and McCarthy, E. F. Jr.: Clinicopathologic features and treatment of osteoid osteoma and osteoblastoma in children and adolescents. *Orthop Clin North Am* 27:559, 1996.)

Osteoblastomas of the spine are best visualized by a CT or MRI scan (Fig. 12–12). In this location, as in the appendicular skeleton, a lesion may vary from 1 to 15 cm, the average size being 3.5 cm. Also, as with osteoblastomas in the long bones, mineralization in spinal lesions is variable, but 50% of spinal osteoblastomas show no mineralization. A CT of spinal osteoblastomas often demonstrates paravertebral muscle atrophy, a feature that causes scoliosis in many patients with lesions in this site.[49]

On rare occasions, both spinal and appendicular osteoblastomas may spread to involve contiguous bones, a feature seen more commonly in so-called *aggressive osteoblastomas.* A very rare osteoblastoma may be multifocal.[50] However, distinguishing a multifocal osteoblastoma from a multifocal vascular neoplasm with reactive bone is extremely difficult. An unusual presentation of osteoblastomas is a subperiosteal location. In this presentation, plain radiographs can be normal.[51]

Osteoblastomas share many histologic features with osteoid osteomas. Irregular anastomosing seams of osteoid or woven bone are lined by a single layer of bland osteoblasts. Occasionally, broad sheets of osteoid are produced that entrap individual cells (Fig. 12–13). A few osteoclasts are evenly scattered adjacent to the osteoid. The seams of osteoid are separated by a loose fibrovascular stroma containing occasional mitotic figures. Additionally, about 45% of osteoblastomas show foci of aneurysmal bone cyst transformation.

An important histologic feature of osteoblastoma is its sharp demarcation from adjacent native bone. However, on rare occasions, osteoblastomas may have multifocal growth centers. Multifocal growth centers should not be regarded as a permeative growth pattern, a feature that is uncharacteristic of osteoblastomas. Although a permeative growth pattern has been suggested as a histologic variable in osteoblastomas, particularly in the small tubular bones,[52] we feel that permeative growth is indicative of osteosarcoma.

Osteoblastomas have three important histologic features that may lead to diagnostic difficulties. First, 6% of osteoblastomas contain foci of a chondroid matrix or mature hyaline cartilage.[53] Second, rare lesions have a "pseudosarcomatous" stroma. Large cells with bizarre hyperchromatic nuclei are scattered in the stroma (Fig. 12–14). The absence of mitotic figures in these atypical cells is the clue to their nonmalignant nature. Third, osteoblastomas

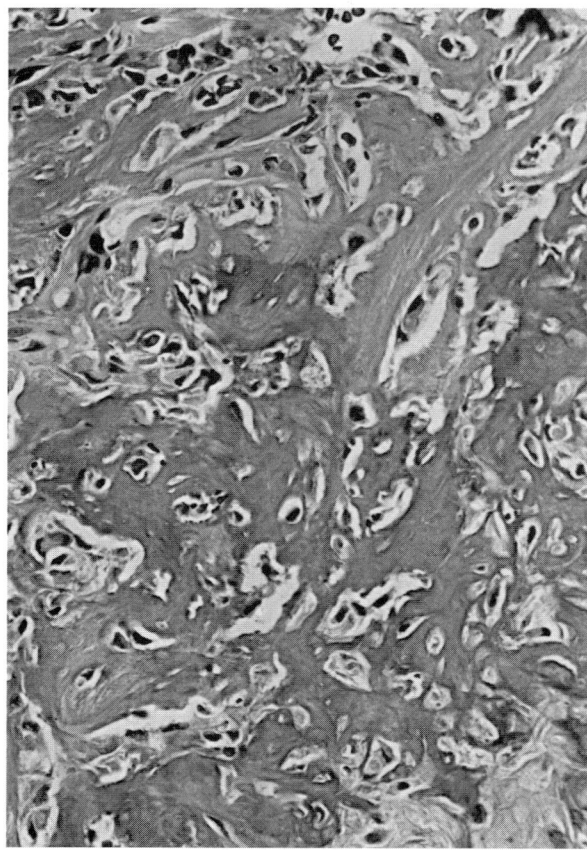

Figure 12-8 ■ Photomicrograph of osteoid osteoma. Seams of new bone are lined by osteoblasts.

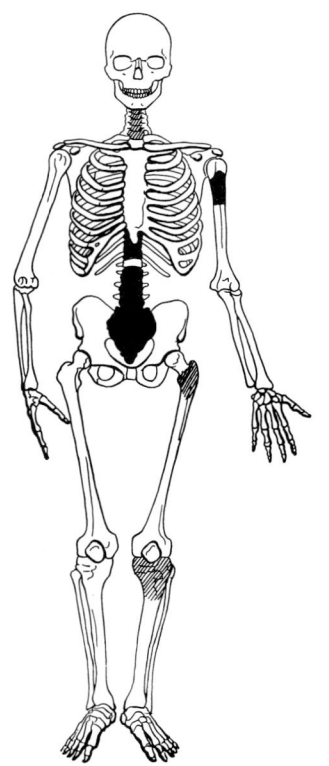

Figure 12-10 ■ Osteoblastoma locations.

may contain large epithelioid osteoblasts (Fig. 12–15). These cells have abundant cytoplasm and a large nucleus with a prominent nucleolus. Although a few epithelioid osteoblasts are present in most osteoblastomas, lesions with over 75% of the osteoblasts showing this feature have been called "aggressive osteoblastomas."

The term *aggressive osteoblastoma* is useful to distinguish diagnostically problematic osteoblastomas from osteosarcomas. This variant of osteoblastoma, which accounts for 10% of all cases, is locally aggressive, but it does not metastasize. Several features characterize these lesions. Radiologically,

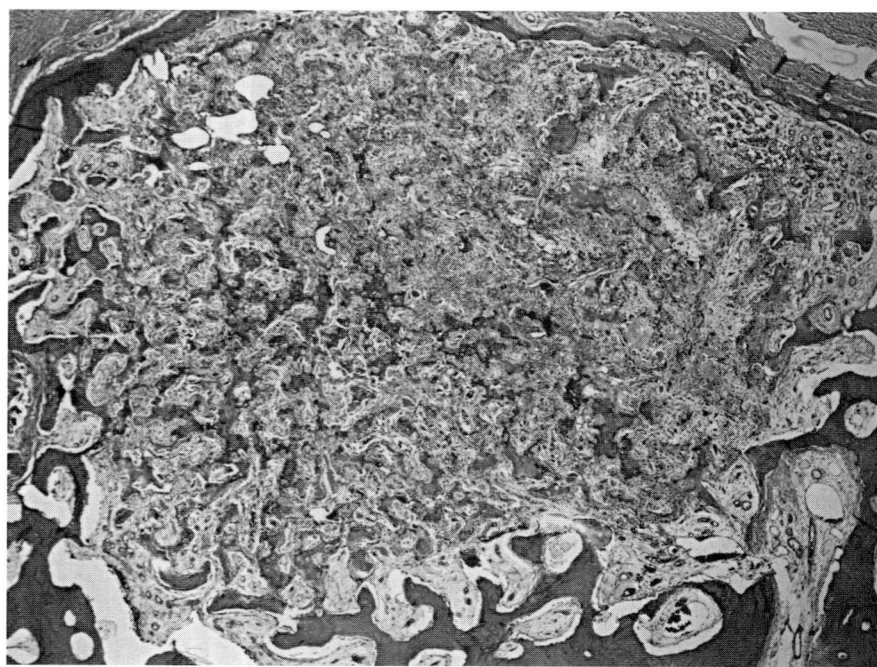

Figure 12-9 ■ Low-power photomicrograph of an osteoid osteoma. The nidus of new bone spicules is well defined and delineated from normal bone and a thin overlying cortex. (From Frassica, F. J., and McCarthy, E. F.: Orthopedic pathology. Miller, M. D., Ed. *Review of Orthopaedics,* 2nd ed. Philadelphia, W. B. Saunders, 1996, p. 300.)

aggressive osteoblastomas tend to be larger. They may also have a destructive growth pattern, and they may spread to adjacent bones.[54] Histologically, many epithelioid osteoblasts are present. In addition, they often have a lace-like pattern of osteoid that mimics osteosarcoma. Finally, mitotic figures, although never atypical, are more numerous than in conventional osteoblastoma.

The principal differential diagnosis for osteoblastoma, particularly aggressive osteoblastoma, is osteoblastic osteosarcoma. Occasionally, it may be difficult to distinguish these lesions because some osteosarcomas contain bland foci that may be indistinguishable from osteoblastoma.[55,56] Adequate sampling is necessary to solve this diagnostic dilemma. An osteoblastoma-like osteosarcoma has areas of destructive permeative growth and areas of sarcomatous stroma that identify it as a malignant neoplasm. In addition, osteosarcomas lack the loose fibrovascular stroma characteristic of osteoblastomas.

Osteoblastomas should be treated by curettage. Although the recurrence rate may be as high as 20%, a repeat curettage usually results in a cure. Although aggressive osteoblastomas have a slightly higher recurrence rate, they should be treated like conventional osteoblastomas.[48]

Osteosarcoma

Osteosarcoma, the most common primary malignant bone tumor, usually affects children and young adults. By defini-

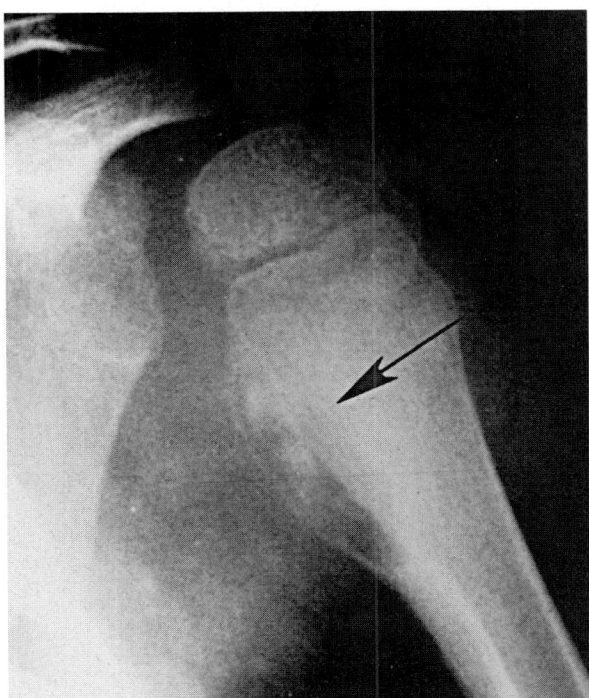

Figure 12-11 ■ Osteoblastoma of the proximal humerus. A well-defined radiolucency *(arrow)* contains fluffy mineralization. (From McCarthy, E. F.: *Differential Diagnosis in Pathology. Bone and Joint Disorders.* New York and Tokyo. Igaku-Shoin, 1996. With permission from Williams & Wilkins.)

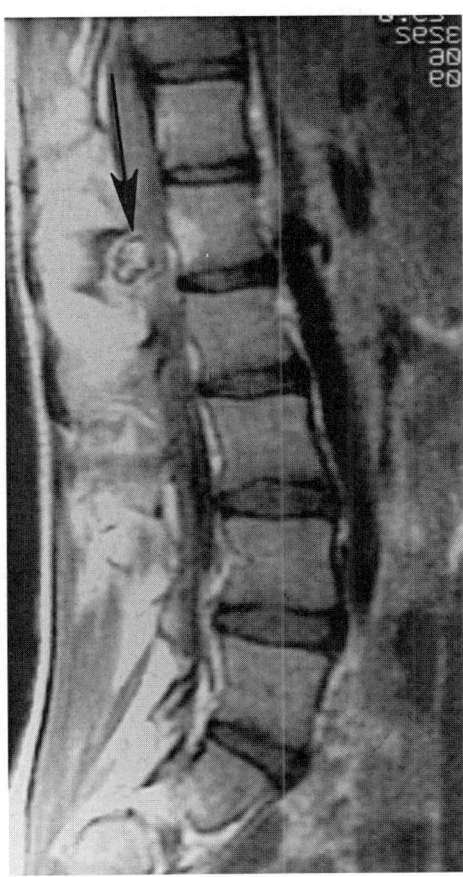

Figure 12-12 ■ An MRI of the spine showing an osteoblastoma of the posterior elements. The lesion shows a well-defined area of increased signal *(arrow)*. (From Frassica, F. J., et al.: Clinicopathologic features and treatment of osteoid osteoma and osteoblastoma in children and adolescents. *Orthop Clin North Am* 27:559, 1996.)

tion, an osteosarcoma is a neoplasm in which osteoid is synthesized by malignant cells. By contrast, malignant neoplasms with extensive reactive bone, an occasional finding in malignant fibrous histiocytomas, Ewing sarcomas, and chondrosarcomas, do not qualify as osteosarcomas.

Osteosarcomas have a wide range of radiographic and histologic patterns. For example, osteosarcomas may be radiolucent or very radiodense. Some originate and grow on the bone surface, and others are confined to the medullary cavity. Histologically, some osteosarcomas show extensive cartilage differentiation, and others contain abundant fibrous tissue. In addition, osteosarcomas may be any histologic grade. For example, some contain many pleomorphic cells and mitotic figures, and others may be difficult to recognize as malignant neoplasms.

Until the early part of the 20th century, any bone tumor that caused increased bone density was called an osteosarcoma. It was not until 1926 that Ernest Codman clearly defined osteosarcoma as a diagnostic entity.[57] His definition, based on clinical, radiographic, and histologic features, was the first attempt to precisely define any bone tumor. Starting in 1951 with the description of parosteal osteosarcoma by Geschickter and Copeland,[58] radiologists, pathologists, and

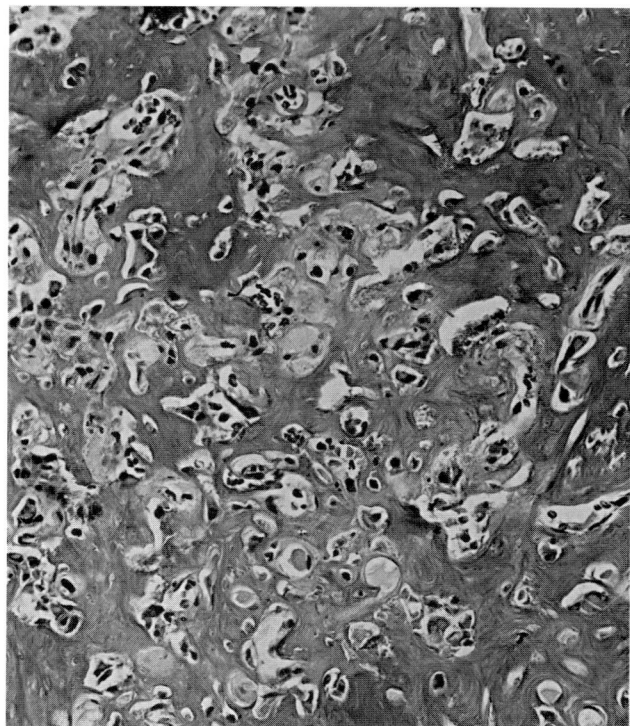

Figure 12-13 ■ Photomicrograph of an osteoblastoma. Sheets of neoplastic osteoid encase the osteoblasts.

Table 12-3 ■ **OSTEOSARCOMA VARIANTS**

Parosteal osteosarcoma
Periosteal osteosarcoma
Well-differentiated intramedullary osteosarcoma
Telangiectatic osteosarcoma
Small cell osteosarcoma
Multifocal osteosarcoma
Intracortical osteosarcoma
High-grade surface osteosarcoma

orthopedic surgeons began to recognize that certain radiographic or histologic features identified important prognostic differences. In addition, some osteosarcomas showed features that led to their being misdiagnosed as other neoplasms. Osteosarcomas with these special features have been identified as specific variants[59] (Fig. 12–16). Eight important osteosarcoma variants now exist, although together they account for only 10% of all osteosarcomas (Table 12–3). In addition to these variants, osteosarcomas with typical histologic features occur in specific clinical settings. These include sarcomas complicating radiation therapy, Paget's disease, bone infarcts, and low-grade cartilage lesions. Osteosarcomas also occur in the soft tissue without bone involvement.

Conventional Osteosarcoma

Conventional osteosarcoma accounts for 90% of all osteosarcomas.[40] It begins in the medullary canal and sometimes penetrates the cortex and invades the adjacent soft tissues. Most patients with conventional osteosarcoma are adolescents or young adults. About 85% of patients are younger than 30 years, the peak incidence being at 20 to 25 years of age. This neoplasm is extremely rare in children younger than 10. Older adults may also develop conventional osteosarcoma, although many have predisposing factors such as Paget's disease or prior radiation therapy. In younger patients, conventional osteosarcoma most commonly occurs around the knee, the distal femur accounting for one third of all cases (Fig. 12–17). By contrast, older patients develop osteosarcomas more commonly in the flat bones. Pain, tenderness, and swelling, rarely occurring for more than a few months, are the usual presenting symptoms.

Some patients may be genetically predisposed to develop osteosarcoma. For example, patients who have familial reti-

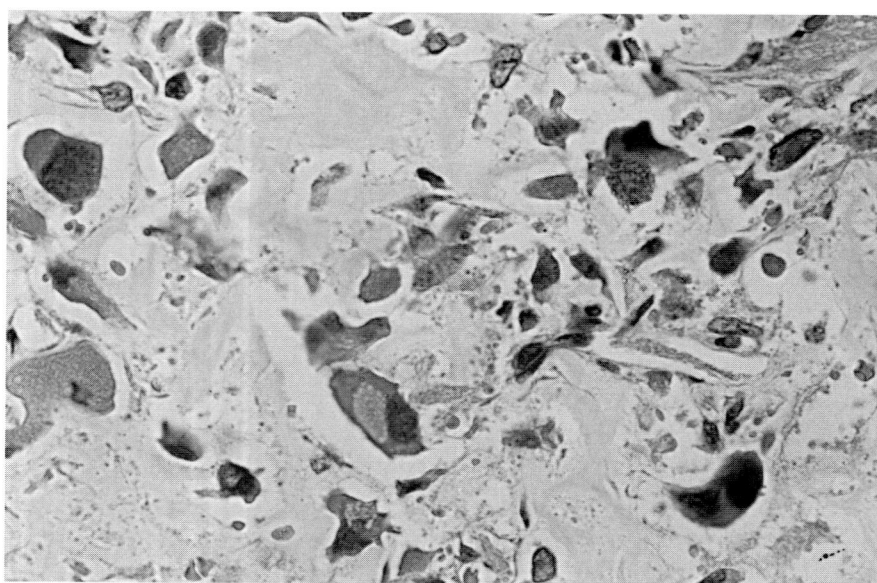

Figure 12-14 ■ Photomicrograph of an osteoblastoma with numerous bizarre atypical cells.

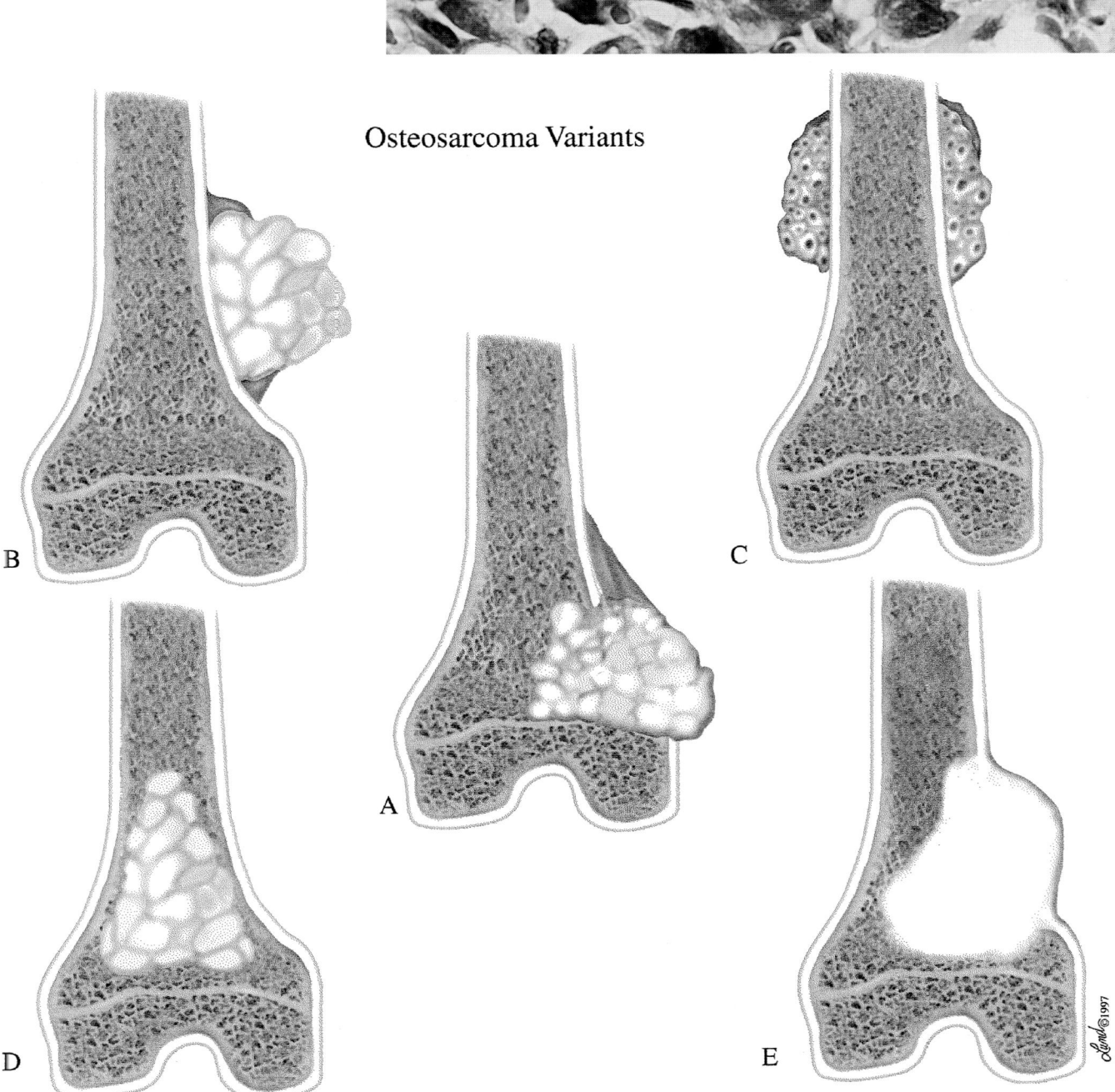

Figure 12-15 ■ Photomicrograph of an aggressive osteoblastoma. Numerous large epithelioid osteoblasts are present.

Figure 12-16 ■ Osteosarcoma variants. **A,** Conventional osteosarcoma. **B,** Parosteal osteosarcoma. **C,** Periosteal osteosarcoma. **D,** Well-differentiated intramedullary osteosarcoma. **E,** Telangiectatic osteosarcoma.

noblastoma have a several hundred-fold increase in the incidence of osteosarcoma. These patients have an inactive retinoblastoma gene, located on chromosome 13, which renders them susceptible to numerous malignancies, including osteosarcoma.[60] In addition to patients with retinoblastoma, patients with the Rothmund-Thomson syndrome are also prone to developing osteosarcoma.[61]

Radiographic Features. The radiographic features of conventional osteosarcoma are diagnostic in two thirds of cases. The lesion is a poorly circumscribed medullary lucency with mottled areas of radiodensity (Fig. 12–18). Occasionally, a lesion may be entirely radiodense. Cortical destruction is usually present, and a focally mineralized soft tissue mass is often present. Benign, periosteal reactive bone forms a Codman's triangle adjacent to the soft tissue mass (Fig. 12–19). In the long bones, conventional osteosarcoma is usually centered in the metaphysis. An open epiphyseal plate is a partial barrier to epiphyseal invasion, although most tumors can focally penetrate this barrier.[62] In skeletally mature patients, the epiphysis is extensively involved. On rare occasions, osteosarcomas may be confined to the epiphysis.[63]

Ancillary radiographic modalities, such as CT or MRI, are not necessary to establish the diagnosis of osteosarcoma. However, they are needed to delineate the extent of disease. Multiplanar MRI images are used to detect skip metastases, which occur in 5 to 10% of patients. The MRI scan also delineates the relationship of the soft tissue component to the neurovascular bundles.

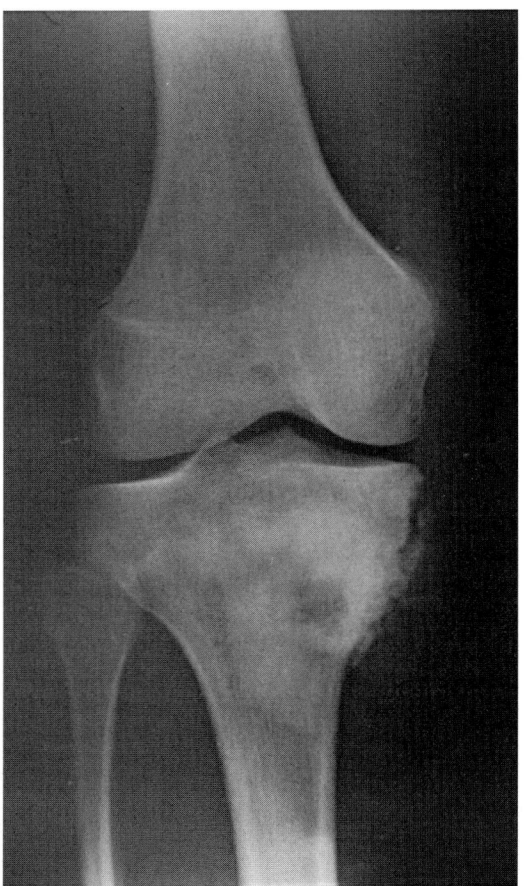

Figure 12-18 ■ Conventional osteosarcoma of proximal tibia. A poorly defined mixed radiolytic and radiodense lesion is associated with a periosteal reaction. (From Frassica, F. J., and McCarthy, E. F.: Orthopaedic pathology. Miller, M. D., Ed. *Review of Orthopaedics,* 2nd ed. Philadelphia, W. B. Saunders, 1996, p. 303.)

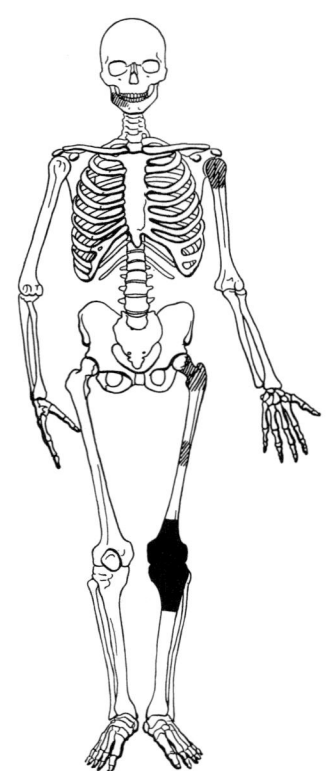

Figure 12-17 ■ Osteosarcoma locations.

Histologic Features. Conventional osteosarcoma is usually an osteoblastic neoplasm. Seams or sheets of eosinophilic osteoid are distributed in a sarcomatous stroma (Fig. 12–20). The stromal cells of conventional osteosarcoma are usually high-grade (Fig. 12–21). They show varying degrees of atypia and numerous mitotic figures. The pattern and distribution of osteoid is often variable. In some areas, osteoid is deposited in fine lace-like seams (Fig. 12–22). In other areas, broad sheets of osteoid may entrap single neoplastic osteoblasts. An unusual pattern of osteoid deposition is entombment of individual marrow fat cells. This pattern may be confused with nonneoplastic fat necrosis (Fig. 12–23).

In addition to osteoblastic areas, other patterns of differentiation are often present in conventional osteosarcoma. For example, chondroblastic areas may be present (Fig. 12–24). These areas contain lobules or islands of cartilage with markedly atypical chondrocytes. A second pattern of differentiation that may be focally present resembles malignant fibrous histiocytoma. In these foci, atypical spindle cells, often arranged in a storiform pattern, are admixed with tumor giant cells. A final pattern focally present in many conventional osteosarcomas is aneurysmal bone cyst change.

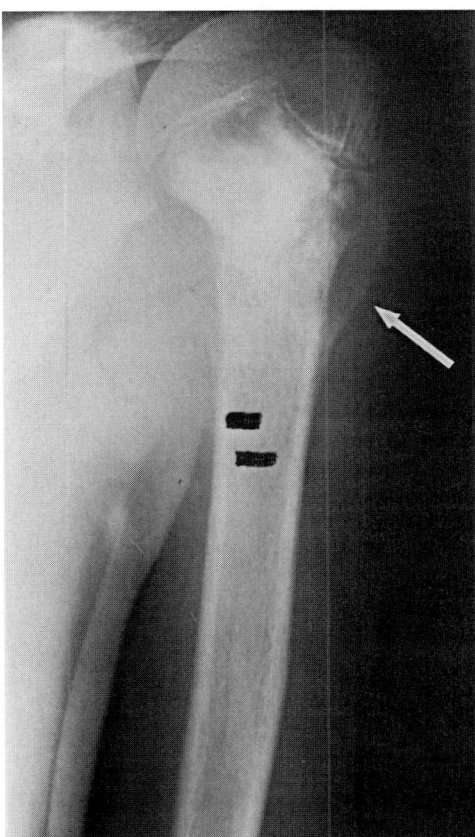

Figure 12-19 ■ Conventional osteosarcoma of the proximal humerus. A Codman's triangle of reactive bone *(arrow)* is present on the lateral cortex.

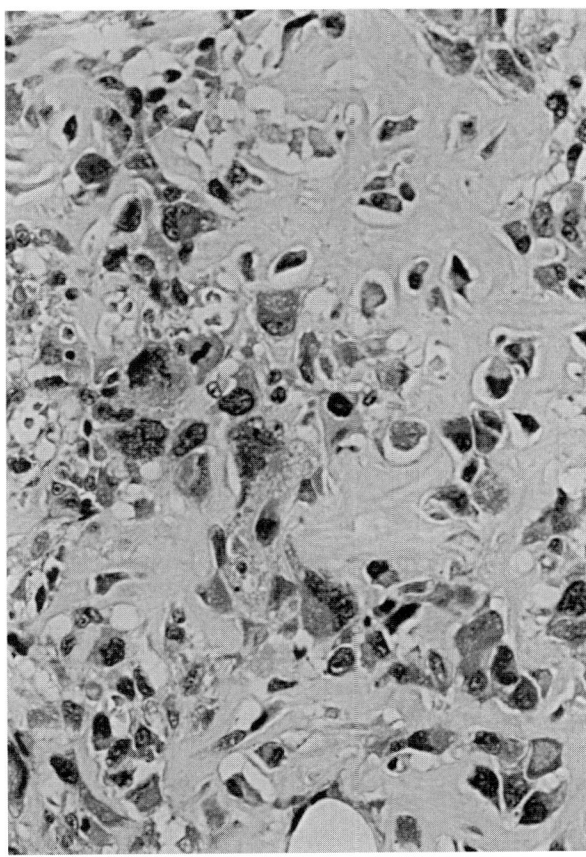

Figure 12-20 ■ Photomicrograph of conventional osteosarcoma. Bizarre pleomorphic cells are present in an osteoid matrix.

In these areas, blood-filled lakes surrounded by fibrous septae are admixed with sarcomatous stroma. Although focal aneurysmal bone cyst areas are often present in conventional osteosarcoma, a lesion with total aneurysmal bone cyst transformation should be regarded as a telangiectatic osteosarcoma.

Occasionally, it may be difficult to distinguish osteoid from hyalinized fibrous tissue. Because special stains cannot distinguish these two substances, only the presence of mineralization can positively identify an eosinophilic extracellular substance as osteoid. Therefore, because mineralization is the key to establishing the diagnosis of osteosarcoma, it is

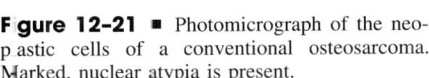

Figure 12-21 ■ Photomicrograph of the neoplastic cells of a conventional osteosarcoma. Marked, nuclear atypia is present.

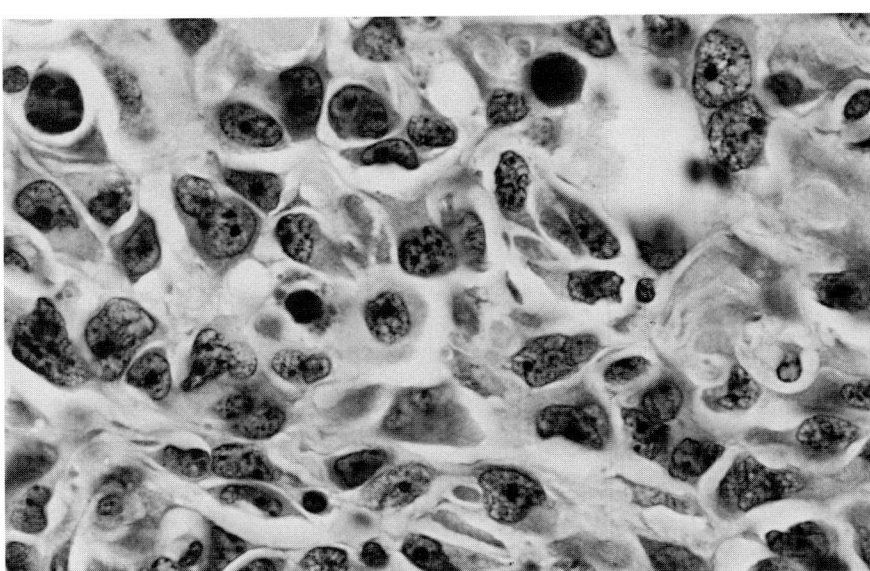

PRIMARY BONE TUMORS

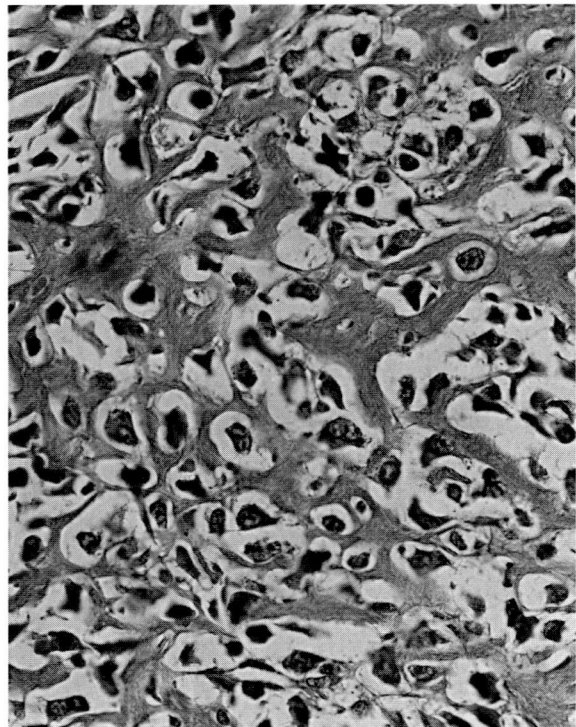

Figure 12-22 ■ Photomicrograph of osteosarcoma showing lace-like deposition of osteoid.

lated mass is attached to the cortex with a broad base (Fig. 12–26). The medullary canal is typically uninvolved but may occasionally show a radiodense process continuous with the surface mass. As the neoplasm grows, it often encircles the shaft and sometimes leaves a thin, lucent cleft between the underlying bone and the neoplasm, the so-called "string sign." Most parosteal osteosarcomas are from 4 to 6 cm in diameter when diagnosed, although some may reach 10 cm or more. Usually, the bony mass is homogeneous. However, lucent areas may be present near the surface. Ill-defined lucent areas deep in the lesion are most likely dedifferentiated areas. The CT scan is the most important imaging tool to determine the relation of the bony mass to the cortex. CT is also useful in determining the extent of soft tissue involvement and to establish the presence of intralesional lucency or medullary invasion.[67]

Histologic Features. Histologically, parosteal osteosarcomas are well-differentiated fibroosseous neoplasms. Broad seams of osteoid lie in a bland, fibrous stroma (Fig. 12–27). The osteoid may mature and develop a lamellar pattern. The hypocellular fibrous stroma usually shows only minimal cytologic atypia (Fig. 12–28). Although parosteal osteosarcomas are always external to the bone, in rare cases a focus of well-differentiated fibroosseous tissue may also be present

extremely important to process some tissue without decalcification. Otherwise, this distinguishing feature may be obliterated, making the diagnosis of osteosarcoma presumptive.

Parosteal Osteosarcoma

Parosteal osteosarcoma was the first osteosarcoma variant to be defined. Although it is the most common variant, it only accounts for 5% of all osteosarcomas. Parosteal osteosarcoma is a low-grade, slow-growing neoplasm that originates from the surface of the cortex and forms a bony mass in the soft tissue. Patients present with a slow-growing painless swelling that is often present a year or more before they seek medical attention. Some have symptoms for as long as 10 years.[64] Although this neoplasm may arise at any age, 75% of patients are between ages 20 and 45. An unusual feature of parosteal osteosarcoma is its predilection for one particular site, the posterior aspect of the distal femur. This location accounts for 73% of patients. The proximal tibia and proximal humerus are the next most frequently involved sites (Fig. 12–25). This neoplasm is extremely rare in the pelvis, spine, skull, and bones of the hands and feet.

Although usually a low-grade, slow-growing neoplasm, parosteal osteosarcoma may dedifferentiate—foci of high-grade osteosarcoma develop within the low-grade areas in 16 to 43% of cases.[65,66] Dedifferentiation may be present at the time of initial diagnosis (primary), or it may develop in recurrent or incompletely excised lesions (secondary).

Radiographic Features. Parosteal osteosarcomas have a characteristic radiographic appearance. A radiodense lobu-

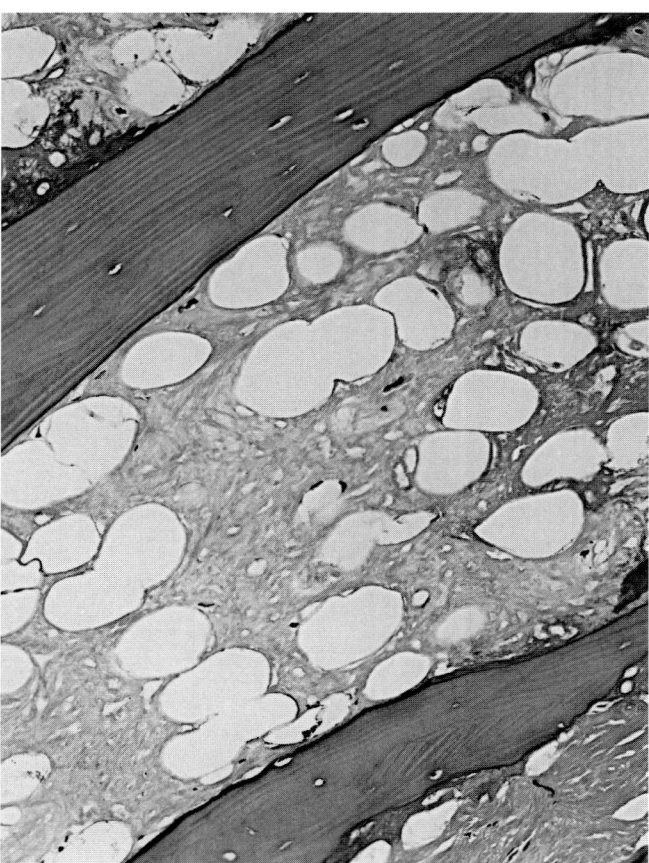

Figure 12-23 ■ Photomicrograph of conventional osteosarcoma. Neoplastic osteoid is entombing marrow fat cells. This microscopic pattern can be confused with fat necrosis in a bone infarct.

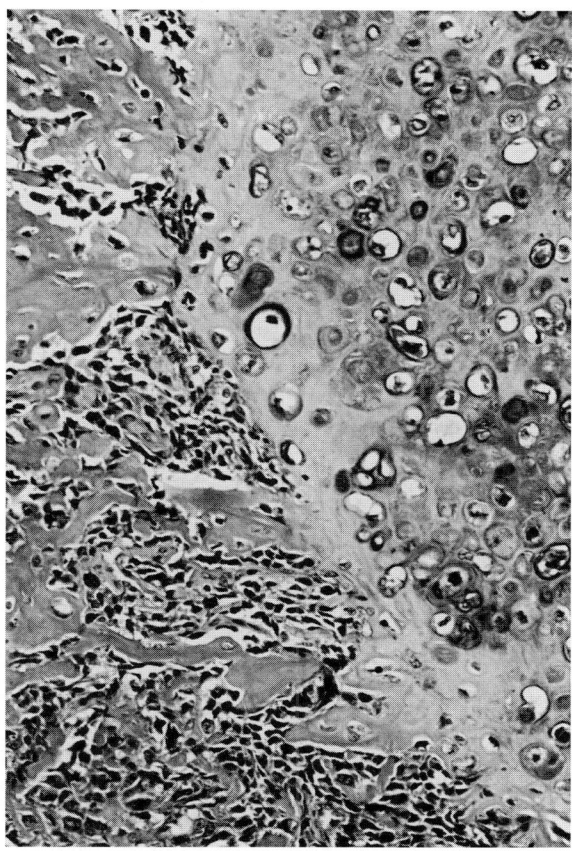

Figure 12-24 ■ Atypical cartilage in a conventional osteosarcoma.

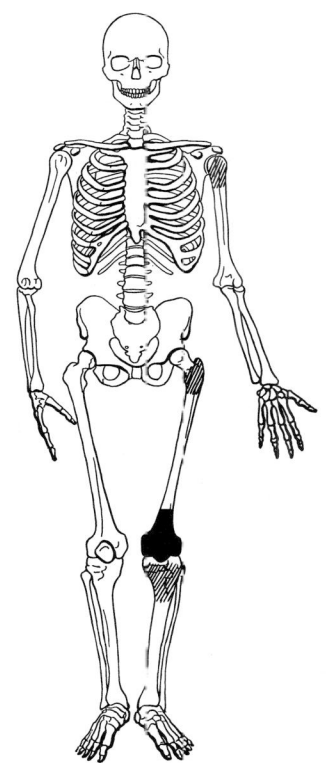

Figure 12-25 ■ Parosteal osteosarcoma locations.

in the medullary canal adjacent to the cortical origin of the soft tissue mass. This medullary component does not change the prognosis. In addition to the fibroosseous tissue, foci of mildly atypical cartilage, corresponding to the radiolucencies, may be present at the periphery of the mass. Dedifferentiation usually develops inside the bony mass. In this event, areas of high-grade osteosarcoma are juxtaposed to the low-grade fibroosseous tissue.

Differential Diagnosis. The most important differential diagnosis of parosteal osteosarcoma is myositis ossificans. Two radiologic features of myositis ossificans help distinguish these lesions. First, in the early stages, myositis ossifi-

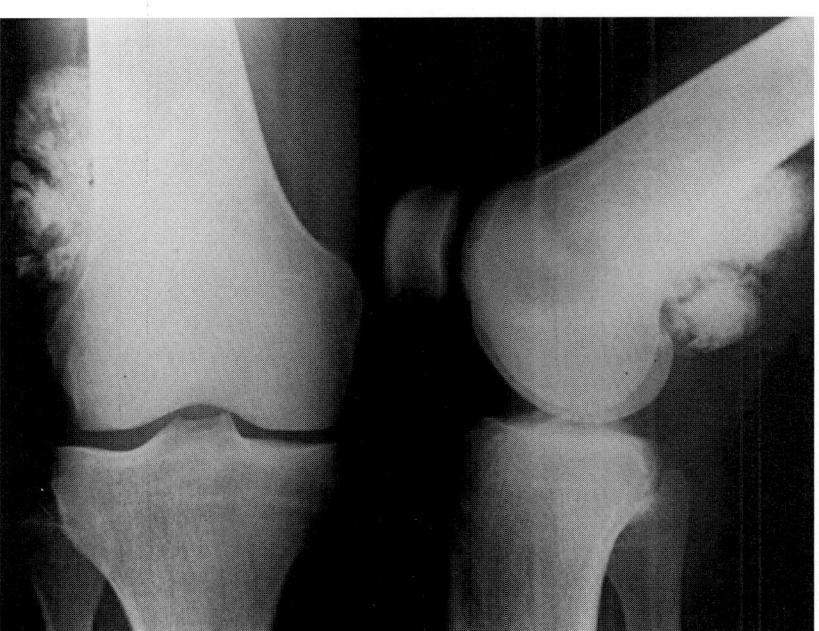

Figure 12-26 ■ Anteroposterior *(left)* and lateral radiographs of parosteal osteosarcoma of the distal femur. A radiodense surface lesion is present on the posterior lateral cortex.

cans has a zonal pattern of mineralization that is absent in parosteal osteosarcoma—mineralization is denser in the periphery of the juxtacortical mass. Second, mature lesions of myositis ossificans have distinct trabecular lines; a neocortex may even be present. By contrast, the mineralization in parosteal osteosarcoma is more homogeneous. Histologic features are also helpful in distinguishing these lesions. Myositis ossificans is a very cellular lesion with a zonal pattern of bone deposition. Parosteal osteosarcoma is less cellular, and the neoplastic bone is uniformly distributed.

Another lesion that may be confused radiographically with parosteal osteosarcoma is an osteochondroma. However, the cortex of the osteochondroma stalk is continuous with the native cortex, a feature that allows communication of the marrow cavity of the bone with that of the osteochondroma. By contrast, the native cortex beneath a parosteal osteosarcoma is uninterrupted.

Periosteal Osteosarcoma

Periosteal osteosarcoma, another surface variant of osteosarcoma, is much rarer than parosteal osteosarcoma. Unlike parosteal osteosarcoma, which extends from the cortex like a bony knob, periosteal osteosarcoma tightly encases the bone like a glove. As with most osteosarcomas, patients are

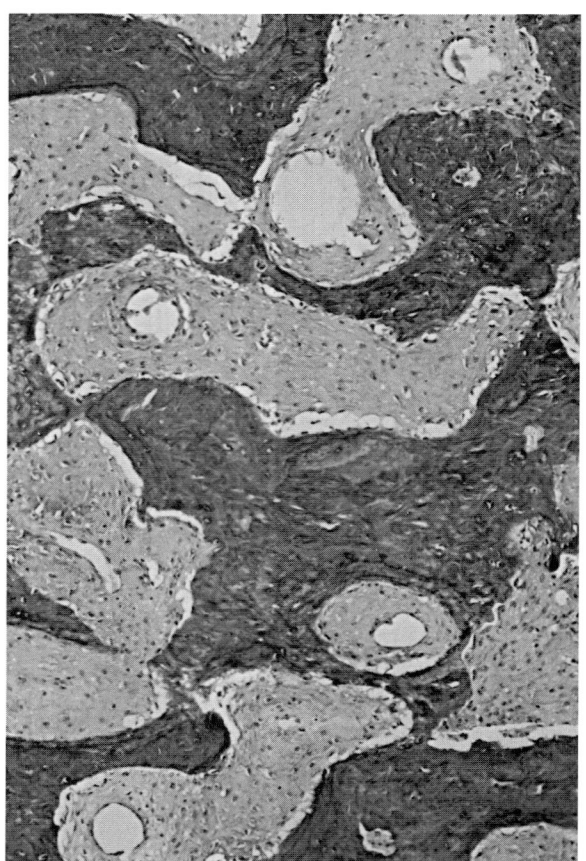

Figure 12-27 ■ Low-power photomicrograph of parosteal osteosarcoma. Broad seams of neoplastic osteoid are present in a bland fibrous background.

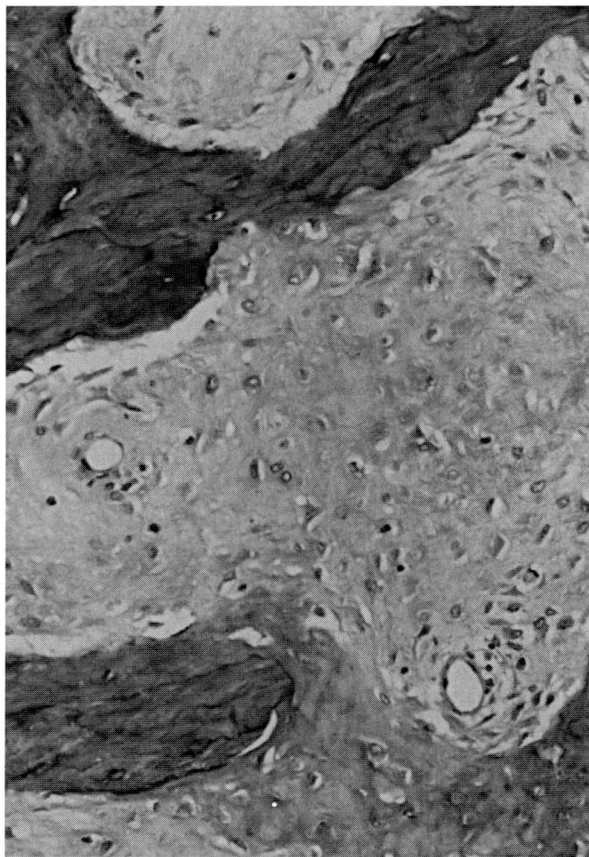

Figure 12-28 ■ High-power photomicrograph of periosteal osteosarcoma. The bland fibrous background is sparsely cellular and contains mildly atypical cells.

usually between 15 and 25 years of age and present with pain.[68] However, unlike other osteosarcomas, which usually develop in the metaphyseal portion of bone, periosteal osteosarcoma tends to involve the diaphysis. The tibia and femur are most frequently affected (Fig. 12-29). Other long bones may also be involved, but involvement of the flat bones is rare.

Radiographically, periosteal osteosarcoma is a circumferential surface mass that is less radiodense than parosteal osteosarcoma. Mineralization occurs as ring-shaped radiodensities or as streaks of reactive bone radiating from the cortex (Fig. 12-30). The cortex may be focally eroded, but the medullary canal is usually not involved.[69]

Periosteal osteosarcoma is a chondroblastic neoplasm. It consists almost entirely of lobules of cellular, atypical cartilage separated by thin bands of fibrous tissue (Fig. 12-31). Careful study of the fibrous bands reveals seams of neoplastic osteoid, usually at the outer surface of the neoplasm. This osteoid, often difficult to find, distinguishes this lesion from a surface chondrosarcoma. The cartilage shows focal calcification, and reactive bone forms between the cartilage lobules.

Intraosseous Well-Differentiated Osteosarcoma

Intraosseous well-differentiated osteosarcoma, also known as low-grade central osteosarcoma, is a rare fibroosseous malignant neoplasm accounting for only 2% of osteosarcomas. This lesion is histologically and prognostically similar to parosteal osteosarcoma but occurs in the medullary canal. Although it is a low-grade neoplasm, about 15% of low-grade intraosseous osteosarcomas dedifferentiate to high-grade osteosarcoma,[70] another similarity to parosteal osteosarcoma. Attesting to the usual slow growth of intraosseous well-differentiated osteosarcoma, symptoms, chiefly pain, are usually present for over a year. Patients range in age from 9 to 83 years, but most are in their 20s. The distal femur and proximal tibia account for about half the reported cases. However, any bone may be involved. Cases have been reported in the skull, spine, and small bones of the hands and feet.

Intraosseous well-differentiated osteosarcoma involves the metaphyseal region of bone and is usually confined to the medullary canal. Although reported lesions have varied in size from 2 to 25 cm in maximum dimension, most are large (average, 9 cm). Radiographically, the amount of matrix formation is variable. Most lesions are radiodense in either a diffuse or mottled pattern (Fig. 12–32). However, about one fourth of lesions are entirely radiolucent (Fig. 12–33). Although this neoplasm is usually poorly circumscribed, a feature reflecting infiltrative growth, it sometimes has a well-defined margin simulating a benign process. On very rare occasions, a well-differentiated osteosarcoma has both an intraosseous and a parosteal growth pattern.

The histologic features of well-differentiated intraosseous osteosarcoma are identical to parosteal osteosarcoma. How-

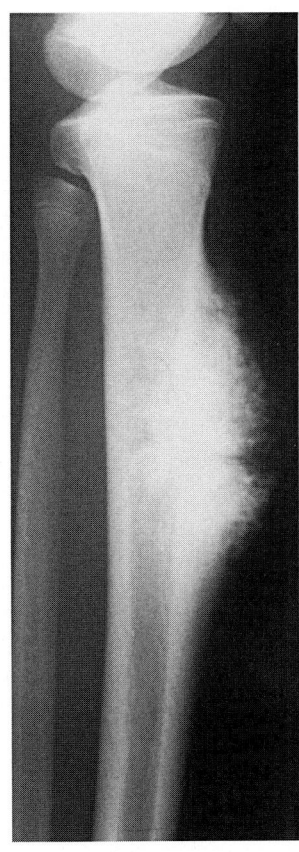 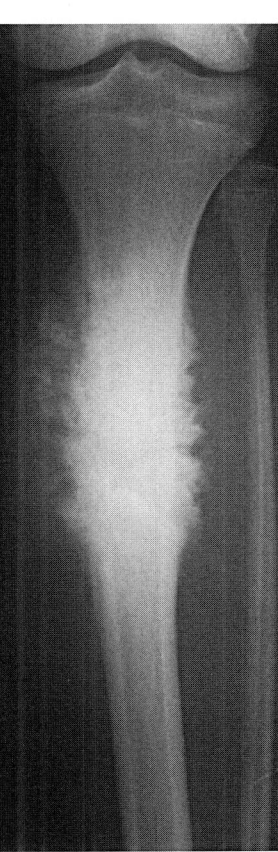

Figure 12-30 ■ Lateral *(left)* and anteroposterior radiographs of periosteal osteosarcoma of the tibia. A well-defined surface mass contains stippled and linear radiodensities.

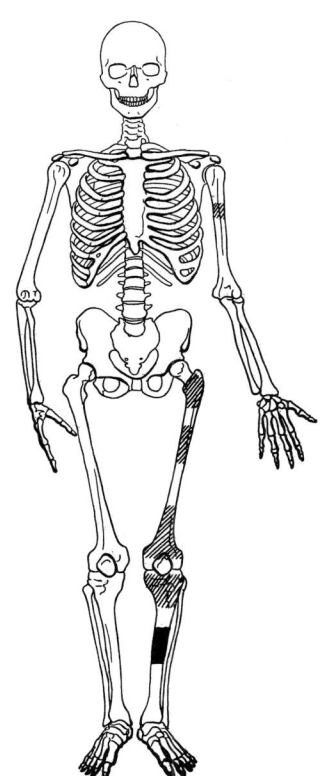

Figure 12-29 ■ Periosteal osteosarcoma locations.

ever, in well-differentiated intraosseous osteosarcoma, the fibroosseous neoplastic tissue grows inside the medullary canal. Seams of neoplastic bone are distributed throughout a bland fibrous stroma (Fig. 12–34). The neoplastic bone is often lamellar and contains remodeling lines, features indicating slow growth and maturation. The seams of neoplastic bone show extensive cross-connections and are arranged in a roughly parallel pattern. The fibrous stroma shows only mild cellular atypia and rare mitotic figures, features that belie the malignant nature of this neoplasm. Occasionally, neoplasms are almost entirely fibrous and contain only scant amounts of neoplastic bone. This histologic pattern corresponds to the purely lytic manifestation occasionally seen on plain radiographs. Like parosteal osteosarcoma, well-differentiated intraosseous osteosarcoma contains occasional islands of atypical cartilage, present in 18% of cases. Careful search through areas of the low-grade fibrous neoplasm is necessary to rule out dedifferentiation to a high-grade osteoblastic osteosarcoma.

An important differential diagnosis of intraosseous well-differentiated osteosarcoma is fibrous dysplasia. Occasionally, distinguishing these lesions is difficult. In fact, many reported cases of malignant transformation of fibrous dysplasia were probably misdiagnosed intraosseous well-differentiated osteosarcomas. Two important distinguishing features

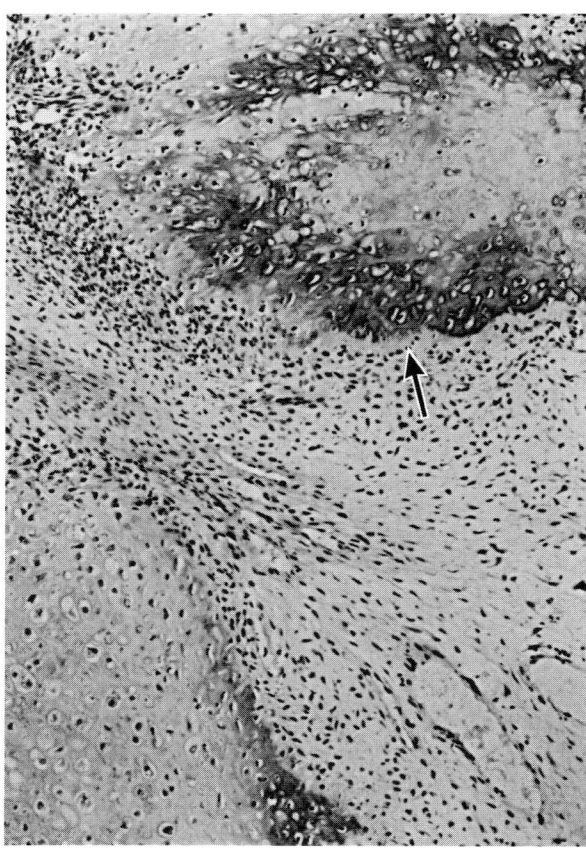

Figure 12-31 ■ Low-power photomicrograph of periosteal osteosarcoma. Atypical cartilage is present in a fibrous background. Mineralizing osteoid is also present *(arrow)*.

Figure 12-32 ■ Oblique *(left)* and anteroposterior radiographs of well-differentiated intraosseous osteosarcoma of the distal tibia. A well-defined intramedullary radiodensity is present in the metaphysis and epiphysis. (From McCarthy, E. F.: *Differential Diagnosis in Pathology. Bone and Joint Disorders.* New York and Tokyo, Igaku-Shoin, 1996. With permission from Williams & Wilkins.)

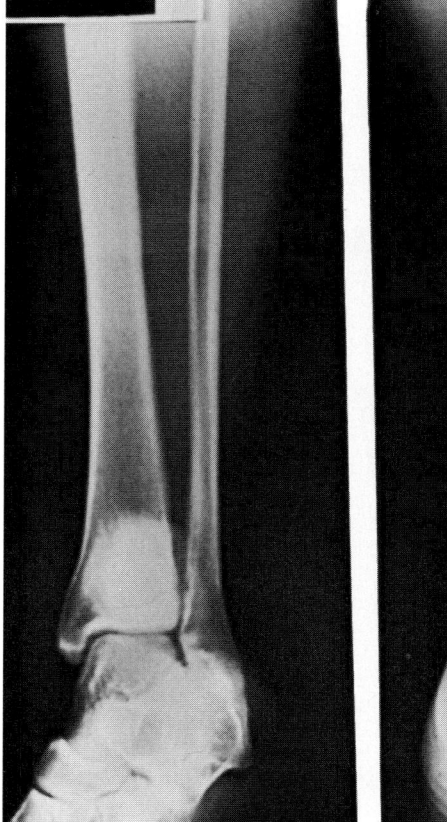
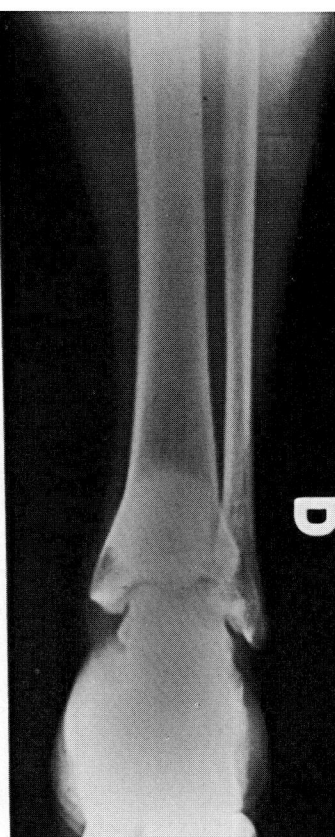

exist. First, the fibrous tissue stroma of fibrous dysplasia, although occasionally very cellular, never shows cytologic atypia. By contrast, mild cellular atypia is characteristic of well-differentiated intraosseous osteosarcoma. Second, the lesional bone in fibrous dysplasia is woven bone and is deposited as thin isolated trabeculae arranged in curved shapes reminiscent of Chinese letters. This differs from the broad interconnected trabeculae, usually containing remodeling lines, of intraosseous well-differentiated osteosarcoma.

Telangiectatic Osteosarcoma

Telangiectatic osteosarcomas are high-grade intramedullary osteosarcomas that have undergone total, or near total aneurysmal bone cyst change.[71] This rare variant, accounting for only 4% of all osteosarcomas, is completely lytic on plain radiographic images. Histologically, these lesions contain many blood-filled spaces, a feature of the aneurysmal bone cyst process.

Although patients may be any age, most, as in conventional osteosarcoma, are in the second decade of life. Pain and rapid swelling are the presenting symptoms. Because this neoplasm is highly destructive, 25% of patients present with pathologic fracture.[72] Over 60% of cases occur in the distal femur or proximal tibia[73] (Fig. 12–35). The humerus is also a common location. Additionally, the osteosarcomas that complicate long-standing Paget's disease are frequently the telangiectatic variant.

Telangiectatic osteosarcomas are lytic lesions with no radiographic mineralization. Therefore, unlike other osteosarcomas, the clue to their osteoid-producing nature is lacking.

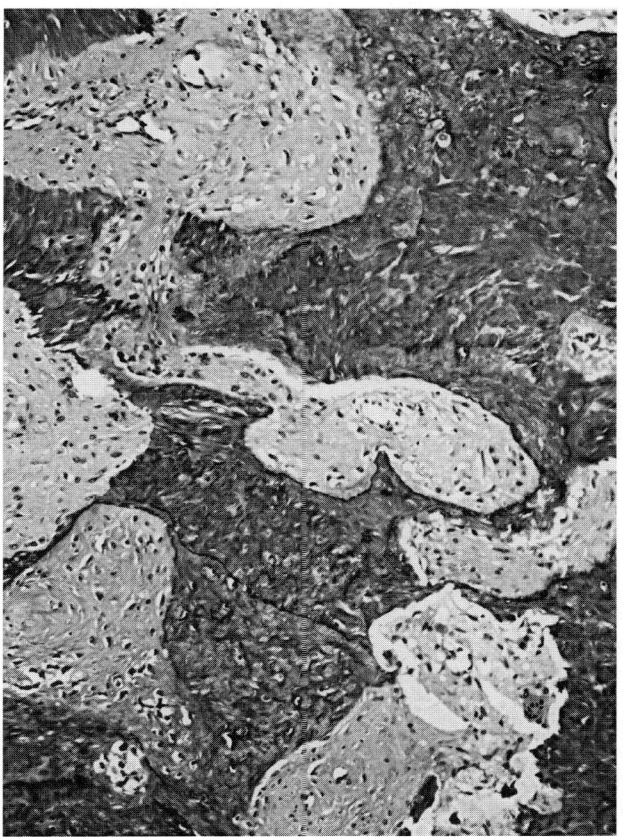

Figure 12-34 ■ Photomicrograph of a well-differentiated intramedullary osteosarcoma. Broad seams of neoplastic bone are present in a bland fibrous background.

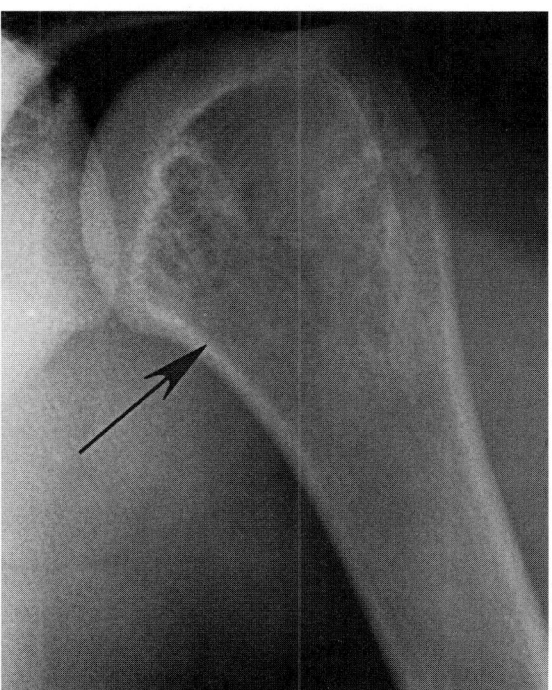

Figure 12-33 ■ Well-differentiated intramedullary osteosarcoma of the proximal humerus. A poorly defined area of radiolucency (arrow) with faint mineralizations is present in the metaphysis.

In fact, the radiographic pattern may be identical to an aneurysmal bone cyst engrafted on a benign process. Extensive cortical expansion or destruction and often a soft tissue mass are seen. A periosteal new bone reaction is present in over 75% of cases (Fig. 12–36). The MRI often shows multiple fluid-filled locules, a pattern identical to aneurysmal bone cyst (Fig. 12–37).

Histologically, telangiectatic osteosarcomas are characterized by many blood-filled cystic cavities and areas of hemorrhagic necrosis. Areas of stroma resembling benign aneurysmal bone cyst are present (Fig. 12–38). These areas are cellular, with numerous mitotic figures. In addition, many benign osteoclast-like giant cells are present, a feature characteristic of almost all telangiectatic osteosarcomas.

The diagnostic feature of telangiectatic osteosarcoma is the presence of areas of high-grade sarcoma (Fig. 12–39). Markedly atypical pleomorphic cells and many atypical mitotic figures are seen. These areas, although only focally present, are easily recognized as malignant and can almost always be found if the entire specimen is meticulously examined histologically. Tumor osteoid may be scarce in telangiectatic osteosarcomas and is often not present in small biopsy specimens. Where present, this osteoid has a fine, lace-like pattern.

Telangiectatic osteosarcoma is difficult to distinguish from an aneurysmal bone cyst, especially if the aneurysmal bone cyst is highly destructive or if it contains abundant reactive bone. However, the reactive bone is deposited in broad seams and is unlike the lace-like osteoid of telangiectatic osteosarcoma. Furthermore, areas of sarcomatous stroma, focally present in telangiectatic osteosarcomas, are absent in aneurysmal bone cyst.

Small Cell Osteosarcoma

Small cell osteosarcoma, another rare osteosarcoma variant, is characterized by seams of neoplastic osteoid variably distributed in sheets of small round blue cells. Therefore, this neoplasm may be confused with other small round blue cell tumors. Patients with small cell osteosarcoma have a clinical presentation similar to those with conventional osteosarcoma. A rare patient may be younger than 5 years or older than 80, but most are in their teens or 20s.[74] Lesions in the distal femur, proximal tibia, and proximal femur account for over half of the reported cases.

Small cell osteosarcomas generally have a very permeative radiographic pattern, a feature similar to Ewing sarcoma (Fig. 12–40). In addition, cortical destruction is common. However, unlike Ewing sarcoma, mineralization, sometimes extensive, is present in small cell osteosarcomas. Often, the mineralization is present in the metaphyseal portion of the lesion and tapers off in the diaphysis, which shows a permeative radiolytic pattern. This zonal distribution of mineralization is a radiographic feature highly suggestive of small cell osteosarcoma.[75]

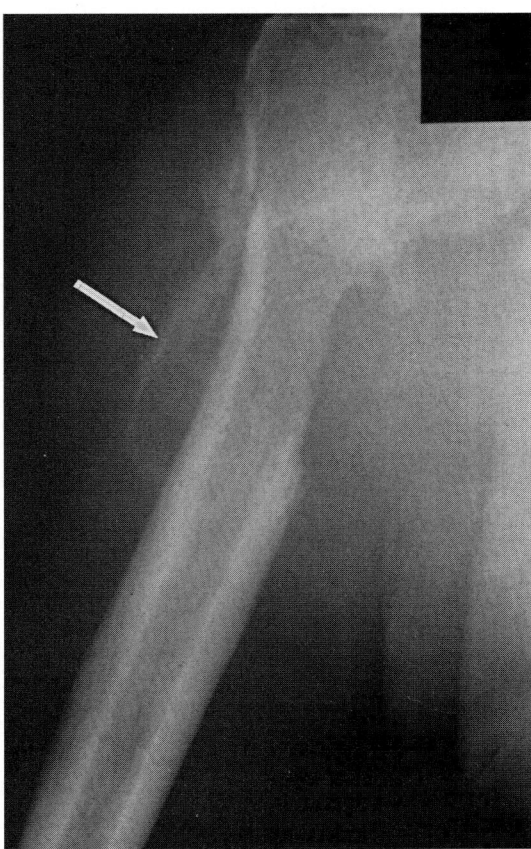

Figure 12-36 ■ Telangiectatic osteosarcoma of the proximal humerus. The lesion is a poorly defined radiolytic area. Abundant reactive periosteal bone is present *(arrow)*.

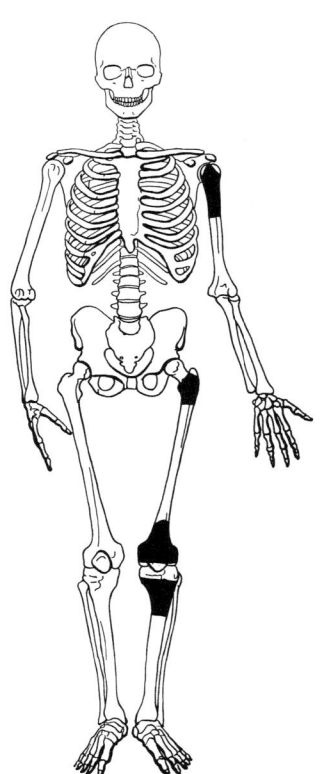

Figure 12-35 ■ Telangiectatic osteosarcoma locations.

Histologically, the neoplastic cells of small cell osteosarcomas resemble those of other small round blue cell tumors. Three histologic patterns are possible.[76] First, the cells of two thirds of small cell osteosarcomas resemble those of Ewing sarcoma (Fig. 12–41). They have round, densely hyperchromatic nuclei with dense, coarsely clumped chromatin. The cytoplasm of these cells is scanty. The second pattern resembles large cell lymphomas. These cells have more abundant cytoplasm and a larger, more vesicular nucleus, often with a prominent nucleolus. The third, but much less common, histologic pattern is densely packed small spindle cells. In addition to the cells, osteoid is variably distributed throughout the stroma, and often it has a lace-like pattern. Foci of atypical cartilage are present in about a third of cases.

Small cell osteosarcoma must be distinguished from other small round blue cell neoplasms. The cells of small cell osteosarcoma do not stain for common leukocyte antigen or B-cell markers and can be thus distinguished from primary lymphoma of bone. However, the cells of small cell osteosarcoma often contain glycogen and sometimes contain neuron-specific enolase.[77] Therefore, stains for these substances do not distinguish small cell osteosarcoma from Ewing sarcoma or peripheral neuroectodermal tumor. These entities can be excluded only by the presence of neoplastic osteoid.

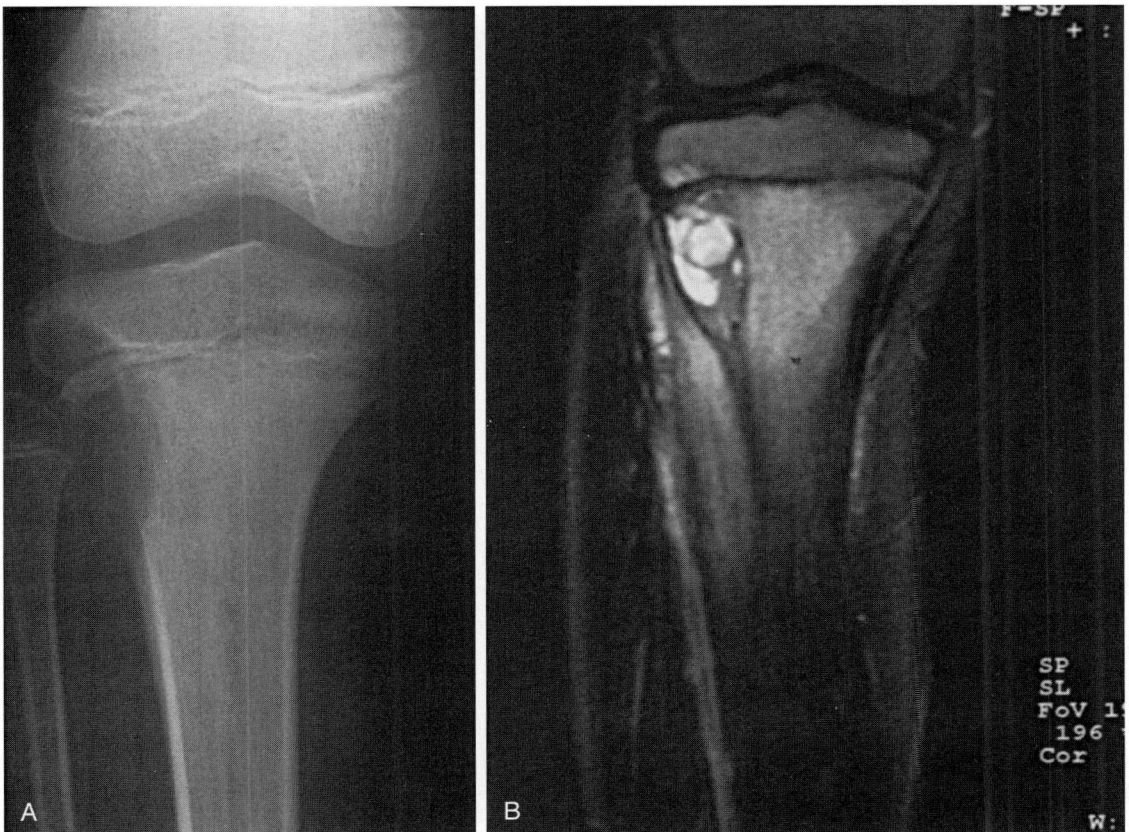

Figure 12-37 ■ Telangiectatic osteosarcoma of proximal tibia. **A,** Plain radiograph showing a lucency in the epiphysis and metaphysis. One cortex is destroyed. **B,** T_2-weighted MRI showing locules of bright signal corresponding to blood.

Multicentric Osteosarcoma

On very rare occasions, a patient may develop osteosarcomas in several bones. This variant, known as multicentric osteosarcoma, has two distinct presentations: synchronous and metachronous.[78]

Osteosarcomas that present synchronously are conventional osteosarcomas. They exhibit the radiographic and histologic features of typical high-grade osteoblastic osteosarcoma. Patients are usually children, and the multiosseous involvement is usually symmetric, each lesion being at about the same stage of development. This variant is rapidly fatal, usually within 1 year.

In contrast to the high-grade features of the synchronous variant, lesions of the metachronous variant show low-grade osteoblastic features. Patients are usually older, in their 20s or 30s, when the first lesions appear. In contrast to the synchronous variant in which lesions occur in typical osteosarcoma locations, lesions of the metachronous variant favor the axial skeleton—the pelvis, spine, shoulder girdle, or skull. Patients with this variant usually have a long clinical course, with new lesions showing up every year or so. Ultimately, however, this variant is also fatal.

Intracortical and High-Grade Surface Osteosarcoma

Intracortical osteosarcoma is a high-grade osteoblastic osteosarcoma with a very distinctive radiographic presentation—the lesion looks almost exactly like an osteoid osteoma.[79,80] Radiographically, this variant is a well-defined intracortical lucency surrounded by a sclerotic rim. The average size is 1.5 cm. Almost all cases involve the femur or tibia of children. Histologically, neoplastic osteoid is associated with atypical stromal cells. Entrapment of islands of native cortex, a reflection of destructive growth, distinguishes this extremely rare lesion from an osteoid osteoma. Although a high-grade sarcoma, the small size and localized growth of intracortical osteosarcoma affords excellent therapeutic results.

High-grade surface osteosarcoma is another very rare variant of osteosarcoma. This neoplasm is histologically indistinguishable from conventional osteosarcoma. However, it arises on the bone surface like parosteal or periosteal osteosarcoma.[81] Although microscopic cortical invasion is present in a majority of cases, this feature is not apparent radiographically. The typical radiographic pattern is a partially mineralized surface mass with adjacent Codman's triangles of reactive bone. Some of these lesions may represent small parosteal osteosarcomas that have been effaced by a dedifferentiated component. The behavior of high-grade surface osteosarcoma is similar to that of conventional osteosarcoma.

Treatment of Osteosarcoma

The treatment of high-grade intramedullary osteosarcomas has evolved considerably over the past 20 years. Prior to the

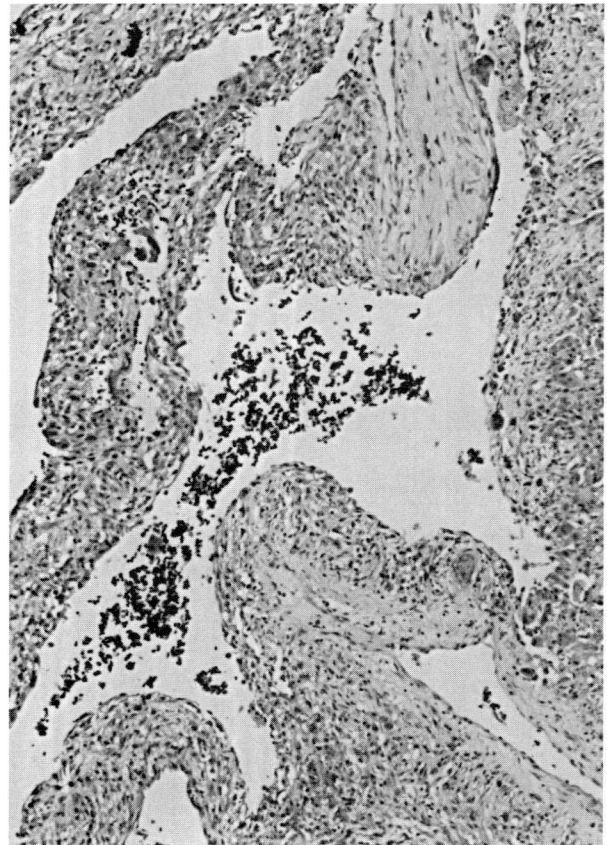

Figure 12-38 ■ Low-power photomicrograph of blood-filled lakes from a telangiectatic osteosarcoma. This pattern is similar to aneurysmal bone cyst.

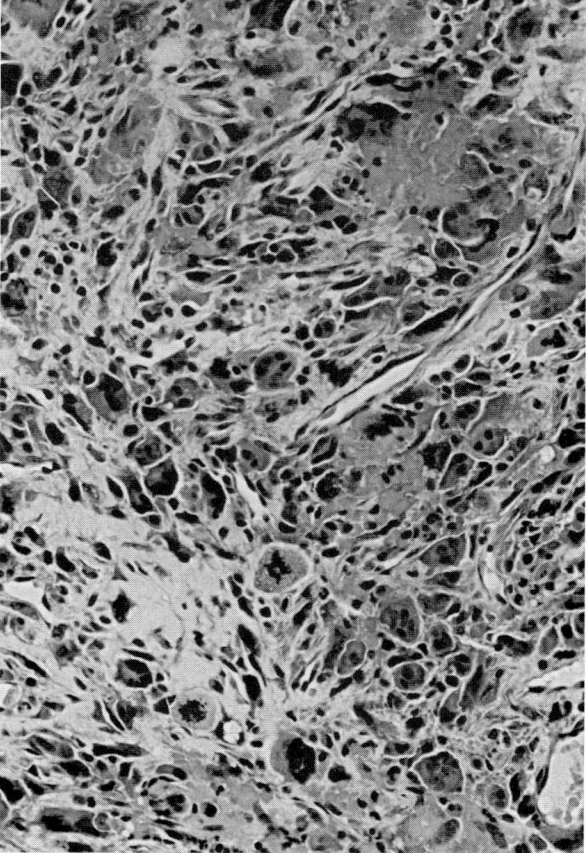

Figure 12-39 ■ Sarcomatous area from telangiectatic osteosarcoma. Bizarre atypical cells are present, as are numerous mitotic figures.

discovery of effective multiagent chemotherapy regimens, the prognosis was dismal. Amputation was the definitive form of treatment, and, unfortunately, pulmonary metastases developed within 2 years in 80 to 90% of cases. Multiagent chemotherapy is now routinely used preoperatively. Ideally, this preoperative therapy, known as *neoadjuvant chemotherapy,* kills 95 to 100% of the tumor. Following neoadjuvant treatment, staging studies are repeated to evaluate the feasibility of limb salvage surgery. About 90% of patients are limb salvage candidates, and the tumor is resected en bloc with a wide margin. Many novel reconstructive techniques are possible, including custom-made prostheses, osteoarticular allografts, allograft-prosthetic composites, and allograft arthrodeses (Fig. 12–42). When the tumor kill is extensive (> 90% of the tumor is necrotic), the prognosis is excellent, with long-term survival of over 70% and a local recurrence rate less than 10%. Maintenance chemotherapy is then given for 6 to 12 months. If localized pulmonary metastases develop, they are removed with one or more thoracotomies.

Parosteal osteosarcomas and well-differentiated intramedullary osteosarcomas are low-grade lesions, and the risk of developing systemic metastases is less than 5%. If the tumor can be removed successfully, almost all patients are cured. Partial removal results in local recurrence. Accordingly, recent trends have favored resecting the entire lesion and reconstructing the limb with a prosthesis or allograft. Che-

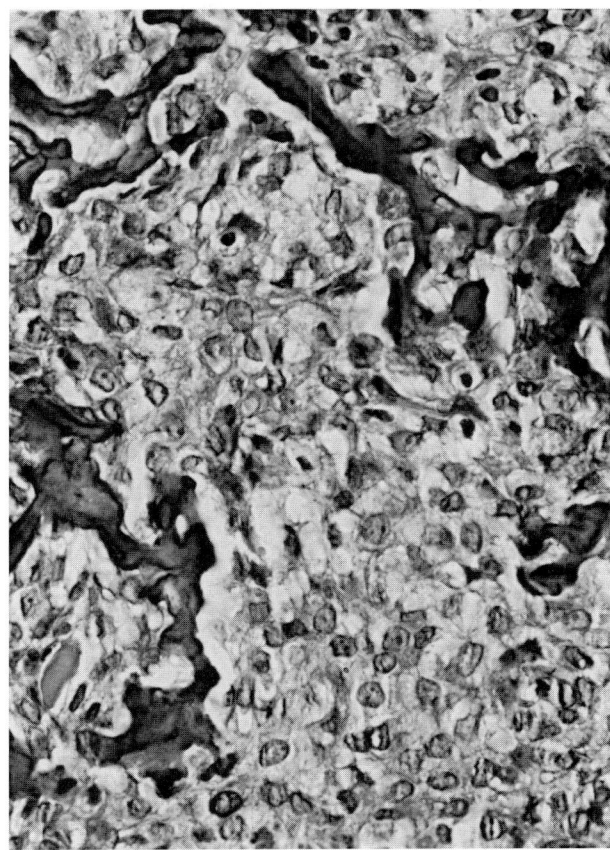

Figure 12–41 ■ Photomicrograph of small cell osteosarcoma. Small round cells are present in sheets, and they are associated with seams of neoplastic osteoid.

motherapy is not utilized either preoperatively or postoperatively.

In contrast to parosteal osteosarcomas, periosteal osteosarcomas and high-grade surface osteosarcomas have a much higher risk of systemic metastases. Both of these high-grade surface lesions are treated similarly to high-grade intramedullary osteosarcomas—preoperative chemotherapy, resection, and postoperative chemotherapy.

Pathologic Evaluation of Resected Osteosarcoma Specimens

The pathologist plays a crucial role in the management of osteosarcoma by quantifying the effect of neoadjuvant chemotherapy.[82,83] The extent of tumor necrosis in the resected specimen correlates with prognosis. For example, a kill percentage of greater than 90% is associated with a 91% survival rate. By contrast, less than 90% tumor necrosis offers only a 14% survival. Based on the amount of tumor necrosis, chemotherapy regimens may be continued or altered.

The percent of necrotic tumor may be estimated by calculating the tumor necrosis present in a slab of the neoplasm that is 0.8 cm thick. The specimen should be bivalved in a plane that displays the greatest amount of neoplasm. This

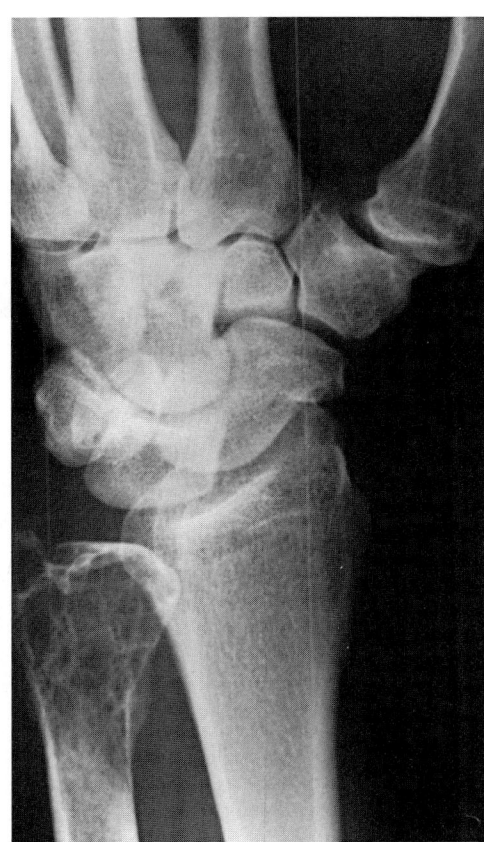

Figure 12–40 ■ Small cell osteosarcoma of the distal ulna. A poorly defined radiolytic area is adjacent to the articular surface.

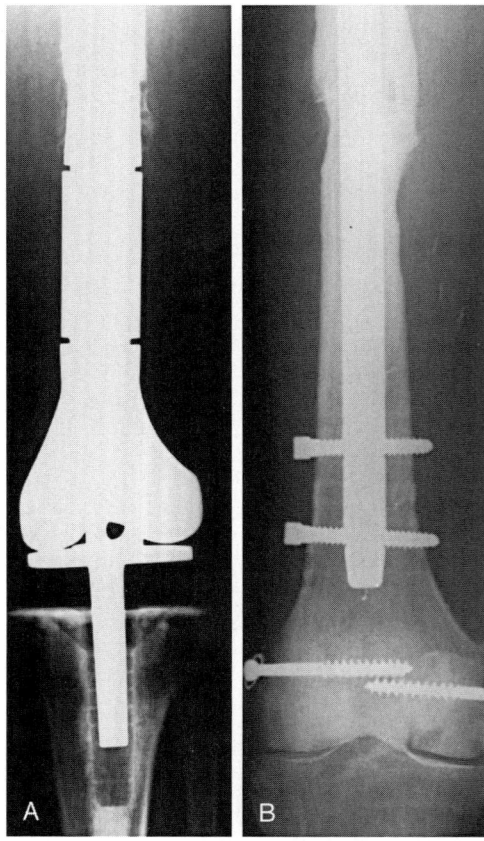

Figure 12–42 ■ Reconstruction options following limb-sparing resection of an osteosarcoma from the distal femur. **A,** A custom-built distal femoral prosthesis. **B,** A distal femoral allograft.

of hyaline cartilage. The first group consists of two benign neoplasms: chondroblastoma and chondromyxoid fibroma. These neoplasms, which probably arise from precursor cells in the epiphyseal plate, occur most commonly in children and are confined to the medullary canal. They occur in distinctive locations relative to the epiphyseal plate—chondroblastoma is centered in the epiphysis, and chondromyxoid fibroma involves the metaphysis. Because the cartilage of these lesions is incompletely differentiated, they are usually poorly mineralized and present as well-defined radiolucencies.

Although only two lesions of incompletely differentiated cartilage exist, lesions of hyaline cartilage are numerous. These lesions are composed of differentiated chondrocytes in an abundant extracellular matrix. Cartilage mineralization is often extensive, a process that leads to the characteristic radiographic feature of most of these lesions—ring-shaped and stippled radiodensities.

Hyaline cartilage lesions may be subclassified into those that arise in the medullary canal and those that arise on the bone surfaces (Fig. 12–45). Benign and malignant lesions occur in both locations. Another process, synovial chondromatosis, also consists of hyaline cartilage but occurs in the soft tissues or inside joints. Although synovial chondromatosis is a metaplastic process rather than a neoplasm, it is also characterized by a ring and stippled pattern of mineralization.

The first step in the diagnosis of hyaline cartilage lesions is to localize the rings and stipples to either the surface or can be determined by correlation with plain radiographs or CT scan. After the specimen is bivalved, a slab may be removed with a parallel saw cut.

First, the slab should be radiographed and then photographed (Fig. 12–43). Then, to plan the microscopic analysis, an image of the specimen should be made on a photocopy machine, preferably in color. A grid is drawn on the photocopy, and the specimen is blocked and labeled according to the grid (Fig. 12–44). Usually, 15 to 30 tissue blocks are required to examine the entire slab histologically.

The next step is the histologic examination of the slides. The amount of tumor necrosis is calculated in each slide and then averaged for the entire neoplasm. Deciding whether a neoplasm is necrotic requires practice. The process is sometimes complicated by the replacement of necrotic tumor by viable granulation tissue. Areas with this reparative tissue should be regarded as necrotic neoplasm. One objective feature indicating necrosis of the neoplastic tissue is loss of nuclear detail.

CARTILAGE LESIONS

Cartilage neoplasms may be divided into two groups: lesions of incompletely differentiated cartilage and lesions

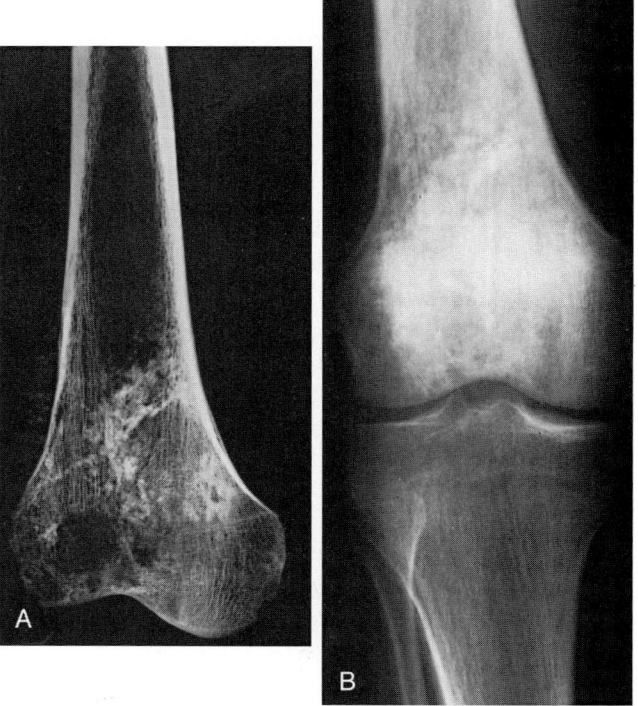

Figure 12–43 ■ Osteosarcoma of the distal femur. **A,** Radiograph of a slab of the resected specimen. **B,** Plain radiograph of the lesion before surgery.

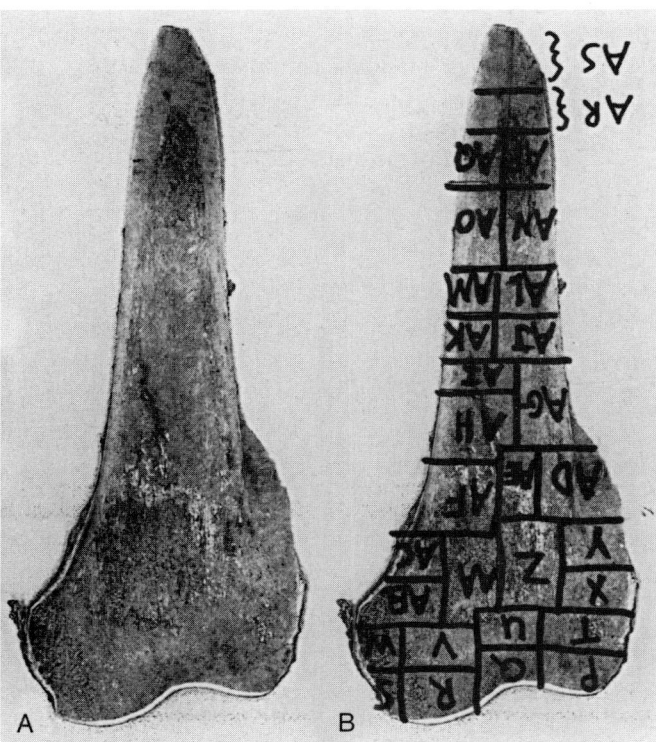

Figure 12-44 ■ Osteosarcoma in the distal femur after resection. **A,** Image of a slab of the specimen made on a photocopy machine. **B,** Same image with a grid corresponding to histologic blocks. The entire slab is examined histologically to quantitate the amount of tumor necrosis.

the medullary canal. The distinction between benign and malignant must be made by a combination of clinical, radiographic, and histologic features. Because the histologic features of benign and low-grade malignant cartilage overlap, the clinical and radiographic features are the key in predicting the behavior of hyaline cartilage lesions.

Chondroblastoma

Chondroblastoma is a rare benign neoplasm of fetal-type cartilage differentiation. Although reported in patients ranging in age from 3 to 72 years, over 50% of lesions occur in patients between the ages of 15 and 25.[84] Approximately 70% of chondroblastomas occur in the long bones, most commonly the proximal humerus, followed by the distal femur and proximal tibia[85] (Fig. 12-46). In the long bones, the center of the lesion is almost always the epiphysis. Other bones commonly involved are the proximal femur, the small bones of the feet, and temporal bone of the skull. Very rarely, multiple sites are involved.[86] Chondroblastoma almost never occurs in the spine. Patients usually present with pain. In addition, because of epiphyseal involvement, joint symptoms, such as stiffness or effusion, are common.

Radiologically, chondroblastoma is usually a well-circumscribed lytic lesion that, when in a long bone, involves the epiphysis (Fig. 12-47). About 50% of lesions extend into the metaphysis, a feature usually seen only when the epiphyseal plate is closed. Most lesions lack a sclerotic rim. Varying degrees of stippled calcification are present in 40% of lesions, the remainder being completely lucent. Chondroblastomas average 4.3 cm in maximal dimension, but they may be as large as 19 cm. Occasionally, they expand or destroy the cortex.

Histologically, chondroblastoma is composed of sheets of stromal cells, scattered multinucleated giant cells, and varying amounts of chondroid matrix (Fig. 12-48). The stromal cells, resembling fetal chondroblasts, are distinctive. They are round with an abundant cytoplasm, and they usually have distinct cytoplasmic membranes. The nuclei are also round and are located in the center of the cytoplasm, imparting a "fried egg" appearance to the cells (Fig. 12-49). The nuclei have faintly clumped chromatin and often have a grooved or folded membrane. Some chondroblastomas have slightly enlarged atypical nuclei. Mitotic figures are rare among the stromal cells. In most chondroblastomas, these stromal cells are positive with the immunohistochemical stain for S-100 protein.[87] In addition to the stromal cells, multinucleated giant cells, often with many nuclei, are scattered unevenly throughout the neoplasm. These giant cells are immunohistochemically distinct from the stromal cells. They lack S-100 positivity but stain for macrophage-associated antigens.[88] This staining characteristic suggests that the giant cells do not form by fusion of stromal cells.

Admixed with the stromal cells and giant cells is a varying amount of faintly bluish extracellular matrix (Fig. 12-50). In addition, foci of overtly cartilaginous matrix are usually present. In these areas, the stromal cells are in discrete lacunae. The matrix may be calcified, usually around individual cells, imparting a "chicken wire" appearance (Fig. 12-51). Reactive bone may also be present in varying amounts. Some chondroblastomas have areas indistinguishable from chondromyxoid fibroma of bone, particularly if the lesion partially involves the metaphysis. In addition, 31% of lesions have foci of aneurysmal bone cyst change.[84]

Chondroblastoma is a benign, slow-growing neoplasm that is best treated with curettage and bone grafting. A recurrence rate of 10 to 20% can be expected following curettage. Most recurrences, which usually develop within 3 years, are successfully treated by a second curettage. Rarely, chondroblastoma is locally destructive. Another rare behavior is pulmonary metastasis, the so-called "benign metastasizing chondroblastoma."[89] Growth of these rare metastatic foci is very slow, and they are usually treated successfully by pulmonary wedge resections.

Chondromyxoid Fibroma

Chondromyxoid fibroma, like chondroblastoma, is also characterized by incomplete cartilage differentiation. However, unlike chondroblastoma, which involves the epiphysis, chondromyxoid fibroma in the long bones always occurs in the metaphysis or metadiaphysis. Most lesions occur in patients younger than 35 years, and the peak incidence (36%

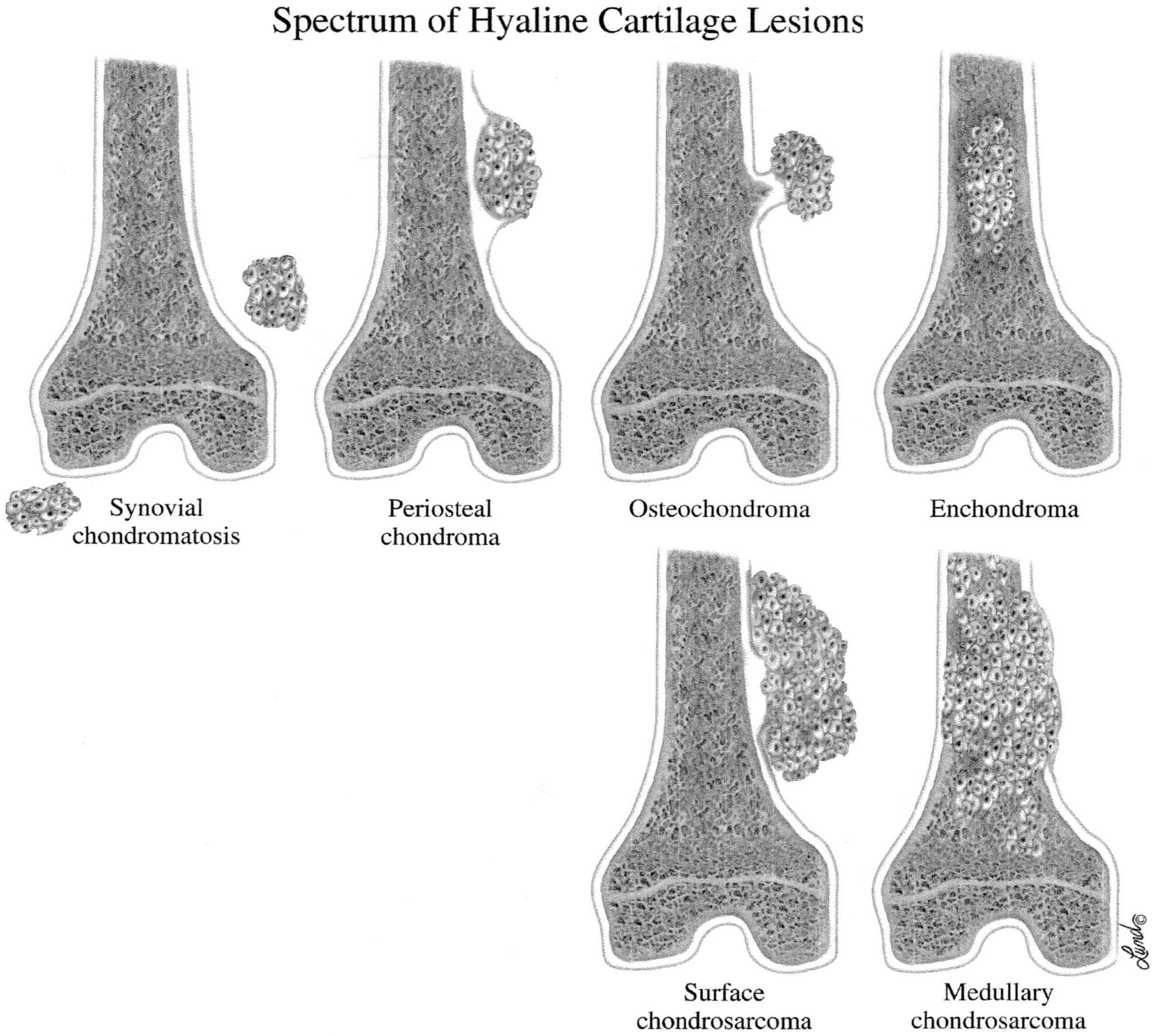

Spectrum of Hyaline Cartilage Lesions

Synovial chondromatosis

Periosteal chondroma

Osteochondroma

Enchondroma

Surface chondrosarcoma

Medullary chondrosarcoma

Figure 12-45 ■ Hyaline cartilage lesions. These lesions are all characterized by stippled and ring-shaped radiodensities. They are located either in the medullary canal or on the bone surface. Correlating the pattern of radiodensities with their location is the first step toward the correct radiographic diagnosis.

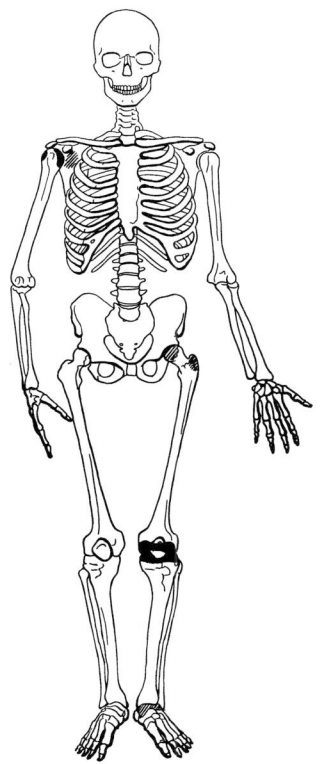

Figure 12-46 ■ Chondroblastoma locations.

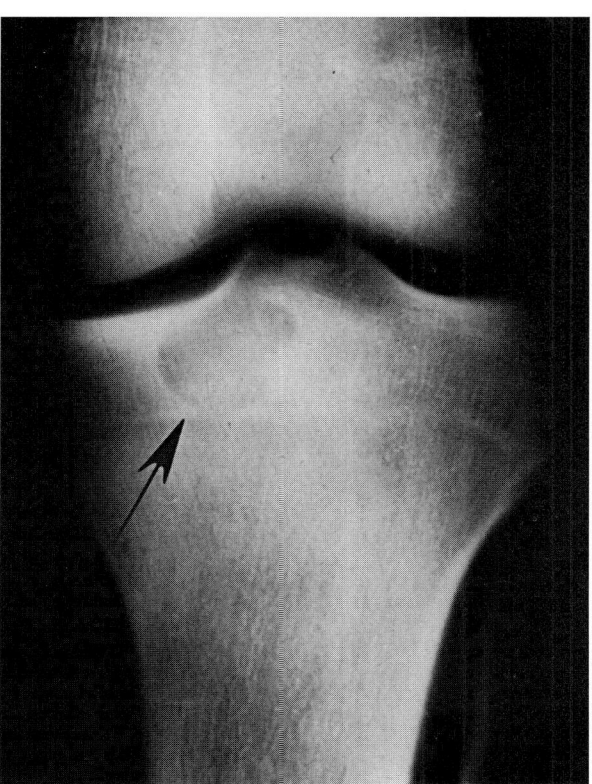

Figure 12-47 ■ Chondroblastoma of the proximal tibial epiphysis. A well-defined lucency is surrounded by a thin sclerotic rim *(arrow)*. (From McCarthy, E. F.: *Differential Diagnosis in Pathology. Bone and Joint Disorders.* New York and Tokyo, Igaku-Shoin, 1996. With permission from Williams & Wilkins.)

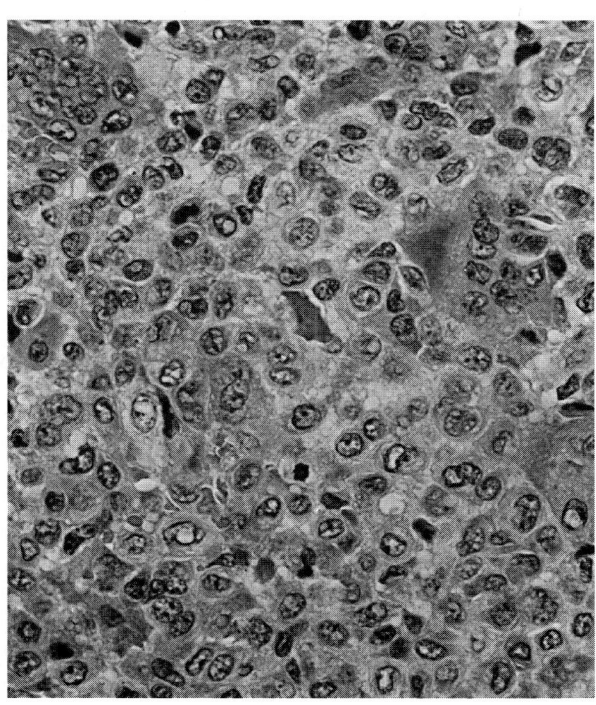

Figure 12-48 ■ Photomicrograph of a chondroblastoma showing multinucleated giant cells admixed with round stromal cells.

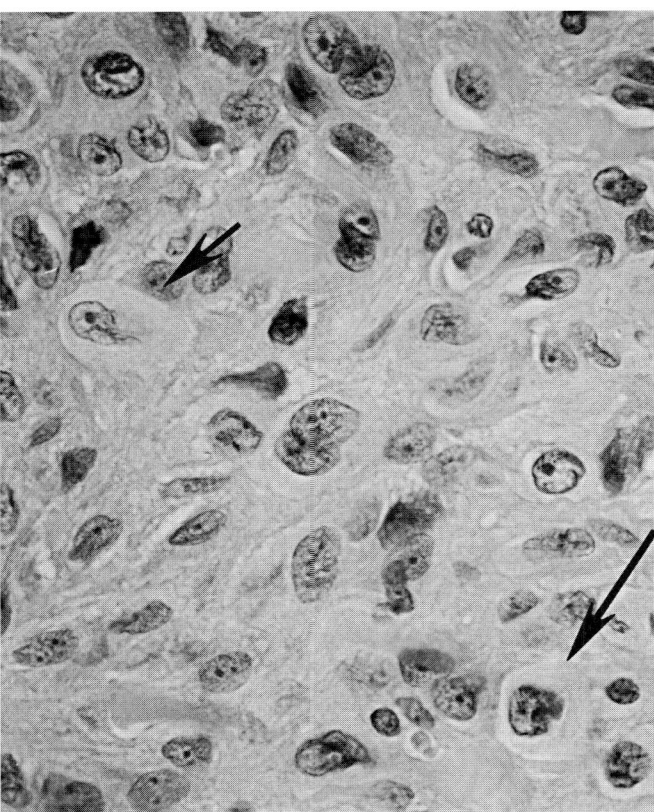

Figure 12-49 ■ High-power photomicrograph of chondroblastoma stromal cells. Round nuclei are present in abundant cytoplasms. Some cells have the characteristic "fried egg" appearance *(arrows)*.

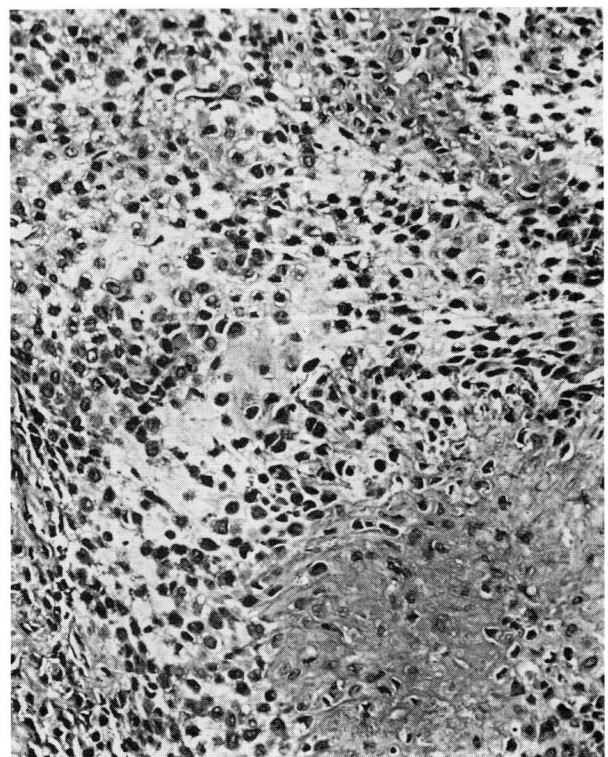

Figure 12-50 ■ Photomicrograph of chondroblastoma showing an area with extensive extracellular chondroid matrix.

Figure 12-51 ■ High-power photomicrograph of a chondroblastoma showing calcification of the matrix. The calcification has a "chicken wire" appearance.

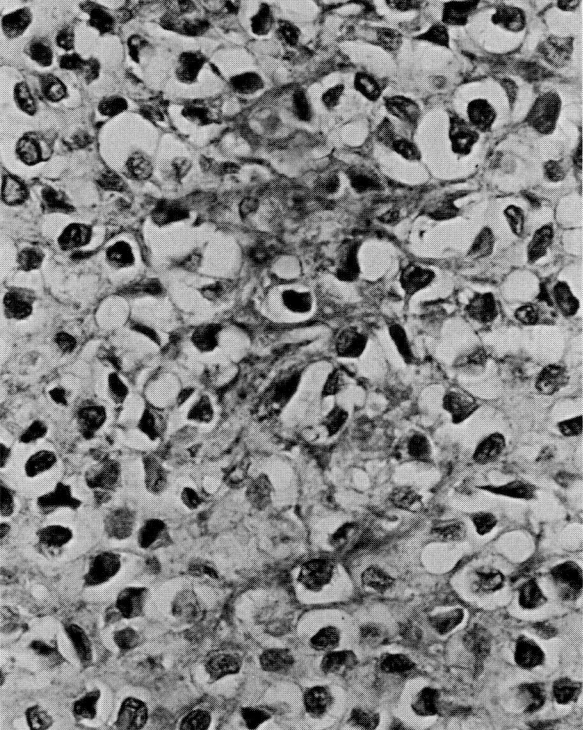

of cases) is in patients between ages 10 and 20.[90,91] However, patients as old as 70 may develop a chondromyxoid fibroma. The distal femur and proximal tibia are the most common sites[92] (Fig. 12–52). Chondromyxoid fibroma is also common in the pelvis and in the bones of the hands and feet. Pain and mild swelling are the usual presenting symptoms. On rare occasions, a chondromyxoid fibroma may be asymptomatic.

Chondromyxoid fibroma, when in a long bone, is a metaphyseal lesion that usually abuts one cortex (Fig. 12–53). Occasionally, lesions involve a portion of the epiphysis if the plate is closed. In all locations, lesions are radiographically well circumscribed and often have a sclerotic margin. Some lesions, particularly in the pelvis, have a multiloculated, "soap bubble" appearance, and some have a scalloped margin (Fig. 12–54). Lesions range in size from 2 to 10 cm in maximal dimension. An important radiographic feature of chondromyxoid fibroma is the rarity of intralesional calcification.

Chondromyxoid fibroma has distinctive histologic features. Elongated or stellate cells are present in an abundant extracellular chondroid matrix (Fig. 12–55). Two important features seen with low-power examination are a lobular growth pattern (Fig. 12–56) and sharp demarcation from the surrounding bone. Cellularity is variable, but each lobule tends to be more cellular at the periphery. The peripheral cells are more spindle shaped and appear to separate the lobules by fibrous bands. The fibrous bands contain blood vessels and often osteoclast-like giant cells. The character of

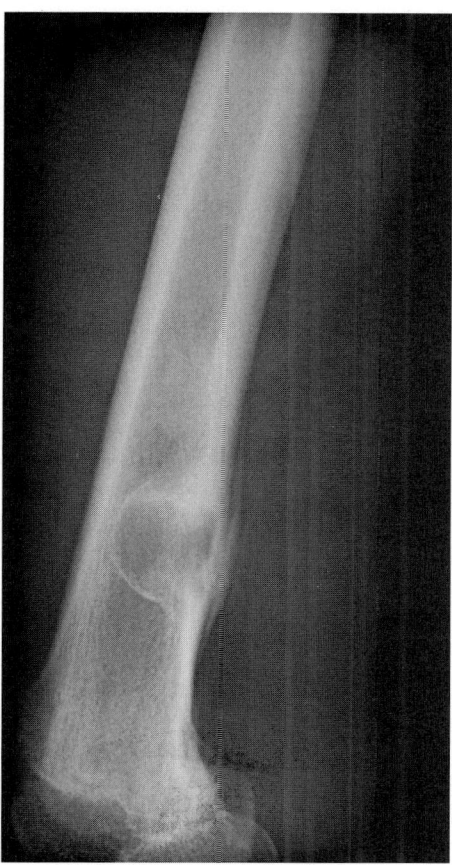

Figure 12-53 ■ Chondromyxoid fibroma of the distal femur. A well-defined metaphyseal radiolucency is surrounded by sclerotic rim. A periosteal reaction is also present. (From Frassica, F. J., and McCarthy E. F.: Orthopaedic pathology. Miller, M. D., Ed. *Review of Orthopaedics,* 2nd ed. Philadelphia, W. B. Saunders, 1996, p. 312.)

the extracellular matrix is also variable. Depending on the amount of proteoglycan secreted, the matrix may be myxoid, or it may have a bluish chondroid hue. However, matrix hyaline cartilage is extremely rare. Faint matrix calcification is present in 14% of cases. In addition, some cases have minimal reactive bone.

The typical cell of a chondromyxoid fibroma is a plump spindle cell or a stellate cell with elongated cytoplasmic processes. They are not present in discrete lacunae but seem to float in the chondroid matrix. The nuclei of the stellate cells are hyperchromatic or have clumped chromatin. Mitotic figures are extremely rare.

A disturbing feature of some chondromyxoid fibromas, present in one third of cases, is cellular pleomorphism. Sometimes the pleomorphism is extreme; large cells contain bizarre atypical nuclei (Fig. 12–57). However, even in lesions with extreme pleomorphism, mitotic figures are very rare. In addition, chondromyxoid fibromas may have areas indistinguishable from chondroblastoma, especially if the lesion extends into the epiphysis. Finally, chondromyxoid fibromas often have areas of aneurysmal bone cyst change.

Some chondromyxoid fibromas may be treated by curettage and bone grafting. This treatment is associated with a

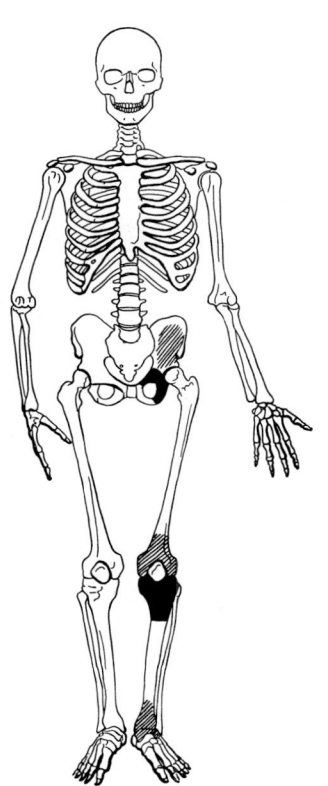

Figure 12-52 ■ Chondromyxoid fibroma locations.

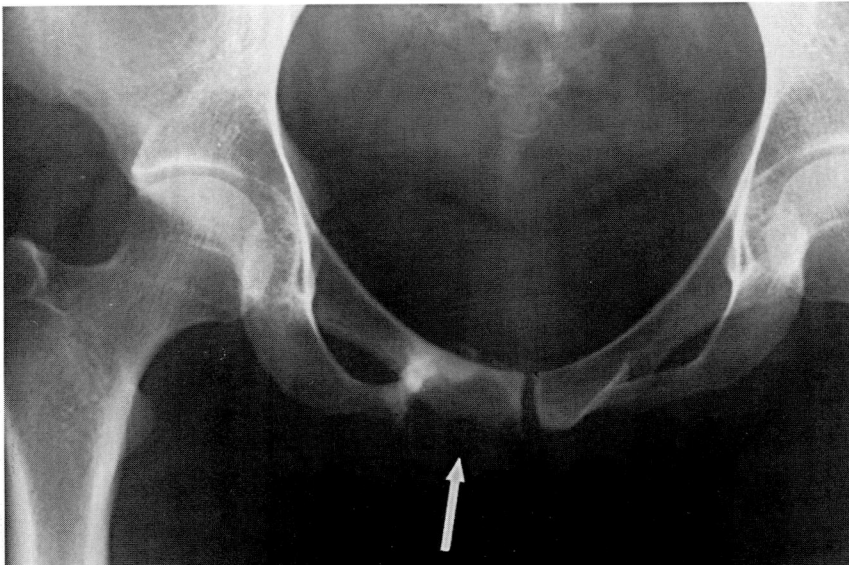

Figure 12-54 ▪ Chondromyxoid fibroma of the pubis. A scalloped radiolytic area is present *(arrow)*, and destruction of one cortex has occurred.

10% recurrence rate, a complication more commonly seen in children. Large destructive or recurrent lesions may need to be treated with en bloc surgical excision, a procedure usually resulting in complete cure. Although no instances of metastases have been reported, chondromyxoid fibromas are locally aggressive. An interesting and rare complication is soft tissue growth of tumor nodules secondary to implantation during surgery.[93]

Chondromyxoid fibroma may be misdiagnosed as a chondrosarcoma, especially if the lesion involves the pelvis. Ra-

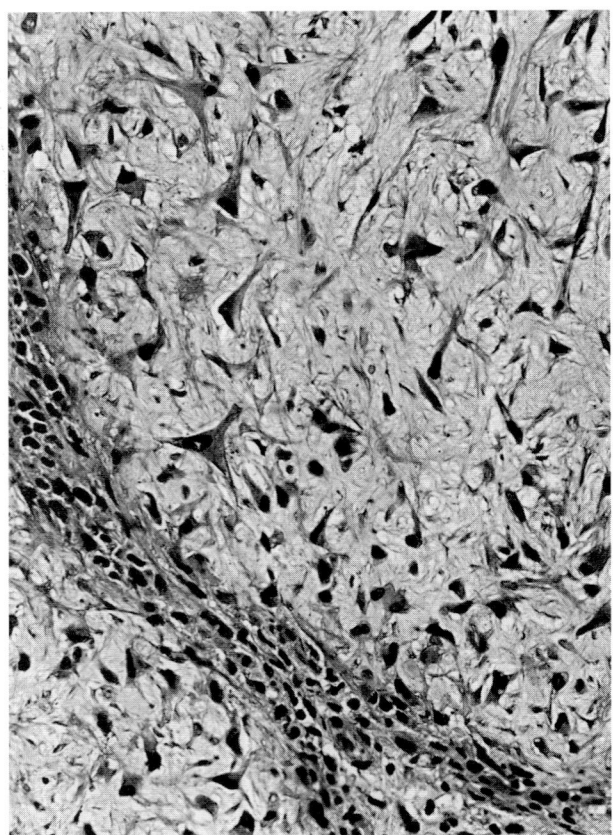

Figure 12-55 ▪ Photomicrograph of chondromyxoid fibroma. Stellate and spindle cells are present in a myxoid matrix.

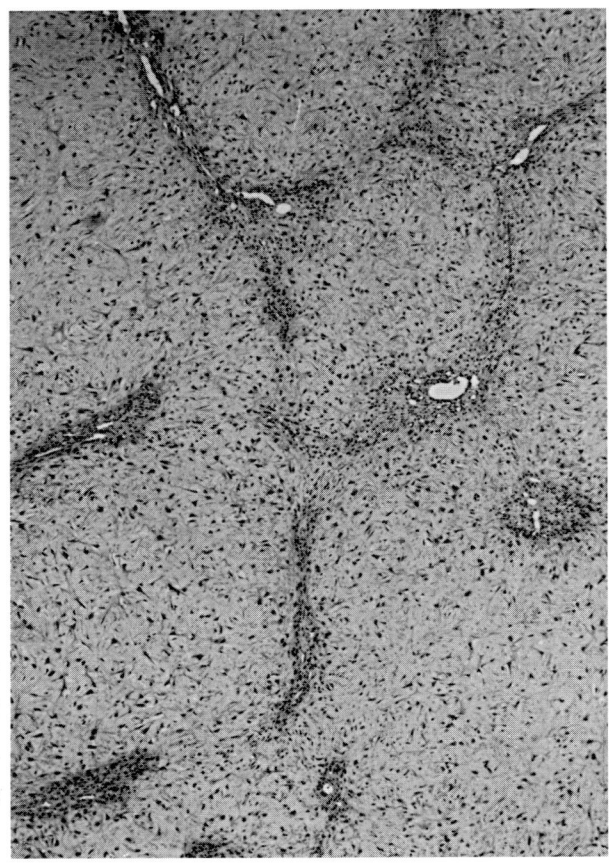

Figure 12-56 ▪ Low-power photomicrograph of chondromyxoid fibroma showing the lobular arrangement. The lobules are separated by fibrous bands.

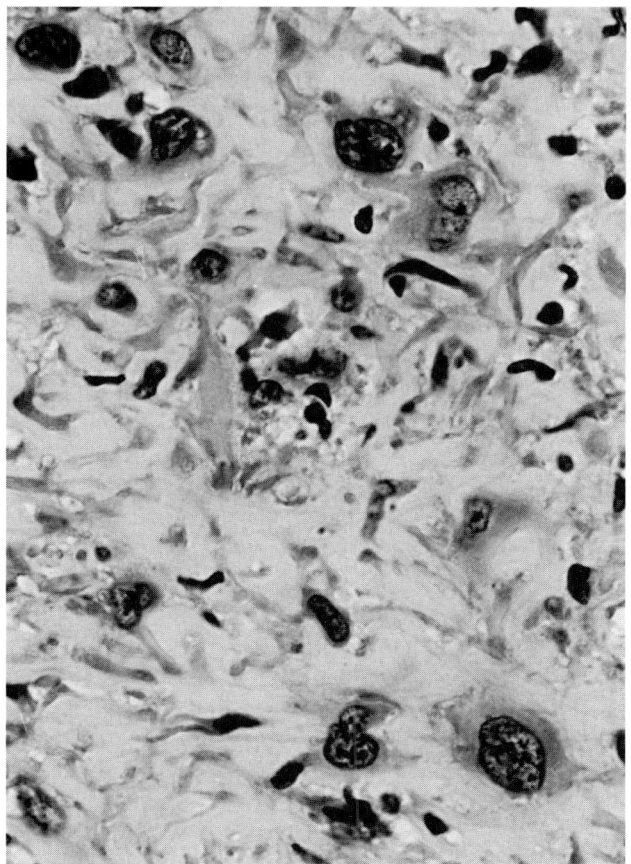

Figure 12-57 ■ High-power photomicrograph of chondromyxoid fibroma showing markedly atypical cells.

the medullary canal of the femur, presumably because of this entrapment mechanism.[94] These rests are undoubtedly present in other bones as well. The cartilaginous islands, subject to the same growth factors as epiphyseal plate cartilage, cease to grow in adulthood.

Enchondromas most commonly involve the tubular bones of the hands and feet (Fig. 12-58). In fact, enchondromas are the most common bone tumor of the hand (Fig. 12-59). The long bones, particularly the tibia, the distal femur, and the proximal humerus, are also common sites. Rarely, the pelvis is involved. Enchondromas are extremely rare in the spine, and they do not occur in bones that form by membranous ossification, such as the calvarium.

Enchondromas in adulthood are usually asymptomatic; they are discovered incidentally on radiographs or bone scans done for other reasons. Large enchondromas or enchondromas in the hand, however, may produce pain from a stress fracture. Enchondromas may be discovered at any age, but most are found between the ages of 15 and 40.

Radiologically, in young patients, enchondromas are well-defined lytic lesions in the central portion of the metaphysis or metadiaphysis. As patients age, the normally radiolucent cartilage begins to calcify and ossify. In older patients, enchondromas show the characteristic mineralization pattern of hyaline cartilage—radiodense rings and stipples (Fig. 12-60). Occasionally, the mineralization is very dense (Fig. 12-61). Characteristically, the clusters of ring-like and stippled mineralization are well defined and can be traced by a continuous line. In adults, enchondromas vary in size from

diologic features help distinguish these lesions. Chondrosarcomas are usually poorly circumscribed and contain calcifications. Often cortical thickening occurs as a result of neoplastic permeation. In contrast to chondrosarcomas, chondromyxoid fibromas are well circumscribed, and mineralization is very rare. Cortical thickening almost never occurs. Histologic features also help distinguish these lesions. Despite the occasional presence of pleomorphic cells, mitotic figures are extremely rare in chondromyxoid fibroma. Also, this neoplasm is sharply demarcated from the native bone. By contrast, mitotic figures are present in high-grade chondrosarcomas, and the neoplastic cartilage permeates the marrow spaces. A final distinguishing feature is that multinucleated giant cells, common in chondromyxoid fibroma, are extremely rare in chondrosarcomas.

Enchondroma

An enchondroma is a hamartomatous proliferation of mature hyaline cartilage in the medullary canal of the metaphysis or metadiaphysis. The origin of this lesion is thought to be a portion of epiphyseal plate entrapped in the metaphysis during bone growth. These lesions are common. Approximately 2% of all people have a small cartilaginous island in

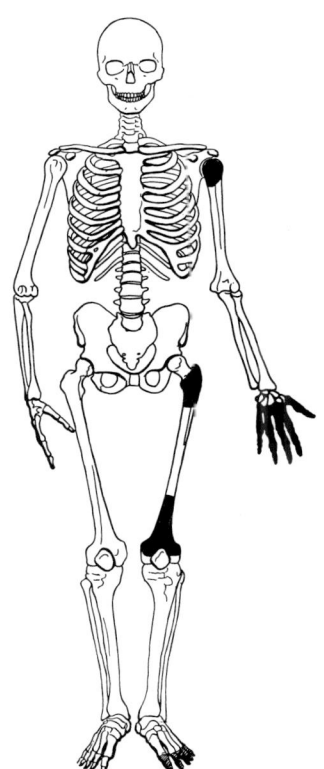

Figure 12-58 ■ Enchondroma locations.

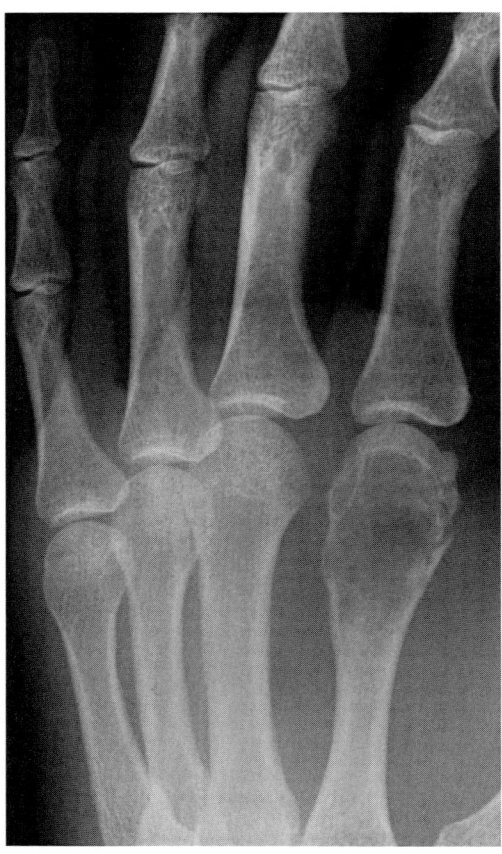

Figure 12-59 ■ An enchondroma of the distal second metacarpal. The lesion is radiolucent with mild expansion of the cortices.

1 cm to almost 10 cm in maximal dimension. Many enchondromas show mild endosteal erosion, or the cortex may be mildly expanded. However, cortical destruction or cortical thickening is not present. In an unusual radiographic presentation, the so-called *enchondroma protuberans,* an eccentric enchondroma bulges the cortex and masquerades as a large sessile osteochondroma[95] (Fig. 12–62). Enchondromas in adults are nongrowing lesions. Serial radiographs at 3-month intervals or a review of old radiographs, if available, is an accurate way to ascertain if the lesion is stationary.

Because the cartilage of an enchondroma may not be fully mineralized, the correct size is difficult to determine by plain radiographs. MRIs, however, accurately assess the extent of the lesion. Characteristically, MRI of an enchondroma shows a well-circumscribed lobular lesion that, because of high water content of the cartilage matrix, is bright on T_2-weighted images. T_1-weighted images show low signal intensity.

Enchondromas also accumulate radionuclide tracer. Therefore, a positive bone scan should be interpreted with caution. Enchondromas, although they are not growing, are constantly remodeling the endochondral bone formed in the cartilage. Therefore, radionuclide uptake, because of this remodeling activity, should not be interpreted as evidence of neoplastic growth.

Enchondromas consist of mature hyaline cartilage lobules of varying cellularity (Fig. 12–63). Some enchondromas are sparsely cellular and contain abundant extracellular matrix. Other enchondromas, particularly those in the hand or those in Ollier's disease, may be highly cellular (see later). These cellular enchondromas often contain chondrocytes with plump or double nuclei. Occasionally, myxoid change or focal necrosis is present.

Two important low-power microscopic features, if present, favor a diagnosis of enchondroma. These features reflect the lack of cartilage growth that is characteristic of enchondromas in adults. First, cartilage lobules are separated by normal marrow (Fig. 12–64). Second, cartilage lobules are partially encased by mature lamellar bone (Fig. 12–65). This latter feature reflects prior endochondral ossification at the periphery of the lobules. An important immunohistochemical feature that reflects lack of growth is a negative Ki-67 stain.[96] Ki-67 is a nuclear antigen present only when cells are in proliferation cycles. Positivity means cellular division even though mitotic figures are not apparent.

Because enchondromas are nongrowing lesions, surgery is not necessary. However, patients should be followed up with serial radiographs to be certain that the lesion is not growing. The incidence of malignant transformation is extremely low. Enchondromas of the hand often present with pathologic fracture and should be treated with curettage.

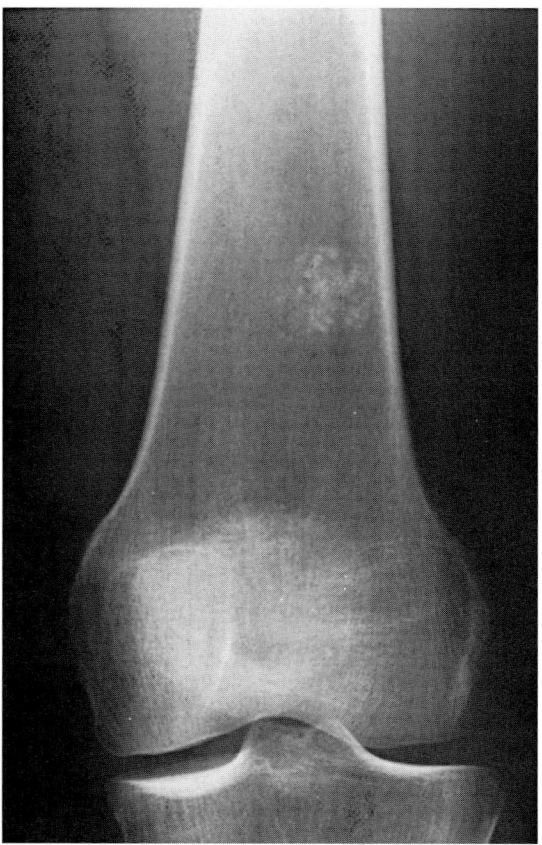

Figure 12-60 ■ A small enchondroma of the distal femur. A well-defined cluster of stippled calcifications is present.

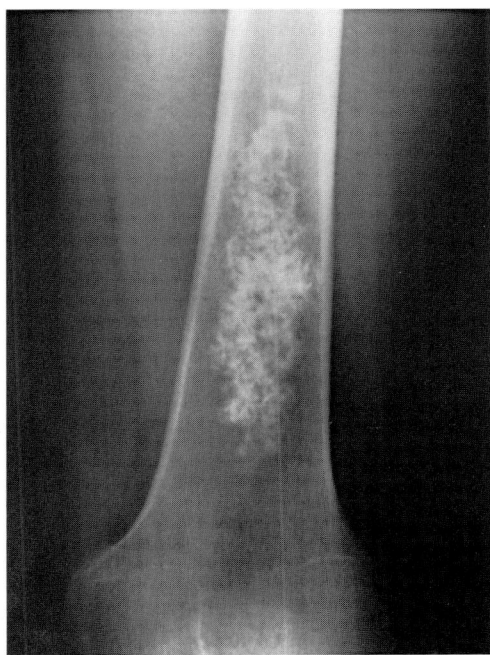

Figure 12-61 ▪ A large enchondroma of the distal femur. A well-defined zone of stippled and ring-shaped radiodensities is present.

Enchondromatosis

Enchondromatosis, also known as *Ollier's disease*, is a rare syndrome characterized by multiple enchondromas and skeletal deformity. A genetic basis for this sporadic developmental disease has not been established, although occurrence in multiple siblings has been documented.[97] The enchondromas in Ollier's disease occur in a few or many bones (Fig. 12–66). Sometimes the disease is limited to the bones of one extremity. Characteristically, abnormalities of the growth plate cause growth deformities, both angular and in length. The cartilage lesions in this disorder are particularly exuberant. Often they markedly expand the cortex (Fig. 12–67).

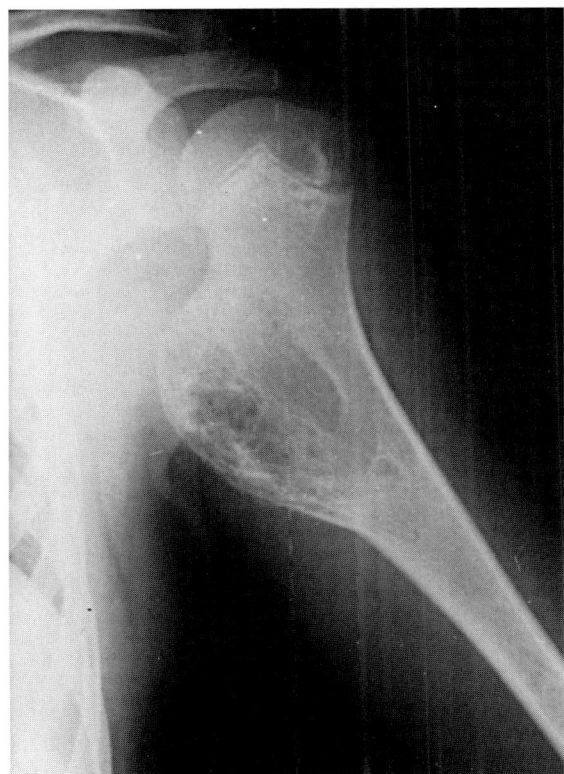

Figure 12-62 ▪ Enchondroma protuberans of the proximal humerus.

Unlike solitary enchondromas, cartilage lesions of Ollier's disease may be located in zones other than the center of the medullary canal. For example, they may be intracortical or subperiosteal. Sometimes even the epiphyses may be involved.

Microscopically, the cartilage of enchondromatosis is very cellular, and chondrocyte atypia also may be present. This atypia, in a solitary long bone enchondroma, would be suspicious for chondrosarcoma. The chondrocyte atypia of en-

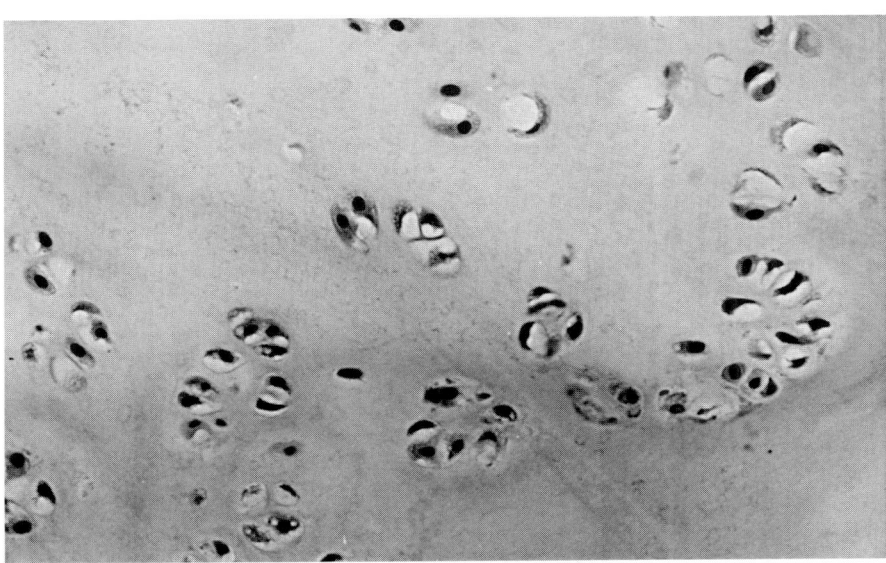

Figure 12-63 ▪ Photomicrograph of an enchondroma. Clones of chondrocytes are present in an extracellular chondroid matrix.

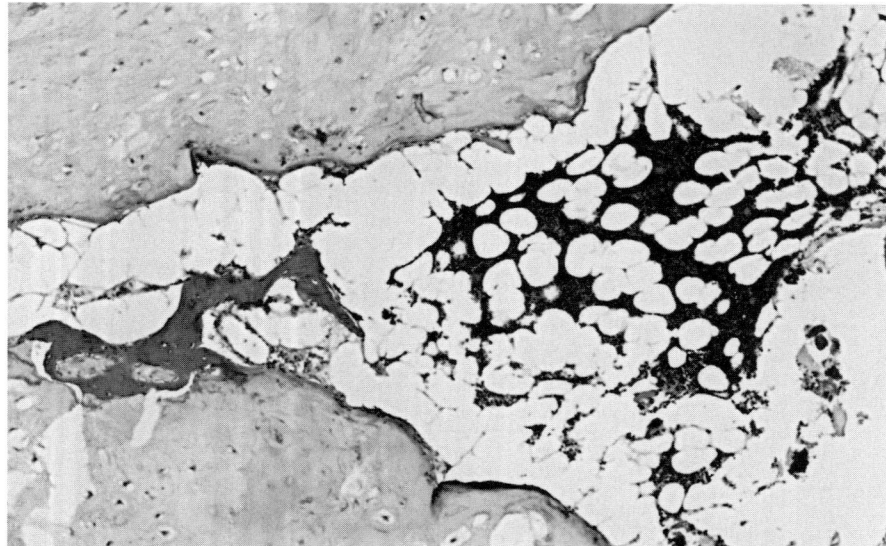

Figure 12-64 ■ Photomicrograph of enchondroma. Lobules of cartilage are separated by normal marrow.

chondromatosis is particularly problematic because 25 to 50% of patients with this syndrome eventually develop a low-grade chondrosarcoma.[98,99] This complication usually occurs when patients are in their 30s or 40s. Making the distinction between an enchondroma of Ollier's disease and a low-grade chondrosarcoma is particularly difficult. Cartilage necrosis and soft tissue invasion favor a diagnosis of chondrosarcoma.

Maffucci syndrome is a rare disease similar to enchondromatosis.[100] However, patients with this syndrome also have soft tissue hemangiomas. Radiographically, vascular

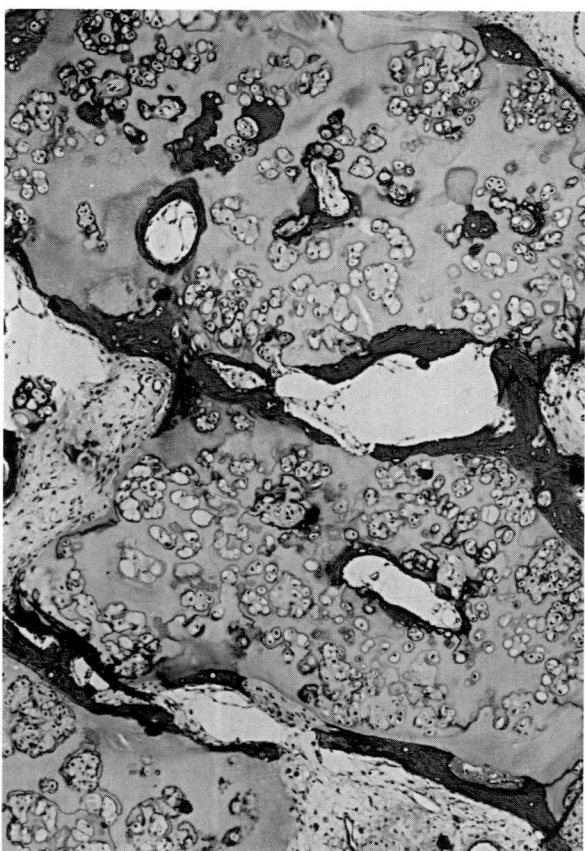

Figure 12-65 ■ Low-power photomicrograph of an enchondroma. Lobules of cartilage are encased by rims of endochondral bone.

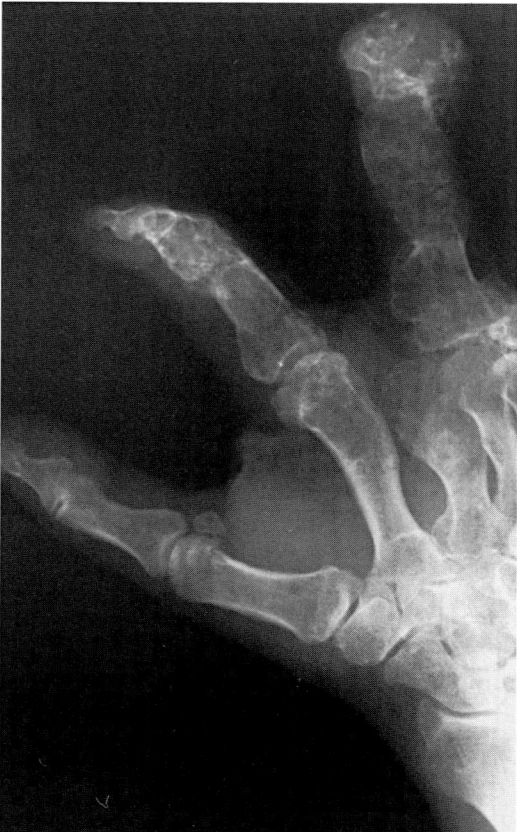

Figure 12-66 ■ Ollier's disease in the hand. Enchondromas extensively involving the second and fourth digits. The third finger has been amputated because of the development of a chondrosarcoma.

phleboliths are apparent in soft tissue adjacent to the enchondromas (Fig. 12–68). Like patients with enchondromatosis, patients with Maffucci syndrome are susceptible to developing malignant neoplasms. In addition to the low-grade chondrosarcomas, patients may also develop malignant brain tumors, liver and pancreatic carcinomas, and other malignancies.

Osteochondroma

Osteochondromas are hamartomatous proliferations of bone and cartilage that arise from the cortex and project into the soft tissue. They are thought to arise from islands of epiphyseal plate cartilage entrapped beneath the periosteum during skeletal growth. The cartilage rests grow and ossify at the same rate as the adjacent bone. When skeletal maturity is reached, osteochondromas stop growing. Osteochondromas are probably the most common tumorous process of bone. The true incidence cannot be calculated because many are asymptomatic. Some are discovered incidentally on radiographs taken for other reasons. Most osteochondromas are solitary.

Symptomatic lesions usually present before age 30. Large osteochondromas present clinically as firm subcutaneous masses. Pain may be caused by fracture of the stalk, nerve impingement, or inflammation of an overlying bursa. Osteo-

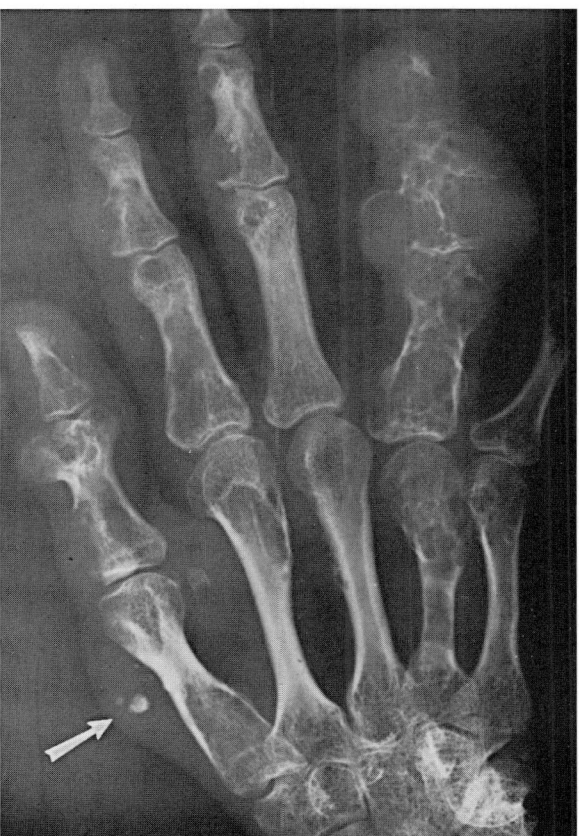

Figure 12-68 ■ Maffucci's syndrome. Enchondromas extensively involve the bones of the hand, and hemangiomas are present in the soft tissues as evidenced by phleboliths (arrow).

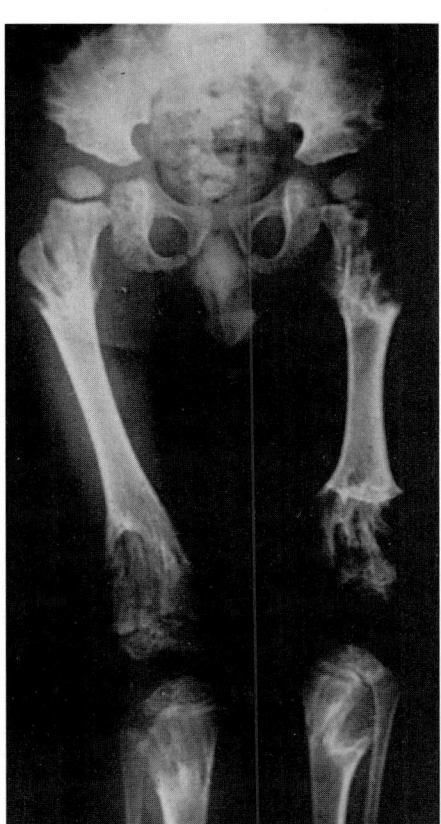

Figure 12-67 ■ Ollier's disease involving the bones of the lower extremities and the pelvis.

chondromas may arise from any bone formed in cartilage, but the distal femur, proximal tibia, proximal humerus, and pelvis are the most common sites (Fig. 12–69).

In addition to developmental osteochondromas, identical bony protrusions may occur as a result of radiotherapy to bone for other reasons during childhood.[101] These lesions, which have a structure similar to developmental osteochondromas, may be diagnosed as long as 16 years after irradiation.

Osteochondromas vary greatly in size and shape. Most are 1 to 3 cm in length (Fig. 12–70). However, some may reach 15 cm or more in maximal dimension (Fig. 12–71). They may be sessile or pediculated. Sessile osteochondromas are gently contoured bony prominences, and pedunculated lesions have a narrow stalk that broadens into a cauliflower-like knob. They arise from the metaphyseal cortex and the soft tissue, always in the direction away from the joint (Fig. 12–72). An important radiographic feature of osteochondromas is the continuity of the cortex of the stalk with the cortex of the bone (Fig. 12–73). Therefore, the marrow cavity of the osteochondroma and the bone are continuous.

The cartilage cap of an osteochondroma is usually entirely radiolucent. However, it may occasionally contain stippled calcifications. In large lesions, cartilage-type calcifications often may be present inside the bony stalk of the osteochondroma. On plain radiographs, the boundary of the calcifications in the cap, together with the stalk, should be well defined and traceable with a continuous line. The cartilage cap is best visualized with MRI[102] or ultrasound.[103] Using these modalities, a cartilage cap thicker than 2 cm should raise the suspicion of a secondary chondrosarcoma.

A diagnostic pitfall in evaluating osteochondromas is the presence of metaplastic cartilage nodules (synovial chondromatosis) in the bursa overlying the osteochondromas.[104] This process, known as *exostosis bursata,* may be mistaken for chondrosarcoma infiltrating the soft tissue. However, unlike in chondrosarcoma, the calcifications are uniform and bounded by a continuous imaginary line (see Chapter 15).

Histologically, an osteochondroma consists of a cartilage cap overlying a stalk of cortical and trabecular bone (Fig. 12–74). The cartilage cap is bounded by a well-defined perichondrium, separating the lesion from the surrounding soft tissue. Often, particularly in large osteochondromas, islands of partially calcified and ossified cartilage are present inside the stalk, indicating cartilage entrapment during growth.

During skeletal growth, the base of the cartilage cap shows chondrocyte proliferation and endochondral ossification similar to an epiphyseal plate. By contrast, an ancient osteochondroma in an older patient may lack a cartilage cap. Most osteochondromas, however, have a cartilage cap 0.5 to 1.5 cm thick. The pathologist should avoid tangential sectioning of the cap during specimen preparation. This error leads to an inaccurate measurement. The cartilage in the cap

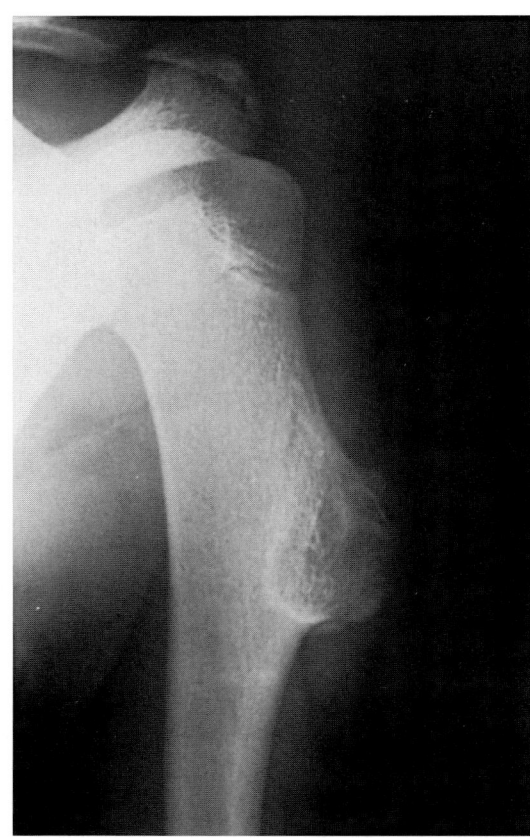

Figure 12–70 ■ Sessile osteosarcoma of the proximal humerus. (From Frassica, F. J., and McCarthy, E. F.: Orthopaedic pathology. Miller, M. D., Ed. *Review of Orthopaedics*, 2nd ed. Philadelphia, W. B. Saunders, 1996.)

is moderately cellular, and the chondrocytes are evenly spaced throughout the matrix. Mild nuclear atypia is occasionally present.

Asymptomatic osteochondromas may be followed without surgical intervention. Symptomatic lesions may be removed surgically. The perichondrium over the osteochondroma must be excised with the lesion; otherwise a recurrence is probable. On very rare occasions, osteochondromas may disappear spontaneously.[105]

The incidence of transformation of a solitary osteochondroma to chondrosarcoma is less than 1%.

A very rare complication of an osteochondroma, in addition to secondary chondrosarcomatous transformation, is dedifferentiation. A high-grade sarcoma, usually a malignant fibrous histiocytoma, develops in the cap. This process is similar to intramedullary, dedifferentiated chondrosarcoma[106] (see later).

Hereditary Multiple Exostosis

Hereditary multiple exostosis, also known as *osteochondromatosis* or *diaphyseal aclasis,* is a skeletal dysplasia characterized by the development of multiple osteochondromas. Patients may have as many as 30 lesions of varying sizes, which are distributed throughout the skeleton. Skeletal

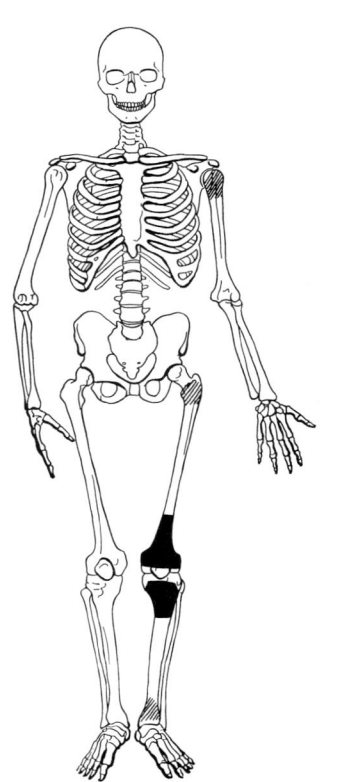

Figure 12–69 ■ Osteochondroma locations.

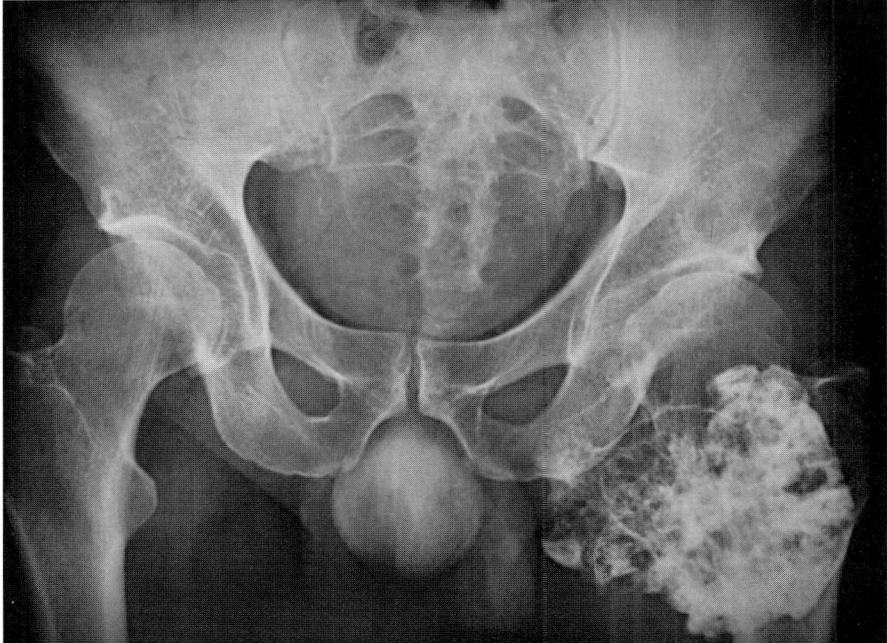

Figure 12-71 ■ Large osteochondroma of the proximal femur. The radiodensity is well defined.

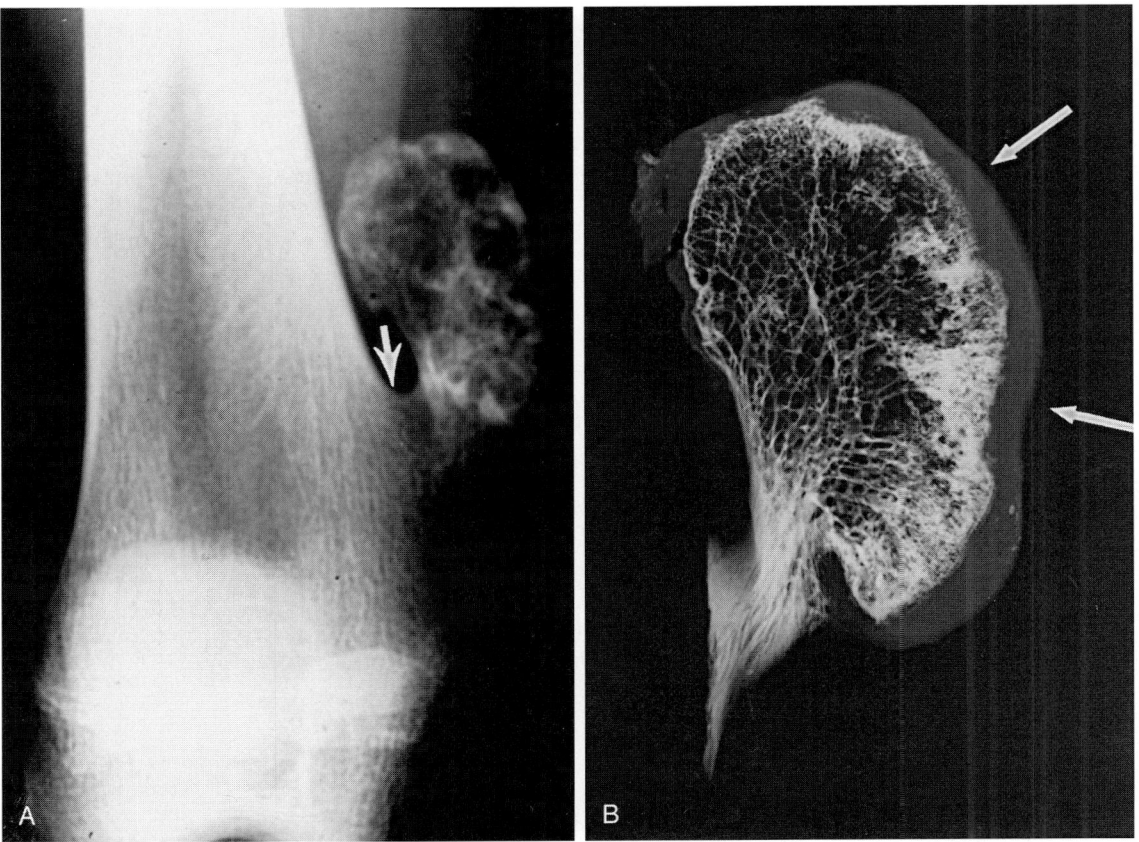

Figure 12-72 ■ Pedunculated osteochondroma of the distal femur. **A,** Plain radiograph showing the continuity of the native cortex with that of the osteochondroma *(arrow).* **B,** Specimen radiograph of the lesion in *panel A.* A uniform cartilage cap is visible *(arrows).*

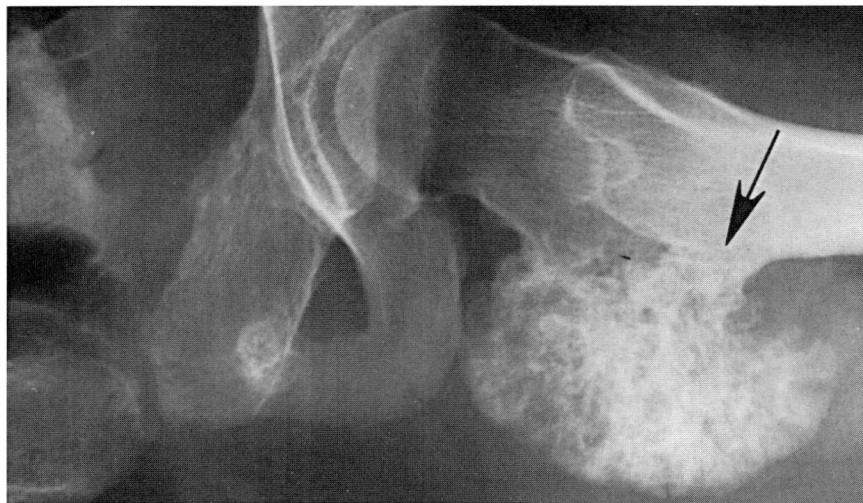

Figure 12–73 ■ A large osteochondroma of the proximal femur. The medullary cavity of the femur is continuous with that of the osteochondroma stalk *(arrow).*

deformity and short stature are also features of this disease. Hereditary multiple exostosis is one of the more common skeletal dysplasias.

The radiologic features of each osteochondroma in this disorder are similar to those of a solitary osteochondroma. However, an occasional osteochondroma in an affected patient grows to a huge size. Deformities occur because of disordered endochondral ossification in the growth plate (Fig. 12–75). These deformities, most prominent in the forearm, knee, and ankle, require frequent orthopedic intervention. Each patient usually requires at least three surgical procedures, including excision of osteochondromas and osteotomies to correct deformity.[107]

The histologic features of each osteochondroma, like the radiologic features, are similar to those of solitary osteochondromas. From 5 to 25% of patients with this syndrome eventually develop a secondary chondrosarcoma, usually in the pelvis.[108]

Periosteal Chondroma

Periosteal chondroma, also known as juxtacortical chondroma, is a benign proliferation of hyaline cartilage on the bone surface beneath the periosteum. Lesions range from 1 to 5 cm in diameter and may involve any bone in the appendicular skeleton, although the proximal or distal femur and the proximal humerus are the most common sites[109–111] (Fig. 12–76). Patients are usually between ages 10 and 30, and they usually present with pain, often for over a year.

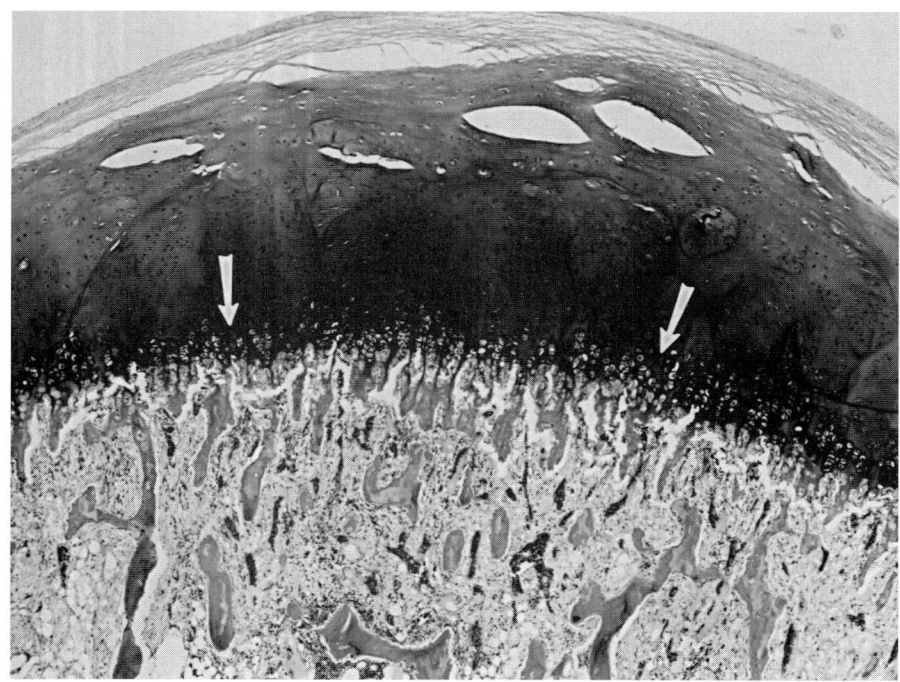

Figure 12–74 ■ Low-power photomicrograph of an osteochondroma showing the cartilage cap. The cap is covered by perichondrium. Endochondral ossification is taking place at the base of the cartilage *(arrows).*

Radiologically, periosteal chondromas, unlike osteochondromas, lack a bony stalk. In a periosteal chondroma, a well-demarcated aggregate of ring-like and stippled densities is directly adjacent to the cortex. The cortex is intact under the cartilaginous mass, although it is usually scalloped or cratered (Fig. 12–77). Buttresses of reactive bone are occasionally present at the margins of the lesion.

Histologically, periosteal chondromas show lobules of hyaline cartilage on the external surface of the cortex beneath the periosteum (Fig. 12–78). Often, networks of reactive and endochondral bone separate the hyaline cartilage lobules. The cartilage is mildly cellular, and sometimes the nuclei are plump and hyperchromatic. Occasionally, the cartilage matrix shows myxoid changes.

Periosteal chondromas are best treated with en bloc excision of the cartilage, including the overlying perichondrium and the underlying cortex. Recurrence, following complete removal, is rare.

Chondrosarcoma

Chondrosarcomas are malignant neoplasms of cartilage-producing cells. Although reactive or benign endochondral bone may be present in these neoplasms, the neoplastic cells do not synthesize osteoid. After osteosarcoma, chondrosarcoma is the second most common primary malignant bone tumor. Unlike most other primary bone tumors, chondrosarcomas tend to occur in older patients, and most often involve the axial skeleton.

Chondrosarcomas may be divided in two major categories: *central chondrosarcomas* and *surface chondrosarcomas*. These occur with equal frequency. Central chondrosarcomas are centered in the medullary canal and occasionally penetrate through the cortex. By contrast, surface chondrosarcomas, also known as peripheral chondrosarcomas, arise on the bone surface and grow into the adjacent soft tissue. A variant of surface chondrosarcoma, known as either periosteal or *juxtacortical chondrosarcoma,* is recognized as a distinct entity.

Some pathologists further subdivide chondrosarcomas into primary and secondary. Primary chondrosarcomas occur de novo, and secondary chondrosarcomas arise in preexisting cartilage lesions. However, this subdivision is probably meaningless. Many, perhaps most, presumed primary chondrosarcomas are secondary chondrosarcomas that have effaced the preexisting lesions.

In addition to central and surface chondrosarcomas, which are composed of hyaline cartilage, three special variants have distinctive histologic features. These variants are clear cell chondrosarcoma, mesenchymal chondrosarcoma, and dedifferentiated chondrosarcoma (Table 12–4).

Chondrosarcomas show a wide range of aggressiveness. Some lesions, although locally aggressive, grow slowly and rarely metastasize. By contrast, other chondrosarcomas are

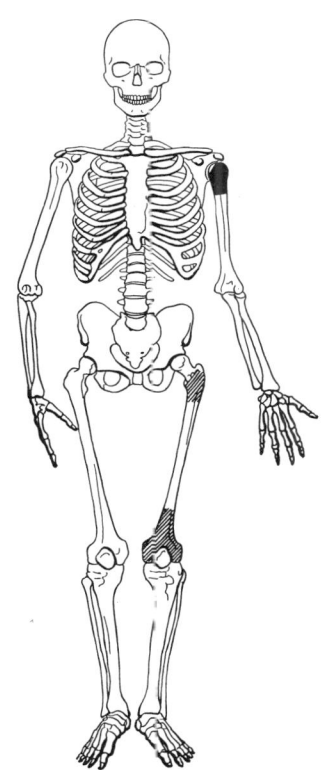

Figure 12-76 ■ Periosteal chondroma locations.

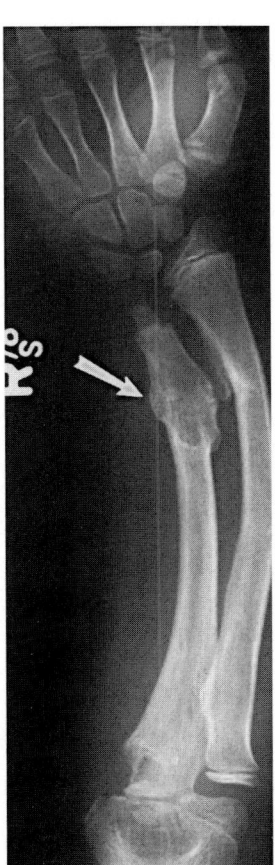

Figure 12-75 ■ Multiple osteochondromatosis. Osteochondromas are present in the distal ulna *(arrow)* and the distal radius. These lesions are causing deformity.

very destructive and metastasize readily. Fortunately, most chondrosarcomas (about 75%) grow slowly.[112] In general, the aggressiveness of a chondrosarcoma can be predicted by its cellularity and degree of nuclear atypia, features known as "histologic grade." Chondrosarcomas, whether central or surface, can be grouped in three histologic grades.[113-117]

Histologic Grading

Grade 1 chondrosarcomas are slow-growing neoplasms. The chondrocytes have small, dark nuclei and scant cytoplasm. Many chondrocytes are arranged in clones, a feature indicating earlier cell division. In addition, each chondrocyte occupies a lacuna in the extracellular matrix. Binucleated cells are present, but mitotic figures are absent. A few cells may have slightly larger nuclei and more cytoplasm. Grade 1 chondrosarcomas have abundant extracellular matrix; therefore, the cellularity is low (Fig. 12–79). Calcification and endochondral ossification are usually present. From 30 to 35% of chondrosarcomas are grade 1 lesions. They almost never metastasize.

Grade 1 cytologic features are present in some enchondromas. Therefore, distinguishing a grade 1 central chondrosarcoma from an enchondroma is extremely difficult. In fact, it

Table 12–4 ■ **CHONDROSARCOMA SUBTYPES**

Central chondrosarcoma
Surface chondrosarcoma
Periosteal chondrosarcoma
Clear cell chondrosarcoma
Mesenchymal chondrosarcoma
Dedifferentiated chondrosarcoma

is probably the most difficult problem in bone pathology. In addition to this diagnostic difficulty with central cartilage lesions, surface chondrosarcoma with grade 1 histology may be difficult to distinguish from extraarticular synovial chondromatosis. Synovial chondromatosis, a metaplastic process, is also characterized by mild cellular atypia. This distinction must be made radiographically.

Grade 2 chondrosarcomas have larger and paler nuclei with visible chromatin. Mild nuclear pleomorphism is present, and the cytoplasm is more abundant. Mitotic figures are extremely rare. Grade 2 chondrosarcomas are more cellular than grade 1 chondrosarcomas, and the increased cellularity is more pronounced at the periphery of the cartilage lobules (Fig. 12–80). In addition, focal myxoid change is often present in the extracellular matrix. From 40 to 50% of chondrosarcomas show grade 2 histology. They are more locally aggressive, and approximately 15 to 20% metastasize.

The histologic features of grade 2 chondrosarcomas, like those of grade 1 lesions, overlap with some benign cartilage lesions. For example, the enchondromas of Ollier's disease, periosteal chondromas, and chondromyxoid fibromas may show similar cytologic atypia.

Grades 1 and 2 chondrosarcomas are considered low grade. By contrast, grade 3 chondrosarcomas are high-grade neoplasms. The chondrocyte nuclei are large and vesicular and often contain a prominent nucleolus. Bizarre, hyperchromatic nuclei are also present. The cytoplasm is abundant, and the cells often assume an elongated spindle shape. Mitotic figures are present, although they are less numerous than high-grade sarcomas of other tissue differentiation, such as osteosarcomas (Fig. 12–81). A mitotic count of 2 per 10 per high-power fields is diagnostic of a grade 3 lesion. The extracellular matrix is sparse and may occasionally be absent. In this case, sheets of rounded or spindle cells without apparent chondroid differentiation are present. About 20% of chondrosarcomas are grade 3 lesions. Seventy percent of these eventually metastasize.

Histologic grade correlates with other measurable parameters. For example, low-grade chondrosarcomas stain focally for Ki-67, a nuclear antigen expressed in the cellular proliferation cycle. High-grade lesions are strongly reactive with this stain.[96] Also, low-grade lesions stain only focally for p53 protein and are diploid. By contrast, high-grade lesions are strongly positive for p53 and are aneuploid.[118]

Central Chondrosarcoma

Central chondrosarcomas develop in the medullary cavity. Approximately 50% of these neoplasms show radiologic or

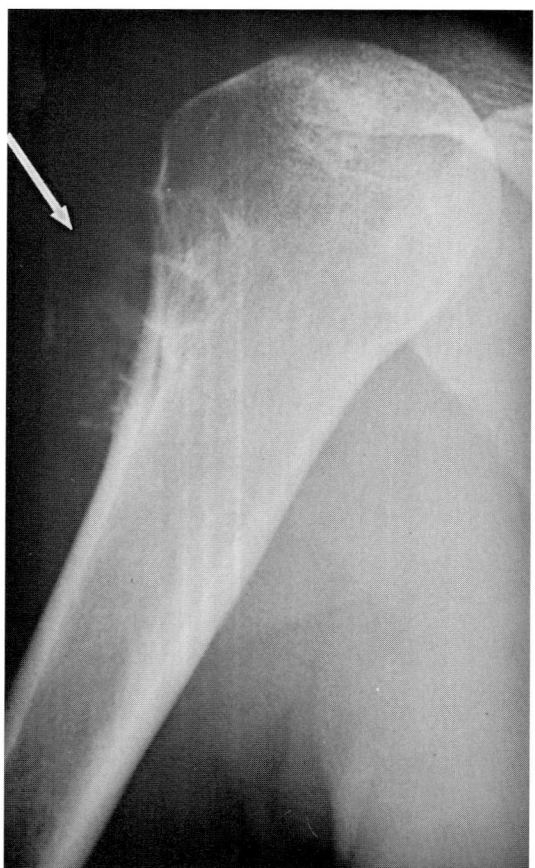

Figure 12–77 ■ Periosteal chondroma of the proximal humerus. A well-defined surface lesion with scalloping of the cortex is present. (From Frassica, F. J., and McCarthy, E. F.: Miller, M. D., Ed. *Review of Orthopaedics*, 2nd ed. Philadelphia, W. B. Saunders, 1996, p. 308.)

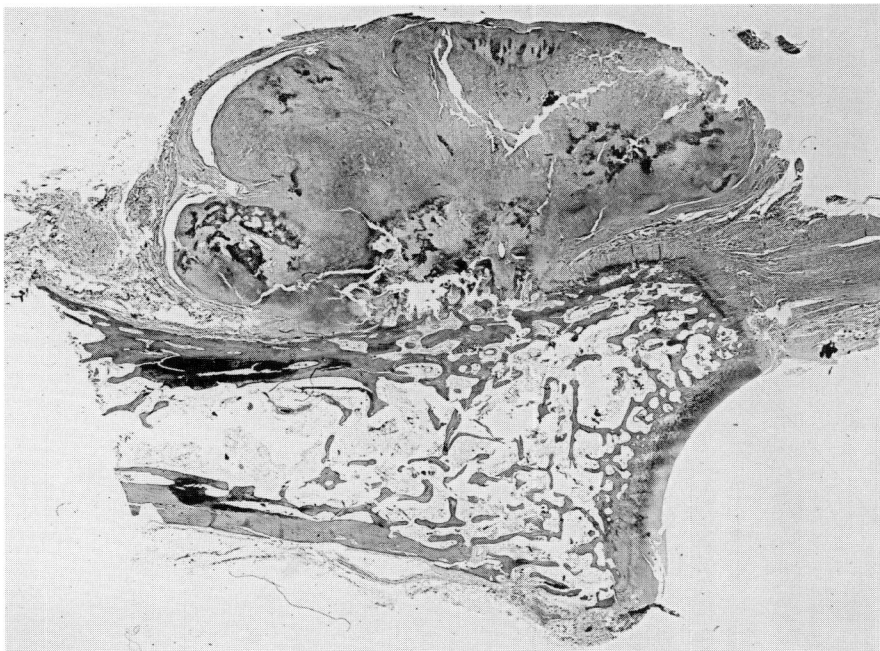

Figure 12-78 ■ Periosteal chondroma of a toe phalanx. A well-defined lobule of cartilage is present on the bone surface. (From McCarthy, E. F.: *Differential Diagnosis in Pathology. Bone and Joint Disorders.* New York and Tokyo, Igaku-Shoin, 1996. With permission from Williams & Wilkins.)

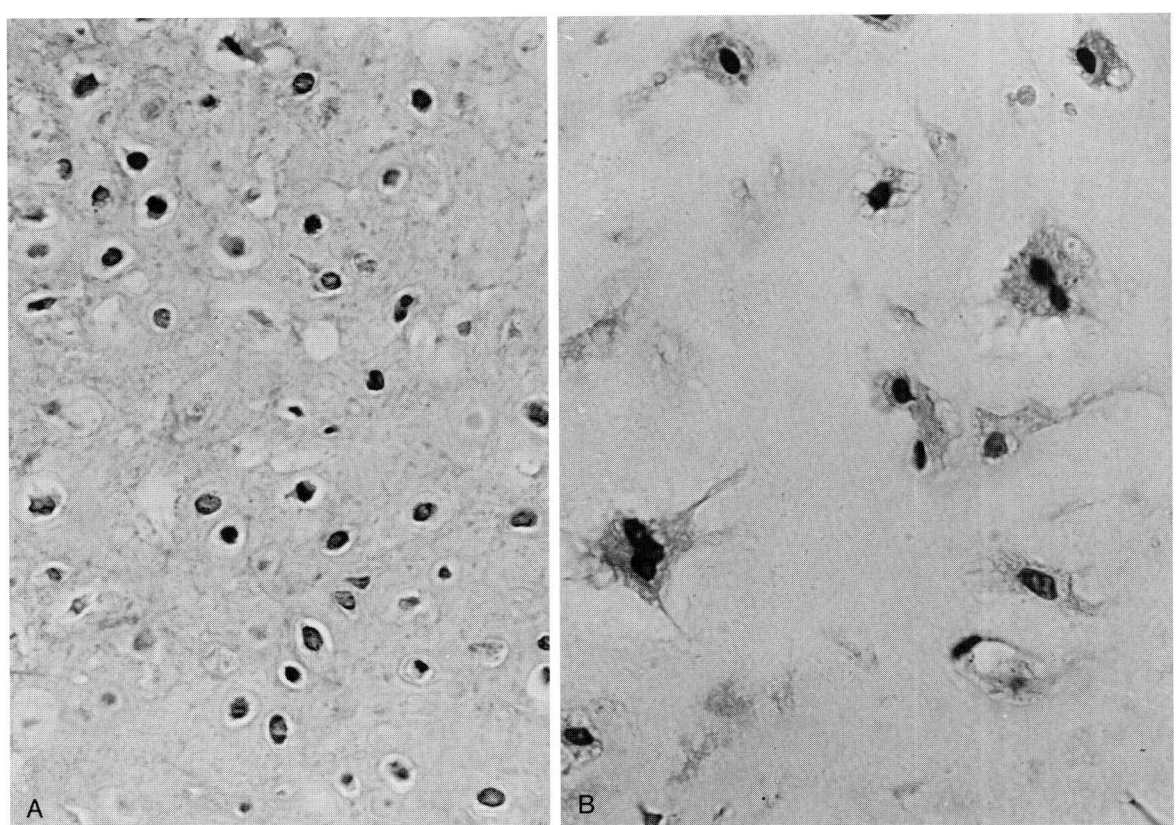

Figure 12-79 ■ Grade 1 cartilage. **A,** Low-power photomicrograph showing chondrocytes in an abundant extracellular matrix. **B,** High-power photomicrograph showing occasional binucleated chondrocytes.

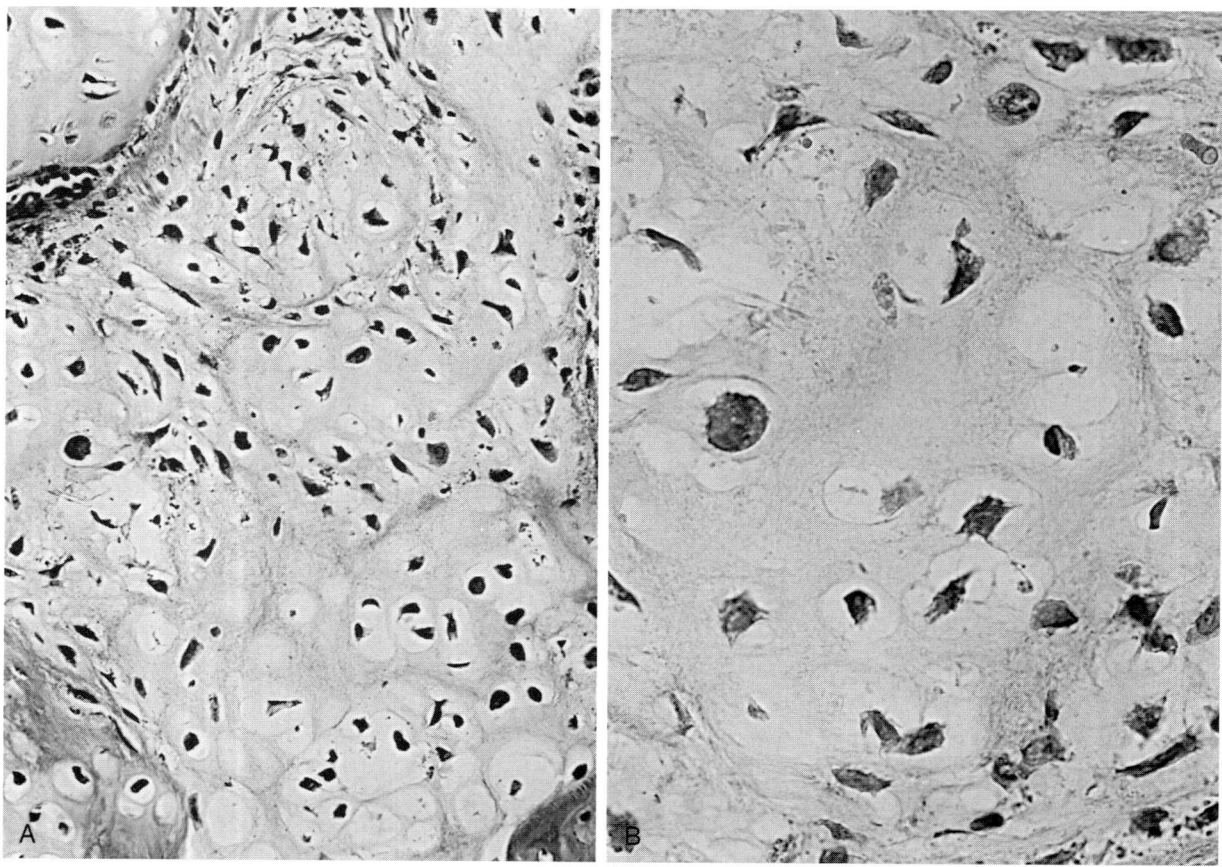

Figure 12-80 ▪ Grade 2 cartilage. **A,** Low-power photomicrograph showing moderately cellular cartilage. **B,** High-power photomicrograph showing atypical chondrocytes.

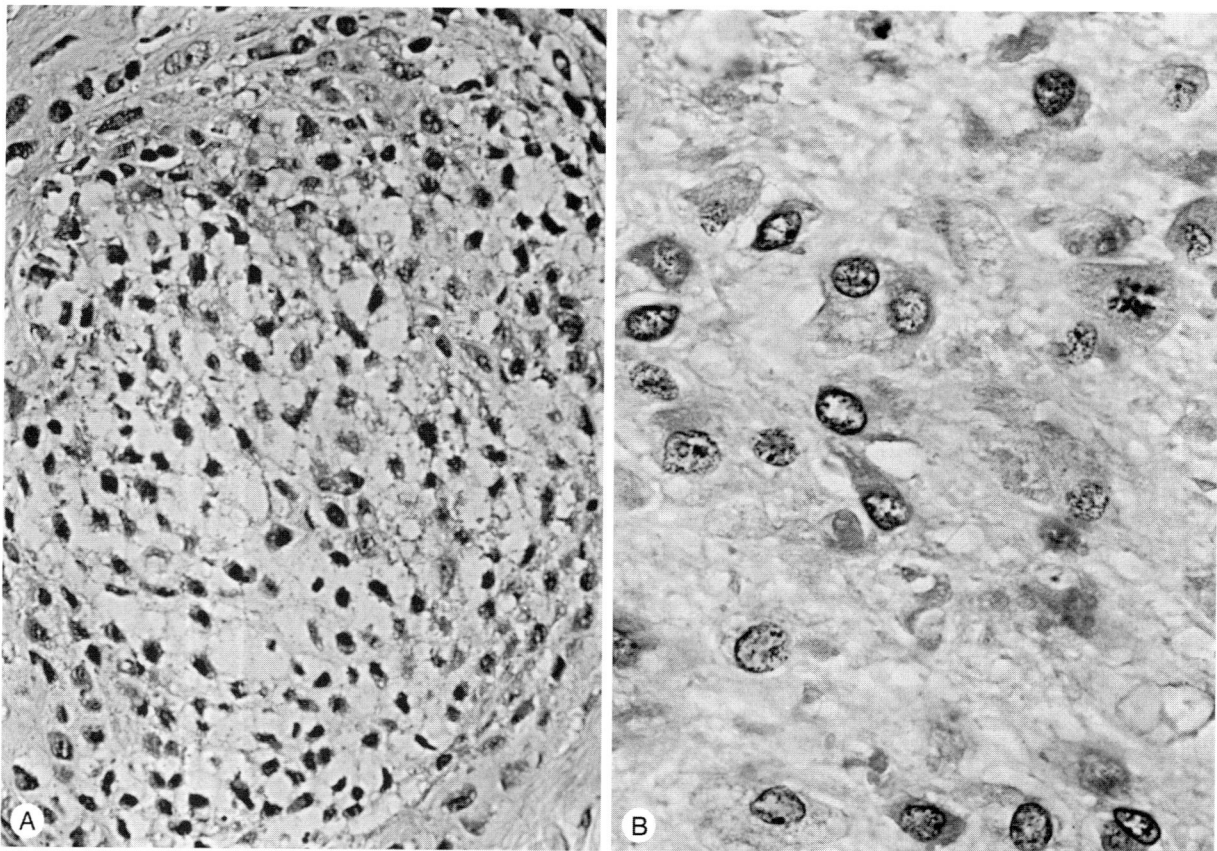

Figure 12-81 ▪ Grade 3 cartilage. **A,** Low-power photomicrograph showing high cellularity. **B,** High-power photomicrograph showing markedly atypical chondrocytes, and a mitotic figure is present.

histologic evidence of a preexisting enchondroma, suggesting that perhaps all central chondrosarcomas arise in enchondromas.[119] Central chondrosarcomas may occur at any age, but most patients are in their 40s or 50s. Unlike enchondromas, which are common in the hands and feet, central chondrosarcomas are very rare in these locations. Otherwise, the preferred sites of central chondrosarcoma parallel those of enchondromas: the proximal humerus, proximal and distal femur, and tibia.

High-Grade Central Chondrosarcoma. High-grade central chondrosarcomas pose few diagnostic problems. Patients have worsening pain. Radiologically, ring-shaped and stippled calcifications are irregularly distributed in the medullary canal, and the boundary of these calcifications usually cannot be traced with a continuous imaginary line. Cortical erosion or expansion also occurs. Sometimes the cortex is thickened, a sign of permeative intracortical growth (Fig. 12–82). Occasionally, a soft tissue mass may be present adjacent to an area of cortical destruction. A biopsy of a high-grade central chondrosarcoma shows grade 3 histologic features.

Low-Grade Central Chondrosarcoma Versus Enchondroma. In contrast to easily diagnosed high-grade chondrosarcomas, low-grade central chondrosarcomas pose a very difficult diagnostic problem—they must be distinguished from enchondromas (Fig. 12–83). Making the correct diagnosis depends on close communication with the clinician and the radiologist before a biopsy is done because enchondromas and low-grade chondrosarcomas are distinguished by how they behave; histologic features overlap considerably. Therefore, a pathologist attempting to analyze a cartilage lesion by histologic features alone may be forced to render a diagnosis of "borderline cartilage neoplasm" or "cartilage neoplasm of uncertain malignant potential." These diagnoses are of no use to the surgeon who must treat the patient. If the behavior of a cartilage lesion is learned by clinical and radiographic features before a biopsy is done, the histologic features can be interpreted in the light of this information.

The behavior of a cartilage lesion is best predicted by asking the question, "Is the lesion growing?" In adults, solitary enchondromas of long bones do not grow, whereas low-grade chondrosarcomas grow slowly. Clinical and radiographic features should be interpreted in the light of this difference. The question of growth is best answered by monthly plain radiographs for 6 months and then at 6-month intervals for 2 years. If the lesion is growing, radiographic features change, and the diagnosis of low-grade chondrosarcoma can be established. The prognosis should not be worsened by a delay of this duration. In addition to follow-up radiographs, efforts should be made to find any previous radiographs of the affected bone. The problem of a worrisome or ambiguous lesion may be clarified if a radiograph, taken years earlier, shows exactly the same lesion.

In addition to radiographic changes over time, the presence of pain is a second important clue indicating growth of a cartilage lesion. However, the orthopedic surgeon must be certain that the pain is due to the neoplasm. Often, unrelated joint pain, particularly of the knee or shoulder prompts radiographic studies that reveal incidental cartilage lesions. Relief of pain by resting the joint or by analgesic injection indicates that the pain is not due to the cartilage lesion.

Another cause of pain associated with a nongrowing cartilage lesion is a stress fracture. Large enchondromas, particularly in weight-bearing bones, may suffer this complication. In this event, a more aggressive neoplasm may be suspected, especially if an MRI study shows marrow and soft tissue edema. With awareness of this complication, the nongrowing nature of a cartilage lesion usually declares itself.

Although considerable overlap exists between the histologic features of enchondromas and low-grade chondrosarcomas, two clues assist in recognizing a growing lesion.[119] These clues are apparent on low-power study and, when present, support a diagnosis of low-grade chondrosarcoma. The first clue is permeation of the bone marrow by cartilage (Fig. 12–84). Islands of hyaline cartilage are directly adjacent to, or encasing, native trabecular bone. Second, cartilage lobules are separated by fibrous bands (Fig. 12–85). This differs from enchondromas, where lobules are separated by bone marrow or endochondral bone. In addition to these two clues, other histologic features support the diagnosis of low-grade chondrosarcoma, although they are often not present. These include penetration of the cortex, myxoid change, necrosis, or fibrosis.[120] Finally, in adult long bone

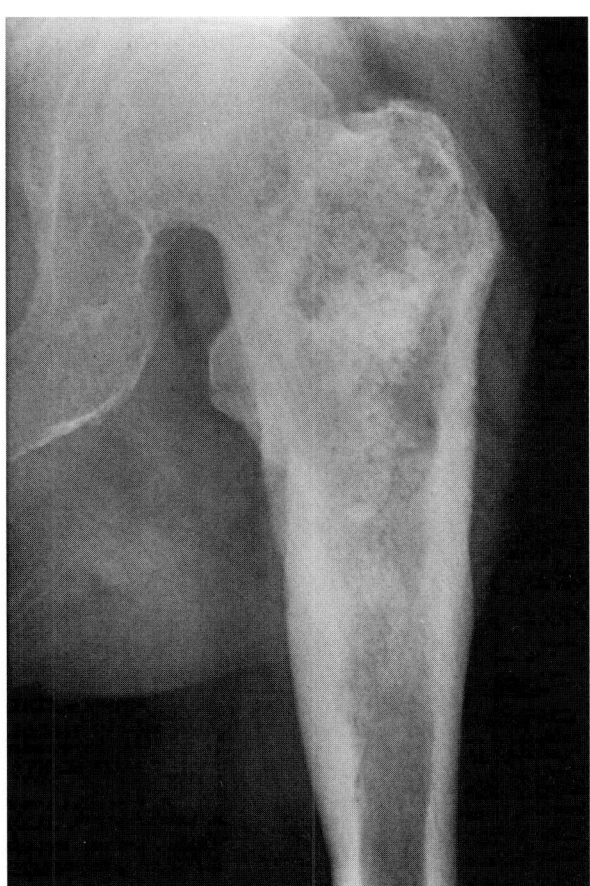

Figure 12-82 ■ Central chondrosarcoma of proximal femur. A poorly defined zone of stippled radiodensities and cortical thickening are present.

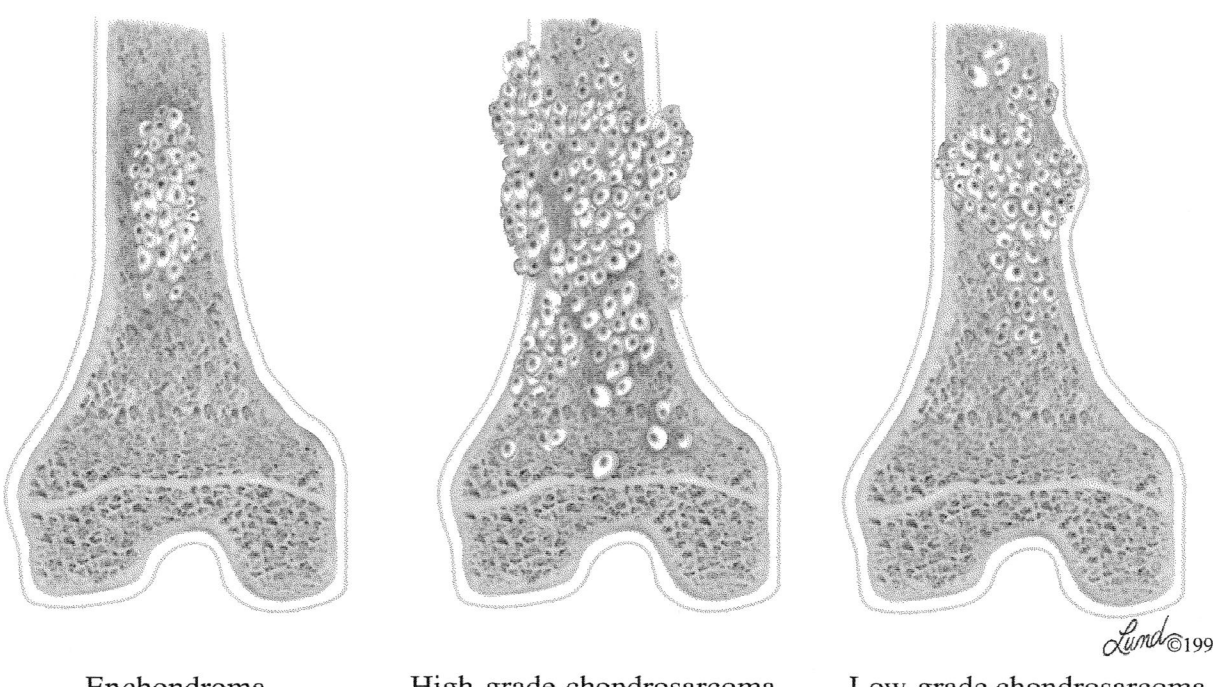

Figure 12-83 ■ Central cartilage lesions. Distinguishing an enchondroma from a low-grade chondrosarcoma poses many diagnostic problems. By contrast, a high-grade central chondrosarcoma usually can be diagnosed with the plain radiograph.

lesions, Ki-67 positivity supports a diagnosis of low-grade chondrosarcoma.[96]

Surface Chondrosarcoma

Surface chondrosarcomas, also called peripheral chondrosarcomas, arise on the bone surface and project into the soft tissue. Some arise in preexisting osteochondromas, as evidenced by remnants of an osteochondroma at the base of the lesion or the occurrence in a patient with hereditary multiple exostosis. Almost all surface chondrosarcomas are low-grade, slow-growing neoplasms. Patients are usually between ages 20 and 40 and present with pain and swelling. Most surface chondrosarcomas arise in the pelvis or proximal femur.

Radiologically, surface chondrosarcomas show lobulated masses of stippled and ring-like calcifications adjacent to the bone surface (Fig. 12-86). Unlike the surface calcifications seen in osteochondromas or periosteal chondromas, these calcifications are not well defined and usually cannot be circumscribed by a continuous line (Fig. 12-87). Surface chondrosarcomas that have arisen in an osteochondroma have distinctive radiographic features. First, an area of radiolucency may be present in the stalk or in the cap of an osteochondroma. This lucent area usually indicates rapidly growing, unmineralized cartilage. Second, irregular, stippled calcifications may develop in the soft tissue overlying an osteochondroma. These differ from the regular, well-defined calcifications of *exostosis bursata*. Third, remnants of a bony stalk may be apparent at the base of the cartilage mass.

Histologically, surface chondrosarcomas consist of lobular masses of cartilage, which vary in size. The cartilage lobules show grade 1 or grade 2 features. These lobules, lacking the stalk of an osteochondroma, are usually directly adjacent to the bone surface. The most important diagnostic feature of surface chondrosarcoma is infiltration of adjacent soft tissues by cartilage lobules.

Juxtacortical Chondrosarcoma

Juxtacortical chondrosarcoma, also called periosteal chondrosarcoma, is a special surface variant.[121,122] This rare neoplasm grows broadly on the bone surface as if confined by the periosteum. However, some soft tissue infiltration is usually present. The underlying cortex is often scalloped or sclerotic. The femur, humerus, and tibia are the most common locations. Juxtacortical chondrosarcoma consists of lobules of low-grade cartilage separated by fibrous bands. The absence of neoplastic osteoid distinguishes this lesion from periosteal osteosarcoma.

Clear Cell Chondrosarcoma

Clear cell chondrosarcomas are rare, low-grade malignant neoplasms that share many radiologic and histologic features with chondroblastomas. Indeed, some clear cell chondrosarcomas contain areas histologically identical to chondroblastoma. Because these neoplasms tend to occur in an older age group than chondroblastomas, the similarities suggest that clear cell chondrosarcomas represent transformed chondroblastomas.

Patients present at any age, but most are between ages 25 and 50, an older age group than most patients with chondroblastoma. Clear cell chondrosarcomas, like chondroblastomas, almost always involve the epiphyseal end of long bones.[123,124] The lesions most commonly occur in the head of the femur, involved in 63% of cases (Fig. 12–88). Other common locations are the proximal humerus and distal femur. Patients usually present with pain that, in 18% of cases, has been present for longer than 5 years. Joint stiffness is also a common symptom.

The radiologic features of clear cell chondrosarcomas are very similar to those of chondroblastomas. They are lytic, well-circumscribed epiphyseal lesions that usually lack a sclerotic rim. Lesions almost always extend into the metaphysis, and cortical thinning and expansion are often present. Most clear cell chondrosarcomas are purely lytic, but fluffy calcification is present in approximately one third of cases.

Histologically, clear cell chondrosarcomas contain sheets of rounded cells with numerous scattered foci of extracellular chondroid matrix. Foci of mature hyaline cartilage also may be present. Like chondroblastomas, the cells of clear cell chondrosarcomas are round with rounded central nuclei and

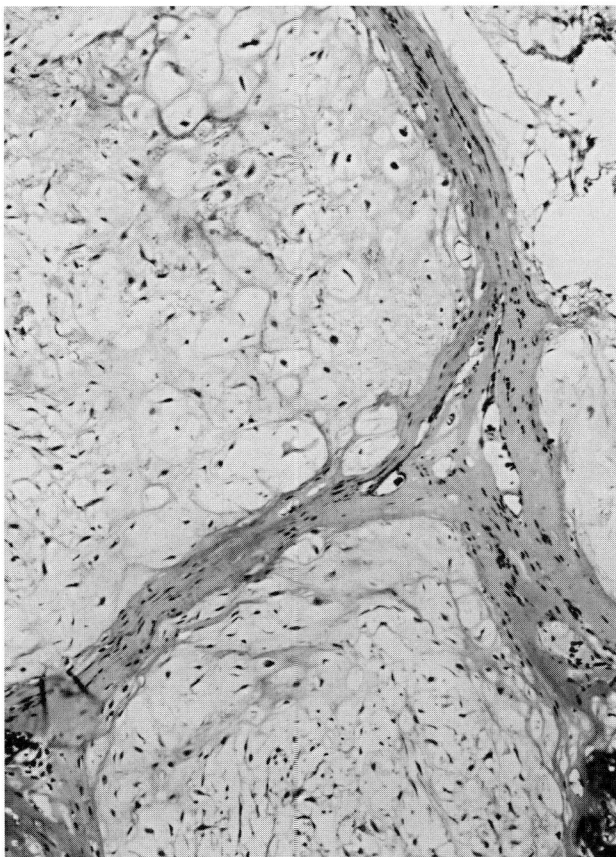

Figure 12–85 ■ Photomicrograph of chondrosarcoma showing lobules of malignant cartilage separated by fibrous bands.

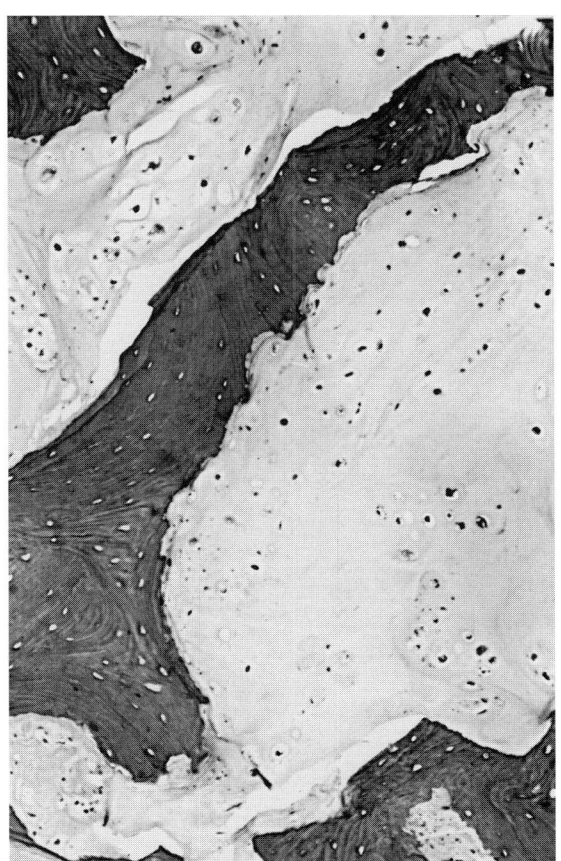

Figure 12–84 ■ Photomicrograph of a chondrosarcoma showing encasement of native bone trabeculae by malignant cartilage.

distinct cytoplasmic membranes. Some cells are in fact identical to chondroblastoma cells. In addition, multinucleated giant cells and reactive bone are also present in clear cell chondrosarcomas. Mitotic figures are rare.

Unlike the stromal cells of a chondroblastoma, however, the cytoplasm of almost all the cells of a clear cell chondrosarcoma is clear (Fig. 12–89). Some cells contain variable amounts of clumped eosinophilic material. Also, the cells are slightly larger than chondroblastoma cells. Approximately 50% of clear cell chondrosarcomas contain foci of conventional, grade 1 chondrosarcoma.

Clear cell chondrosarcomas, although malignant, are slow growing. En bloc surgical excision is the preferred treatment. If surgical margins are clear, the prognosis is excellent.

Mesenchymal Chondrosarcoma

Mesenchymal chondrosarcomas are small round blue cell neoplasms with foci of cartilage differentiation. This rare chondrosarcoma variant is the cartilaginous equivalent to small cell osteosarcoma.

This malignant neoplasm may occur at any age, but most patients are between ages 10 and 40. The most common sites are the bones of the face, ribs, pelvis, and femur.[125] In addition to these bony sites, about one half of the reported

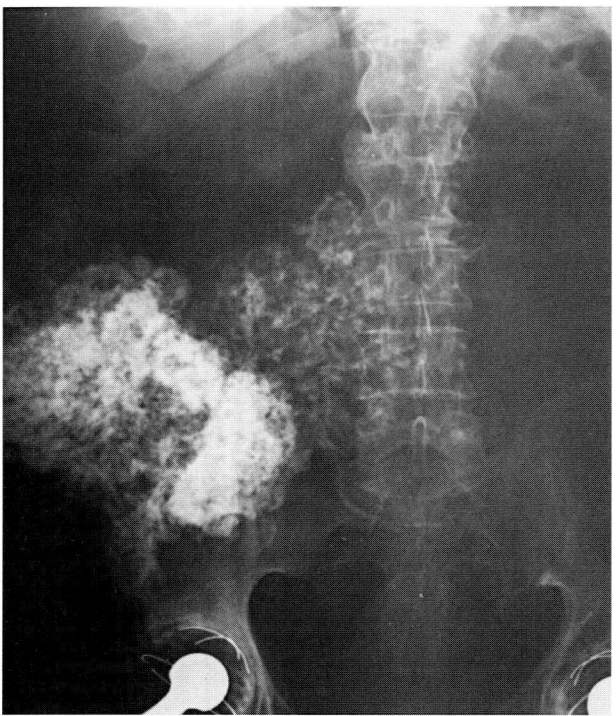

Figure 12-86 ■ A surface chondrosarcoma of the ilium. A huge mass of mineralizing cartilage is present.

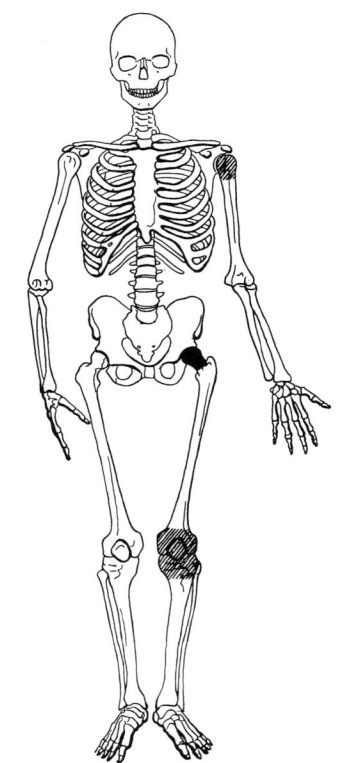

Figure 12-88 ■ Clear cell chondrosarcoma locations.

cases of mesenchymal chondrosarcomas develop in the soft tissues.

Radiologically, mesenchymal chondrosarcomas are poorly circumscribed lytic lesions. Faint stippled calcifications may be present. In the soft tissues, a poorly circumscribed collection of ring-shaped and stippled calcification is present.

The principal histologic feature of mesenchymal chondrosarcoma is sheets of small round cells with scant cytoplasm. Sometimes the cells are spindle shaped. These cells are often arranged in a manner suggestive of hemangiopericytoma. Admixed with the small round cells are small foci of hyaline cartilage. These foci are sharply demarcated from the surrounding cells and show focal calcification and endochondral bone formation. An important immunohistochemical feature of mesenchymal chondrosarcoma is positive staining with the O13 antibody.[126] This antibody identifies CD99, the MIC2 gene product. This product is also a marker for the

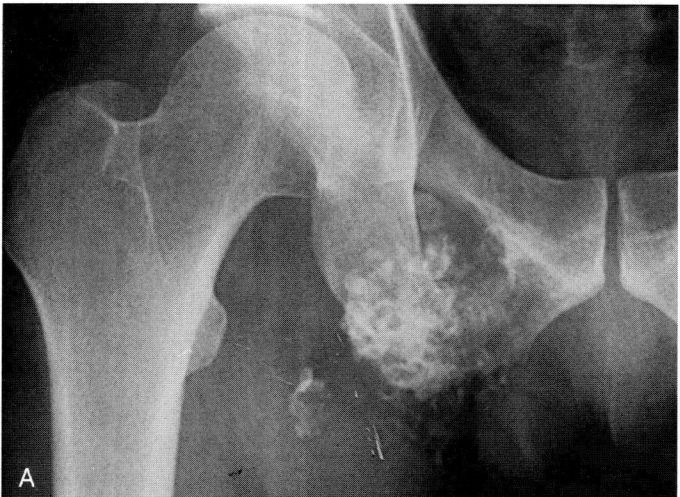
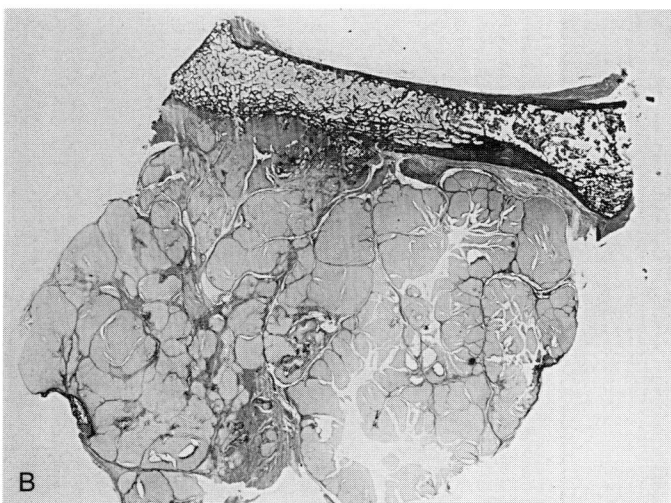

Figure 12-87 ■ Surface chondrosarcoma of the ischium. **A,** Plain radiograph showing a poorly defined zone of ring-shaped radiodensities. **B,** Low-power photomicrograph showing lobules of cartilage on the bone surface. (From McCarthy, E. F.: *Differential Diagnosis in Pathology. Bone and Joint Disorders.* New York and Tokyo, Igaku-Shoin, 1996. With permission from Williams & Wilkins.)

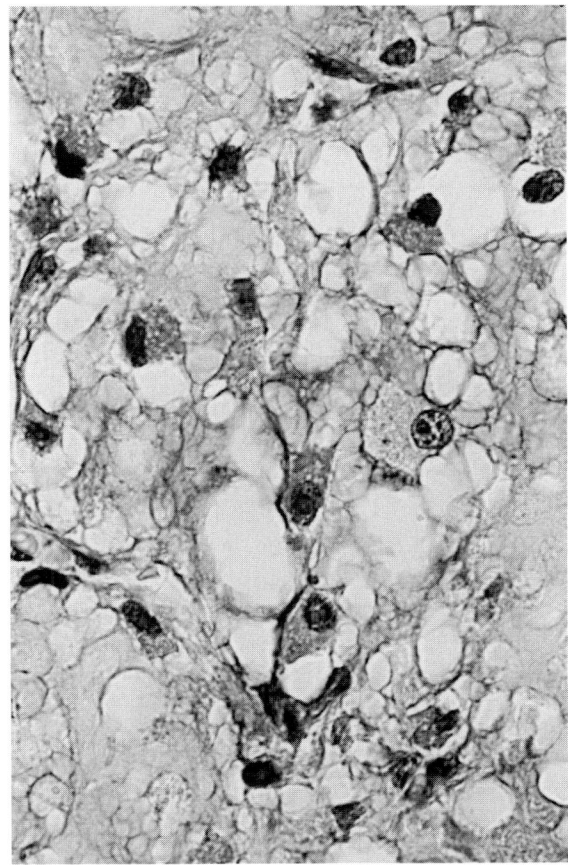

Figure 12-89 ■ Photomicrograph of clear cell chondrosarcoma. Numerous cells with a clear cytoplasm are disbursed in an extracellular chondroid matrix.

Ewing sarcoma/peripheral neuroectodermal tumor (PNET) group of neoplasms.

Mesenchymal chondrosarcoma is an aggressive neoplasm. Patients whose lesions are unresectable respond temporarily to radiation and chemotherapy. However, 70% of patients die 5 to 22 years after treatment.

Dedifferentiated Chondrosarcoma

Dedifferentiated chondrosarcomas, accounting for 11% of chondrosarcomas, are highly malignant neoplasms characterized by a high-grade sarcoma developing in association with a low-grade cartilage lesion, either an enchondroma or a low-grade chondrosarcoma. Whether the high-grade sarcoma develops from a clone of cartilage cells or from a noncartilaginous cell line is not known. However, enchondromas show no cell division, and it is unlikely that nondividing cells can dedifferentiate. Therefore, the high-grade component probably develops from another tissue element. Although enchondromas usually show increased uptake on radionuclide scans, tracer accumulates because of remodeling and reparative change, not because of growth of the lesion. This reparative tissue is the likely source of the high-grade neoplasm. A similar event may occur in the reparative tissue surrounding a bone infarct. Thus, the name *dedifferentiated chondrosarcoma* is a misnomer. It is not a chondrosarcoma, and dedifferentiation has not taken place.

Dedifferentiated chondrosarcomas present with pain, usually of only a few months' duration, and some patients present with a pathologic fracture. Patients are usually adults between the ages of 30 and 60. Rarely, young adults may be affected. The pelvis is the most common location, followed by the femur and the humerus[127,128] (Fig. 12–90).

Dedifferentiated chondrosarcomas have a distinctive radiographic pattern. A destructive radiolytic area is superimposed over a focus of radiodensity (Fig. 12–91). The radiodensity is a well-circumscribed group of stippled calcifications, a feature characteristic of cartilage. Sometimes the calcifications are poorly circumscribed. The superimposed radiolytic area is poorly circumscribed, usually with expansion or destruction of the cortex. An adjacent soft tissue mass, best visualized with MRI, is sometimes present. Occasionally, the radiolytic component obliterates most of the radiodensities.

Histologically, dedifferentiated chondrosarcomas have two distinct components—well-defined nodules of hyaline cartilage and a high-grade sarcoma. The cartilage is consistent with an enchondroma or, rarely, a low-grade chondrosarcoma. The high-grade lesion is usually a malignant fibrous histiocytoma or an osteosarcoma (Fig. 12–92). Other reported differentiations have been angiosarcoma, rhabdomyosarcoma,[129] and a lesion identical to conventional giant cell tumor.[130]

Dedifferentiated chondrosarcomas should be treated with

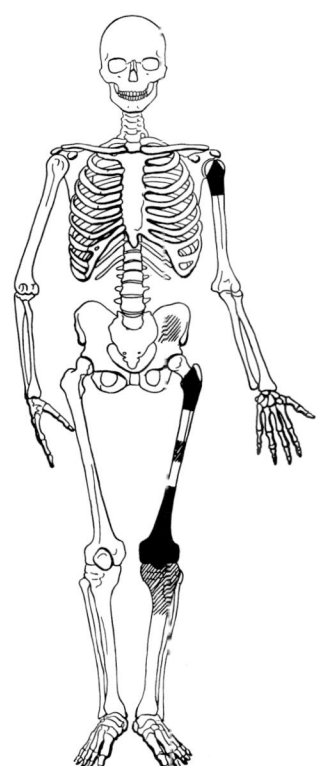

Figure 12-90 ■ Dedifferentiated chondrosarcoma locations.

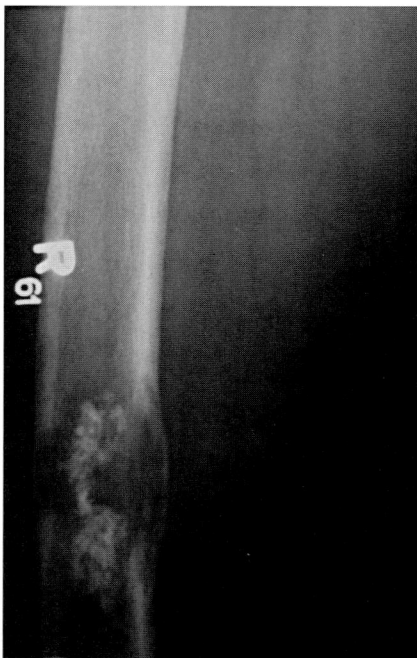

Figure 12-91 ■ Dedifferentiated chondrosarcoma of the femur. A well-defined zone of radiodensity is surrounded by a poorly defined area of radiolucency. (From Frassica, F. J., and McCarthy, E. F.: Miller, M. D., Ed. *Review of Orthopaedics*, 2nd ed. Philadelphia, W. B. Saunders, 1996, p. 314.)

teal osteoclastic resorption during metaphyseal remodeling. This exaggerated resorptive process often begins at the site of tendon insertions.[131] Small lesions, known as fibrous cortical defects, result from the same process. Although they form in the metaphysis, lesions migrate into the diaphysis as the bone grows.

Nonossifying fibromas most commonly involve the distal femur and the distal or proximal tibia, sites that account for 80% of lesions. The flat bones, the small bones of the hands and feet, the spine, and the craniofacial skeleton are not affected. Lesions in these locations with similar histologic features are best regarded as benign fibrous histiocytomas. Many nonossifying fibromas are asymptomatic and are discovered incidentally on radiographs taken for other reasons. Undoubtedly, many are never diagnosed. Large nonossifying fibromas may cause pain, and some present with pathologic fracture. Symptoms, when present, usually develop when patients are in their midteens. The development of a nonossifying fibroma before age 5 is extremely rare. A syndrome of multiple nonossifying fibromas and cutaneous café au lait spots is known as the Jaffe-Campanacci syndrome.[132]

Radiographically, nonossifying fibromas are lytic metaphyseal lesions. Characteristically, lesions are eccentric in the medullary canal and are juxtaposed to one cortex (Fig. 12–93). In addition, the margins are scalloped, and a scle-

chemotherapy and limb-sparing radical surgery or amputation. The prognosis is extremely poor. Metastases, always identical to the high-grade component, are often present at the time of diagnosis. Ninety percent of patients die within 2 years.

Treatment of Chondrosarcomas

The treatment of chondrosarcomas depends on the type and grade of the tumor. In general, grade 1 and grade 2 neoplasms do not respond to chemotherapy or radiation therapy. Therefore, surgery is the mainstay of treatment. Plain radiographs and the MRI scan are used to design surgical margins so that the entire lesion and a cuff of normal tissue can be removed.

In patients with grade 3 lesions (including dedifferentiated chondrosarcoma and mesenchymal chondrosarcoma), preoperative and postoperative chemotherapy can be used to help reduce the risk of local and systemic failure. Unfortunately, no universally effective regimens similar to those for osteosarcoma and Ewing sarcoma exist.

FIBROUS LESIONS

Nonossifying Fibroma

Nonossifying fibromas are common developmental proliferations of fibrous tissue that occur in the metaphyseal region of long bones. Although the cause of these lesions is unknown, they are probably caused by exaggerated subperios-

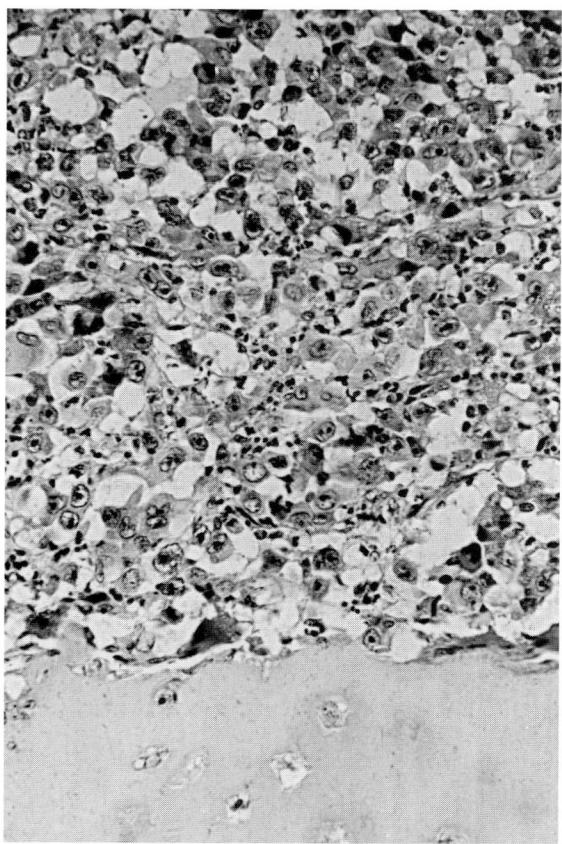

Figure 12-92 ■ Photomicrograph of dedifferentiated chondrosarcoma. An area of hyaline cartilage is adjacent to a sheet of atypical bizarre malignant cells.

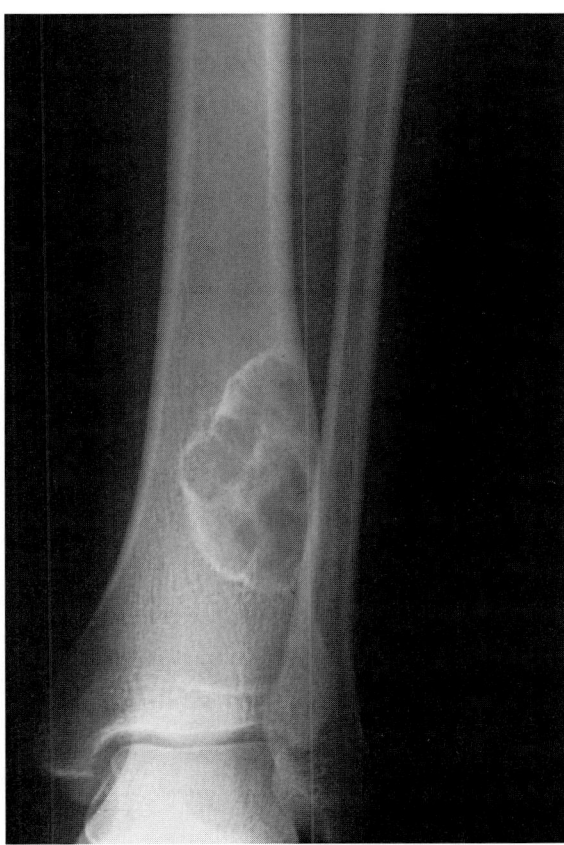

Figure 12-93 ■ Nonossifying fibroma of the distal tibia. A well-defined zone of radiolucency is present adjacent to the metaphyseal cortex. It is surrounded by a rim of sclerotic bone.

in the medullary canal. This tissue proliferates during skeletal growth and, in some cases, continues to grow during adulthood. Bone involvement in fibrous dysplasia exhibits a wide spectrum of severity. In about 80% of cases, only a small focus of one bone is affected, a presentation known as monostotic fibrous dysplasia. Multiple bones are involved in the remainder of patients, the so-called polyostotic fibrous dysplasia. In this presentation, fibrous dysplasia may involve long segments of bone, and it may cause significant cortical expansion. Occasionally, polyostotic fibrous dysplasia involves only one extremity.

Fibrous dysplasia may occur in any bone. In the axial skeleton, the craniofacial bones and ribs are the most common sites. The tibia and proximal femur are the preferred sites in the appendicular skeleton. Fibrous dysplasia is often asymptomatic—lesions are discovered on plain radiographs taken for other reasons. Although lesions develop during skeletal growth, 25% of cases are not diagnosed until after age 30.

Some patients with severe polyostotic fibrous dysplasia also have pigmented skin lesions and endocrine abnormalities. Patients with this syndrome, known as the McCune-Albright syndrome, have severely deformed bones and are usually symptomatic before age 10. The skin lesions are macular café au lait spots that have jagged "coast of Maine"

rotic rim is present. Nonossifying fibromas in older patients often have intralesional radiodensity, a manifestation of healing. Small lesions, from 1 to 2 cm, are regarded as fibrous cortical defects. Alternatively, some lesions reach 7 cm in maximal diameter and cause cortical expansion.

Histologically, nonossifying fibromas consist of a spindle cell stroma with scattered small multinucleated giant cells, although the giant cells may be scarce. Characteristically, the spindle cells are arranged in a whorled or storiform pattern (Fig. 12–94). Occasionally, the stroma is very cellular, and the spindle cells often have plump hyperchromatic nuclei. In some larger lesions, a moderate number of typical mitotic figures are present. In addition to the giant cells and stromal cells, foam cells and occasional hemosiderin-laden macrophages are present. This feature has led some authors to call this lesion a fibroxanthoma. Reactive bone is common, especially in older lesions.

Small asymptomatic nonossifying fibromas need no therapy. Most heal spontaneously over several years. Larger lesions, particularly those that expand the cortex or present with pathologic fracture, should be treated by curettage and bone grafting. Recurrence after treatment is very rare.

Fibrous Dysplasia

Fibrous dysplasia is a common skeletal lesion characterized by a hamartomatous proliferation of fibroosseous tissue

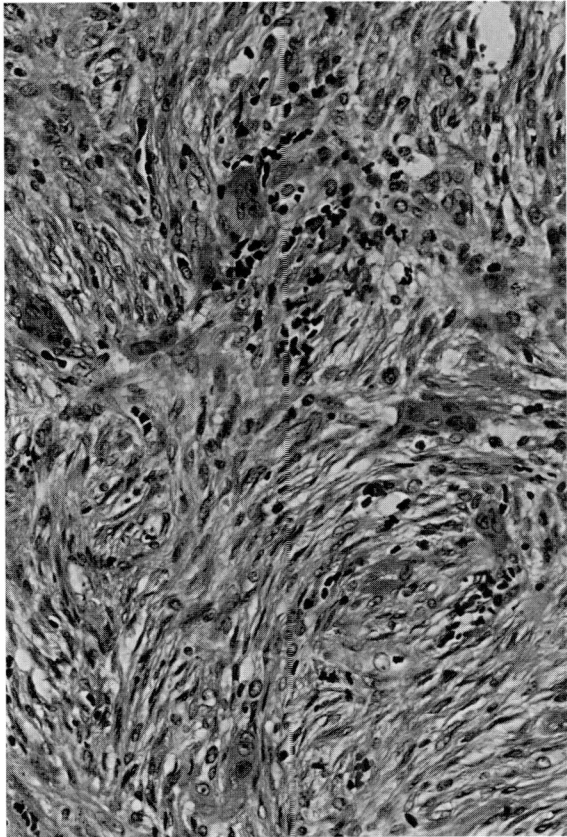

Figure 12-94 ■ Photomicrograph of nonossifying fibroma. A few multinucleated giant cells are present in a fibrous tissue background. The fibroblasts are arranged in a storiform pattern.

edges. These contrast with the smoothly contoured "coast of California" café au lait spots of neurofibromatosis. In the McCune-Albright syndrome, the skin lesions are often confined to one extremity. Some patients with this syndrome also have soft tissue myxomas. The McCune-Albright syndrome is now known to be a genetic mutation caused by a mosaic state of an activating mutation in the *GNAS 1* gene. This gene codes for an adenosinediphosphate-dependent G protein.[133] In addition, overexpression of the C-fos protooncogene has been noted in the bones of some patients with polyostotic fibrous dysplasia.[134]

The radiologic features of fibrous dysplasia are often diagnostic. In the appendicular skeleton, fibrous dysplasia is typically an elongated lesion with symmetric cortical thinning and expansion—the characteristic "long lesion in a long bone" (Fig. 12–95). On rare occasions, fibrous dysplasia may grow as a bubble-like expansion of one cortex, a pattern known as fibrous dysplasia protuberans.[135] Although most lesions have a "ground glass" texture, some may be entirely radiolytic; others may be radiodense (Fig. 12–96). The spectrum of radiodensity reflects the amount of dysplastic bone in the lesional tissue. In severely involved weight-

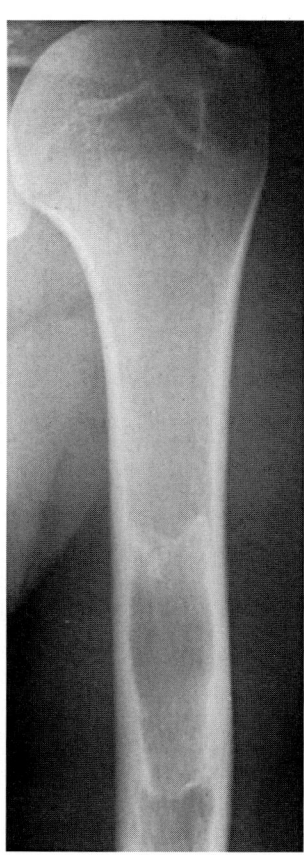

Figure 12-96 ■ A small lesion of fibrous dysplasia present in the proximal humerus. The distal portion of the lesion has a "ground-glass" appearance.

bearing bones, deformity due to multiple fractures is common (Fig. 12–97). In the femoral neck, the so-called "shepherd's crook" deformity may result from this process (Fig. 12–98). On occasion, lesions of fibrous dysplasia appear to rapidly increase in size. This change is due to cystic degeneration or to aneurysmal bone cyst transformation.

Histologically, fibrous dysplasia shows irregular seams of woven new bone in a cellular fibrous stroma. The seams of bone are thin and disconnected and are arranged in curved shapes reminiscent of Chinese letters or "alphabet soup" (Fig. 12–99). Although osteoblasts are occasionally adjacent to the seams of woven bone, orderly osteoblastic rimming, characteristic of reactive or neoplastic bone, is not present (Fig. 12–100). The amount of woven bone is variable. In some areas, only the fibrous stroma is present. A careful search in these areas usually reveals scant traces of osteoid production. Alternatively, bone may be abundant and show evidence of remodeling into lamellar bone.

In some lesions of fibrous dysplasia, particularly those that involve the craniofacial bones, the osteoid is deposited as round globules resembling cementum[136] (Fig. 12–101). Some pathologists regard these lesions as *fibrous cementomas* or *cementoossifying fibromas*.[137] A more appropriate term is *cementomatous variant of fibrous dysplasia*.

Hyaline cartilage nodules are present in some lesions of

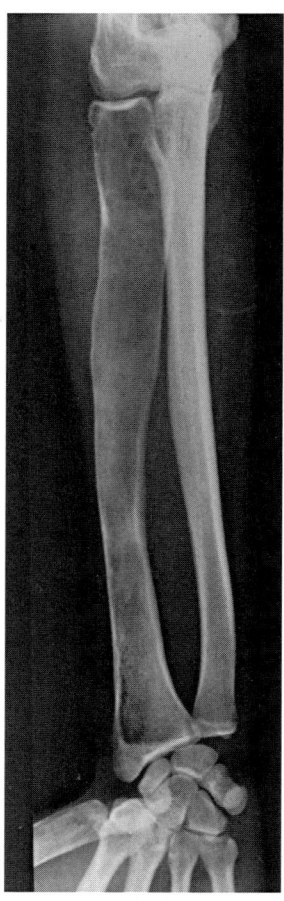

Figure 12-95 ■ Fibrous dysplasia of the radius. This lesion typifies a long lesion in a long bone. A fusiform expansion of the proximal two thirds of the radius is present. The lesion has a "ground-glass" texture. (From Frassica, F. J., and McCarthy, E. F.: Orthopaedic pathology. Miller, M. D., Ed. *Review of Orthopaedics*, 2nd ed. Philadelphia, W. B. Saunders, 1996, p. 332.)

PRIMARY BONE TUMORS   247

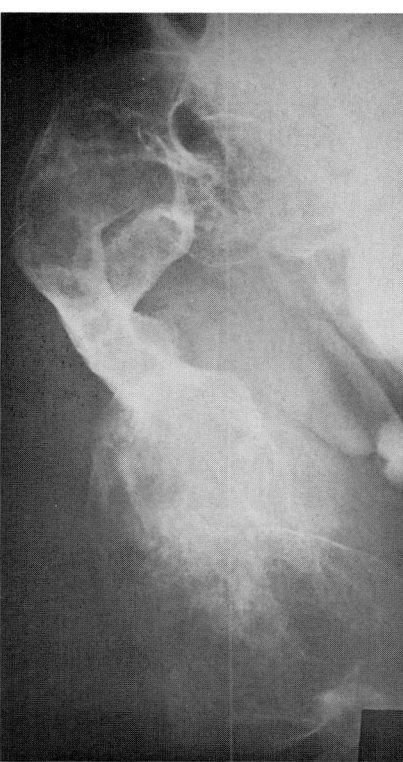

Figure 12-97 ■ Extensive fibrous dysplasia of the entire femur in a patient with the McCune-Albright syndrome.

fibrous dysplasia. Endochondral ossification occurs at the periphery of these nodules, a process that results in dysplastic fibroosseous tissue rather than normal bone. Sometimes the cartilage is massive, and the lesion may be mistaken for a chondrosarcoma.[138] However, the cartilage of fibrous dysplasia rarely shows cytologic atypia. Some pathologists recognize an entity called *fibrocartilaginous mesenchymoma of bone*, a lesion with a more cellular and slightly atypical fibrous stroma.[139] An alternative view is that fibrocartilaginous mesenchymoma is fibrous dysplasia with cartilage.

Treatment is unnecessary for asymptomatic lesions of fibrous dysplasia, which have no potential for pathologic fracture. Large or symptomatic lesions may be treated by curettage and bone grafting. Recurrences are the result of incomplete removal of lesional tissue. Rare instances of malignant transformation of fibrous dysplasia have been reported. However, some of these cases were probably postradiation sarcomas, and some may have been osteosarcomas originally but were misdiagnosed as fibrous dysplasia. True malignant transformation of fibrous dysplasia is extremely rare.

Fibrous dysplasia has two important differential diagnoses: well-differentiated intraosseous osteosarcoma and, in the tibia, osteofibrous dysplasia. Well-differentiated intraosseous osteosarcoma is also a fibroosseous lesion. However, unlike the disconnected spicules of woven bone in fibrous dysplasia, the bone spicules in well-differentiated intraosseous osteosarcoma are broad and connected. Usually the bone is lamellar, unlike the predominantly woven bone of fibrous dysplasia. Another distinguishing feature of well-differentiated intraosseous osteosarcoma is mild cellular atypia. By contrast, the stroma of fibrous dysplasia, although often very cellular, is never atypical.

Fibrous dysplasia in the tibia may be confused with osteofibrous dysplasia. However, the characteristic radiographic features of osteofibrous dysplasia—intracortical lucencies and anterior tibial bowing—are not present in fibrous dysplasia. Also, orderly osteoblastic rimming of bone, characteristic of osteofibrous dysplasia, is absent in fibrous dysplasia.

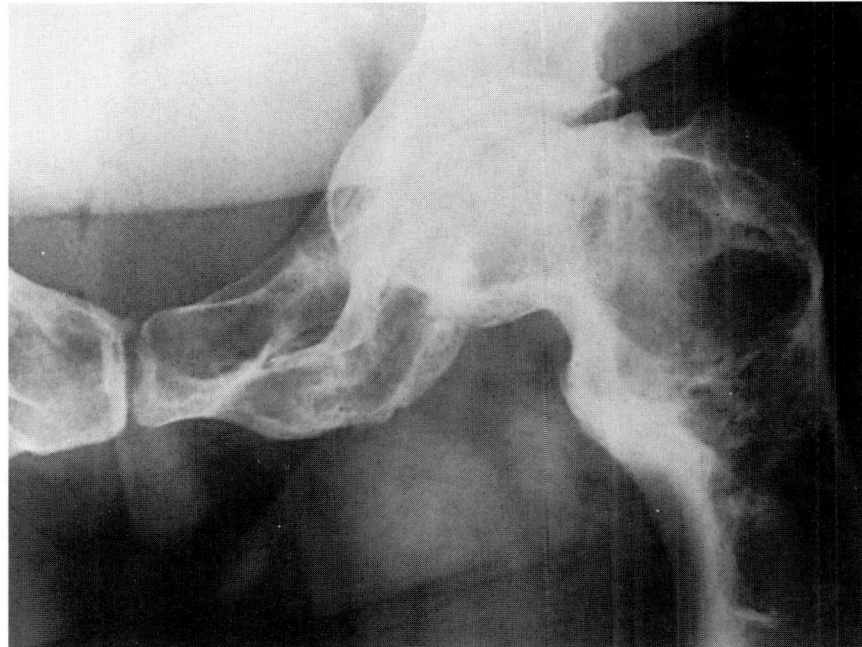

Figure 12-98 ■ Fibrous dysplasia of the proximal femur and pelvis. The proximal femur has a "shepherd's crook" deformity.

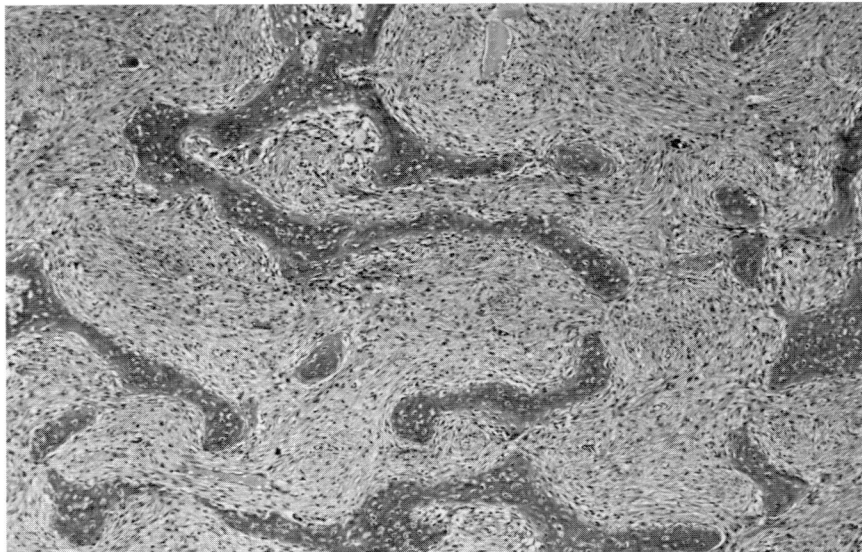

Figure 12-99 ■ Low-power photomicrograph of fibrous dysplasia showing curved trabeculae of new bone in a fibrous background. There is the so-called "Chinese letter" pattern of new bone.

Benign Fibrous Histiocytoma of Bone

Some pathologists recognize an entity called benign fibrous histiocytoma of bone.[140-143] This lesion is histologically characterized by a storiform arrangement of spindle cells, scattered foam cells, and giant cells. However, this histologic pattern, when in the metaphysis, is more properly regarded as a nonossifying fibroma. In the epiphysis, where most cases have been reported, this histologic pattern most probably represents involutional change in a conventional giant cell tumor. Therefore, benign fibrous histiocytoma is best regarded as a histologic pattern rather than a distinct bone neoplasm.

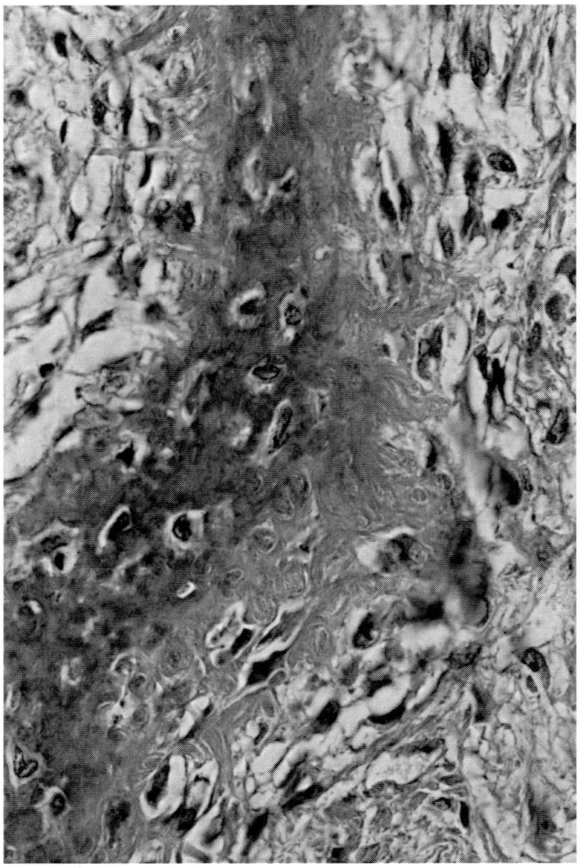

Desmoplastic Fibroma

Desmoplastic fibromas, the intraosseous equivalent of soft tissue fibromatosis, are extremely rare neoplasms that most

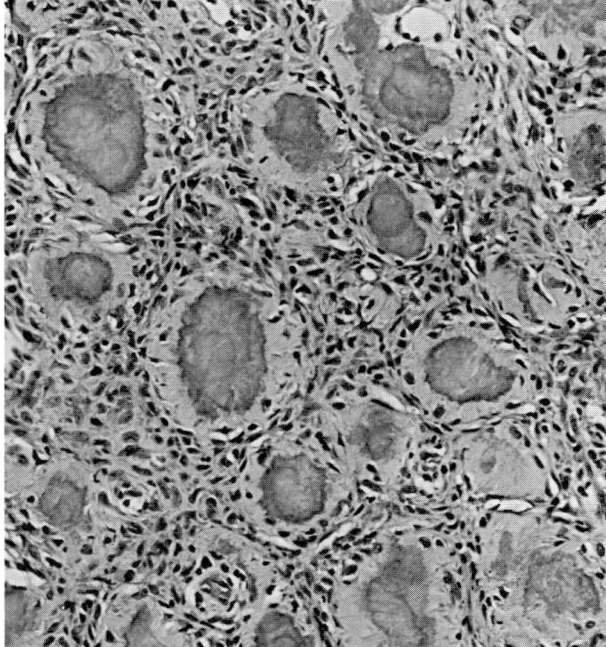

Figure 12-100 ■ High-power photomicrograph of fibrous dysplasia. The new bone is not lined by osteoblasts.

Figure 12-101 ■ Photomicrograph of fibrous dysplasia showing numerous cementum-like bodies. This histologic pattern is common in lesions of the skull and face.

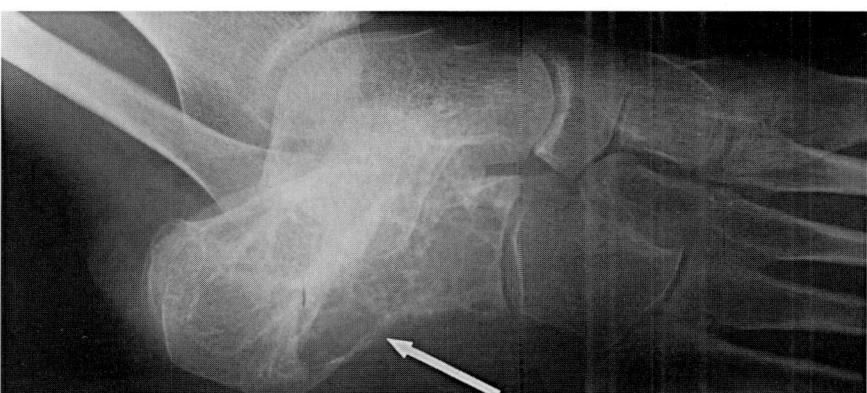

Figure 12-102 ■ Desmoplastic fibroma of the calcaneus. A poorly defined radiolytic lesion is present *(arrow)*. It has a soap bubble appearance.

commonly involve the jaw, femur, and tibia. Although patients may be any age, almost one half are between 10 and 20 years.[144] Patients present with pain, often for several years, which suggests lesional growth. On rare occasions, desmoplastic fibromas may be incidental findings.[145]

Desmoplastic fibromas are radiolytic lesions, usually well defined and centered in the metaphyseal portion of the bone[146] (Fig. 12-102). A multicystic, expansile pattern is typical. The cortex is often focally destroyed, and a soft tissue mass, best visualized on MRI, may be present. Twelve percent of patients present with a pathologic fracture.[147] Histologically, desmoplastic fibromas show a patternless proliferation of benign-appearing fibroblasts with a densely collagenized stroma (Fig. 12-103). The fibroblasts have bland, oval, or elongated nuclei, usually without a nucleolus, and mitotic figures are extremely rare. The fibroblastic proliferation has an infiltrative growth pattern, often entrapping native trabeculae. Desmoplastic fibromas are locally aggressive neoplasms that do not metastasize. However, 50% of lesions recur after curettage. Therefore, wide surgical excision with negative margins is the preferred treatment. Patients with extensive bone involvement may require amputation.

Fibrosarcoma of Bone

Fibrosarcomas of bone are neoplasms of varying malignant potential that may occur de novo in bone or, in 25% of cases, as a complication of other conditions such as Paget's disease or radiation osteitis. Like desmoplastic fibromas, these neoplasms are also rare. Many cases originally diagnosed as fibrosarcoma have been reclassified as malignant fibrous histiocytoma. Patients may be any age, and they present with pain. Any bone may be involved, but the femur, tibia, and pelvis are the most common sites.[148,149]

Fibrosarcomas, although also radiolytic lesions, are usually poorly defined (Fig. 12-104). The lytic process typically involves the central portion of the medullary canal, although occasional lesions may be centered on the cortex and have a significant soft tissue mass.

Histologically, a fibrosarcoma may be difficult to distinguish from a desmoplastic fibroma. However, two important histologic differences exist. First, unlike the spindle cells of a desmoplastic fibroma, which are haphazardly arranged, the spindle cells of a fibrosarcoma are usually arranged in bundles (Fig. 12-105). Sometimes, the bundles interlace to form

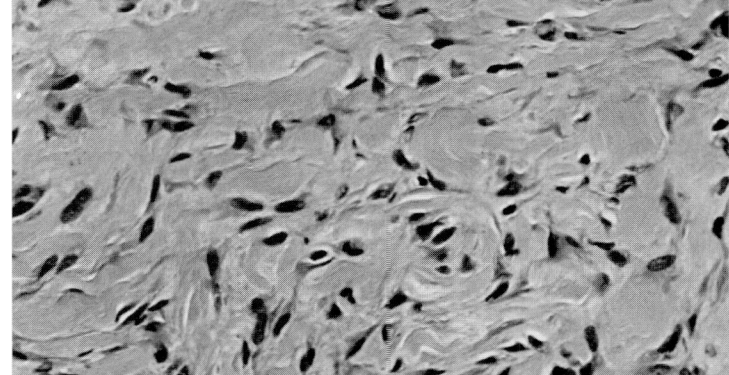

Figure 12-103 ■ Photomicrograph of desmoplastic fibroma. Small fibroblasts are present in a highly collagenized extracellular matrix.

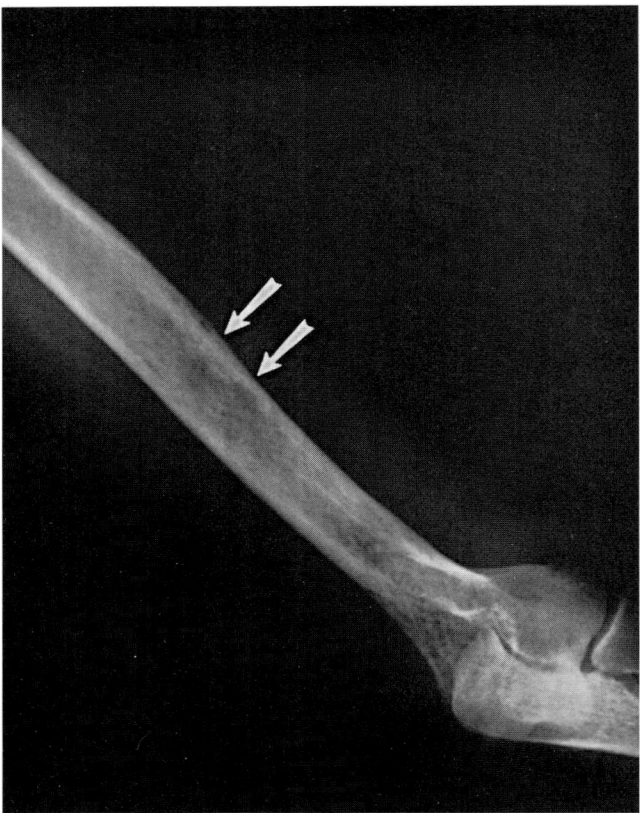

Figure 12-104 ■ Fibrosarcoma of the humerus. The lesion is a poorly defined lytic area with a permeative growth pattern *(arrows)*. (From Frassica, F. J., and McCarthy, E. F.: Miller, M. D., Ed. *Review of Orthopaedics,* 2nd ed. Philadelphia, W. B. Saunders, 1996, p. 316.)

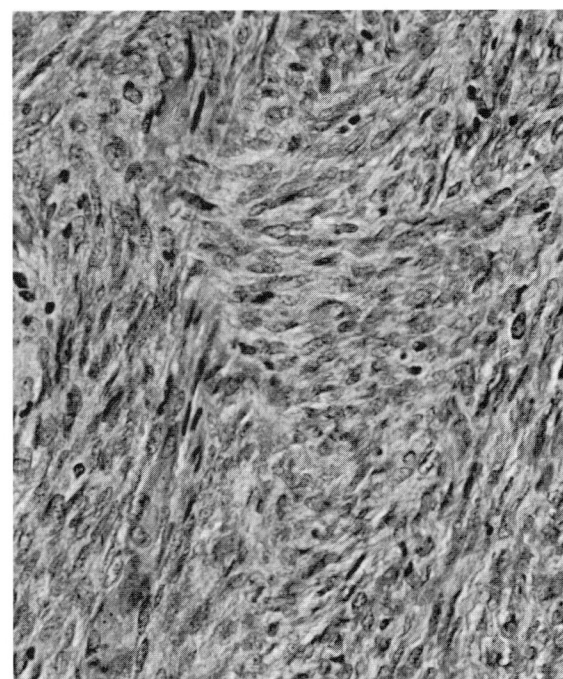

Figure 12-105 ■ Photomicrograph of fibrosarcoma. Cellular fibroblasts are arranged in a herringbone pattern.

a "herringbone" pattern. In addition, a focal storiform pattern may be present, although lesions with an extensive storiform pattern should be classified as malignant fibrous histiocytomas. Second, the fibroblasts of a fibrosarcoma, in contrast to those of a desmoplastic fibroma, show a spectrum of nuclear atypia. Even a low-grade (grade 1) fibrosarcoma, a lesion that closely resembles a desmoplastic fibroma, shows some nuclear atypia. Many nuclei contain nucleoli, and, in addition, some mitotic figures are present (1 to 4 per 10 high-power fields). At the other end of the spectrum, a high-grade (grade 3) fibrosarcoma shows marked nuclear typia and many mitoses. In addition, a high-grade fibrosarcoma may contain focal myxoid areas.

Fibrosarcomas should be treated with wide surgical excision, or if negative margins cannot be attained, amputation. The prognosis correlates with histologic grade. Many patients (83%) with low-grade lesions survive 10 years. However, those patients with high-grade fibrosarcomas have only a 34% 10-year survival. Fibrosarcomas that are centered on the cortex rather than the medullary canal have a somewhat better prognosis.

Malignant Fibrous Histiocytoma

Malignant fibrous histiocytomas are high-grade sarcomas with fibrohistiocytic differentiation. In addition to occurrence in bone as a primary lesion, this neoplasm is the most common sarcoma to complicate preexisting osseous lesions, such as radiation damage, Paget's disease, and cartilaginous neoplasms. In addition, malignant fibrous histiocytomas may,

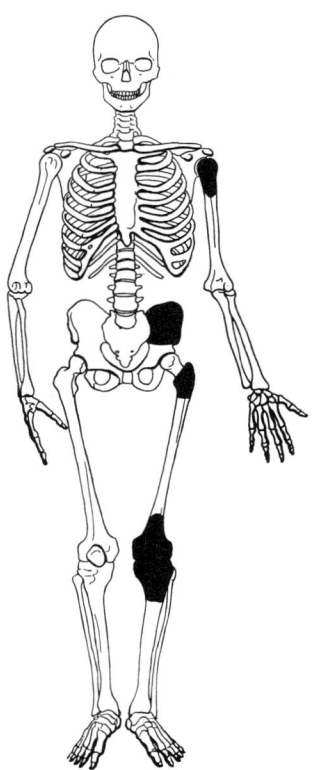

Figure 12-106 ■ Malignant fibrous histiocytoma locations.

on rare occasions, occur as a complication of a bone infarct.[150-152] In this situation, the sarcoma probably develops in the reparative granulation tissue at the margin of the infarct.

Primary malignant fibrous histiocytomas may involve any bone.[153] However, the femur is the most common site (one third of cases), followed by the tibia and humerus (Fig. 12–106). Patients range in age from 6 to 81 years, but more than 50% of cases occur in patients older than 40 years.[154] Patients present with pain, and 67% present with swelling or a mass. Some patients present with a pathologic fracture.

Radiographically, malignant fibrous histiocytomas are poorly defined radiolytic lesions, often with extensive cortical destruction (Fig. 12–107). A periosteal new bone reaction is unusual. MRI often shows an associated soft tissue mass. Malignant fibrous histiocytoma most commonly involves the metaphyseal region of bone. However, secondary involvement of the epiphysis is common.

Malignant fibrous histiocytomas are composed of spindle cells, histiocytic cells, or an intermingled combination of the two in varying proportions (Fig. 12–108). The spindle cells are arranged in a storiform pattern, the most characteristic feature of malignant fibrous histiocytoma.[140,155] The nuclei are oval and vesicular, with mild to moderate pleomorphism. Occasionally, broad bands of osteoid-like collagen separate the stromal cells, a feature that may lead to the misdiagnosis

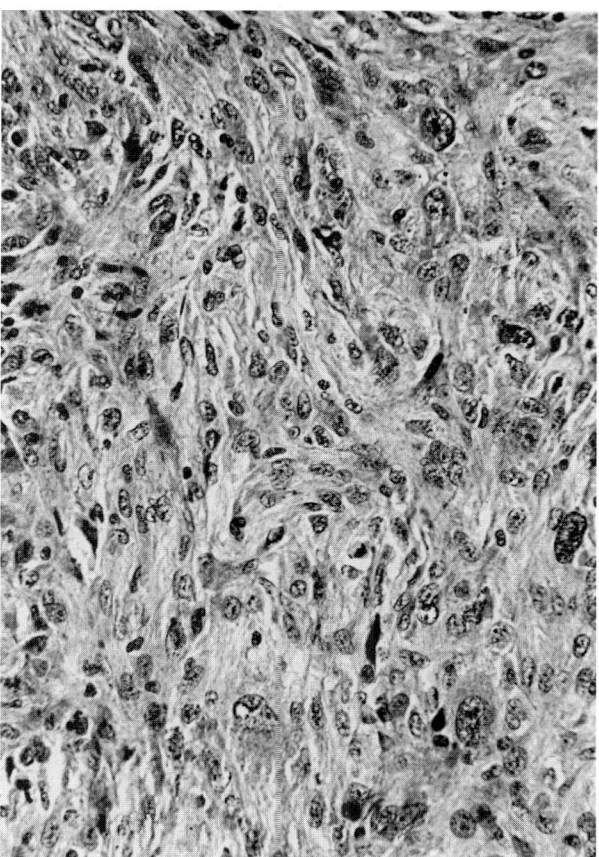

Figure 12-108 ■ Photomicrograph of a malignant fibrous histiocytoma, showing the pleomorphic-storiform pattern.

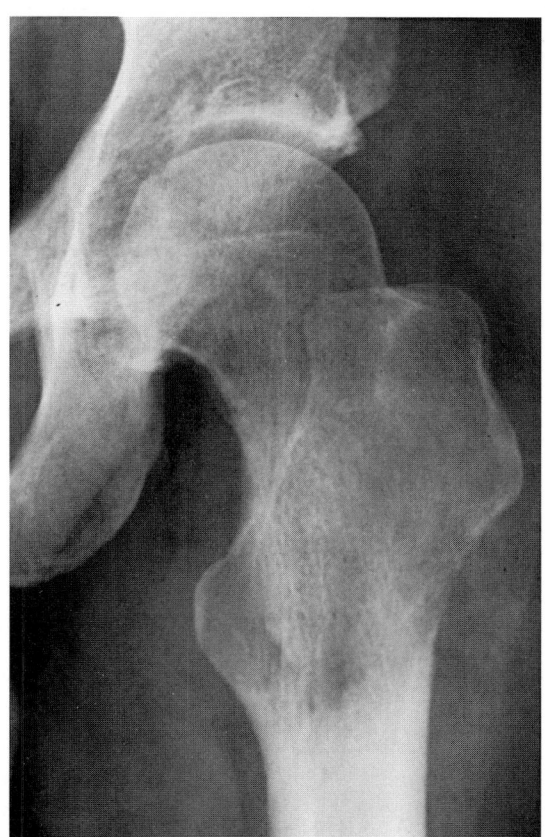

Figure 12-107 ■ A malignant fibrous histiocytoma of the proximal femur. A poorly defined radiolytic area is present in the intertrochanteric region.

of osteosarcoma. However, mineralization, the only absolute diagnostic feature of osteoid, is not present. Therefore, undecalcified neoplastic tissue must always be examined to rule out mineralization. At the other end of the spectrum, malignant fibrous histiocytomas may have a histiocytic differentiation (Fig. 12–109). In contrast to the uniform spindle cells, the histiocytic cells are usually pleomorphic and bizarre. These cells are rounded and have large oval or lobulated nuclei, often with a prominent eosinophilic nucleolus. Some of the histiocytic cells contain hemosiderin or lipid. Lesions with predominantly histiocytic differentiation contain multinucleated giant cells with bizarre nuclei. Bland, osteoclast-like giant cells may infrequently be present.

Malignant fibrous histiocytomas may have a variety of secondary histologic features.[156] First, some may have a heavy inflammatory cell infiltrate, a feature that may lead to the misdiagnosis of Hodgkin's disease. Second, large areas of myxoid stroma may be present, a change that is also seen in malignant fibrous histiocytomas of soft tissue. Some have a very collagenized stroma. Finally, neoplastic cells may be arranged in an organoid pattern around branching vascular spaces, a pattern reminiscent of hemangiopericytoma.

Twenty-eight percent of malignant fibrous histiocytomas of bone are associated with precursor lesions, mandating a careful radiologic and histologic search for such entities as

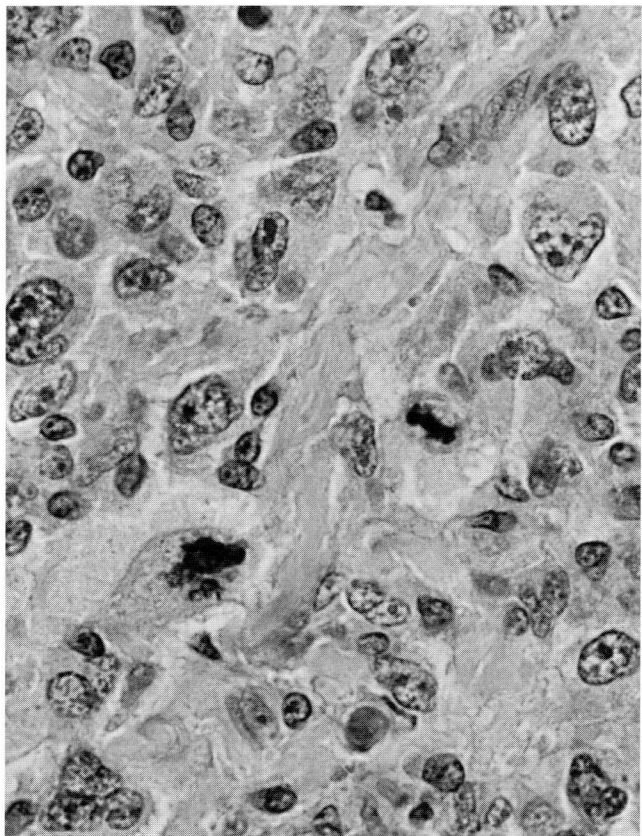

Figure 12-109 ▪ Photomicrograph of a malignant fibrous histiocytoma. These cells resemble histiocytes.

Paget's disease, a bone infarct, prior radiation damage, or cartilage.

Treatment of Fibrosarcoma and Malignant Fibrous Histiocytoma

The treatment of high-grade malignant fibrous lesions of bone (fibrosarcoma and malignant fibrous histiocytoma) is similar. In both lesions, the risk of local failure is high unless the entire tumor and a cuff of normal tissue is removed. Pulmonary metastases develop in up to 30 to 40% of patients. Patients are treated in a fashion similar to osteosarcoma patients—wide resection and preoperative and postoperative chemotherapy. Unfortunately, the chemotherapy regimens are less effective than those for osteosarcoma and Ewing sarcoma.

GIANT CELL TUMOR OF BONE

Giant cell tumor of bone, sometimes referred to as conventional giant cell tumor, is a benign locally aggressive neoplasm that usually affects young adults; about two thirds of patients are between ages 20 and 40. Giant cell tumors may occasionally occur in the elderly—a patient 74 years old has been documented.[157] However, these neoplasms are extremely rare in growing children. Fewer than 2% of giant cell tumors affect patients under age 15.

Giant cell tumors occur most commonly in the distal femur, proximal tibia, and distal radius (Fig. 12–110). These locations account for about 65% of cases. Other common locations include the pelvis, vertebral bodies, and proximal femur. Patients almost always present with pain, and a few present with a pathologic fracture. On rare occasions, giant cell tumor may be multicentric; as many as nine foci may occur either synchronously or metachronously.[158,159]

Giant cell tumors, when they occur in the long bones, have a diagnostic radiographic pattern (Fig. 12–111). A well-defined lytic lesion involves both the epiphysis and the metaphysis and almost always extends to the subchondral bone. The epiphyseal plate is almost always closed. Although well circumscribed, giant cell tumors usually lack a sclerotic rim. At least one cortex is thin and may also be expanded or destroyed. In the flat bones, giant cell tumors are also well-defined lytic lesions without a sclerotic rim.

Histologically, giant cell tumors consist of multinucleated giant cells admixed with mononuclear stromal cells (Fig. 12–112). The stromal cells are polygonal or slightly elongated (Fig. 12–113). Mitotic figures in the stromal cells are numerous. The multinucleated giant cells, often numerous, resemble osteoclasts. Formerly, particularly in the British literature, giant cell tumors were called osteoclastomas because of the abundance of these cells. Mature cartilage or chondroid matrix is not present in giant cell tumors.

Immunohistochemical studies of giant cell tumors have

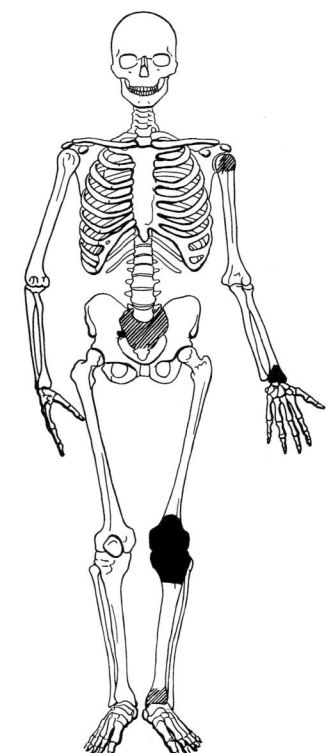

Figure 12-110 ▪ Giant cell tumor locations.

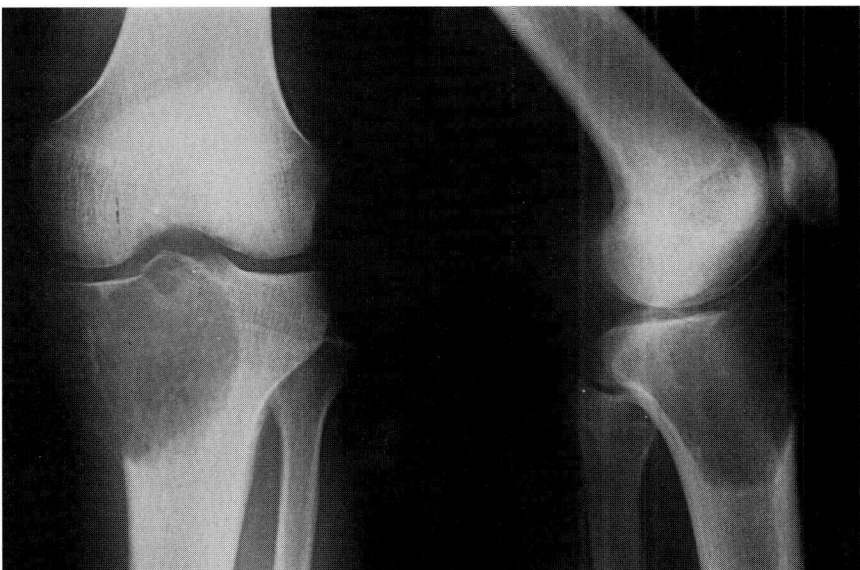

Figure 12-111 ■ Anteroposterior *(left)* and lateral radiographs of giant cell tumor of the proximal tibia. A well-defined area of radiolucency is present and involves the epiphysis and metaphysis.

clarified the relationship of the stromal cells to the giant cells.[160,161] These studies suggest that two populations of stromal cells exist. One population, thought to be the neoplastic component, consists of spindle-shaped cells. The other population consists of the polygonal cell, which resembles a macrophage. These two populations are immunohistochemically distinguishable—the polygonal cells stain for macrophage-associated antigens, particularly CD11a, CD18 and CD13, whereas the spindle cells do not. Many antigen profiles have supported this distinction. However, we have found this differential staining to be most striking with the

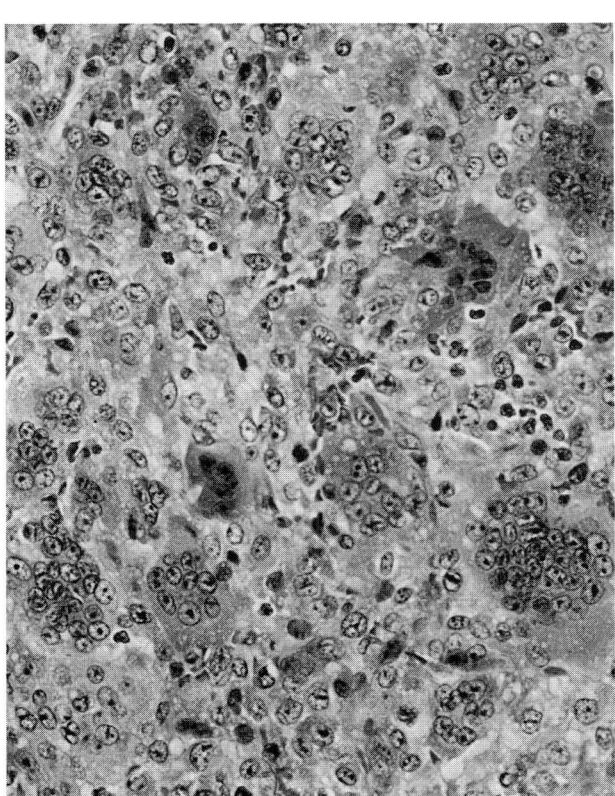

Figure 12-112 ■ Photomicrograph of giant cell tumor showing multiple giant cells admixed with stromal cells.

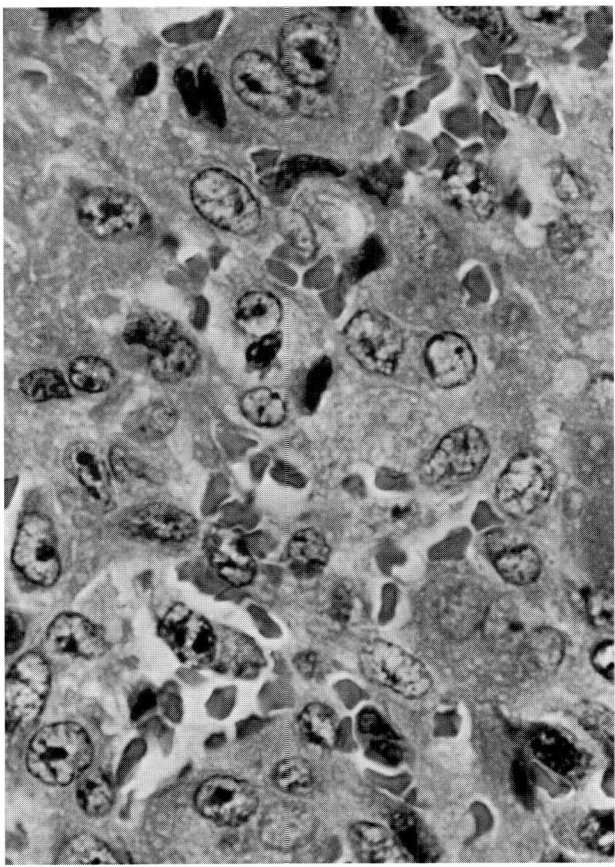

Figure 12-113 ■ High-power photomicrograph of giant cell tumor stromal cells. The stromal cells have vesicular nuclei with prominent nucleoli.

KP1 stain. With this stain, the giant cells stain identically to the macrophage-like cells. This strongly suggests that the giant cells originate from fusion of the macrophage-like cells and not the neoplastic spindle cells. Giant cells also stain for acid phosphatase, a reaction also exhibited by bone-resorbing osteoclasts. These histochemical observations suggest that giant cells are of macrophage origin and are very similar to true osteoclasts. However, they do not result from fusion of the neoplastic cells.

In addition to the typical histologic features of giant cells and stromal cells, giant cell tumors frequently undergo secondary histologic changes, and these changes often lead to diagnostic confusion (Fig. 12–114). First, focal necrosis is common; only the ghosts of the stromal cells and giant cells may be seen. On rare occasions, an entire neoplasm may be necrotic. Second, giant cell tumors may have areas of fibrohistiocytic reparative tissue (Fig. 12–115). Spindle cells in a storiform pattern may be mixed with foam cells. In these areas, reactive bone formation is common. Senescent giant cell tumors may be composed entirely of this reparative tissue, and diagnostic giant cells and stromal cells may be absent. Probably many examples of the entity "benign fibrous histiocytoma of bone" are ancient giant cell tumors that have been effaced by this fibrohistiocytic reaction. Finally, giant cell tumors may have focal areas of aneurysmal bone cyst that may obscure the giant cells and stroma. If these secondary changes—necrosis, fibrosis with reactive

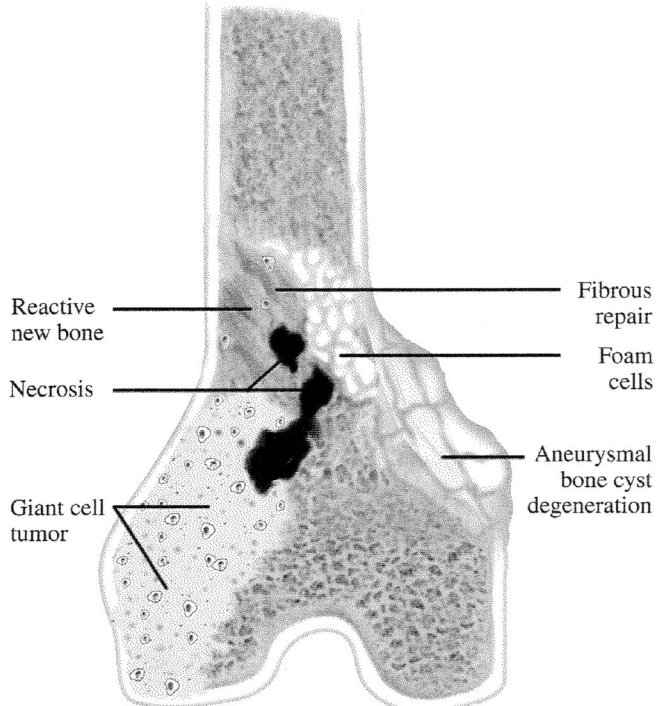

Figure 12-114 ■ Secondary histologic changes that can occur in a giant cell tumor. These changes include reactive new bone, fibrohistiocytic repair tissue, foam cells, necrosis, and aneurysmal bone cyst degeneration.

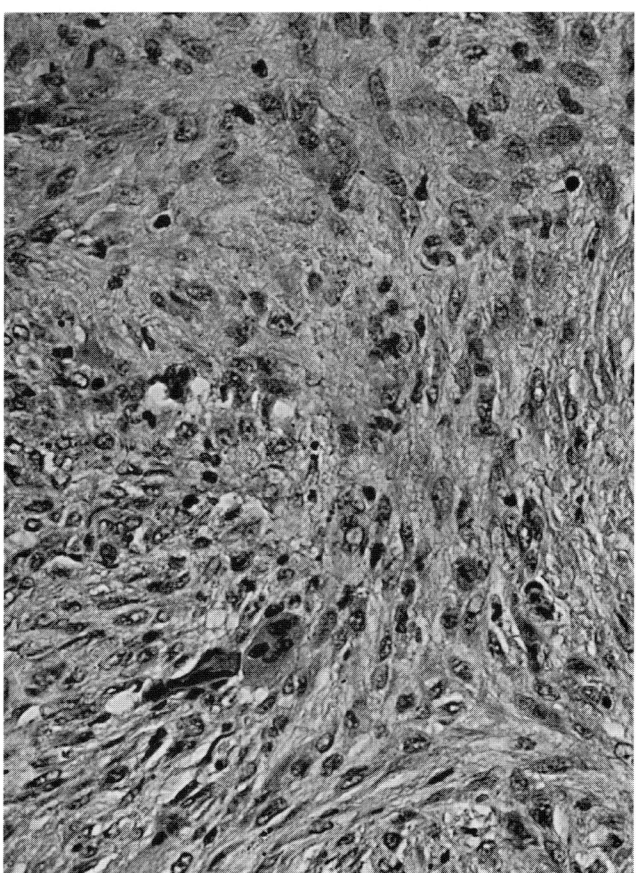

Figure 12-115 ■ Photomicrograph of a fibrohistiocytic area in a giant cell tumor. These areas, which resemble nonossifying fibroma, are common in giant cell tumors.

bone, or aneurysmal bone cyst—predominate, the pathologist must rely on characteristic radiographic features to make the diagnosis of giant cell tumor.

Attempts to identify prognostic features, particularly the likelihood of recurrence, have met with variable success. Formerly, cytologic grading of stromal cells was thought to predict behavior of giant cell tumors. However, this practice is subjective and did not correlate with recurrence. Furthermore, the proliferation index and vascular density of giant cell tumors does not correlate with prognosis.[162] Recently, histomorphometric study of giant cell tumors has identified some cellular features that correlate with aggressive behavior.[163] However, this cumbersome tool is not clinically practical. Other investigators have studied telomerase activity,[164] metalloproteinase expression,[165] and transforming growth factor β in giant cell tumors.[166] These studies may contribute to our understanding the behavior of this neoplasm.

Some benign giant cell tumors have a deceptively ominous appearance. Lesions may have a very cellular stroma, and the cells contain plump, slightly hyperchromatic nuclei. Mitotic figures may be numerous. In addition, many giant cell tumors, 40% in some series, show evidence of vascular invasion. Plugs of both stromal cells and giant cells are present in vascular lumina adjacent to the neoplasm (Fig.

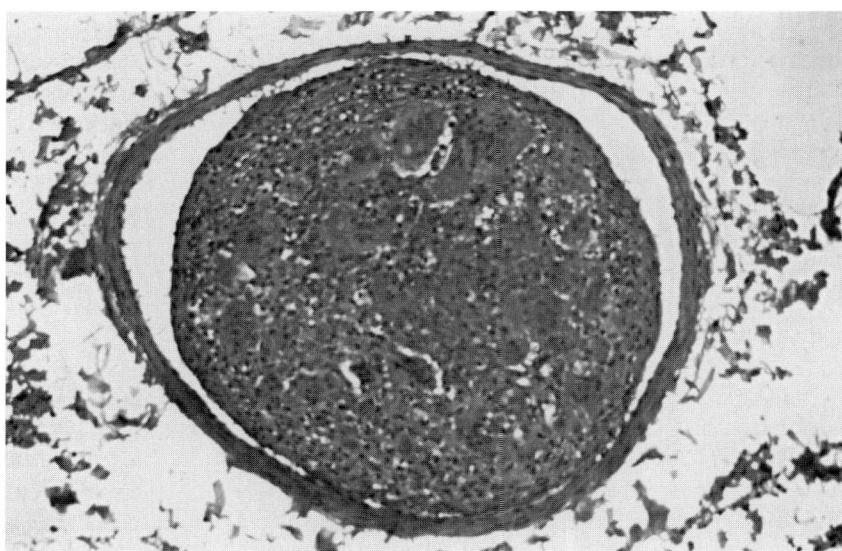

Figure 12-116 ■ Photomicrograph of an embolus of giant cell tumor in a vessel adjacent to a lesion in the hand.

12–116). Vascular invasion is not associated with a worse prognosis, although it may be the mechanism of "benign metastasis."

Benign Metastasizing Giant Cell Tumor

A rare behavior of conventional giant cell tumor, present in 1 to 2% of cases, is pulmonary metastasis, the so-called benign metastasizing giant cell tumor. The pulmonary metastases are usually detected a few years after surgery and probably result from tumor embolization. In these unusual cases, the primary bone lesion is identical in all clinical, radiologic, and histologic respects to other conventional giant cell tumors.[167] Also, the pulmonary metastases are histologically benign. This complication does not indicate an unfavorable prognosis.[168] Pulmonary lesions grow very slowly and may be surgically resected.[169] In fact, some pulmonary lesions remain stationary or even resolve. However, approximately 10% of patients with these "benign" lung metastases die of their disease.

Malignant Giant Cell Tumor

Malignant giant cell tumor is a high-grade sarcoma developing in association with conventional giant cell tumor. This combination, when identifiable at the time of the initial presentation, is known as primary malignant giant cell tumor.[170] Alternatively, secondary malignant giant cell tumor is the late development of a sarcoma after radiotherapy or a curettage of a giant cell tumor. Both manifestations of malignant giant cell tumor are extremely rare and account for about 7% of all giant cell tumors. Primary malignant giant cell tumors probably are manifestations of *dedifferentiation,* similar to that seen in parosteal osteosarcoma or chordomas.[171] By contrast, secondary sarcomatous development in an irradiated giant cell tumor may be radiation induced. The risk of malignant transformation in an irradiated giant cell tumor averages 20%.[172] Reported time intervals until the development of sarcoma have been 4 to 39 years. As expected, patients with secondary malignant giant cell tumors are older than those with conventional giant cell tumors, the peak incidence being in the 5th decade of life. Both primary and secondary malignant giant cell tumors develop in locations typical of conventional giant cell tumor.

Malignant giant cell tumors, both primary and secondary, occur in the same radiographic setting as the conventional variant—the epiphyseal end of a long bone (Fig. 12–117). The radiographic pattern of a primary malignant giant cell tumor may be identical to a conventional lesion. Most, however, are poorly circumscribed. A large volume of sarcomatous tissue may cause significant cortical destruction and soft tissue invasion. By contrast, secondary malignant giant cell tumors, occurring years after the original lesion, have a more destructive pattern. The location at the end of a long bone may be the only clue to its relationship to the original conventional giant cell tumor.

Histologically, primary malignant giant cell tumors are biphasic neoplasms. Islands of conventional giant cell tumor are juxtaposed to a high-grade sarcoma. The sarcomatous component is usually a malignant fibrous histiocytoma, although occasionally an osteosarcoma is present. The sarcomatous component may compose less than 20% of the volume of the neoplasm, emphasizing that conventional giant cell tumors must be generously sampled for histologic study.

Treatment of Giant Cell Tumor of Bone

Although 90% of conventional giant cell tumors never metastasize, they are very difficult to treat because of their local invasiveness. In the past, treatment with curettage and bone grafting led to a local recurrence rate of 30 to 40%.[157] In the past 10 years, the treatment strategy has evolved to

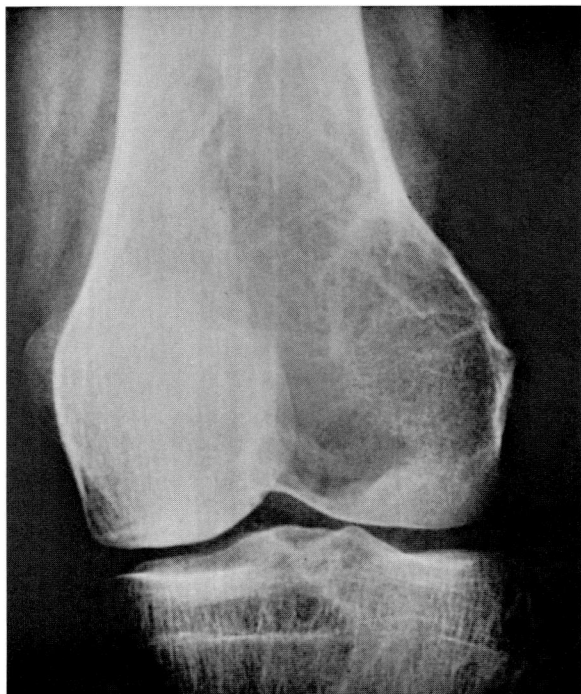

Figure 12-117 ■ Malignant giant cell tumor of the distal femur. A poorly defined radiolucent area is present in a typical giant cell tumor location. (From McCarthy, E. F.: *Differential Diagnosis in Pathology. Bone and Joint Disorders.* New York and Tokyo, Igaku-Shoin, 1996. With permission from Williams & Wilkins.)

include wide exteriorization of the cortex, curettage with hand and power instruments, chemical cauterization with phenol, and reconstruction with subchondral cancellous bone grafts and methyl methacrylate. Internal fixation is often necessary. Wide exteriorization involves removing all the cortical bone over the lesion so that the surgeon does not have to work around any corners during curettage. The gross lesional tissue is removed with hand curettes, and then the remaining bone is burred down with power instruments to extend the curettage. This procedure removes the small (1- to 2-mm) pockets of the neoplasm. If the lesion has extended to within 1 cm of the articular cartilage, this area is reconstructed with cancellous graft. The large remaining defect is filled with cement to prevent fracture and allow early motion. With this technique, which allows very extensive curettage, the local failure rate is less than 10%. The risk of arthritis is small if the cement is placed more than 1 cm from the articular surfaces.

LYMPHOMA OF BONE

Malignant lymphomas may secondarily involve bone marrow as a manifestation of disseminated disease. For example, bone marrow may be involved in disseminated small lymphocytic lymphomas and in many small cleaved cell lymphomas. In these low-grade lymphomas, bone involvement does not necessarily carry a poor prognosis, and plain radiographs do not often show osseous abnormalities. In addition, secondary bone involvement may occur in patients with stage IV, high-grade lymphomas. However, bone involvement in these patients indicates a poor prognosis.

In contrast to secondary osseous involvement, a malignant lymphoma may present in bone without evidence of nodal and visceral disease. Patients with this disease, known as *primary malignant lymphoma of bone,* have a more favorable prognosis than those with secondary bone involvement. Primary malignant lymphomas of bone may occur at any age; patients range in age from 1.5 to 86.0 years, the mean being 46.0 years.[173] Any bone may be involved, and 29% of patients have multiple osseous sites. The mandible, maxilla, femur, pelvis, and spine are the most common locations (Fig. 12–118). Patients present with pain, often for longer than a year's duration. Some patients with a lymphoma at the epiphyseal end of a bone present with joint effusion secondary to neoplastic involvement of joint structures.

Malignant lymphomas are characteristically diffusely permeative lytic lesions that often involve a large segment of the affected bone. Lesions have varying amounts of intraosseous reactive bone, which imparts a mottled appearance. Occasionally, a lesion may have extensive osteosclerosis, a feature that often results in misdiagnosis as other lesions, particularly Paget's disease (Fig. 12–119). In some cases, lymphomas may completely destroy a segment of bone. In these cases, only a soft tissue mass, visible on MRI scan, is present.

Malignant lymphomas of bone are usually diffuse, large cell, noncleaved lymphomas (Fig. 12–120). The neoplastic

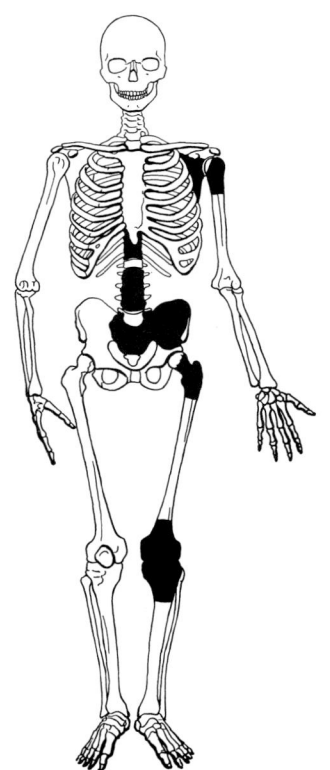

Figure 12-118 ■ Lymphoma of bone locations.

cells are usually uniform, with a large round nucleus and clumped chromatin; cytoplasm is scant. However, some osseous lymphomas have cells with cleaved or even multilobed nuclei.[174] Also, in rare cases, the cells may be pleomorphic and have abundant cytoplasm, a pattern consistent with immunoblastic lymphoma. Osseous lymphomas in children may be the lymphoblastic type and have small cells with round nuclei and fine chromatin.

Most lymphomas of bone have associated histologic features that make diagnosis difficult. First, many contain a dense population of inflammatory cells, most of which are T lymphocytes; neutrophils may also be present (Fig. 12-121). This inflammatory infiltrate may obscure the lymphoma cells and lead to the incorrect diagnosis of osteomyelitis. Second, lymphoma of bone may contain loose or dense fibrous tissue that entraps the neoplastic cells in a pseudoorganoid pattern. This pattern may lead to the misdiagnosis of metastatic carcinoma. Lesions with extensive fibrosis often have abundant reactive bone. Third, the lymphoma cells may, although rarely, have a spindle shape. These cells may be arranged in a storiform pattern and masquerade as a sarcoma. Finally, some lymphomas have cells with clear cytoplasm and signet-ring nuclei, a pattern that may also be confused with metastatic carcinoma.

Malignant lymphomas of bone are almost always B-cell neoplasms. Lymphoid origin is confirmed by a CD45 (leuko-

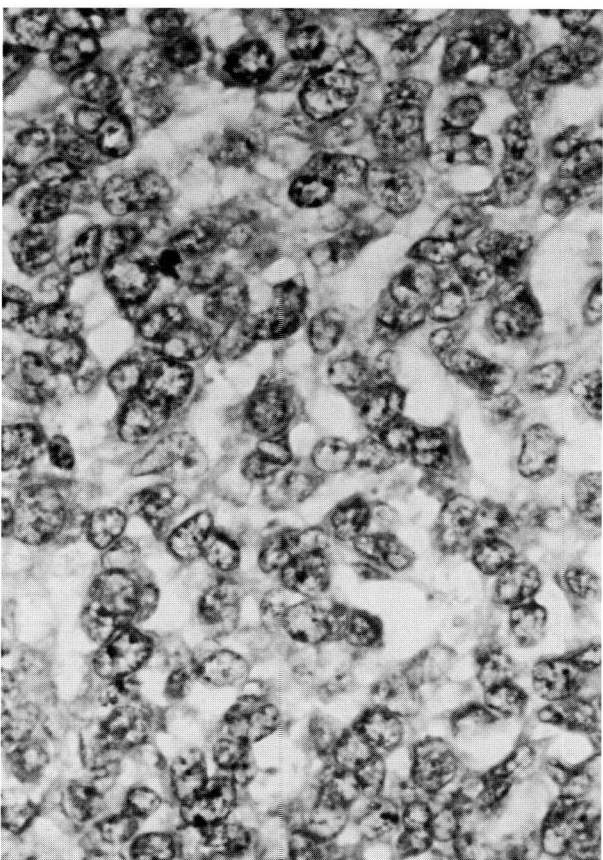

Figure 12-120 ■ Photomicrograph of lymphoma of bone. Most primary lymphomas of bone are large, noncleaved, B-cell lymphomas.

cyte common antigen) stain. The B-cell lineage is confirmed by a CD10 (L26) stain. This latter stain differentiates the neoplastic cells from the inflammatory infiltrate, which usually consists of many T lymphocytes. Occasionally, anaplastic osseous lymphomas with cells containing multilobed nuclei stain with the Ki-1 antigen.[175] These Ki-1–positive cells also contain CD45 and epithelial membrane antigen. Glycogen is absent from lymphoma cells.

Lymphomas of bone, without nodal or visceral disease, have a favorable prognosis. Generally, younger patients do better. Irradiation, with adjuvant chemotherapy, yields a 5-year survival of 50 to 88%. Patients with multifocal osseous disease but without soft tissue involvement also do well, 40% surviving 5 years.

HODGKIN'S DISEASE OF BONE

Bones may be secondarily involved in disseminated Hodgkin's disease, a process similar to bone involvement in the late stages of lymphomas. In Hodgkin's disease, radiologic evidence of bone involvement is present in 13% of advanced cases.[176] The incidence at autopsy is much higher.[177] Bone marrow involvement without radiologic change may occur in 15% of advanced cases.[178] In disseminated (stage IV) disease, bone involvement is due to hematog-

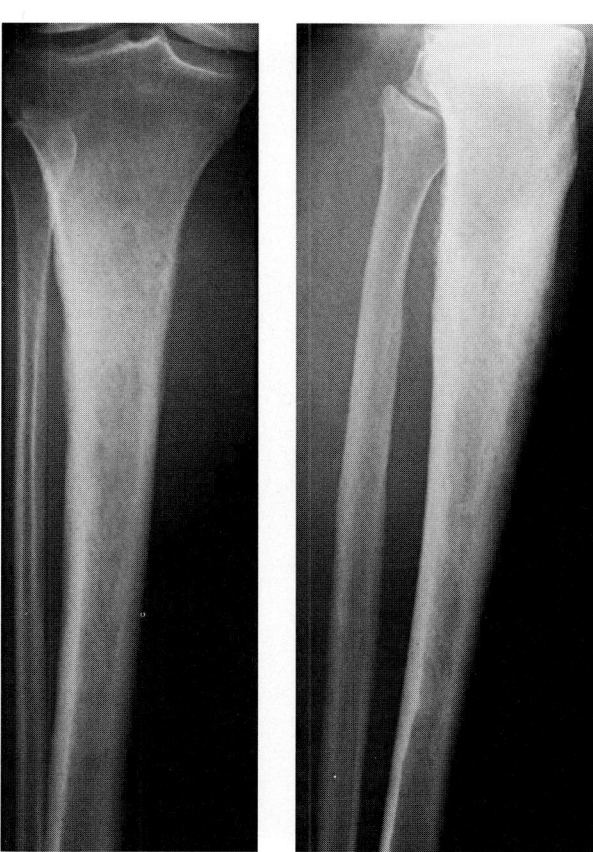

Figure 12-119 ■ Anteroposterior *(left)* and lateral radiographs of lymphoma of the tibial metaphysis and diaphysis. Extensive irregular bone sclerosis is present. This lesion was originally diagnosed as Paget's disease.

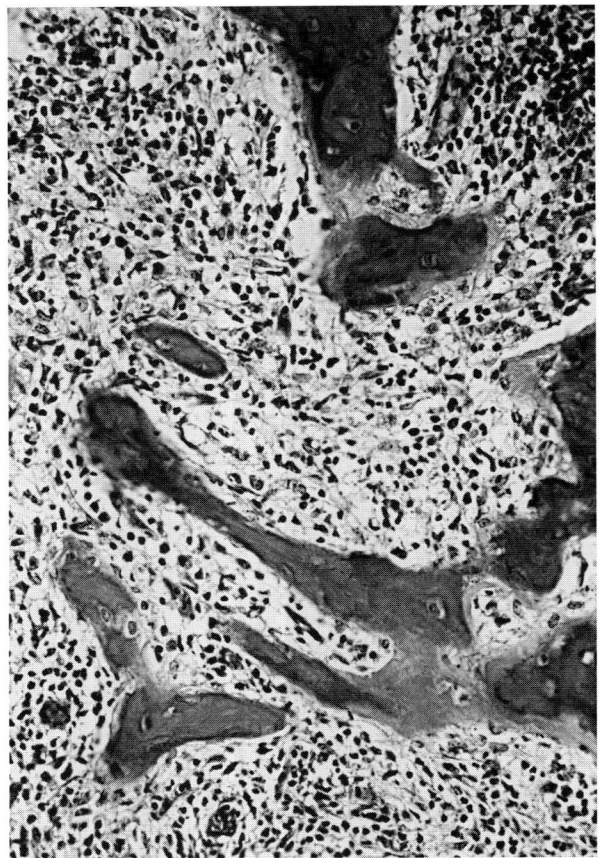

Figure 12-121 ■ Lymphoma of bone with extensive reactive new bone formation.

positive staining for CD15 and CD30 and negative staining for CD45 and T-cell and B-cell markers. By contrast, the Langerhans' cells of eosinophilic granuloma are positive for S-100 protein. By exclusion, if the immunohistochemical stains for S-100 protein, CD15, and CD30 are negative, osteomyelitis is the probable diagnosis.

Hodgkin's disease in bone with only limited nodal disease responds to combined aggressive radiotherapy and chemotherapy. Most patients survive at least 3 years. By contrast, patients with bone involvement secondary to disseminated Hodgkin's disease have a very poor prognosis. Their survival is usually less than a year.

EWING SARCOMA/PERIPHERAL NEUROECTODERMAL TUMOR

Ewing sarcoma and its differentiated subtype, peripheral neuroectodermal tumor (PNET) of bone, are the most malignant of all the primary bone tumors. They are the most common tumors in the group called "small round blue cell tumors."[180] Other neoplasms in this group are primary lymphomas of bone, small cell osteosarcoma, and mesenchymal chondrosarcoma. A genetic abnormality that distinguishes Ewing sarcoma from other neoplasms is a characteristic chromosomal translocation—t(11;22)(q24;12).[181] Other

enous spread. Bone involvement also may occur as a result of direct invasion from an adjacent lymph node (stage IE). Secondary bone involvement by Hodgkin's disease usually produces lytic lesions, although blastic and mixed lesions also occur. The sites most frequently involved are in the axial skeleton: the spine, pelvis, ribs, and proximal femurs.

On rare occasions, Hodgkin's disease presents in bone without obvious lymph node involvement. Only 21 cases of this presentation have been documented.[179] After close clinical and radiologic study, however, many of these cases also had adjacent nodal disease, a finding that suggests that bones were secondarily involved by contiguous spread from nodal disease. The bones most frequently involved were the sternum, femur, vertebrae, tibia, and humerus. The bone lesions were usually lytic, and the age range was from 5 to 83 years, the average age being 31 (Fig. 12–122).

In most cases, the Hodgkin's disease associated with bone involvement is the nodular sclerosing or mixed cellularity type. Histologically, Reed-Sternberg cells and mononuclear variants are present in a polymorphous background that includes lymphocytes, plasma cells, eosinophils, and fibrous tissue. This mixture of cells may be mistaken for chronic osteomyelitis or eosinophilic granuloma. Immunohistochemical studies are often necessary to distinguish these lesions. The presence of Reed-Sternberg cells may be confirmed by

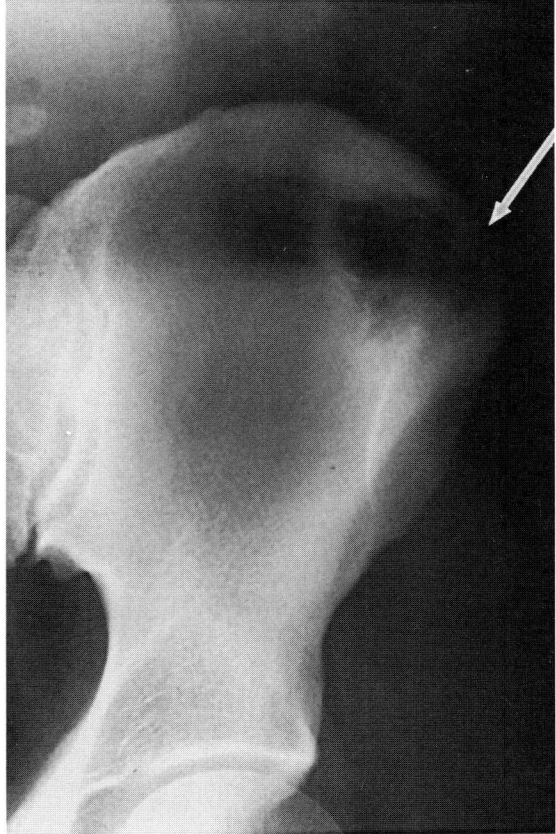

Figure 12-122 ■ Hodgkin's disease of bone in the ilium. A zone of radiolucency is surrounded by sclerotic bone (arrow).

small round blue cell tumors, such as embryonal rhabdomyosarcoma and neuroblastoma, are not primary osseous tumors but may involve bone secondarily.

Ewing sarcoma is not uncommon. It accounts for as many as 15% of all primary malignant bone tumors and is the fourth most common bone malignancy after myeloma, osteosarcoma, and chondrosarcoma.[182] Ewing sarcoma occurs in patients younger than those with all other primary malignant bone tumors. Although patients range from 5 months to 47 years old, 85% of patients are between ages 5 and 20.[183] Any bone may be affected, but involvement of the femur and pelvis accounts for one third of cases (Fig. 12–123). The fibula is commonly involved by PNET of bone. A characteristic presentation of both Ewing sarcoma and PNET is a very large soft tissue mass adjacent to the involved bone. Patients present with pain, and many present with signs and symptoms that mimic acute osteomyelitis: fever, leukocytosis, and an elevated sedimentation rate. Occasionally, patients present with a pathologic fracture.

The very aggressive growth of Ewing sarcoma and PNET is evident radiographically. Both neoplasms show a highly permeative growth pattern with a periosteal new bone reaction. The periosteal reaction may be the "onion skin" or the "sunburst" pattern (Fig. 12–124). The diaphysis of bone is the usual location; however, the metaphysis is also sometimes affected (Fig. 12–125). The intraosseous component of some lesions may be so highly permeative that plain radiographs may be interpreted as normal. In these cases, a minimal periosteal reaction may be the only clue to the

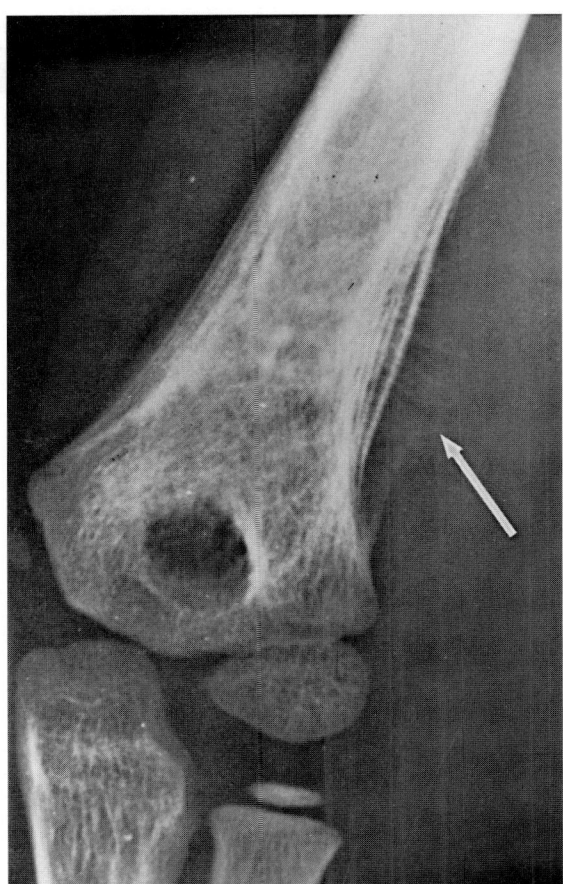

Figure 12-124 ■ Ewing sarcoma of the distal humerus. A poorly defined lytic lesion is present. Both an onion skin and a sunburst pattern of periosteal bone reaction can be seen (arrow).

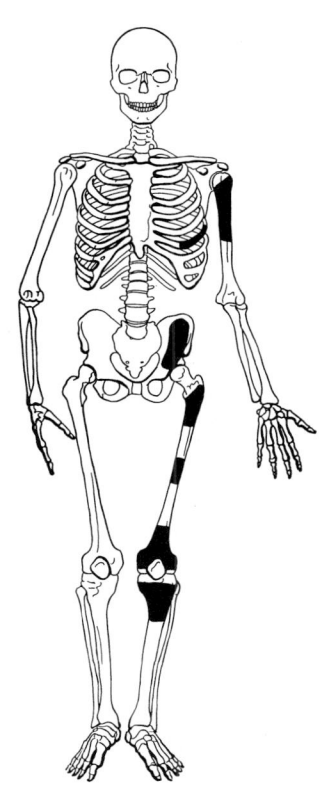

Figure 12-123 ■ Ewing sarcoma locations.

presence of a neoplasm. An MRI or a bone scan, however, reveals long segments of marrow involvement. In addition, the MRI often reveals an adjacent soft tissue mass. In about one third of cases, Ewing sarcoma and PNET provoke intramedullary reactive bone and appear focally radiodense. This pattern may mimic an osteosarcoma.[184]

Histologically, Ewing sarcoma and PNET consist of broad fields of small uniform round cells with scant cytoplasm (Fig. 12–126). The nuclei are round and contain fine chromatin. Nucleoli are usually inconspicuous (Fig. 12–127). Often, a second population of cells is scattered amid the primary cells. These cells are smaller and have an eosinophilic cytoplasm and a dense hyperchromatic nucleus[183] (Fig. 12–128). Occasionally, the cells of some Ewing sarcomas have larger nuclei and prominent nucleoli but are otherwise identical to typical cases. Neoplasms with these nuclear features have been called the "large cell variant" of Ewing sarcoma.[185]

A common feature of tumors in the Ewing/PNET group is broad sheets of geographic necrosis, often with cuffs of viable cells around blood vessels. In addition, some tumors have a lobular pattern due to the entrapment of cell clusters by fibrous bands. An interesting characteristic artifact in Ewing/PNET neoplasms is the so-called "Azzopardi

260 PRIMARY BONE TUMORS

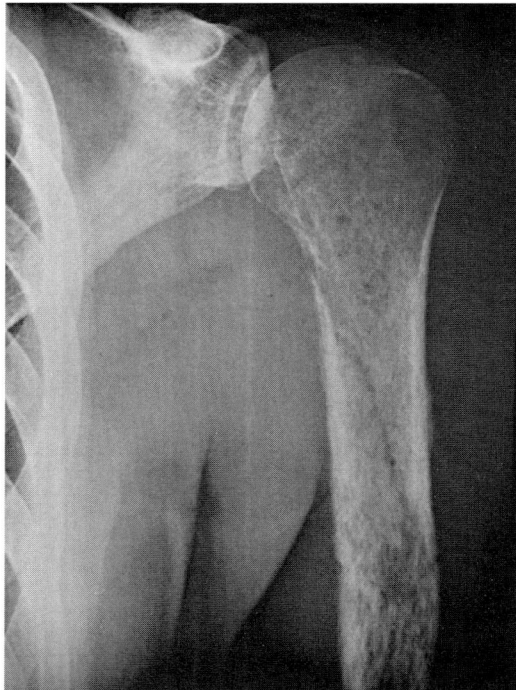

Figure 12–125 ■ Ewing sarcoma of the proximal humerus. The lesion shows an extensive permeative growth pattern. (From McCarthy, E. F.: *Differential Diagnosis in Pathology. Bone and Joint Disorders.* New York and Tokyo, Igaku-Shoin, 1996. With permission from Williams & Wilkins).

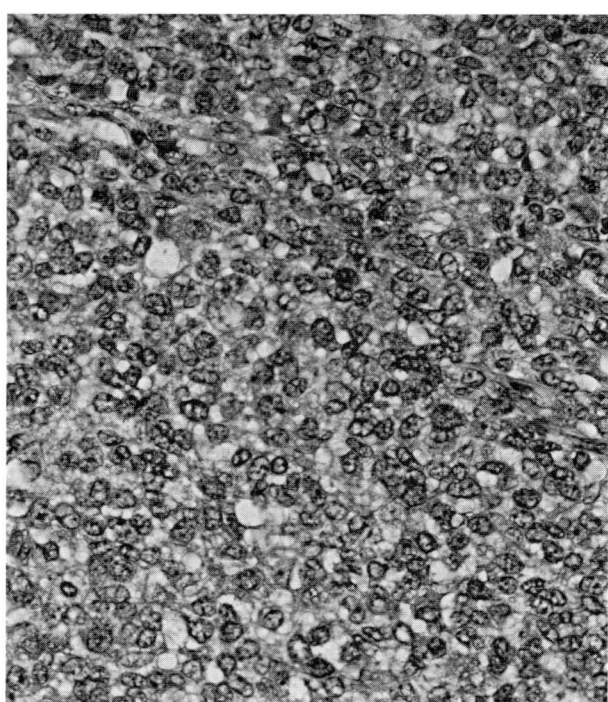

Figure 12–126 ■ Photomicrograph of Ewing sarcoma. Sheets of small round blue cells are present.

phenomenon"—neoplasms contain streams of hematoxyphilic material that represent crushed nuclei.

Two additional features are present in PNET. First, the cells are often arranged in poorly formed rosettes that surround a faintly eosinophilic fibrillary material (Fig. 12–129). Second, the cells may form a lobular pattern and be separated by loose fibrous tissue.

Immunohistochemistry

When James Ewing described this neoplasm in 1921, he postulated a vascular origin for it and labeled it a "diffuse endothelioma."[14] However, the scant amount of cytoplasm led most pathologists to suspect that Ewing sarcoma was a completely undifferentiated neoplasm. The presence of cytoplasmic glycogen, present in about 75% of Ewing sarcomas, was the only way to differentiate this neoplasm from other small round blue cell tumors.

Immunohistochemistry techniques have proved extremely useful in the diagnosis of Ewing sarcoma and PNET. Positivity for the immunostain neuron-specific enolase (NSE) in some Ewing sarcomas has identified a subset of neoplasms called PNETs.[185,186] As a result, Ewing sarcoma (with negative NSE stains) is felt to be an undifferentiated variant of PNET, a neoplasm with neural differentiation.

Another immunohistochemical stain is extremely important in diagnosing Ewing sarcoma/PNET. This stain identifies an abnormal gene product. Numerous genetic abnormalities have been identified in Ewing sarcoma. One abnormality with diagnostic usefulness is the overexpression of the *MIC2* gene. *MIC2* is a pseudoautosomal gene mapping to the short arm of the X chromosome. The product of this gene is a membrane glycoprotein, p30/32 MIC2, which has been designated CD99. This glycoprotein, located on the

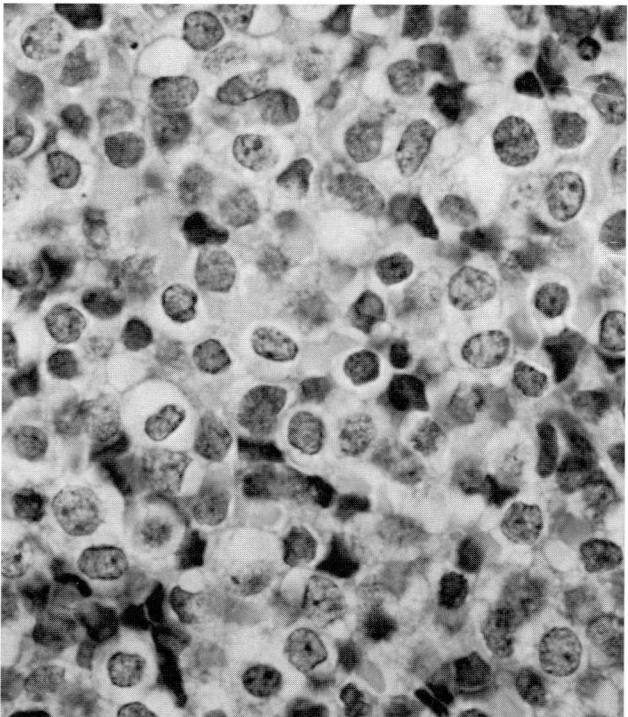

Figure 12–127 ■ High-power photomicrograph of Ewing sarcoma cells. The cells contain rounded nuclei with a faint chromatin pattern and a small nucleolus.

cell surface, is involved in cell adhesion processes.[187] It can be immunohistochemically identified with several monoclonal antibodies, particularly O13 and 12E7. In the appropriate clinical setting, positivity with these antibodies is a marker for tumors in the Ewing/PNET group. However, other neoplasms, including lymphoblastic lymphoma, Wilms' tumor, mesenchymal chondrosarcoma, small cell osteosarcoma, and some synovial sarcomas, also express this glycoprotein.

Neoplasms in the Ewing sarcoma/PNET group have a very poor prognosis. It was once considered a nonsurgical disease similar to malignant lymphoma; however, now most oncologists advocate ablative surgery with adjuvant or neoadjuvant chemotherapy. Lesions in the appendicular skeleton are most amenable to resection. A 5-year survival of 55% is expected following complete resection and chemotherapy. Patients with metastasis at the time of initial presentation, representing 20% of cases, have a worse prognosis, the 5-year survival being only 30%. The most important prognostic factor is location of the primary lesion. Involvement of the pelvis has the worst prognosis, followed by lesions in the proximal femur. Other factors associated with a poor prognosis are large lesions and those with extensive soft tissue involvement. PNET of bone has a slightly worse prognosis than classic Ewing sarcoma.

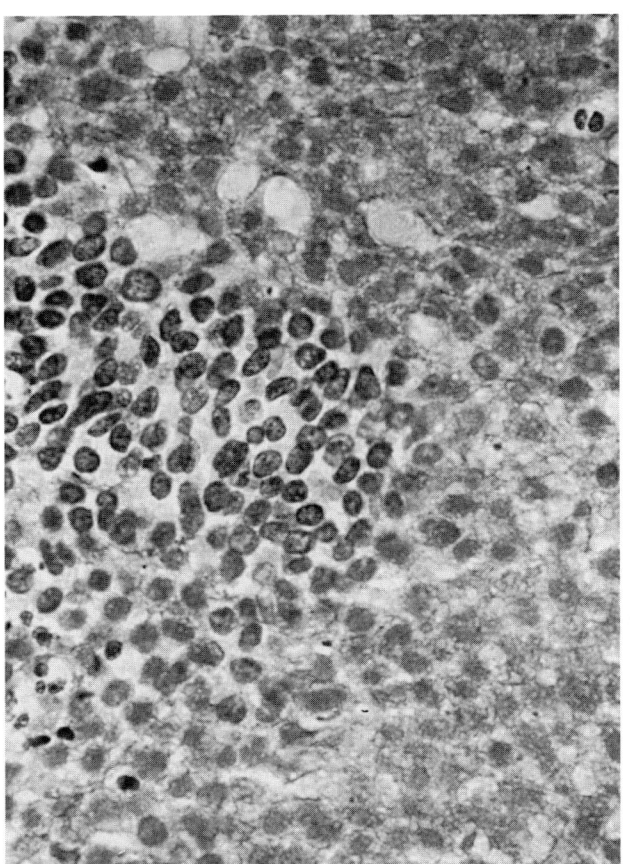

Figure 12-128 ■ Photomicrograph of Ewing sarcoma showing light and dark cells. The dark cells are most probably a secondary degenerative change.

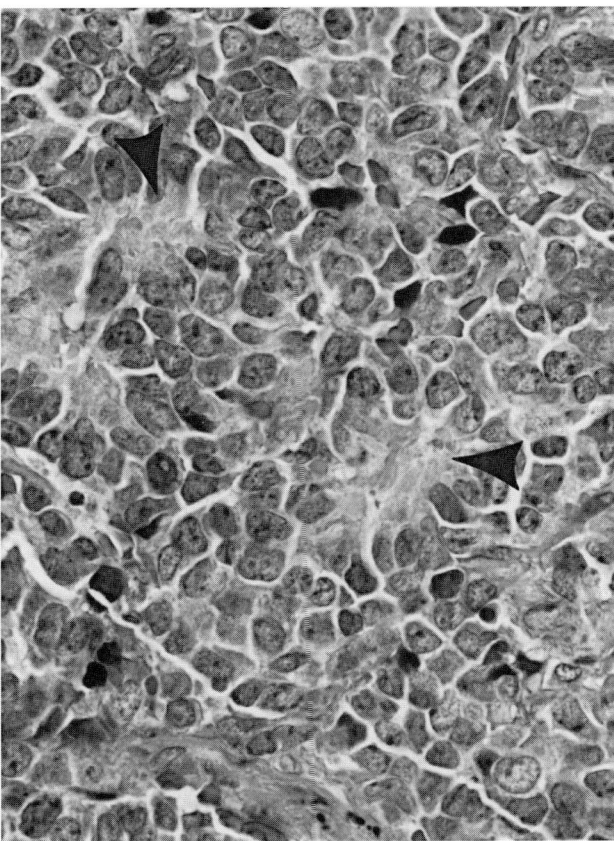

Figure 12-129 ■ Photomicrograph of a PNET. Some of the cells are arranged in pseudorosettes *(arrowheads)*.

OSTEOFIBROUS DYSPLASIA

Osteofibrous dysplasia is a fibroosseous proliferation that affects the bones of children, almost always before they are 10 years old. The distinctive feature of this lesion is its predilection for one site—the anterior cortex of the tibia. Osteofibrous dysplasia is not rare. In addition to sporadic reports of one or two cases, the nine collections of this lesion published to date document 219 cases.[188-196] Additional cases are undoubtedly misdiagnosed as fibrous dysplasia or congenital tibial bowing, and because some lesions are asymptomatic, they are not diagnosed at all.

Osteofibrous dysplasia was first described by Frangenhein in 1921 as congenital osteitis fibrosa.[197] In 1936, Compere noted a relationship between this lesion, which he called localized osteitis fibrosa, and congenital pseudarthrosis.[198] This relationship was further explored by Aegerter in 1950, who believed that this tibial lesion was a form of fibrous dysplasia.[199] He postulated that the tibial process was a manifestation of neurofibromatosis, a genetic disease, sometimes complicated by congenital pseudarthrosis. In 1966, Kempson's accurate histologic and electron microscopic study distinguished this process from fibrous dysplasia.[200] He called this lesion "ossifying fibroma of long bones" because of histologic similarity to ossifying fibroma of the facial bones. However, it was not until Campanacci's description of 35 cases in 1976[201] that the clinical, radiographic, and histologic spectrum of this disorder was defined. Campanacci called this lesion osteofibrous dysplasia to emphasize its nonneoplastic nature.

Osteofibrous dysplasia has a distinct clinical presentation. This disorder is almost exclusively limited to the tibia, and most patients present between the ages of 5 and 10 years. On rare occasions, a lesion may not be recognized until the patient is approximately age 30. Patients typically present with painless swelling over the midtibia. Anterior bowing is often present.

The distinctive radiologic feature of osteofibrous dysplasia is multiloculated intracortical lucencies, which are almost always centered on the anterior diaphyseal cortex (Fig. 12–130). Varying amounts of sclerotic bone are usually present. Radiographs reveal a spectrum of severity. In some cases, lesions are small (1 to 2 cm) and remain stationary. Other lesions involve most of the tibial shaft (Fig. 12–131). Often, in these severe cases, the lesions expand and coalesce until skeletal growth is complete. In as many as 17% of cases, the ipsilateral fibula is also focally involved.[191] In addition, a pseudarthrosis develops in 12 to 33% of cases.[196,190]

Histologically, osteofibrous dysplasia is characterized by irregular new bone trabeculae amidst cellular fibrous tissue, a pattern reminiscent of fibrous dysplasia. However, unlike the trabeculae of fibrous dysplasia, which seem to appear de

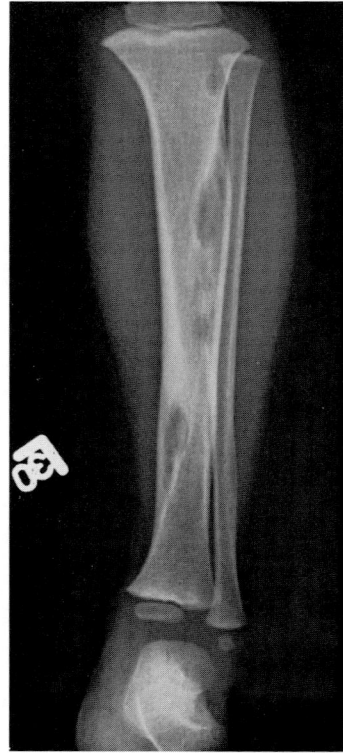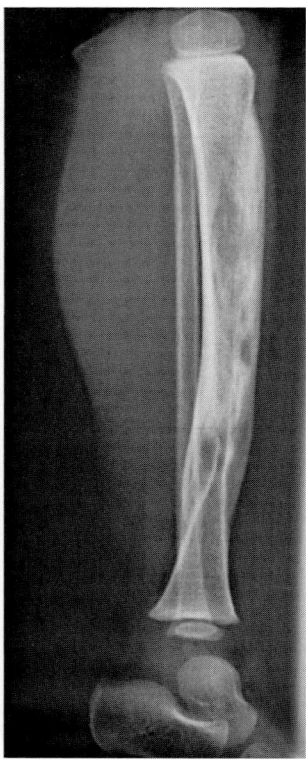

Figure 12-131 ■ Anteroposterior *(left)* and lateral radiographs of osteofibrous dysplasia involving most of the tibial shaft.

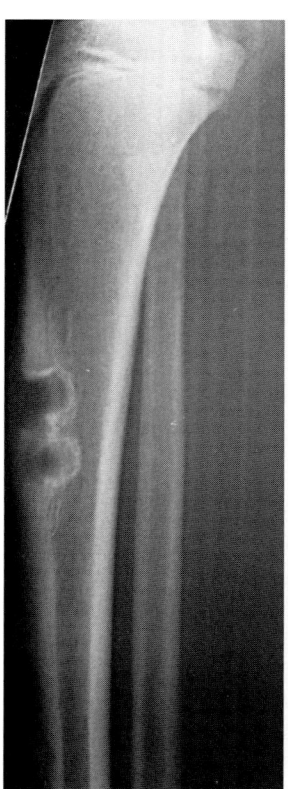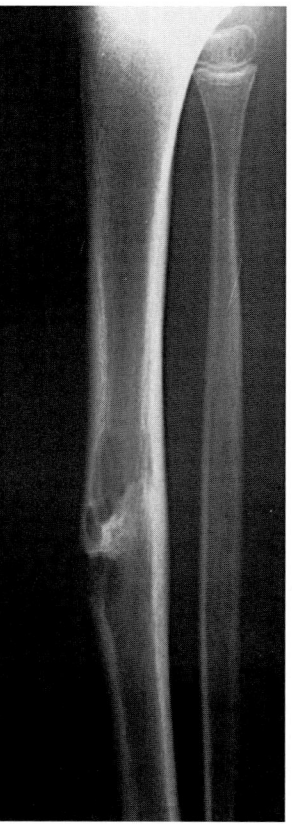

Figure 12-130 ■ Two examples of osteofibrous dysplasia. The lesions are present on the anterior tibial cortex. They are scalloped lesions with sclerotic rims.

novo in the fibrous stroma, the trabeculae of osteofibrous dysplasia are lined by plump osteoblasts (Fig. 12–132). The trabeculae of osteofibrous dysplasia are arranged in a zonal pattern. The center of the lesion is predominantly fibrous, whereas the periphery contains more new bone. This zonal pattern is not a feature of fibrous dysplasia. The most distinctive histologic feature of osteofibrous dysplasia is keratin-positive cells. Ninety-three percent of lesions contain scattered spindle cells, which stain immunocytochemically for cytokeratin.[191] Having no other epithelial features, these cells are not apparent with a routine hematoxylin and eosin stain.

Osteofibrous dysplasia is a nonneoplastic, self-limited process. Lesions grow slowly until skeletal maturity, and thereafter they stabilize. Small lesions sometimes disappear spontaneously. Large lesions, even those that have resulted in architectural deformity, stop growing. Therefore, surgical removal of these lesions should be avoided. Curettage during the proliferative phase is almost always followed by recurrence. Surgery should be reserved for those lesions with severe deformity or pseudarthrosis.

The predilection of osteofibrous dysplasia for the tibia and the presence of keratin-positive cells have led to considerable speculation about the relationship of osteofibrous dysplasia to adamantinoma.[189,193] Adamantinomas also occur almost exclusively in the tibia and also contain keratin-positive cells, although to a much greater degree. Moreover, adamantinomas often contain fibroosseous tissue identical to the characteristic tissue of osteofibrous dysplasia. The exact nature of this relationship is uncertain. However, despite many similarities, the behavior of these two lesions is quite different. Adamantinomas are malignant neoplasms that occur in patients who are almost always older than age 20.[189] Although some radiographic similarities to osteofibrous dysplasia can be seen, areas of cortical destruction and involvement of the medullary canal are common. In addition, a soft tissue mass is often present, and metastases occur in about 30% of cases. Furthermore, no case of transformation of osteofibrous dysplasia to an adamantinoma has been reported.

ADAMANTINOMA

Adamantinoma is a very rare neoplasm. Patients range in age from 3 to 72, but most are in their 20s and 30s. Almost all lesions occur in the midshaft of the tibia, and in 10% of cases, the ipsilateral fibula is involved (Fig. 12–133). On rare occasions, other long bones, such as the femur, humerus, and ulna, may be involved. This neoplasm also has been reported in the pretibial soft tissues.[202] Patients usually complain of pain and swelling, often of long duration. Approximately one third of patients have had symptoms for longer than 5 years. One reported patient had symptoms for 50 years.[203]

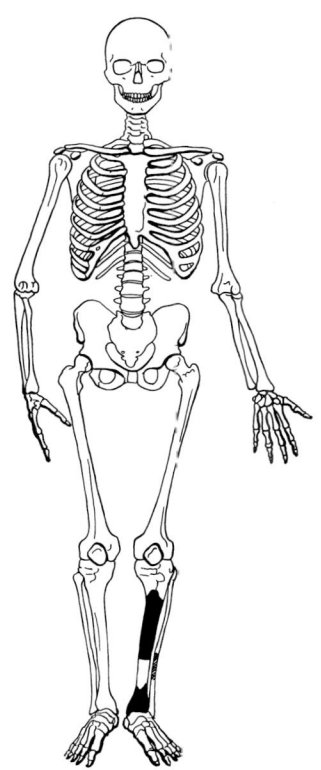

Figure 12–133 ■ Adamantinoma locations.

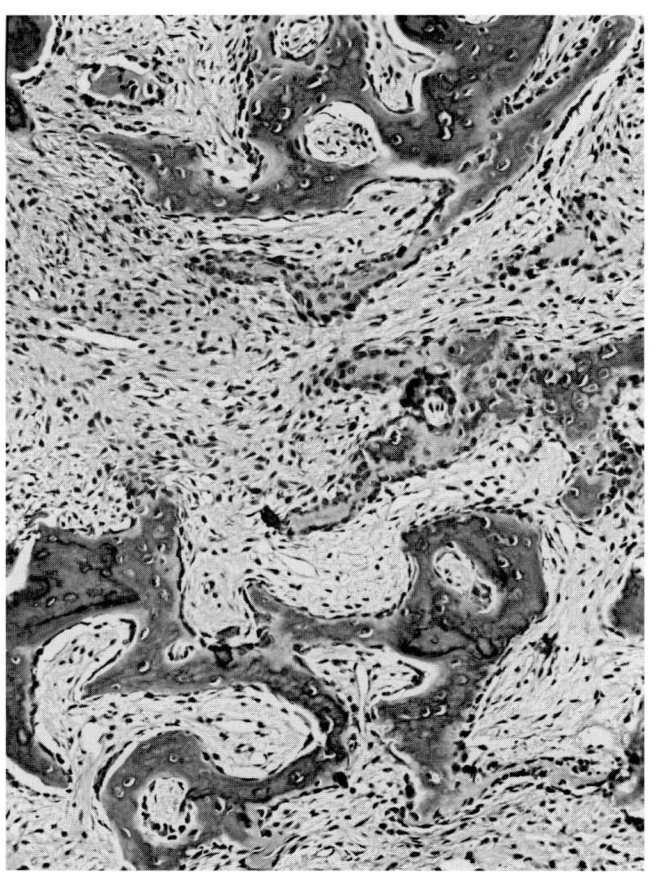

Figure 12–132 ■ Photomicrograph of osteofibrous dysplasia. New bone spicules lined by osteoblasts are present in a fibrous matrix.

Adamantinomas share some radiologic features with osteofibrous dysplasia.[204] For example, adamantinomas are also cortical-based lesions, and 90% of cases involve the diaphysis. In addition, like osteofibrous dysplasia, adamantinomas show multiloculated lytic areas surrounded by dense reactive bone. Often, the lesion appears multifocal and involves long segments of the tibial shaft. However, two radiographic features help distinguish adamantinomas from osteofibrous dysplasia. The first, seen in 10% of cases, is cortical penetration and involvement of soft tissues. Second, most cases of adamantinoma show one or more foci of medullary canal involvement, a feature not usually seen in osteofibrous dysplasia (Fig. 12–134).

Histologically, adamantinomas consist of various patterns of epithelial cells in a fibrous and fibroosseous stroma. The most common pattern is nests of basaloid epithelial cells with peripheral palisading, a feature similar to basal cell carcinoma of the skin (Fig. 12–135). Cystic spaces of various sizes often develop within the epithelial nests. Another common pattern of the epithelial cells is a spindle shape—cords of elongated cells with plump nuclei are surrounded by a more hyalinized stroma (Fig. 12–136). Occasionally, the stroma may be cellular with a gradual differentiation to epithelial cells. A third epithelial pattern in adamantinoma, tubule formation, resembles glands or vascular spaces. The tubules, present in a fibrous background, are formed by a single layer of small cuboidal cells that line anastomosing spaces. Finally, a rare squamoid pattern of the epithelium may be present. Clusters of cells with large eosinophilic

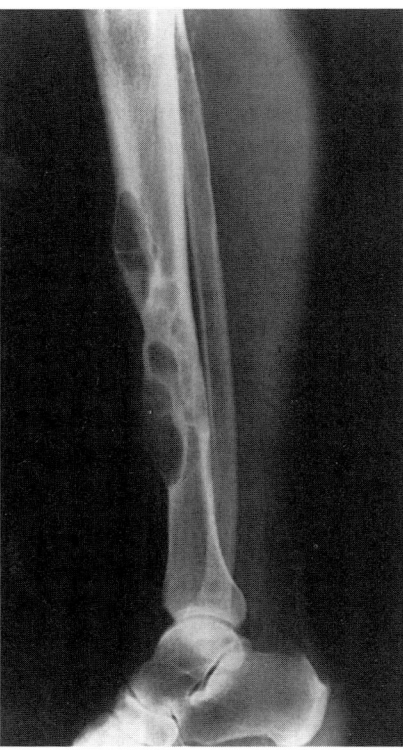

Figure 12-134 ■ Adamantinoma of the tibia. Multiple zones of bone destruction are involving the medullary canal.

cytoplasms and rounded or pyknotic nuclei are nested in the spindle cell background. In all histologic patterns, the epithelial cells stain strongly for cytokeratin. Occasionally, the spindle cell element is focally keratin positive.

The epithelial cells of adamantinomas, although occasionally hyperchromatic, are cytologically bland. They lack pleomorphism, and mitotic figures are rare. These bland features, in addition to a typical radiographic pattern, distinguish adamantinoma from metastatic carcinoma. In addition to the histologic patterns described here, adamantinoma may have areas in which the epithelial cells are not apparent. These areas are morphologically identical to osteofibrous dysplasia, mandating a complete tissue sampling of an osteofibrous dysplasia-like lesion to rule out adamantinoma.[205]

Adamantinomas are low-grade malignant neoplasms. They should be treated by wide segmental resection or amputation. About 25% of patients develop metastases after surgical ablation. Metastasis may occur as late as 16 years after surgery.[206]

Differentiated Adamantinoma

Recently, a new point on the osteofibrous dysplasia–adamantinoma spectrum was identified. Some lesions, clinically and radiographically identical to severe osteofibrous dysplasia, contain discrete nests of epithelial cells, although they are not as prominent as in adamantinomas. These lesions, called differentiated adamantinomas, may represent burned out cases of severe osteofibrous dysplasia.[188,189] Alternatively, they may represent an intermediate stage between osteofibrous dysplasia and classic adamantinoma (Fig. 12–137).

Formerly, lesions that are now regarded as differentiated adamantinomas were grouped with classical adamantinomas. Often, they were regarded as "osteofibrous dysplasia-like" adamantinomas. They occur in a similar age group, and they involve long segments of the tibia. As a result, they were often treated aggressively, similar to adamantinoma. However, differentiated adamantinomas are indolent lesions. Sometimes they are asymptomatic and do not grow at all. Radiographically, they lack cortical destruction and soft tissue infiltration. Therefore, differentiated adamantinomas may be treated conservatively. Surgery should be reserved to correct deformities or stabilize pathologic fractures.

VASCULAR NEOPLASMS

The nomenclature of vasoformative bone lesions has been confusing. Terms such as *epithelioid hemangioma* and *hemangioendothelial sarcoma* create artificial categories that can possibly lead to improper therapy. Vascular lesions of bone are best subdivided into three major categories: hemangioma,

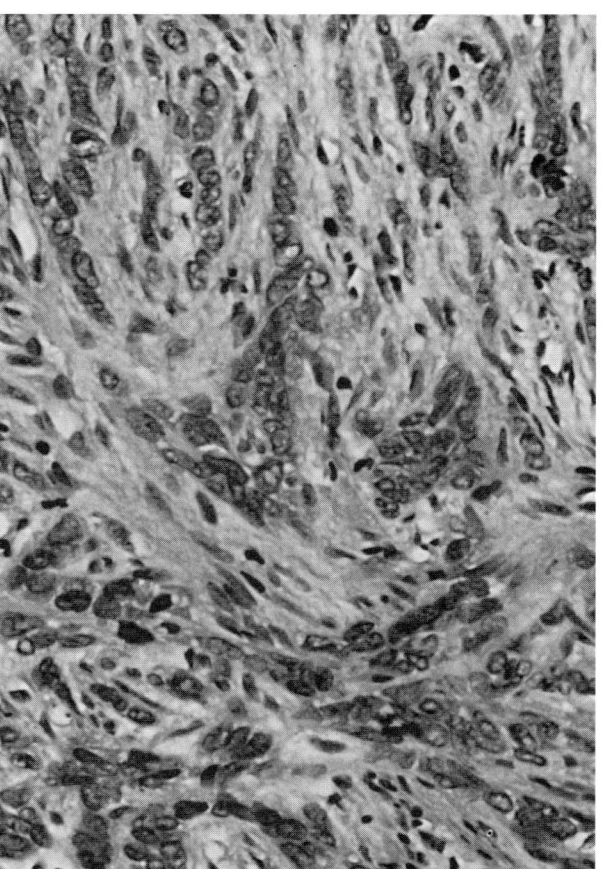

Figure 12-135 ■ Photomicrograph of adamantinoma showing clusters of epithelial cells in a fibrous background.

epithelioid hemangioendothelioma, and angiosarcoma. Hemangiopericytoma also involves bones, but this entity is very rare and is not discussed in this chapter.[207]

Hemangioma

Hemangiomas in the skeleton may be solitary or multiple. Solitary hemangiomas usually affect a vertebral body or the calvarium. Small lesions can be found at autopsy in 11% of carefully examined spines.[208] Most spinal hemangiomas are asymptomatic and are discovered incidentally on radiographs taken for other reasons. Some patients, however, present with back pain due to a compression fracture. Hemangioma of the calvarium usually presents as a slowly growing mass. Hemangiomas may be discovered at any age, but most patients are in their 40s.[209]

Radiographically, vertebral hemangiomas are lytic lesions with coarse vertical striations, the so-called "jail bar" pattern (Fig. 12-138). These dense striations on cross-sectional CT images appear as spots of dense bone. Lesions in the calvarium bulge the outer cortical table and have a "sunburst" appearance of reactive bone.

Cystic angiomatosis is a syndrome of multiple hemangiomas of bone and, occasionally, extraosseous sites.[210] The lesions are hamartomatous proliferations of simple endothe-

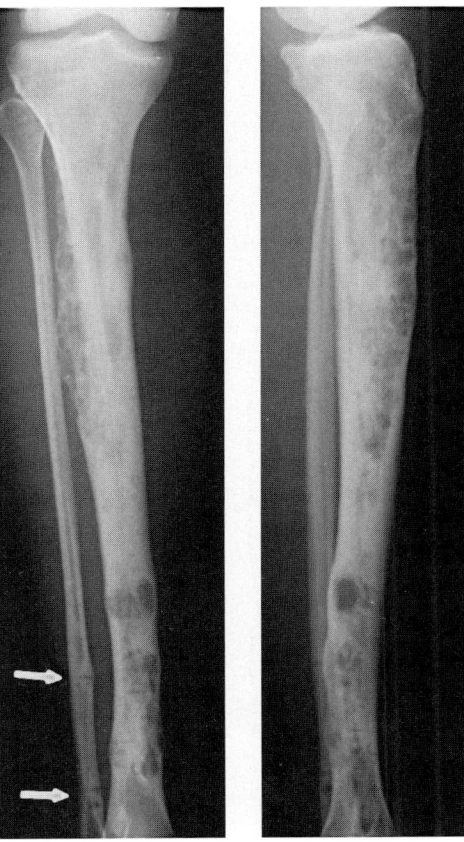

Figure 12-137 ■ Anteroposterior *(left)* and lateral radiographs of differentiated adamantinoma of the entire tibial shaft. This multiloculated lesion has been stationary for many years. Small foci of fibular involvement are also present *(arrows)*. This lesion should be treated conservatively.

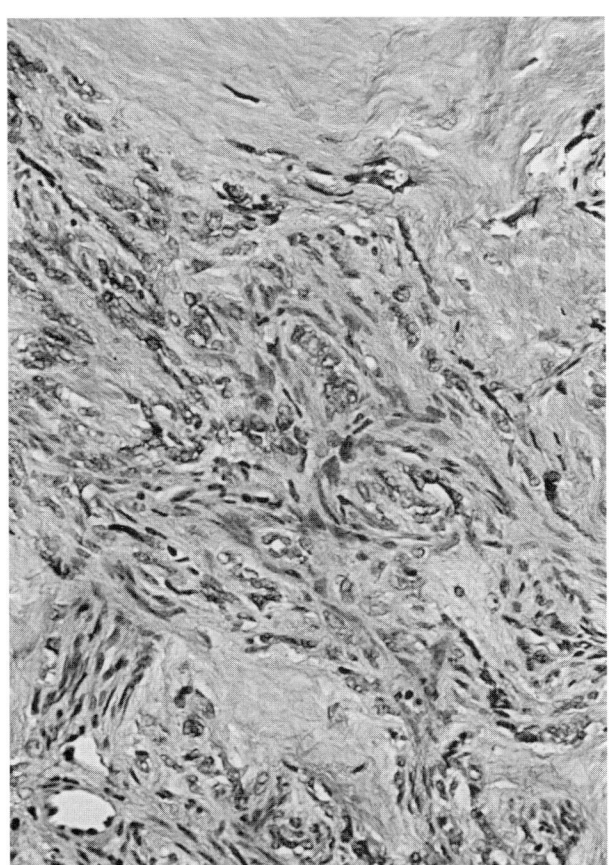

Figure 12-136 ■ Photomicrograph of adamantinoma. The epithelial cells are spindle shaped.

lial-lined spaces, similar to hemangiomas in other locations. Patients may have as many as 20 lesions, and any bone may be affected.[211] Usually, like solitary hemangiomas, cystic angiomatosis is usually asymptomatic, and lesions are found on radiographs taken for other reasons. Occasionally, patients present with a pathologic fracture, and some present with symptoms of an extraosseous hemangioma. Extraosseous sites may be the soft tissue, liver, or spleen. Patients are usually diagnosed before age 20, but some may go undiagnosed until late adulthood. Occasionally, the disease runs in families. Cystic angiomatosis characteristically produces multiple round or oval radiolytic defects, often with a sclerotic rim. The cortex may be expanded, but a periosteal reaction is characteristically absent (Fig. 12-139). On rare occasions, lesions may be poorly circumscribed. Occasionally, because of extensive reactive bone stimulation, lesions may be radiodense and mimic osteoblastic metastases.[212] Radiodense lesions are more common in older patients, suggesting that some lesions heal spontaneously over the years.

Cystic angiomatosis shows microscopic features identical to those of solitary hemangioma of bone. Multiple blood-filled cavities, separated by marrow elements or loose fibrous tissue, surround bone trabeculae (Fig. 12-140). The cavities

266 PRIMARY BONE TUMORS

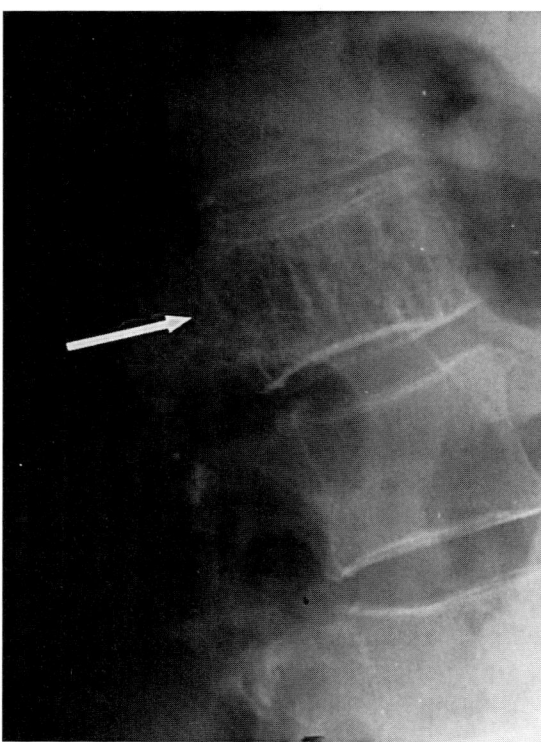

Figure 12-138 ■ Hemangioma of a vertebra. Prominent vertical striations *(arrow)* impart a "jail door" appearance. (From Frassica, F. J., and McCarthy, E. F.: Miller, M. D., Ed. *Review of Orthopaedics,* 2nd ed. Philadelphia, W. B. Saunders, 1996, p. 320.)

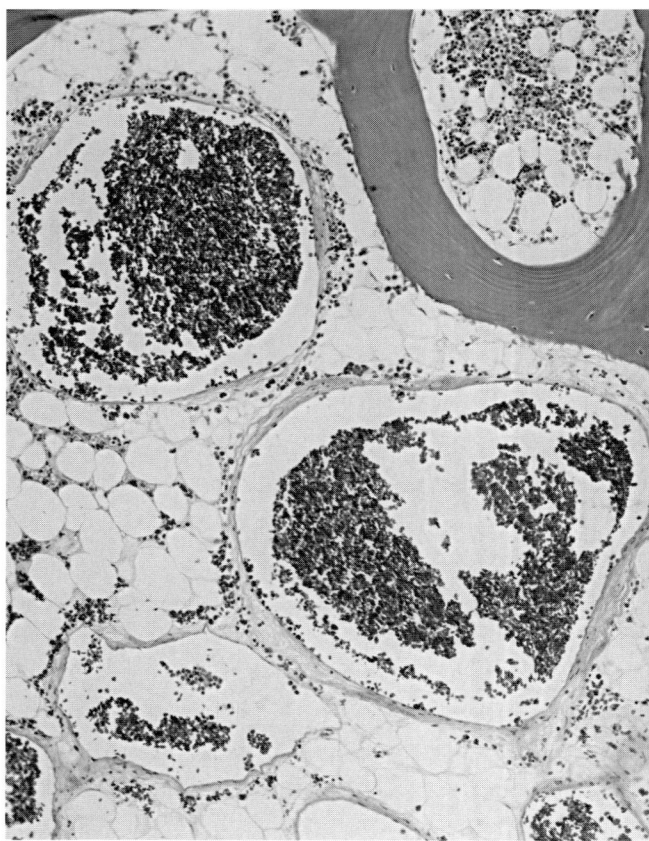

Figure 12-140 ■ Low-power photomicrograph of hemangioma of bone. Numerous dilated endothelial-lined blood filled spaces are present.

may be dilated as in a cavernous hemangioma, or they may be small as in capillary hemangioma. The spaces are lined by a single layer of flattened endothelial cells. The intervening trabeculae may be thickened by successive layers of appositional bone, a microscopic feature correlating with radiodensity.

Cystic angiomatosis, if confined to bone, is a benign condition. Although occasional lesions grow slowly, most are nonprogressive. Lesions with established or impending pathologic fracture may be treated with local excision or

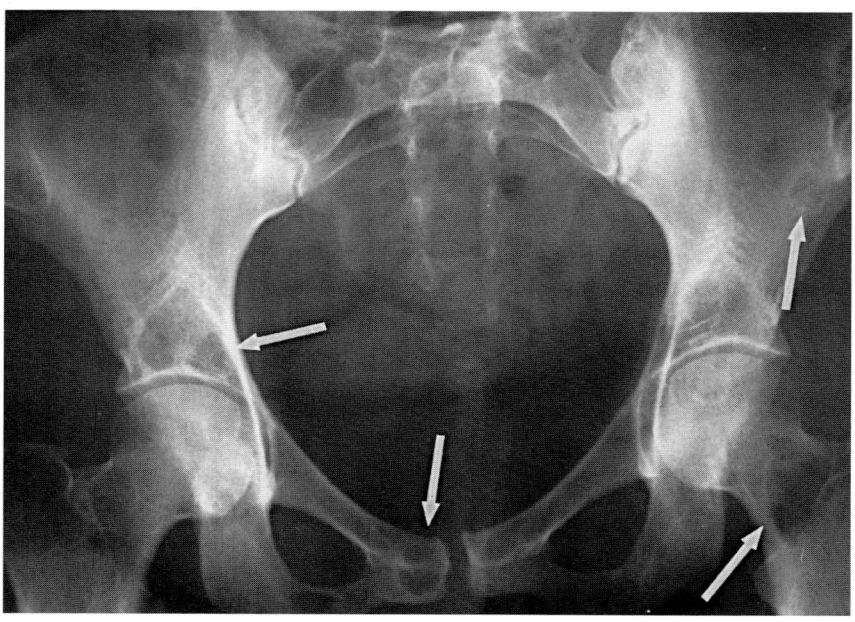

Figure 12-139 ■ Cystic angiomatosis. Numerous lytic lesions are present throughout the pelvis and proximal femurs *(arrows)*. (From McCarthy, E. F.: *Differential Diagnosis in Pathology. Bone and Joint Disorders.* New York and Tokyo, Igaku-Shoin, 1996. With permission from Williams & Wilkins.)

low-dose radiotherapy. Occasionally, lesions regress spontaneously. Patients with cystic angiomatosis of bone should be examined for extraosseous hemangiomas, particularly in abdominal or thoracic viscera. These patients have a worse prognosis, sometimes suffering intraabdominal or intrathoracic hemorrhage. A splenectomy is often necessary.

Epithelioid Hemangioendothelioma

Epithelioid hemangioendotheliomas are indolent neoplasms characterized by the proliferation of plump, histiocytoid endothelial cells.[213] Most epithelioid hemangioendotheliomas of bone are diagnosed in patients between ages 10 and 30, although older patients may also develop this lesion. The femur, pelvis, and tibia are the most common sites.[214] Patients usually present with pain or pathologic fracture. A distinctive feature of epithelioid hemangioendothelioma, present in 64% of patients, is involvement of multiple sites. Curiously, multicentric lesions tend to involve the bones of one extremity. Although any bone may be involved, the bones of the lower extremity are favored sites. Like cystic angiomatosis, this process may involve extraosseous sites, such as the soft tissues or lung, where it is known as intravascular bronchioalveolar tumor.

Epithelioid hemangioendothelioma of bone is usually a well-circumscribed radiolytic defect ranging in size from 2.5 to 15 cm in maximal dimension. A mildly sclerotic border is sometimes present. On rare occasions, lesions may be predominantly sclerotic (Fig. 12–141). Cortical expansion and extension into the soft tissue may occasionally occur.

Epithelioid hemangioendotheliomas of bone are characterized by nests, cords, or sheets of plump, round, or polygonal cells with abundant eosinophilic cytoplasm. Their nuclei are round and moderately hyperchromatic. These "histiocytoid"

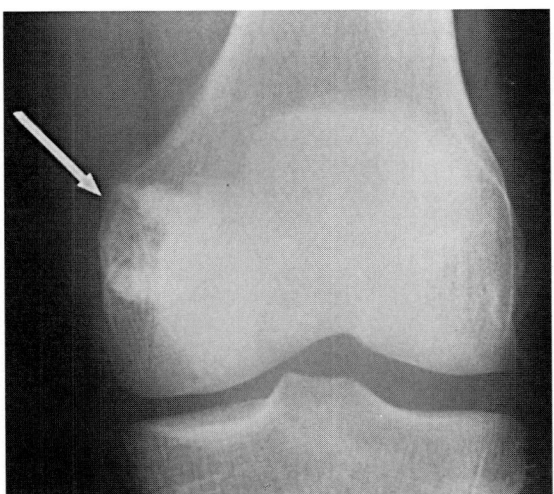

Figure 12–141 ■ Epithelioid hemangioendothelioma of the distal femur. The lesion is a well-defined zone of radiolysis and radiodensity *(arrow)*. (From McCarthy, E. F.: *Differential Diagnosis in Pathology. Bone and Joint Disorders*. New York and Tokyo, Igaku-Shoin, 1996. With permission from Williams & Wilkins.)

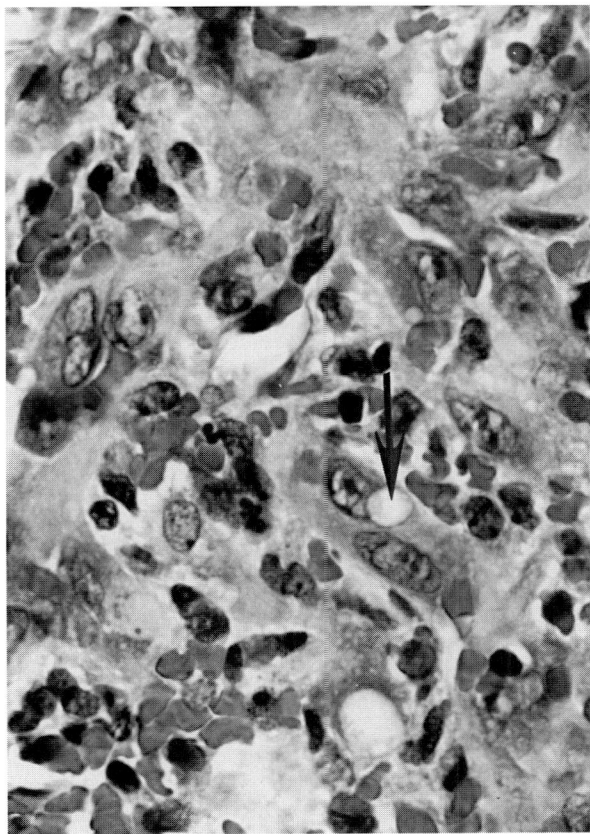

Figure 12–142 ■ Photomicrograph of epithelioid hemangioendothelioma. Numerous epithelioid cells are admixed with extravasated blood. Some of the epithelioid cells show cytoplasmic lumina *(arrow)*.

cells, which show little pleomorphism, often contain intracytoplasmic lumina, which may coalesce with similar structures in an adjacent cell (Fig. 12–142). Often, the cell nests form well-developed vascular lumina that contain red cells (Fig. 12–143). In some areas, the clusters of histiocytoid endothelial cells are separated by a fibrovascular stroma containing lymphocytes, plasma cells, and, often, many eosinophils. The well-formed neoplastic vessels in the fibrous stroma have the appearance of granulation tissue. Occasionally, the stroma may contain abundant hyaline or chondroid matrix, which compresses the entrapped endothelial cells. Epithelioid hemangioendothelioma of bone typically shows little or no mitotic activity. In addition, areas of necrosis are common. Immunohistochemical stains for factor VIII are usually positive, although not necessarily in all tumor cells.

Epithelioid hemangioendotheliomas of bone are slow-growing neoplasms with a protracted clinical course. Lesions should be totally removed, either by complete curettage or by limb-sparing resection. Radiotherapy may be of value if complete excision is impossible. Lesions with more than mild mitotic activity may be more aggressive. Patients with epithelioid hemangioendothelioma should be evaluated for multifocal lesions. These patients have an equally good, perhaps better, prognosis. Rare reports of metastasis of epithelioid hemangioendothelioma may be cases of multifocal lesions rather than metastases.

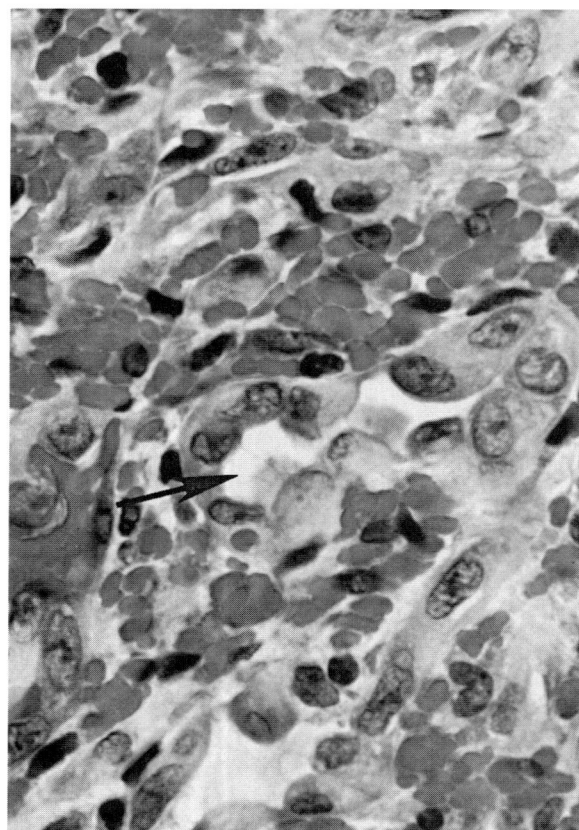

Figure 12–143 ▪ Photomicrograph of epithelioid hemangioendothelioma. Some of the neoplastic cells form a vascular lumen *(arrow)*.

Angiosarcoma of Bone

Angiosarcomas of bone are very rare, highly malignant neoplasms that occur in patients from age 10 to 70. However, most patients are older than 30. Pain lasting several weeks to a few months is the usual presenting symptom. Angiosarcomas most commonly involve the femur and tibia.

Angiosarcomas of bone show a radiographic pattern of an aggressive, high-grade malignant bone tumor (Fig. 12–144). Lesions are radiolytic with poorly defined margins, and cortical expansion and cortical destruction are usually present.

Histologically, these lesions show anastomosing blood-filled clefts and slits (Fig. 12–145). These spaces are lined by large cells with abundant eosinophilic cytoplasm. Unlike the uniform cells of epithelioid hemangioendotheliomas, the cells of angiosarcomas show marked pleomorphism. Large, bizarre, hyperchromatic nuclei are common, and mitotic figures are numerous. Papillary tufts of the pleomorphic cells often project into the neoplastic vascular lumina.

CHORDOMA

Chordomas, thought to arise from notochordal rests, are slow-growing malignant neoplasms that occur exclusively along the spinal axis.[215,216] The two ends of the spinal axis, inside the skull and the sacrococcygeal region, are the most common locations (Fig. 12–146). Half of all chordomas arise in the sacrococcygeal region, where they present with pain and, occasionally, bladder dysfunction. At the other end of the spine, intracranial chordomas, accounting for 40% of lesions, involve bones at the base of the skull. When chordomas occur in this region, patients present with headache and neurologic impairment. The remaining 10% of chordomas involve the vertebral column. These locations correlate with the distribution of notochordal rests found by meticulous study of adult and developing spines.[217] Most patients with a chordoma are older than 40, although intracranial lesions occur in somewhat younger patients.

Radiologically, sacral chordomas are intraosseous destructive lesions that often expand into the soft tissues (Fig. 12–147). Sometimes these neoplasms present as midline paraspinal or intrapelvic masses with minimal or no bone destruction. Chordomas are best studied with the CT scan. Intracranial chordomas may destroy the sella turcica, and they often invade the petrous or sphenoid bone. Occasionally, intracranial chordomas calcify, a feature rarely present in chordomas of the sacrum and spine.

The histologic features of chordomas are distinctive. On low-power microscopic examination, a lobular growth pattern, similar to cartilage neoplasms, is apparent. Cords and

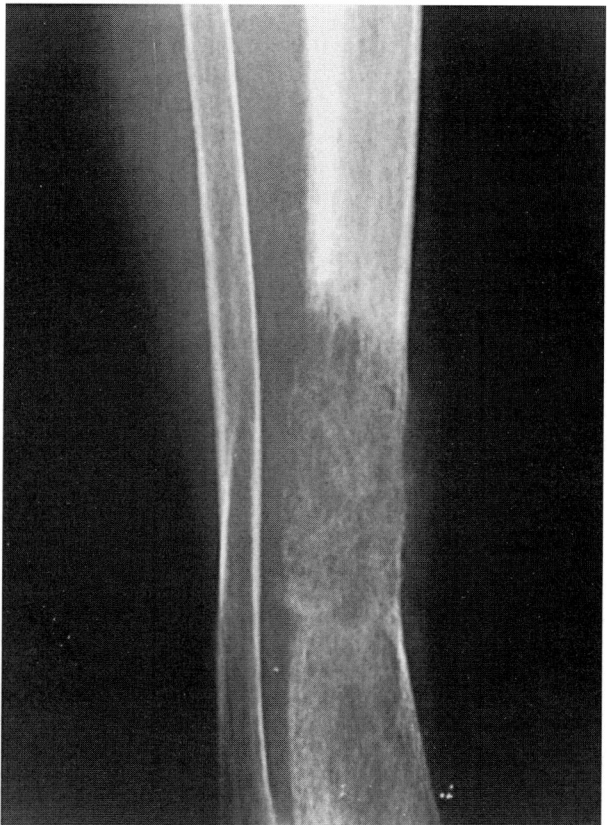

Figure 12–144 ▪ Hemangiosarcoma of the distal tibia. A poorly defined and permeative radiolytic lesion is present in the bone shaft. (From McCarthy, E. F.: *Differential Diagnosis in Pathology. Bone and Joint Disorders.* New York and Tokyo, Igaku-Shoin, 1996. With permission from Williams & Wilkins.)

sheets of cells are embedded in an abundant, pale extracellular matrix (Fig. 12–148). Higher-power study reveals two types of cells. One type is a square to oblong cell with a round central nucleus and an eosinophilic cytoplasm (Fig. 12–149). The other type contains a round nucleus but has a bubbly cytoplasm (physaliferous cell) (Fig. 12–150). Chordomas show little nuclear pleomorphism, and mitotic figures are rare.

Two histologic variants or chordoma are recognized. The first is chondroid chordoma—approximately one fourth of intracranial chordomas show areas that resemble hyaline cartilage.[218] The second variant, known as dedifferentiated chordoma, occurs almost exclusively in the sacrococcygeal region.[219,220] In this rare biphasic neoplasm, a high-grade sarcoma, usually a malignant fibrous histiocytoma, is associated with a histologically typical chordoma. The high-grade component usually develops after multiple recurrences of a conventional chordoma.

Immunohistochemical stains facilitate the diagnosis of chordomas. They are epithelial neoplasms and are strongly positive for cytokeratin. Stains for epithelial membrane antigen and S-100 protein are also positive. However, the stain for S-100 protein is usually only weakly positive. Even the cells in the chondroid areas of chondroid chordomas stain with these epithelial markers, suggesting that this tissue is not true cartilage.

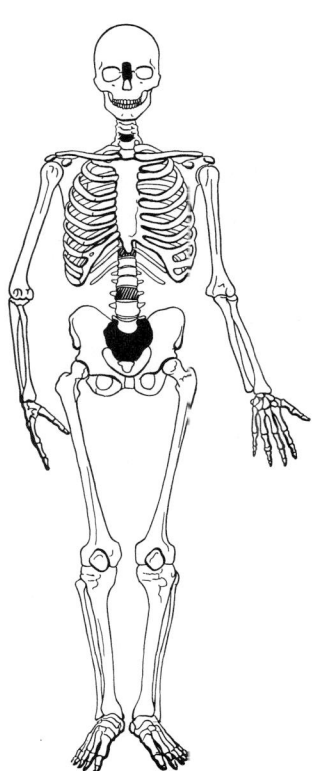

Figure 12-146 ■ Chordoma locations.

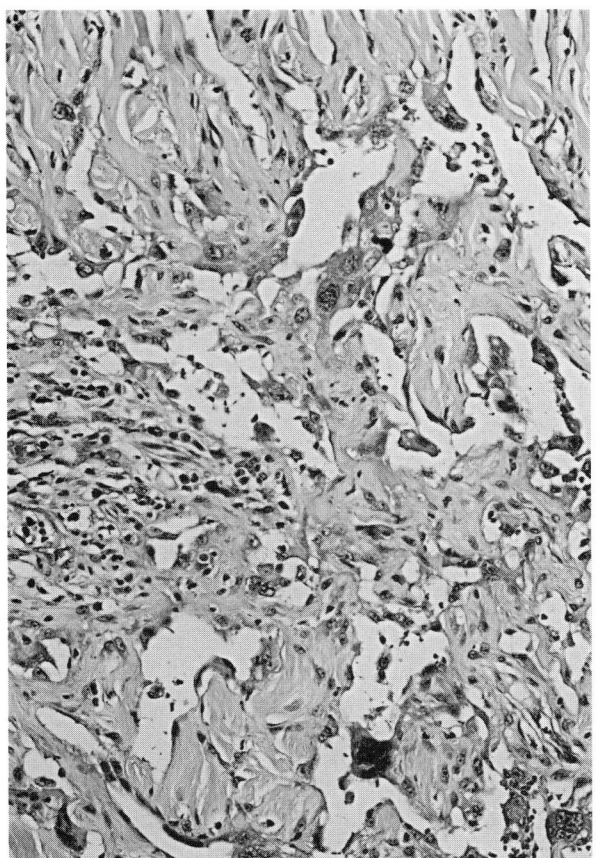

Figure 12-145 ■ Photomicrograph of hemangiosarcoma. Vascular slits are lined by atypical pleomorphic cells.

Chordomas must be distinguished from other spinal neoplasms. The presence of cytokeratin rules out chondrosarcoma. Metastatic adenocarcinoma may be ruled out by the presence of S-100 protein and acid mucin, substances found in chordomas but not in metastatic carcinomas. Also, chordomas do not form glandular lumens. One difficult problem is distinguishing a small chordoma from a large notochordal rest. These lesions are histologically and immunohistochemically identical. In this situation, only evidence of destructive growth can identify a chordoma

Chordomas are aggressive neoplasms that can rarely be completely excised. Removal often requires sacrifice of the cauda equina. Palliative debulking, followed by radiation therapy is the most common therapy. Typically, patients suffer multiple recurrences. Metastasis, usually to the lungs, skin, or bones, occurs in 32% of sacral or vertebral chordomas.[221] More than 90% of patients die within 10 years. The presence of chondroid differentiation is associated with a better prognosis; the mean survival is 15 years. By contrast, dedifferentiated chordoma is rapidly fatal.

SARCOMAS ARISING IN IRRADIATED BONE (POSTRADIATION SARCOMAS)

Patients who have undergone ionizing irradiation may, on rare occasions, develop a sarcoma in the irradiated field. The latency period is defined as the time interval between the completion of the irradiation and the discovery of the sarcoma. Cahan and colleagues[222] and Arlen and others[223] have

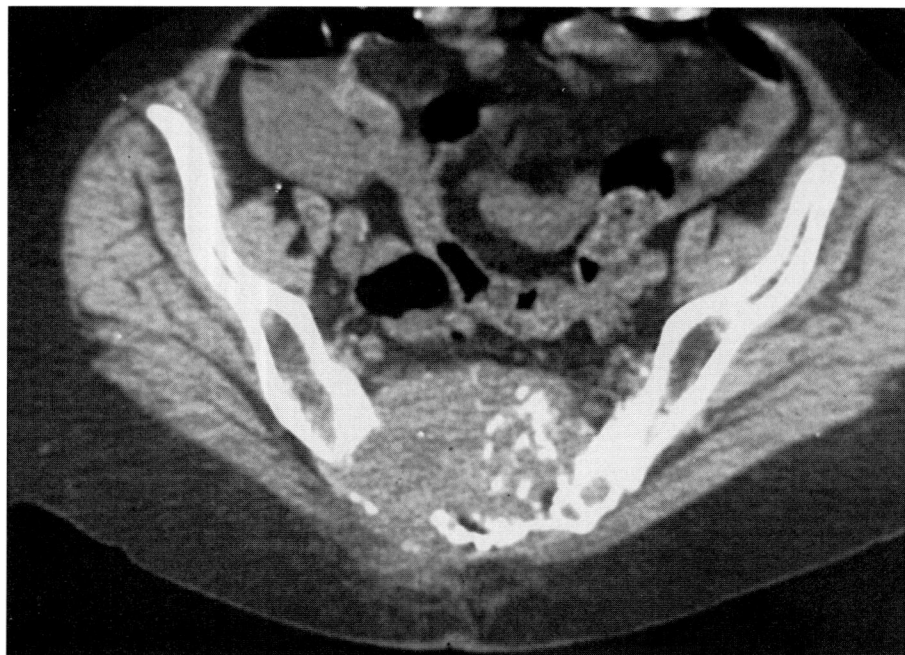

Figure 12-147 ■ Computed tomography scan of a sacral chordoma. This destructive lesion contains intralesional radiodensities. (From Frassica, F. J., and McCarthy, E. F.: Miller, M. D., Ed. *Review of Orthopaedics,* 2nd ed. Philadelphia, W. B. Saunders, 1996, p. 319.)

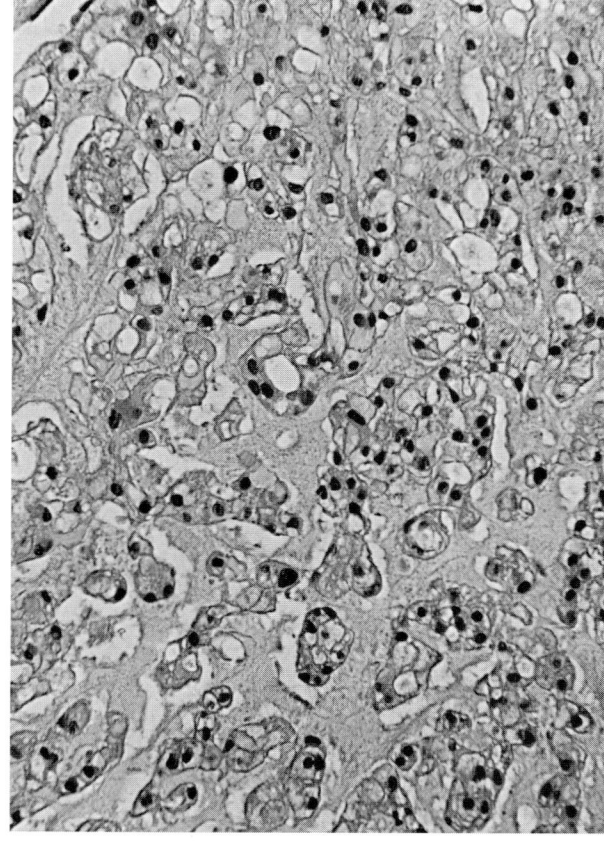

Figure 12-148 ■ Photomicrograph of a chordoma. Clusters of epithelioid cells are present in an abundant extracellular matrix.

outlined the criteria to establish the diagnosis of postradiation sarcoma. First, biopsy evidence of normal bone or an unrelated neoplasm must be documented. Second, the sarcoma must be in the radiated field. Third, a latency period of at least 2 years must occur. And finally, the sarcoma must be documented histologically.

In the past, most patients who have developed a postradiation sarcoma had received the irradiation for a benign bone tumor, such as a giant cell tumor or a chondroblastoma, or for skin lesions, such as acne or psoriasis. The typical latency period is 5 to 20 years. The trend has now shifted such that few patients receive irradiation for benign lesions. Most patients now with postradiation sarcomas have received the irradiation for malignant diseases such as breast cancer, Hodgkin's disease, and Ewing sarcoma. If the patients receive intensive chemotherapy (especially alkylating agents such as cyclophosphamide), the risk of postradiation sarcoma is probably higher and the latency period shorter. The dose of irradiation is generally 4000 to 6000 cGy. Modern radiotherapy techniques (megavoltage) have the same risk of inducing malignancy as the older techniques (orthovoltage).

Patients generally present with intense pain over the site of the lesion. Plain radiographs may be normal, but cross-sectional imaging studies show cortical bone destruction and the presence of a soft tissue mass. Histologically, these

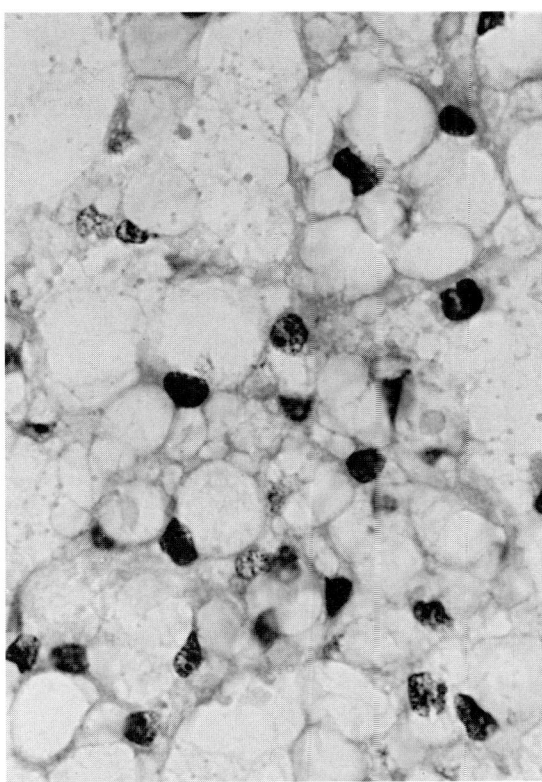

Figure 12-150 ■ Photomicrograph of the physaliferous cells of a chordoma.

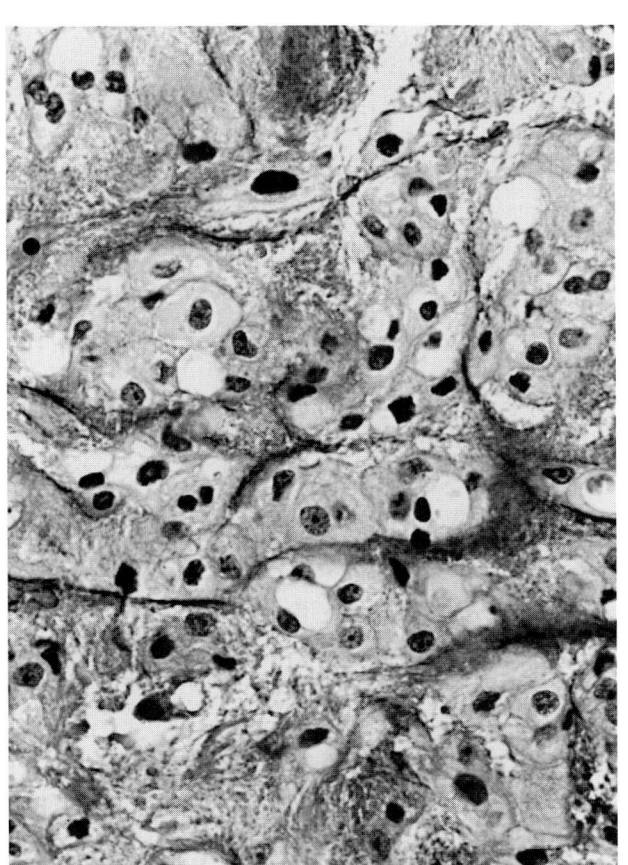

Figure 12-149 ■ One histologic pattern of chordoma. Clusters of epithelioid cells that have vesicular nuclei in a sharply defined cytoplasm.

lesions are usually high-grade malignant fibrous histiocytomas, although high-grade osteosarcomas and fibrosarcomas may also occur.

Postradiation sarcomas are lethal tumors. Commonly, they affect the older age groups in whom high-dose chemotherapy is not feasible. Most patients require amputation surgery, and the prognosis is poor, with a long-term survival of about 20%.

REFERENCES

1. Brothwell, D.: The evidence for neoplasms. Brothwell, D. R., and Sandison, A. T. Eds. *Diseases in Antiquity*. Chicago, IL, Charles Thomas, 1967, pp. 320–345.
2. Abernethy, J.: *Surgical Observations on Tumors*. London, Longmand and Rees, 1804.
3. Boyer, A.: *The Lectures of Boyer Upon Diseases of Bone, Arranged into a Systemic Treatise by A. Richerand*. Philadelphia, James Humphreys, Paris, Baillière, 1805.
4. Dupuytren, G.: Lecons Orales de Clinique Chirurgicale Faites a l'Hôtel-Dieu de Paris [Abstract]. Paris, Baillière, 1839.
5. Hey, W.: *Practical Observations in Surgery, Illustrated with Cases*. London, Cadell and Davies, 1803.
6. Cooper, A., and Travers, B.: *Surgical Essays, Part I*. London: Cox and Son, 1818, p. 186.
7. Majno, G., and Joris, I.: The microscope in the history of pathology. With a note on the pathology of fat cells. *Virch Arch Pathol Anat* 360:273–286, 1973.
8. Bracegirdle, B.: J. J. Lister and the establishment of histology. *Med Hist* 21:187–191, 1977.
9. Muller, J.: *Über den feinern Bau und die Formen der Krankhaften Geschwülste*. Berlin, G. Reimer, 1838.

10. Lebert, H.: *Physiologie Pathologique au Recharches Cliniques, Expérimentales et Microscopiques.* Paris, J. B. Baillière, 1845.
11. Beale, L. S.: *The Microscope in its Application to Practical Medicine.* Philadelphia, Lindsay and Blakiston, 1867, p. 34.
12. Gross, S.: Sarcoma of the long bones; based upon a study of one hundred and sixty-five cases. *Am J Med Sci* 78:17, 1879.
13. Ewing, J.: *Neoplastic Diseases.* Philadelphia, W. B. Saunders, 1919.
14. Ewing, J.: Diffuse endothelioma of bone. *Proc N Y Pathol Soc* 21:17–24, 1921.
15. Bloodgood, J. C.: The conservative treatment of giant-cell sarcoma, with the study of bone transplantation. *Ann Surg* 56:210–239, 1912.
16. Codman, E. A.: The method of procedure of the Registry of Bone Sarcoma. *Surg Gynecol Obstet* 38:712–721, 1924.
17. Enneking, W. F., Spanier, S. S., and Goodman, M. A.: A system for the surgical staging of musculoskeletal sarcoma. *Clin Orthop* 153:106, 1980.
18. Greenspan, A.: Bone island (enostosis): Current concept—a review. *Skeletal Radiol* 24:111–115, 1995.
19. Greenspan, A., Steiner, G., and Knutzon, R.: Bone island (enostosis): Clinical significance and radiologic and pathologic correlations. *Skeletal Radiol* 20:85–90, 1991.
20. Greenspan, A., and Klein, M. J.: Giant bone island. *Skeletal Radiol* 25:67–69, 1996.
21. Gold, R. H., Mirra, J. M., Remotti, F. and Pignatti, G.: Case report 527. *Skeletal Radiol* 18:129, 1989.
22. Sickles, E. A., Genant, H. K., and Hoffer, P. B.: Increased localization of ^{99m}Tc-pyrophosphate in a bone island: Case report. *J Nucl Med* 17:113–115, 1976.
23. Onitsuka, H.: Roentgenologic aspects of bone islands. *Radiology* 123:607–612, 1977.
24. Earwaker, J.: Paranasal sinus osteomas: A review of 46 cases. *Skeletal Radiol* 22:417–423, 1993.
25. Peyser, A. B., Makley, J. T., Callewart, C. C., Brackett, B., Carter, J. R., and Abdul-Karim, F. W.: Osteoma of the long bones and the spine. A study of eleven patients and a review of the literature. *J Bone Joint Surg* 78A:1172–1180, 1996.
26. Geschickter, C. F., and Copeland, M. M.: Osteoma. *Tumors of Bone.* Philadelphia, J. B. Lippincott, 1949, pp. 630–636.
27. Schajowicz, F.: Osteoma. *Tumors and Tumorlike Lesions of Bone and Joints.* New York, Springer, 1981, pp. 25–34.
28. Savic, D. L. J., and Djeric, D. R.: Indications for the surgical treatment of osteomas of the frontal and ethmoid sinuses. *Clin Otolaryngol* 15:397, 1990.
29. Campanacci, M.: Osteoma. *Bone and Soft Tissue Tumors.* New York, Springer, 1990, pp. 349–354.
30. O'Connell, J. X., Rosenthal, D. I., Mankin, H. J., and Rosenberg, A. E.: Solitary osteoma of a long bone. A case report. *Bone Joint Surg* 75A:1830–1834, 1993.
31. Klein, M. H., and Shankman, S.: Osteoid osteoma: Radiologic and pathologic correlation. *Skeletal Radiol* 21:23–31, 1992.
32. Greenspan, A.: Benign bone-forming lesions: osteoma, osteoid osteoma, and osteoblastoma. *Skeletal Radiol* 22:485–500, 1993.
33. Kaweblum, M., Lehman, W. B., Bash, J., Strongwater, A., and Grant, A. D.: Osteoid osteoma under the age of five years. The difficulty of diagnosis. *Clin Orthop* 296:218–224, 1993.
34. Strach, E. H.: Osteoid osteoma. *Br Med J* 1:1031, 1953.
35. Makley, J. T., and Dunn, M. J.: Prostaglandin synthesis by osteoid osteoma. *Lancet* 2:42, 1982.
36. Keim, H. A., and Reina, E. G.: Osteoid-osteoma as a cause of scoliosis. *J Bone Joint Surg Am* 57:159–163, 1975.
37. Norman, A., and Dorfman, H. D.: Osteoid-osteoma inducing overgrowth and deformity of bone. *Clin Orthop* 110:233–238, 1975.
38. Bauer, T. W., Zehr, R. J., Belhobek, G. H., and Marks, K. E.: Juxta-articular osteoid osteoma. *Am J Surg Pathol* 15:381–387, 1991.
39. Biebuyck, J. C., Katz, L. D., and McCauley, T.: Soft tissue edema in osteoid osteoma. *Skeletal Radiol* 22:37–41, 1993.
40. Schai, P., Friederich, N., Kruger, A., Jundt, G., Herbe, E., and Buess, P.: Discrete synchronous multifocal osteoid osteoma of the humerus. *Skeletal Radiol* 25:667–670, 1996.
41. Greenspan, A., Elguezabal, A., and Bryk, D.: Multifocal osteoid osteoma: A case report and review of the literature. *AJR Am J Roentgenol* 121:103–106, 1974.
42. Ayala, A. G., Murray, J. A., Erling, M. A., and Raymond, A. K.: Osteoid-osteoma: Intraoperative tetracycline-fluorescence demonstration of the nidus. *J Bone Joint Surg* 68A:747–751, 1986.
43. Ghelman, B., Thompson, F. M., and Arnold, W. D.: Intraoperative radioactive localization of an osteoid-osteoma. Case report. *J Bone Joint Surg* 63A:826–827, 1981.
44. Sim, F. H., Dahlin, D. C., and Beabout, J. W.: Osteoid-osteoma: Diagnostic problems. *J Bone Joint Surg* 57A:154–160, 1975.
45. deBerg, J. C., Pattynama, P. M. T., Obermann, W. R., Bode, P. J., Vielvoye, G. J., and Taminiau, A. H. M.: Percutaneous computed-tomography-guided thermocoagulation for osteoid osteomas. *Lancet* 346:350–351, 1995.
46. Kneisl, J. S., and Simon, M. A.: Medical management compared with operative treatment for osteoid-osteoma. *J Bone Joint Surg* 74A:179–185, 1992.
47. Mirra, J. M., Theros, E., Smasson, J., Cove, K., and Paladugu, R.: A case of osteoblastoma associated with severe systemic toxicity. *Am J Surg Pathol* 3:463–471, 1979.
48. Lucas, D. R., Unni, K. K., McLeod, R. A., O'Connor, M. I., and Sim, F. H.: Osteoblastoma: Clinicopathologic study of 306 cases. *Hum Pathol* 25:117–134, 1994.
49. Saifuddin, A., Sherazi, Z., Shaikh, M. I., Natali, C., Ransford, A. O., and Pringle, J. A. S.: Spinal osteoblastoma: Relationship between paravertebral muscle abnormalities and scoliosis. *Skeletal Radiol* 25:531–535, 1996.
50. O'Connell, J. X., Rosenthal, D. I., Mankin, H. J., Gudger, G. K., Dickersin, G. R., Schiller, A. L., and Rosenberg, A. E.: A unique multifocal osteoblastoma-like tumor of the bones of a single lower extremity. *J Bone Joint Surg* 75A:597–602, 1993.
51. Goldman, R. L.: The periosteal counterpart of benign osteoblastoma. *Am J Clin Pathol* 56:73–78, 1971.
52. Rocca, C. D., and Huvos, A. G.: Osteoblastoma: Varied histologic presentations with a benign clinical course. An analysis of 55 cases. *Am J Surg Pathol* 20:841–850, 1996.
53. Bertoni, F., Unni, K. K., Lucas, D. R., and McLeod, R. A.: Osteoblastoma with cartilaginous matrix. An unusual morphologic presentation in 18 cases. *Am J Surg Pathol* 17:69–74, 1993.
54. Dorfman, H. D., and Weiss, S. W.: Borderline osteoblastic tumors: Problems in the differential diagnosis of aggressive osteoblastoma and low-grade osteosarcoma. *Semin Diagn Pathol* 1:215–234, 1984.
55. Bertoni, F., Unni, K. K., McLeod, R. A., and Dahlin, D. C.: Osteosarcoma resembling osteoblastoma. *Cancer* 55:416–426, 1985.
56. Bertoni, F., Bacchini, P., Donati, D., Martini, A., Picci, P., and Campanacci, M.: Osteoblastoma-like osteosarcoma. The Rizzoli Institute experience. *Modern Pathol* 6:707–716, 1993.
57. Codman, E. A.: The registry of bone sarcoma. *Surg Gynecol Obstet* 42:381–393, 1926.
58. Geschickter, C. F., and Copeland, M. M.: Parosteal osteoma of bone. A new entity. *Ann Surg* 133:790, 1951.
59. Dahlin, D. C., and Unni, K. K.: Osteosarcoma of bone and its important recognizable varieties. *Am J Surg Pathol* 11:61–72, 1977.
60. Benedict, W. F., Fung, Y. K., and Murphree, A. L.: The gene responsible for the development of retinoblastoma and osteosarcoma. *Cancer* 62:1691–1694, 1988.
61. Sim, F. H., DeVries, E. M. G., Miser, J. S., and Unni, K. K.: Case report 760. *Skeletal Radiol* 21:543–545, 1992.
62. Simon, M. A., and Bos, G. D.: Epiphyseal extension of metaphyseal osteosarcoma in skeletally immature individuals. *J Bone Joint Dis* 62A:195–204, 1980.
63. Tsuneyoshi, M., and Dorfman, H. D.: Epiphyseal osteosarcoma: Distinguishing features from clear cell chondrosarcoma, chondroblastoma, and epiphyseal enchondroma. *Hum Pathol* 18:644–651, 1987.
64. Unni, K. K., Dahlin, D. C., Beabout, J. W., and Ivins, J. C.: Parosteal osteogenic sarcoma. *Cancer* 37:2466–2475, 1976.
65. Sheth, D. S., Yasko, A. W., Raymond, A. K., Ayala, A. G., Carrasco, C. H., Benjamin, R. S., Jaffe, N., and Murray, J. A.: Conventional and dedifferentiated parosteal osteosarcoma. Diagnosis, treatment and outcome. *Cancer* 78:2136–2145, 1996.
66. Raymond, A. K., Ayala, A. G., Carrasco, C. H., Benjamin, R. S., and Murray, J. A.: Parosteal osteosarcoma vs. dedifferentiated: Preoperative identification [Abstract]. *Lab Invest* 54:53-A, 1986.
67. Hudson, T. M., Springfield, D. S., Benjamin, M., Bertoni, F., and Present, D. A.: Computed tomography of parosteal osteosarcoma. *AJR Am J Roentgenol* 144:961–965, 1985.
68. Unni, K. K., Dahlin, D. C., and Beabout, J. W.: Periosteal osteogenic sarcoma. *Cancer* 37:2476–2485, 1976.
69. deSantos, L. A., Murray, J. A., Finklestein, J. B., Spjut, H. J., and Ayala, A. G.: The radiographic spectrum of periosteal osteosarcoma. *Radiology* 127:123–129, 1978.

70. Kurt, A.-M., Unni, K. K., McLeod, R. A., and Pritchard, D. J.: Low-grade intraosseous osteosarcoma. *Cancer* 65:1418–1428, 1990.
71. Matsuno, T., Unni, K. K., McLeod, R. A., and Dahlin, D. C.: Telangiectatic osteogenic sarcoma. *Cancer* 38:2538–2547, 1976.
72. Vanel, D., Tcheng, S., Contesso, G., Zafrani, B., Kalifa, C., Dubousset, J., and Kron, P.: The radiological appearances of telangiectatic osteosarcoma. A study of 14 cases. *Skeletal Radiol* 16:196–200, 1987.
73. Huvos, A. G., Rosen, G., Bretsky, S. S., and Butler, A.: Telangiectatic osteogenic sarcoma: A clinicopathologic study of 124 patients. *Cancer* 49:1679–1689, 1982.
74. Sim, F. H., Unni, K. K., Beabout, J. W., and Dahlin, D. C.: Osteosarcoma with small cells simulating Ewing's tumor. *J Bone Joint Surg* 61A:207–215, 1979.
75. Edeiken, J., Raymond, A. K., Ayala, A. G., Benjamin, R. S., Murray, J. A., and Carrasco, H. C.: Small-cell osteosarcoma. *Skeletal Radiol* 16:621–628, 1987.
76. Ayala, A. G., Ro, J. Y., and Raymond, A. K.: Small cell osteosarcoma. A clinicopathologic study of 27 cases. *Cancer* 64:2162–2173, 1989.
77. Devaney, K., Vinh, T. N., and Sweet, D. E.: Small cell osteosarcoma of bone. An immunohistochemical study with differential diagnostic considerations. *Hum Pathol* 24:1211–1225, 1993.
78. Mahoney, J. P., Spanier, S. S., and Morris, J. L.: Multifocal osteosarcoma: A case report with review of the literature. *Cancer* 44:1897–1907, 1979.
79. Kyriakos, M.: Intracortical osteosarcoma. *Cancer* 46:2525–2533, 1980.
80. Vigorita, V. J., Jones, J. K., Ghelman, B., and Marcove, R. C.: Intracortical osteosarcoma. *Am J Surg Pathol* 8:65–71, 1984.
81. Wold, L. E., Unni, K. K., Beabout, J. W., and Pritchard, D. J.: High-grade surface osteosarcomas. *Am J Surg Pathol* 8:181–186, 1984.
82. Raymond, A. K., and Ayala, A. G.: Specimen management after osteosarcoma chemotherapy. Unni K. K., Ed. *Bone Tumors*. New York, Churchill-Livingstone, 1988, pp. 157–181.
83. Raymond, A. K., Chawla, S. P., Carrasco, C. H., et al: Osteosarcoma chemotherapy effect. A prognostic factor. *Semin Diagn Pathol* 4:212–236, 1987.
84. Turcotte, R. E., Kurt, A.-M., Sim, F. H., Unni, K. K., and McLeod, R. A.: Chondroblastoma. *Hum Pathol* 24:944–949, 1993.
85. Bloem, J. L., and Mulder, J. D.: Chondroblastoma: A clinical and radiological study of 104 cases. *Skeletal Radiol* 14:1–9, 1985.
86. Kyriakos, M., Land, V. J., Penning, H. L., and Parker, S. G.: Metastatic chondroblastoma. Report of a fatal case with a review of the literature on atypical, aggressive, and malignant chondroblastoma. *Cancer* 55:1770–1789, 1985.
87. Monda, L., and Wick, M. R.: S-100 protein immunostaining in the differential diagnosis of chondroblastoma. *Hum Pathol* 16:287–293, 1985.
88. Brecher, M. E., and Simon, M. A.: Chondroblastoma: An immunohistochemical study. *Hum Pathol* 19:1043–1047, 1988.
89. Roberts, P. F., and Taylor, J. G.: Multifocal benign chondroblastomas: Report of a case. *Hum Pathol* 11:296–298, 1980.
90. Zillmer, D. A., and Dorfman, H. D.: Chondromyxoid fibroma of bone: Thirty-six cases with clinicopathologic correlation. *Hum Pathol* 20:952–964, 1989.
91. Gherlinzoni, F., Rock, M., and Picci, P.: Chondromyxoid fibroma. The experience at the Istituto Ortopedico Rizzoli. *J Bone Joint Surg* 65A:198–204, 1983.
92. Wilson, A. J., Kyriakos, M., and Ackerman, L. V.: Chondromyxoid fibroma: Radiographic appearance in 38 cases and in a review of the literature. *Musculoskeletal Radiol* 179:513–522, 1991.
93. Kyriakos, M.: Soft tissue implantation of chondromyxoid fibroma. *Am J Surg Pathol* 3:363–372, 1979.
94. Scherer, E.: Exostosen, Enchondrome und ihre Beziehung zum Periost. *Frankfurt Ztschr Path* 36:587, 1928.
95. Caballes, R. L.: Enchondroma protuberans masquerading as osteochondroma. *Hum Pathol* 13:734–739, 1982.
96. Weinstein, L. J., and McCarthy, E. F.: Ki-67 immunostaining as a tool in the diagnosis of central cartilage lesions. *Iowa Orthop J* 16:39–45, 1996.
97. Lamy, M.: Trois cas de maladie d'Ollier dans une fratrie. *Bull Mèm Soc Mèd Hôp Paris* 70:62–70, 1954.
98. Schwartz, H. S., Zimmerman, N. B., Simon, M. A., Wroble, R. R., Millar, E. A., and Bonfiglio, M.: The malignant potential of enchondromatosis. *J Bone Joint Surg* 69A:269–274, 1987.
99. Liu, J., Hudkins, P. G., Swee, R. G., and Unni, K. K.: Bone sarcomas associated with Ollier's disease. *Cancer* 59:1376–1385, 1987.
100. Lewis, R. J., and Ketcham, A. S.: Maffucci's syndrome: Functional and neoplastic significance. *J Bone Joint Surg* 55A:1465–1479, 1973.
101. Libshitz, H. I., and Cohen, M. A.: Radiation-induced osteochondromas. *Radiology* 142:643–647, 1982.
102. Cohen, E. K., Kressel, H. Y., Frank, T. S., et al: Hyaline cartilage-origin bone and soft-tissue neoplasms: MR appearance and histologic correlation. *Radiology* 167:477–481, 1988.
103. Malghem, J., Vande Berg, B., Noel, H., and Maldague, B.: Benign osteochondromas and exostotic chondrosarcomas: Evaluation of cartilage cap thickness by ultrasound. *Skeletal Radiol* 21:33–37, 1992.
104. Borges, A. M., Huvos, A. G., and Smith, J.: Bursa formation and synovial chondrometaplasia associated with osteochondromas. *Am J Clin Pathol* 75:648–653, 1981.
105. Montgomery, D. M., and LaMont, R. L.: Resolving solitary osteochondromas. A report of two cases and literature review. *Orthopedics* 12:861–863, 1989.
106. Bertoni, F., Bacchini, P., Picci, P., Pignatti, G., Gherlinzoni, F., and Campanacci, M.: Dedifferentiated peripheral chondrosarcomas. *Cancer* 63:2954–2059, 1989.
107. Shapiro, F., Simon, S., and Glimcher, M. J.: Hereditary multiple exostoses. *J Bone Joint Surg* 61A:815–824, 1979.
108. Garrison, R. C., Unni, K. K., McLeod, R. A., Pritchard, D. J., and Dahlin, D. C.: Chondrosarcoma arising in osteochondroma. *Cancer* 49:1890–1897, 1982.
109. Boriani, S., Bacchini, P., Bertoni, F., and Campanacci, M.: Periosteal chondroma. A review of twenty cases. *J Bone Joint Surg* 65A:205–212, 1983.
110. Bauer, T. W., Dorfman, H. D., and Latham, J. T. Jr.: Periosteal chondroma. A clinicopathologic study of 23 cases. *Am J Surg Pathol* 6:631–637, 1982.
111. Nojima, T., Unni, K. K., McLeod, R. A., and Pritchard, D. J.: Periosteal chondroma and periosteal chondrosarcoma. *Am J Surg Pathol* 9:666–677, 1985.
112. Dorfman, H. D.: Chondrosarcoma variants. *Radiology Today* 2:165–170, 1983.
113. Kreicbergs, A., Boquist, L., Borssen, B., and Larsson, S.: Prognostic factors in chondrosarcoma: A comparative study of cellular DNA content and clinicopathologic features. *Cancer* 50:577–583, 1982.
114. Gitelis, S., Bertoni, F., Picci, P., and Campanacci, M.: Chondrosarcoma of bone. The experience at the Instituto Ortopedico Rizzoli. *J Bone Joint Surg* 63A:1248–1256, 1981.
115. Evans, H. L., Ayala, A. G., and Romsdahl, M. M.: Prognostic factors in chondrosarcoma of bone. A clinicopathologic analysis with emphasis on histologic grading. *Cancer* 40:818–831, 1977.
116. Sanerkin, N. G.: The diagnosis and grading of chondrosarcoma of bone. A combined cytologic and histologic approach. *Cancer* 45:582–594, 1980.
117. Pritchard, D. J., Lunke, R. J., Taylor, W. F., Dahlin, D. C., and Medley, B. E.: Chondrosarcoma: A cliniccpathologic and statistical analysis. *Cancer* 45:149–157, 1980.
118. Coughlan, B., Feliz, A., Ishida, T., Czerniak, B., and Dorfman, H. D.: p53 expression and DNA ploidy of cartilage lesions. *Hum Pathol* 26:620–624, 1995.
119. Mirra, J. M., Gold, R., Downs, J., and Eckardt, J. J.: A new histologic approach to the differentiation of enchondroma and chondrosarcoma of the bones. A clinicopathologic analysis of 51 cases. *Clin Orthop* 201:214–237, 1985.
120. Schiller, A. L.: Diagnosis of borderline cartilage lesions of bone. *Semin Diagn Pathol* 2:42–62, 1985.
121. Schajowicz, F.: Juxtacortical chondrosarcoma. *J Bone Joint Surg* 59B:473–480, 1977.
122. Bertoni, F., Boriani, S., Laus, M., and Campanacci, M.: Periosteal chondrosarcoma and periosteal osteosarcoma. Two distinct entities. *J Bone Joint Surg* 64B:370–376, 1982.
123. Present, D., Bacchini, P., Pignatti, G., Picci, P., Bertoni, F., and Campanacci, M.: Clear cell chondrosarcoma of bone. A report of 8 cases. *Skeletal Radiol* 20:187–191, 1991.
124. Bjornsson, J., Unni, K. K., Dahlin, D. C., Beabout, J. W., and Sim, F. H.: Clear cell chondrosarcoma of bone. Observations in 47 cases. *Am J Surg Pathol* 8:223–230, 1984.
125. Nakashima, Y., Unni, K. K., Shives, T. C., Swee, R. G., and Dahlin, D. C.: Mesenchymal chondrosarcoma of bone and soft tissue. *Cancer* 57:2444–2453, 1986.
126. Granter, S. R., Renshaw, A. A., Fletcher, C. D. M., Bhan, A. K., and Rosenberg, A. E.: CD99 reactivity in mesenchymal chondrosarcoma. *Hum Pathol* 27:1273–1276, 1996.

127. Frassica, F. J., Unni, K. K., Beabout, J. W., and Sim, F. H.: Dedifferentiated chondrosarcoma. A report of the clinicopathological features and treatment of seventy-eight cases. *Bone Joint Surg* 68A:1197–1205, 1986.
128. McCarthy, E. F., and Dorfman, H. D.: Chondrosarcoma of bone with dedifferentiation. A study of eighteen cases. *Hum Pathol* 13:36–40, 1982.
129. Reith, J. D., Bauer, T. W., Fischler, D. F., Joyce, M. J., and Marks, K. E.: Dedifferentiated chondrosarcoma with rhabdomyosarcomatous differentiation. *Am J Surg Pathol* 20:293–298, 1996.
130. Ishida, T., Dorfman, H. D., and Habermann, E. T.: Dedifferentiated chondrosarcoma of humerus with giant cell tumor-like features. *Skeletal Radiol* 24:76–80, 1995.
131. Ritschl, P., Karnel, F., and Hajek, P.: Fibrous metaphyseal defects—determination of their origin and natural history using a radiomorphological study. *Skeletal Radiol* 17:8–15, 1988.
132. Mirra, J. M., Gold, R. H., and Rand, F.: Disseminated nonossifying fibromas in association with café-au-lait spots (Jaffe-Campanacci syndrome). *Clin Orthop* 168:192–205, 1982.
133. Weinstein, L. S., Shenker, A., Gejman, P. V., Merino, M. J., Friedman, E., and Spiegel, A. M.: Activating mutations of the stimulatory G protein in the McCune-Albright syndrome. *N Engl J Med* 325:1688–1695, 1991.
134. Candelier, G. A., Glorieux, F. H., Prud'homme, J., and St.-Arnaud, R.: Increased expression of the c-fos proto-oncogene in bone from patients with fibrous dysplasia. *N Engl J Med* 332:1546–1551, 1995.
135. Dorfman, H. D., Ishida, T., and Tsuneyoshi, M.: Exophytic variant of fibrous dysplasia (fibrous dysplasia protuberans). *Hum Pathol* 25:1234–1237, 1994.
136. Sissons, H. A., Steiner, G. C., and Dorfman, H. D.: Calcified spherules in fibro-osseous lesions of bone. *Arch Pathol Lab Med* 117:284–290, 1993.
137. Voytek, T. M., Ro, J. Y., Edeiken, J., and Ayala, A. G.: Fibrous dysplasia and cemento-ossifying fibroma. A histologic spectrum. *Am J Surg Pathol* 19:775–781, 1995.
138. Ishida, T., and Dorfman, H. D.: Massive chondroid differentiation in fibrous dysplasia of bone (fibrocartilaginous dysplasia). *Am J Surg Pathol* 17:924–930, 1993.
139. Bulychova, I. V., Unni, K. K., Bertoni, F., and Beabout, J. W.: Fibrocartilaginous mesenchymoma of bone. *Am J Surg Pathol* 17:830–836, 1993.
140. Bertoni, F., Calderoni, P., Bacchini, P., Sudanese, A., Baldini, N., Present, D., and Campanacci, M.: Benign fibrous histiocytoma of bone. *J Bone Joint Surg* 68A:1225–1230, 1986.
141. Clarke, B. E., Xipell, J. M., and Thomas, D. P.: Benign fibrous histiocytoma of bone. *Am J Surg Pathol* 9:806–814, 1985.
142. Hamada, T., Ito, H., Araki, Y., Fujii, K., Inoue, M., and Ishida, O.: Benign fibrous histiocytoma of the femur: Review of three cases. *Skeletal Radiol* 25:25–29, 1996.
143. Matsuno, T.: Benign fibrous histiocytoma involving the ends of long bone. *Skeletal Radiol* 19:561–566, 1990.
144. Inwards, C. Y., Unni, K. K., Beabout, J. W., and Sim, F. H.: Desmoplastic fibroma of bone. *Cancer* 68:1978–1983, 1991.
145. Taconis, W. K., Schutte, H. E., and van der Heul, R. O.: Desmoplastic fibroma of bone: A report of 18 cases. *Skeletal Radiol* 23:283–288, 1994.
146. Young, J. W., Aisner, S. C., Levine, A. M., Resnik, C. S., and Dorfman, H. D.: Computed tomography of desmoid tumors of bone: Desmoplastic fibroma. *Skeletal Radiol* 17:333–337, 1988.
147. Bohm, P., Krober, S., Greschniok, A., Laniado, M., and Kaiserling, E.: Desmoplastic fibroma of the bone. A report of two patients, review of the literature, and therapeutic implications. *Cancer* 78:1011–1023, 1996.
148. Bertoni, F., Capanna, R., Calderoni, P., Patrizia, B., and Campanacci, M.: Primary central (medullary) fibrosarcoma of bone. *Semin Diagn Pathol* 1:185–198, 1984.
149. Larsson, S.-E., Lorentzon, R., and Boquist, L.: Fibrosarcoma of bone. A demographic, clinical and histopathological study of all cases recorded in the Swedish Cancer Registry from 1958 to 1968. *J Bone Joint Surg* 58B:412–425, 1976.
150. Galli, S. J., Weintraub, H. P., and Proppe, K. H.: Malignant fibrous histiocytoma and pleomorphic sarcoma in association with medullary bone infarcts. *Cancer* 41:607–619, 1978.
151. Frierson, H. F., Fechner, R. E., Stallings, R. G., and Wang, G.-J.: Malignant fibrous histiocytoma in bone infarct. Association with sickle cell trait and alcohol abuse. *Cancer* 59:496–500, 1987.
152. Mirra, J. M., Gold, R. H., and Marafiote, R.: Malignant (fibrous) histiocytoma arising in association with a bone infarct in sickle-cell disease: Coincidence or cause-and-effect. *Cancer* 39:186–194, 1977.
153. Capanna, R., Bertoni, F., Bacchini, P., Bacci, G., Guerra, A., and Campanacci, M.: Malignant fibrous histiocytoma of bone. The experience at the Rizzoli Institute: Report of 90 cases. *Cancer* 54:177–187, 1984.
154. Nishida, J., Sim, F. H., Wenger, D. E., and Unni, K. K.: Malignant fibrous histiocytoma of bone. A clinicopathologic study of 81 patients. *Cancer* 79:482–493, 1997.
155. Huvos, A. G., Heilweil, M., and Bretsky, S. S.: The pathology of malignant fibrous histiocytoma of bone. *Am J Surg Pathol* 9:853–871, 1985.
156. McCarthy, E. F., Matsuno, T., and Dorfman, H. D.: Malignant fibrous histiocytoma of bone: A study of 35 cases. *Human Pathol* 10:57–70, 1979.
157. McDonald, D. J., Sim, F. H., McLeod, R. A., and Dahlin, D. C.: Giant-cell tumor of bone. *J Bone Joint Surg* 68A:235–242, 1986.
158. Sim, F. H., Dahlin, D. C., and Beabout, J. W.: Multicentric giant-cell tumor of bone. *J Bone Joint Surg* 59A:1052–1060, 1977.
159. Hindman, B. W., Seeger, L. L., Stanley, P., Forrester, D. M., Schwinn, C. P., and Tan, S. Z.: Multicentric giant cell tumor: Report of five new cases. *Skeletal Radiol* 23:187–190, 1994.
160. Aqel, N. M., Pringle, J. A. S., and Horton, M. A.: Cellular heterogeneity in giant cell tumour of bone (osteoclastoma): An immunohistological study of 16 cases. *Histopathology* 13:675–685, 1988.
161. Brecher, M. E., Franklin, W. A., and Simon, M. A.: Immunohistochemical study of mononuclear phagocyte antigens in giant cell tumor of bone. *Am J Pathol* 125:252–257, 1986.
162. Sulh, M. A., Greco, M. A., Jiang, T., Goswami, S. B., Present, D., and Steiner, G.: Proliferation index and vascular density of giant cell tumors of bone. Are they prognostic markers? *Cancer* 77:2044–2051, 1996.
163. Fornasier, V. L., Protzner, K., Zhang, I., and Mason, L.: The prognostic significance of histomorphometry and immunohistochemistry in giant cell tumors of bone. *Hum Pathol* 27:754–760, 1996.
164. Schwartz, H. S., Juliao, S. F., Sciadini, M. F., Miller, L. K., and Butler, M. G.: Telomerase activity and oncogenesis in giant cell tumor of bone. *Cancer* 75:1094–1099, 1995.
165. Schoedel, K. E., Greco, M. A., Stetler-Stevenson, W. G., Ohori, N. P., Goswami, S., Present, D., and Steiner, G. C.: Expression of metalloproteinases and tissue inhibitors of metalloproteinases in giant cell tumor of bone: An immunohistochemical study with clinical correlation. *Hum Pathol* 27:1144–1148, 1996.
166. Teot, L. A., O'Keefe, R. J., Rosier, R. N., O'Connell, J. X., Fox, E. J., and Hicks, D. G.: Extraosseous primary and recurrent giant cell tumors: Transforming growth factor-β 1 and -β 2 expression may explain metaplastic bone formation. *Hum Pathol* 27:625–632, 1996.
167. Rock, M. G., Pritchard, D. J., and Unni, K. K.: Metastases from histologically benign giant-cell tumor of bone. *J Bone Joint Surg* 66A:269–274, 1984.
168. Vanel, D., Contesso, G., Rebibo, G., Zafrani, B., and Masselot, J.: Benign giant-cell tumours of bone with pulmonary metastases and favourable prognosis. Report on two cases and review of the literature. *Skeletal Radiol* 10:221–226, 1983.
169. Katz, E., Nyska, M., Okon, E., Zajicek, G., and Robin, G.: Growth rate analysis of lung metastases from histologically benign giant cell tumor of bone. *Cancer* 59:1831–1836, 1987.
170. Nascimento, A. G., Huvos, A. G., and Marcove, R. C.: Primary malignant giant cell tumor of bone. A study of eight cases and review of the literature. *Cancer* 44:1393–1402, 1979.
171. Meis, J. M., Dorfman, H. D., Nathanson, S. D., Haggar, A. M., and Wu, K. K.: Primary malignant giant cell tumor of bone: "Dedifferentiated" giant cell tumor. *Modern Pathol* 2:541–546, 1989.
172. Rock, M. G., Sim, F. H., Unni, K. K., Witrak, G. A., Frassica, F. J., Schray, M. F., Beabout, J. W., and Dahlin, D. C.: Secondary malignant giant-cell tumor of bone. Clinicopathological assessment of nineteen patients. *J Bone Joint Surg* 68A:1073–1078, 1986.
173. Ostrowski, M. L., Unni, K. K., Banks, P. M., Shives, T. C., Evans, R. G., and O'Connell, M. J.: Malignant lymphoma of bone. *Cancer* 58:2646–2655, 1986.
174. Pettit, C. K., Zukerberg, L. R., Gray, M. H., Ferry, J. A., Rosenberg, A. E., Harmon, D. C., and Harris, N. L.: Primary lymphoma of bone. A B-cell neoplasm with a high frequency of multilobated cells. *Am J Surg Pathol* 14:329–334, 1990.
175. Chan, J. K. C., Ng, C. S., Hui, P. K., Leung, W. T., Sin, V. C., Lam,

T. K., Chick, K. W., and Lam, W. Y.: Anaplastic large cell Ki-1 lymphoma of bone. *Cancer* 68:2186–2191, 1991.
176. Newcomer, L. N., Silverstein, M. B., Cadman, E. C., Farber, L. R., Bertino, J. R., and Prosnitz, L. R.: Bone involvement in Hodgkin's disease. *Cancer* 49:338–342, 1982.
177. Horan, F. T.: Bone involvement in Hodgkin's disease. A survey of 201 cases. *Br J Surg* 56:277–281, 1969.
178. O'Carroll, D. I., McKenna, R. W., and Brunnig, R. D.: Bone marrow manifestations of Hodgkin's disease. *Cancer* 38:1717–1728, 1976.
179. Ozdemirli, M., Mankin, H. J., Aisenberg, A. C., and Harris, N. L.: Hodgkin's disease presenting as a solitary bone tumor. A report of four cases and review of the literature. *Cancer* 77:79–88, 1996.
180. Triche, T. J., and Askin, F. B.: Neuroblastoma and the differential diagnosis of small-, round-, blue-cell tumors. *Hum Pathol* 14:569–594, 1983.
181. Scotlandi, K., Serra, M., Manara, M. C., Benini, S., Sarti, M., Maurici, D., Lollini, P. L., Picci, P., Bertoni, F., and Baldini, N.: Immunostaining of the p30/32^{MIC2} antigen and molecular detection of EWS rearrangements for the diagnosis of Ewing's sarcoma and peripheral neuroectodermal tumor. *Hum Pathol* 27:408–416, 1996.
182. Jurgens, H. F.: Ewing's sarcoma and peripheral primitive neuroectodermal tumor. *Curr Opin Oncol* 6:391–396, 1994.
183. Kissane, J. M., Askin, F. B., Foulkes, M., Stratton, L. B., and Shirley, S. F.: Ewing's sarcoma of bone: Clinicopathologic aspects of 303 cases from the Intergroup Ewing's Sarcoma Study. *Hum Pathol* 14:773–779, 1983.
184. Shirley, S. K., Gilula, L. A., Siegal, G. P., Foulkes, M. A., Kissane, J. M., and Askin, F. B.: Roentgenographic-pathologic correlation of diffuse sclerosis in Ewing sarcoma of bone. *Skeletal Radiol* 12:69–78, 1984.
185. Landanyi, M., Heinemann, F. S., Huvos, A. G., Rao, P. H., Chen, Q., and Jhanwar, S. C.: Neural differentiation in small round cell tumors of bone and soft tissue with the translocation t(11;22)(q24;q12): An immunohistochemical study of 11 cases. *Hum Pathol* 21:1245–1251, 1990.
186. Tsokos, M., Linnoila, R. I., Chandra, R. S., and Triche, T. J.: Neuron-specific enolase in the diagnosis of neuroblastoma and other small, round-cell tumors in children. *Hum Pathol* 15:575–584, 1984.
187. Llombart-Bosch, A., Contesso, G., and Peydro-Olaya, A.: Histology, immunohistochemistry, and electron microscopy of small round cell tumors of bone. *Semin Diagn Pathol* 13:153–170, 1996.
188. Ishida, T., Iijima, F., Kikuchi, F., Kitagawa, T., Tanida, T., Imamura, T., and Machinami, R.: A clinicopathological and immunohistochemical study of osteofibrous dysplasia, differentiated adamantinoma, and adamantinoma of long bones. *Skeletal Radiol* 21:493–502, 1992.
189. Czerniak, B., Rojas-Corona, R. R., and Dorfman, H. D.: Morphologic diversity of long bone adamantinoma. The concept of differentiated (regressing) adamantinoma and its relationship to osteofibrous dysplasia. *Cancer* 64:2319–2334, 1989.
190. Park, Y.-K., Unni, K. K., McLeod, R. A., and Pritchard, D. J.: Osteofibrous dysplasia: Clinicopathologic study of 80 cases. *Hum Pathol* 24:1339–1347, 1993.
191. Sweet, D. E., Vinh, T. N., and Devaney, K.: Cortical osteofibrous dysplasia of long bone and its relationship to adamantinoma. *Am J Surg Pathol* 16:282–290, 1992.
192. Komiya, S., and Inoue, A.: Aggressive bone tumorous lesion in infancy: osteofibrous dysplasia of the tibia and fibula. *J Pediatr Orthop* 13:577–581, 1993.
193. Springfield, D. S., Rosenberg, A. E., Mankin, H. J., and Mindell, E. R.: Relationship between osteofibrous dysplasia and adamantinoma. *Clin Orthop* 309:234–244, 1994.
194. Blackwell, J. B., McCarthy, S. W., Xipell, J. M., Vernon-Roberts, B., and Duhig, R. E. T.: Osteofibrous dysplasia of the tibia and fibula. *Pathology* 20:227–233, 1988.
195. Nakashima, Y., Yamamuro, T., Fujiwara, Y., Kotoura, Y., Mori, E., and Hamashima, Y.: Osteofibrous dysplasia (ossifying fibroma of long bones): A study of 12 cases. *Cancer* 52:909–914, 1983.
196. Campanacci, M., and Laus, M.: Osteofibrous dysplasia of the tibia and fibula. *J Bone Joint Surg Am* 63:367–375, 1981.
197. Frangenheim, P.: Angeborene ostitis fibrosa als Ursache einer intrauterinen Unterschenkelfractur. *Arch Klin Chir* 117:22–29, 1921.
198. Compere, E. L.: Localized osteitis fibrosa in the newborn and congenital pseudoarthrosis. *J Bone Joint Surg* 18:513–525, 1936.
199. Aegerter, E. E.: The possible relationship of neurofibromatosis, congenital pseudoarthrosis, and fibrous dysplasia. *J Bone Joint Surg* 32A:618–626, 1950.
200. Kempson, R. L.: Ossifying fibroma of the long bones. *Arch Pathol* 82:218–233, 1966.
201. Campanacci, M.: Osteofibrous dysplasia of long bones—a new clinical entity. *Ital J Orthop Traumatol* 2:221–237, 1976.
202. Mills, S. E., and Rosai, J.: Adamantinoma of the pretibial soft tissue. Clinicopathologic features, differential diagnosis, and possible relationship to intraosseous disease. *Am J Clin Pathol* 83:108–114, 1985.
203. Keeney, G. L., Unni, K. K., Beabout, J. W., and Pritchard, D. J.: Adamantinoma of long bones. A clinicopathologic study of 85 cases. *Cancer* 64:730–737, 1989.
204. Campanacci, M., Giunti, A., Bertoni, F., Laus, M., and Gitelis, S.: Adamantinoma of the long bones. The experience at the Istituto Ortopedico Rizzoli. *Am J Surg Pathol* 5:533–542, 1981.
205. Weiss, S. W., and Dorfman, H. D.: Adamantinoma of long bone. An analysis of nine new cases with emphasis on metastasizing lesions and fibrous dysplasia-like changes. *Hum Pathol* 8:141–153, 1977.
206. Cohn, B. T., Brahms, M. A., and Froimson, A. I.: Metastasis of adamantinoma sixteen years after knee disarticulation. Report of a case. *J Bone Joint Surg Am* 48:772–776, 1986.
207. Wold, L. E., Unni, K. K., Cooper, K. L., Sim, F. H., and Dahlin, D. C.: Hemangiopericytoma of bone. *Am J Surg Pathol* 6:53–58, 1982.
208. Schmorl, G., and Junghanns, H.: *The Human Spine in Health and Disease*, 2nd ed. New York, Grune & Stratton, 1971, p. 325.
209. Wold, L. E., Swee, R. G., and Sim, F. H.: Vascular lesions of bone. *Pathol Annu* 20:101–137, 1985.
210. Schajowicz, F., Aiello, C. L., Francone, M. V., and Giannini, R. E.: Cystic angiomatosis (Hamartous haemolymphangiomatosis) of bone. *J Bone Joint Surg* 60B:100–105, 1978.
211. Graham, D. Y., Gonzales, J., and Kothari, S. M.: Diffuse skeletal angiomatosis. *Skeletal Radiol* 2:131–135, 1978.
212. Ishida, T., Dorfman, H. D., Steiner, G. C., and Norman, A.: Cystic angiomatosis of bone with sclerotic changes mimicking osteoblastic metastases. *Skeletal Radiol* 23:247–252, 1994.
213. Tsuneyoshi, M., Dorfman, H. D., and Bauer, T. W.: Epithelioid hemangioendothelioma of bone. A clinicopathologic, ultrastructural, and immunohistochemical study. *Am J Surg Pathol* 10:754–764, 1986.
214. Kleer, C. G., Unni, K. K., and McLeod, R. A.: Epithelioid hemangioendothelioma of bone. *Am J Surg Pathol* 20:1301–1311, 1996.
215. Smith, J., Ludwig, R. L., and Marcove, R. C.: Sacrococcygeal chordoma. A clinicoradiological study of 60 patients. *Skeletal Radiol* 16:37–44, 1987.
216. Volpe, R., and Mazabraud, A.: A clinicopathologic review of 25 cases of chordoma (a pleomorphic and metastasizing neoplasm). *Am J Surg Pathol* 7:161–170, 1983.
217. Horwitz, T.: Chordal ectopia and its possible relation to chordoma. *Arch Pathol* 31:354–362, 1941.
218. Wojno, K. J., Hruban, R. H., Garin-Chesa, P., and Huvos, A. G.: Chondroid chordomas and low-grade chondrosarcomas of the craniospinal axis. *Am J Surg Pathol* 16:1144–1152, 1992.
219. Hruban, R. H., May, M., Marcove, R. C., and Huvos, A. G.: Lumbosacral chordoma with high-grade malignant cartilaginous and spindle cell components. *Am J Surg Pathol* 14:384–389, 1990.
220. Meis, J. M., Raymond, A. K., Evans, H. L., Charles, R. E., and Giraldo, A. A.: "Dedifferentiated" chordoma. A clinicopathologic and immunohistochemical study of three cases. *Am J Surg Pathol* 11:516–525, 1987.
221. Chambers, P. W., and Schwinn, C. P.: Chordoma. A clinicopathologic study of metastasis. *Am J Clin Pathol* 72:765–776, 1979.
222. Cahan, W. G., Woodward, H. Q., Higinbotham, N., et al.: Sarcoma arising in irradiated bone. *Cancer* 1:3–29, 1948.
223. Arlen, M., Higinbotham, N. L., Huvos, A., Marcove, R., et al.: Radiation induced sarcoma of bone. *Cancer* 28:1087–1099, 1971.

CHAPTER 13
Bone Cysts

Bone cysts are fluid-filled cavities with a connective tissue lining and varying numbers of septae. Three important types of bone cyst exist, and each contains a characteristic fluid. The first is the unicameral bone cyst, also known as a simple bone cyst. This type of cyst results from a temporary failure of bone formation during skeletal growth. The unicameral bone cyst usually has a single chamber and is filled with yellow, serous-like fluid. The second type of cyst, the aneurysmal bone cyst, results from a focal hemodynamic alteration in normal bone or in a preexisting bone lesion. An aneurysmal bone cyst contains many locules filled with blood. The third type of cyst is the subchondral cyst. Cysts in this category include osteoarthritic cysts, intraosseous ganglia, and post-traumatic cysts. Subarticular cysts occur adjacent to joints and contain mucoid or jelly-like material.

Bone cysts are radiolucent lesions and may therefore masquerade as solid neoplasms. However, magnetic resonance imaging (MRI), which readily shows their fluid content, has become an important tool in the diagnosis of these lesions. Although the fluid-filled nature of these cysts may now be recognized preoperatively, the pathologist must pay careful attention to the cyst's radiographic setting and the characteristics of its fluid to make the correct diagnosis (Table 13–1).

In addition to unicameral bone cysts, aneurysmal bone cysts, and subchondral cysts, cavities may form in bone as a result of other less common processes. One example is liquefaction of an intraosseous lipoma. Another is trauma to the distal phalanx, which may cause an intraosseous epidermal inclusion cyst.

UNICAMERAL BONE CYST

A unicameral bone cyst forms in childhood as a result of temporary cessation of medullary bone formation by the epiphyseal plate. This developmental failure results in a single-chambered, fluid-filled cyst in the metaphyseal portion of the bone. While the cyst is forming, a so-called "active" lesion, the cavity is adjacent to the epiphyseal plate. After medullary bone formation resumes, the cyst migrates into the diaphysis and is separated from the epiphyseal plate by normal cancellous bone. Although the etiology of the unicameral bone cyst is unknown, several causes have been suggested, including an intraosseous hematoma, a necrotic lipoma, lymphatic or venous obstruction, and intraosseous synovial rests. An important clinical feature of this lesion is

Table 13–1 ■ **BONE CYSTS: RADIOGRAPHIC SETTINGS AND FLUID CHARACTERISTICS**

Cyst Type	Radiographic Setting	Common Locations	Fluid Characteristics
Unicameral bone cyst	Symmetric, metaphyseal lucency	Proximal humerus, proximal femur	Clear, yellow, serous
Aneurysmal bone cyst	Asymmetric, "aneurysmal" metaphyseal lucency	Distal femur, proximal tibia	Bloody
Subchondral cysts			
Osteoarthritic cyst	Epiphyseal; arthritic change	Knee and hip	Mucoid
Intraosseous ganglion	Epiphyseal; no arthritic change	Distal and proximal tibia, distal ulna	Mucoid
Traumatic cyst	Epiphyseal; osteochondral defect	Talus, proximal tibia	Mucoid
Intraosseous lipoma	Metaphyseal lucency	Calcaneus	Oily, liquid fat
Epidermal inclusion cyst	Distal phalanx lucency	Fingers, toes	Keratinaceous debris

its predilection for two locations: the proximal humerus (51% of cases) and the proximal femur (28% of cases). The ilium[1] and calcaneus[2] are also sites that are often affected.

Clinical Features

Unicameral bone cysts are not uncommon: An orthopedic surgeon may see two or three new cases each year. Most patients are children or adolescents. In fact, 85% of lesions are diagnosed in patients younger than 20 years. The walls of a unicameral bone cyst are very thin, so many patients present with a pathologic fracture. Nonfractured lesions often present as incidental findings during radiologic studies for other conditions. Undoubtedly, many unicameral bone cysts are never diagnosed because most lesions are asymptomatic.

Radiologic Features

Unicameral bone cysts are usually diagnosed radiologically. Plain radiographs show a central and symmetric radiolytic lesion present in the metaphysis (Fig. 13–1). Intersecting lines of radiodensity, corresponding to ridges on the inner wall of the cyst, traverse the radiolytic zone. The cortices are often thin and expanded. With actively growing

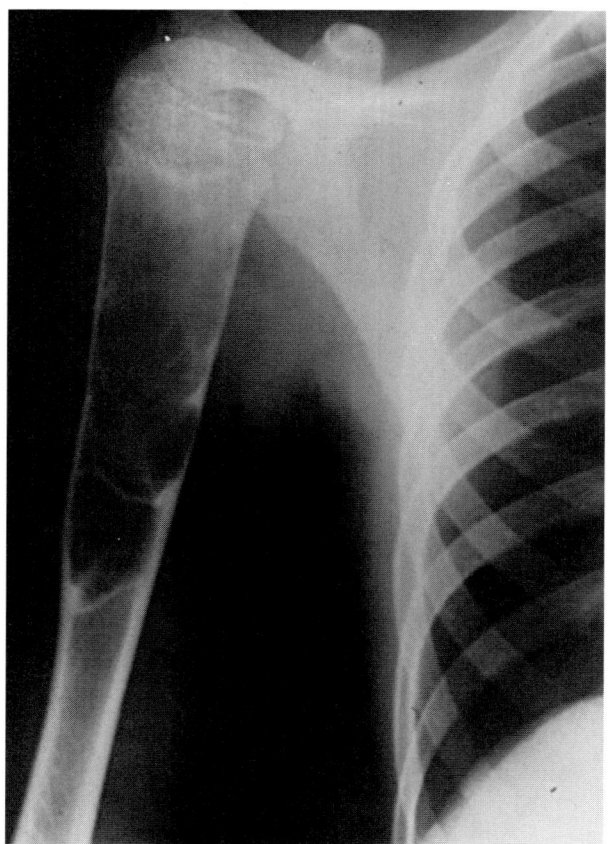

Figure 13-1 ■ Unicameral bone cyst of the proximal humerus. The lesion is a long, symmetric radiolucency in the metaphysis. Uniform thinning of the cortices has occurred.

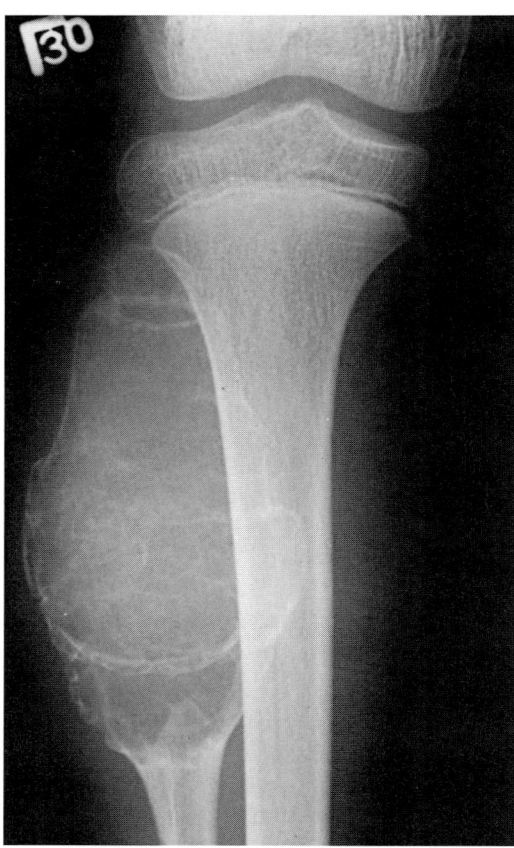

Figure 13-2 ■ Unicameral bone cyst of the proximal fibula. This is an active lesion because the lucency abuts the epiphyseal plate.

cysts, the lytic area abuts the epiphyseal plate (Fig. 13–2). Very rarely, an active cyst penetrates the plate and involves the epiphysis.[3] Inactive cysts are separated from the epiphyseal plate by normal cancellous bone (Fig. 13–3). A unicameral bone cyst is characteristically equal to or slightly greater in diameter than the epiphyseal plate. However, depending on the duration of activity, the length may vary from 3 to 13 cm. In about 20% of cases, a fractured cortical fragment falls into the distal portion of the cyst, producing the *"fallen leaf"* sign[4] (Fig. 13–4). In addition, some unicameral bone cysts contain faint granular or ring-shaped radiodensities.

Usually an MRI confirms the diagnosis of a simple bone cyst. The study shows a well-defined zone of very bright, uniform signal in T_2-weighted images (Fig. 13–5). This finding confirms the high water content of the lesion. The signal from this zone is much less intense in T_1-weighted images.

Pathology

To the surgeon's eye, a unicameral bone cyst is a single-chambered cavity filled with clear yellow serous fluid. Little soft tissue is present in the cyst. Only a fibrous tissue membrane, 1 to 5 mm thick, lines the cyst wall, although occasionally thin fibrous septae traverse the cavity (Fig.

13–6). Therefore, the pathologist should be aware that the amount of tissue removed by complete curettage of the cyst contents is extremely small compared with the size of the lesion seen on radiographs. Often, only one tissue cassette is needed to process the entire contents of a large cyst for histologic study. Lack of awareness of this normal discrepancy between the amount of tissue removed and the size of the lesion may lead to the misinterpretation that the lesion is solid.

Histologically, the lining membrane of unicameral bone cyst consists of bland fibrous tissue and occasional spicules of reactive bone (Fig. 13–7). A few osteoclast-like giant cells are usually present. In addition, approximately 10% of lesions contain cementum-like spherules in the lining membrane (Fig. 13–8). These eosinophilic bodies are thought to be either old fibrin coagula or osteoid. They frequently calcify and correspond to the granular densities seen on plain radiographs.[5,6]

Because unicameral bone cysts often fracture, reparative changes may mimic the tissue of an aneurysmal bone cyst (Fig. 13–9). In fractured lesions, the fluid is usually bloody, and granulation tissue and fracture callus are abundant. Careful attention to the radiographic setting is necessary to prevent misdiagnosis as an aneurysmal bone cyst.

Treatment

Unicameral bone cysts are best treated after they have moved away from the epiphyseal plate. Most lesions, particularly those with few fibrous septae, can be healed with

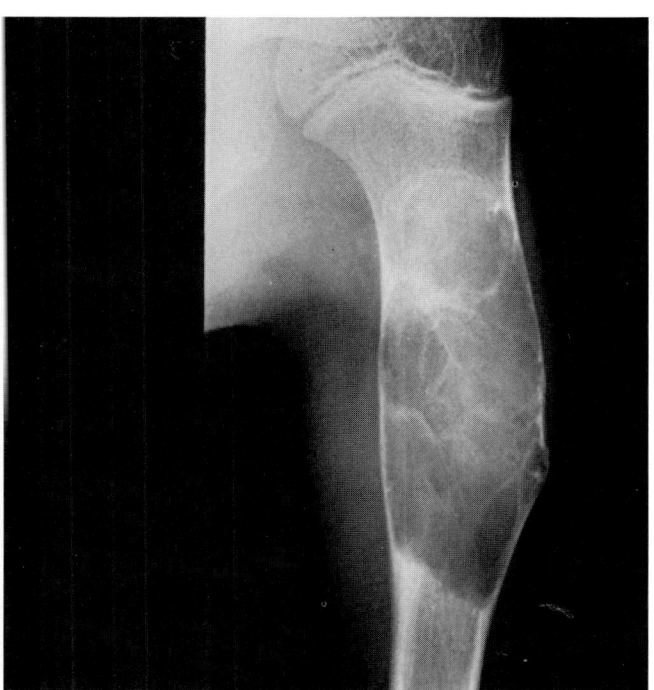

Figure 13-3 ■ Unicameral bone cyst of the humerus. This is an inactive lesion because a zone of normal cancellous bone separates the lytic lesion from the epiphyseal plate.

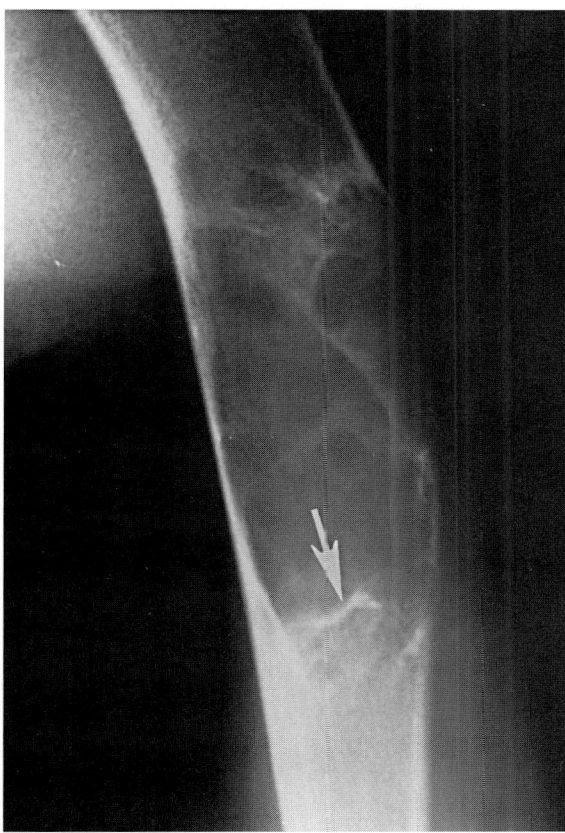

Figure 13-4 ■ This unicameral bone cyst of the humerus illustrates the "fallen leaf sign" *(arrow)*.

cortical drilling followed by intralesional injection of cortisone or other sclerosing agents.[7–9] Curettage and bone grafting, necessary only in rare cases, result in a 12% recurrence rate.[10] Occasionally, a pathologic fracture stimulates spontaneous healing.

ANEURYSMAL BONE CYST

Aneurysmal bone cyst is a destructive, expansile bone lesion characterized by a reactive proliferation of connective tissue containing multiple blood-filled cavities. Probably because of local hemodynamic disturbances, the process arises de novo in bone or is engrafted onto preexisting bone lesions, histologically identifiable in 30% of cases.[11] The incidence of an underlying preexisting lesion may be higher because the aneurysmal bone cyst process can totally efface the histologic features of the original lesion. In this event, the clinical and radiographic setting may be the only clue to the preexisting lesion. Neoplasms most frequently associated with aneurysmal bone cyst are chondroblastoma, giant cell tumor, chondromyxoid fibroma, and fibrous dysplasia. Aneurysmal bone cyst changes may also be engrafted on malignant neoplasms, such as osteosarcoma or metastatic prostate carcinoma. In addition to developing de novo or in neoplasms, aneurysmal bone cysts may develop as a result of a

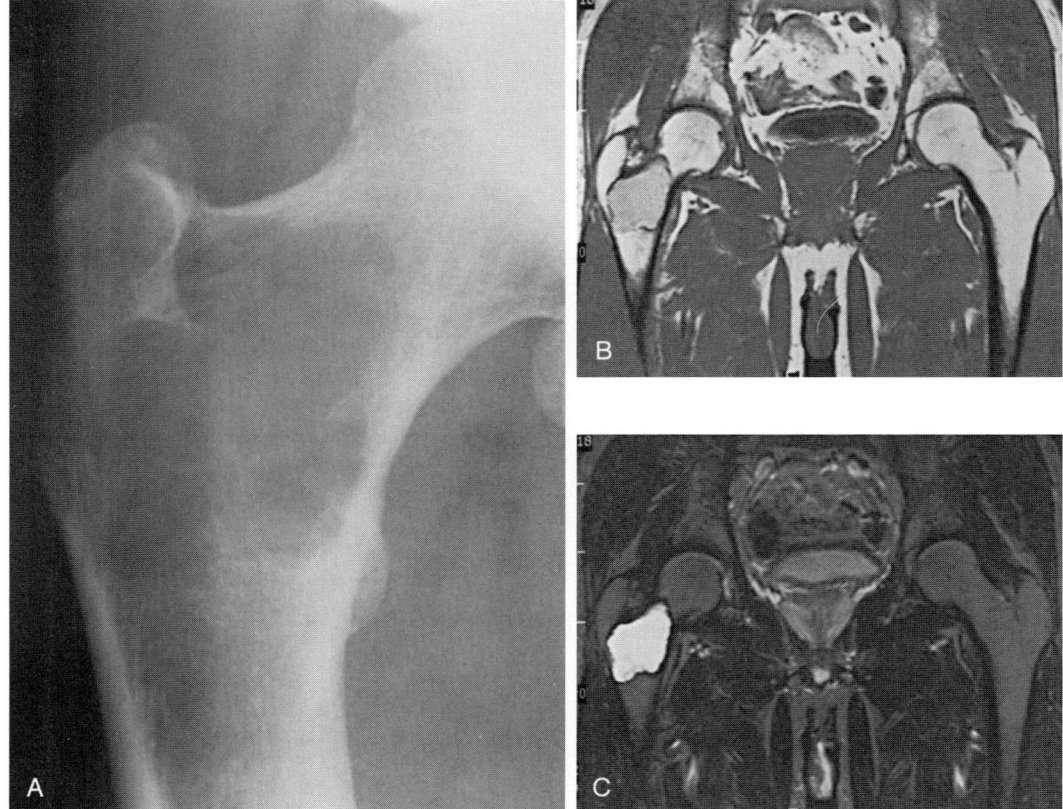

Figure 13-5 ■ Unicameral bone cyst of the proximal femur (its second most common location). **A,** The lesion is a well-circumscribed radiolucent area in the intertrochanteric region. **B,** A T_1-weighted MRI showing an intermediate signal from the lesion. **C,** A T_2-weighted MRI. This sequence is strongly suggestive of a cyst—a well-circumscribed zone of uniformly very bright signal from the lesion.

traumatic subperiosteal hematoma[12] or after a surgical procedure on bone.

Clinical Presentation

Aneurysmal bone cysts occur at any age, although 60 to 86% of patients are younger than 20.[13,14] The distal femur and proximal tibia are the most common locations, followed by the posterior elements of the vertebrae. Any bone, however, including the cranium and facial bones, may be involved. In the long bones, the metaphysis is the most commonly affected area. Aneurysmal bone cysts exhibit two growth patterns rarely seen in other bone lesions: contiguous involvement of adjacent bones, particularly in spinal lesions, and the extension of the process across an open growth plate.[15]

Radiologic Features

Aneurysmal bone cysts have a wide range of radiographic appearances. Some have a benign radiologic pattern with well-circumscribed margins, although they usually lack a sclerotic rim (Fig. 13–10). By contrast, other aneurysmal bone cysts have an aggressive, permeative pattern (Fig. 13–11). These lesions show marked cortical expansion, and sometimes a soft tissue mass, which is best visualized with MRI, is present. These aggressive radiographic features, along with rapid clinical growth, often mimic a malignant neoplasm. The MRI of aneurysmal bone cysts shows multiple fluid-filled cavities. These cavities often show distinct fluid lines representing the interface between blood and serum, a feature best seen on T_2-weighted images (Fig. 13–12).[16]

Pathology

At surgery, the gross appearance of an aneurysmal bone cyst is a pulsatile mass with multiple blood-filled cavities. Heavy bleeding often follows a biopsy, and curettage produces abundant spongy soft tissue. The characteristic microscopic feature of aneurysmal bone cyst, best seen on low-power examination, is multiple blood-filled cavities of varying sizes (Fig. 13–13). The cavities lack an endothelial lining, and the stroma of the intervening septae consists of proliferating fibroblasts and scattered multinucleated giant cells (Fig. 13–14). Reactive bone, usually in broad bands, and fibromyxoid cartilage are often abundant (Fig. 13–15). The stromal cells sometimes show many mitotic figures; however, the stromal cells are uniform, and atypical mitoses are not present (Fig. 13–16).

BONE CYSTS 281

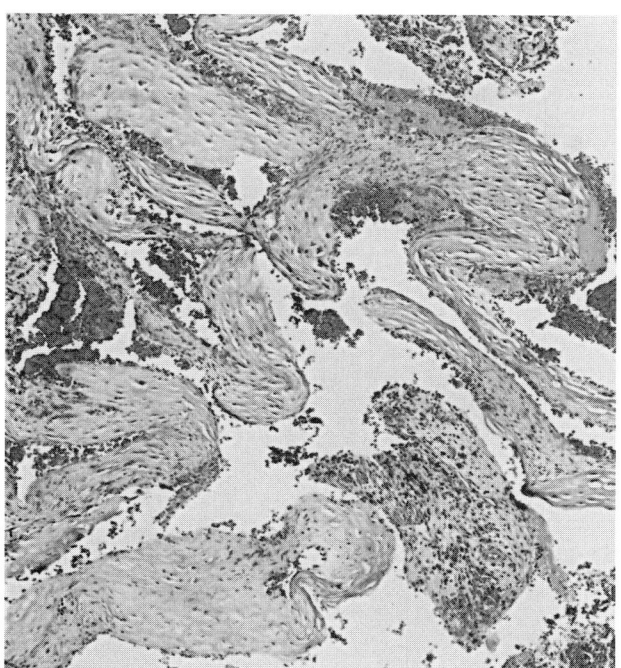

Figure 13-6 ■ Curettings from a unicameral bone cyst. This tissue represents the entire cyst contents.

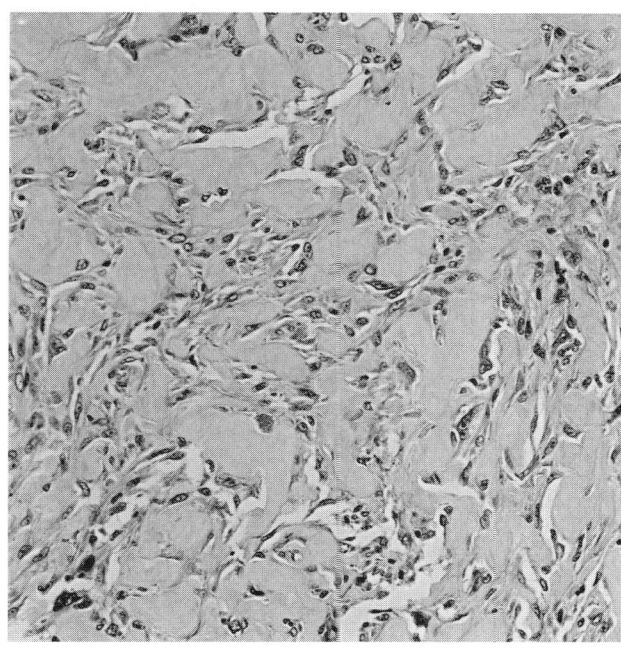

Figure 13-8 ■ Cementum-like bodies in the lining of a unicameral bone cyst.

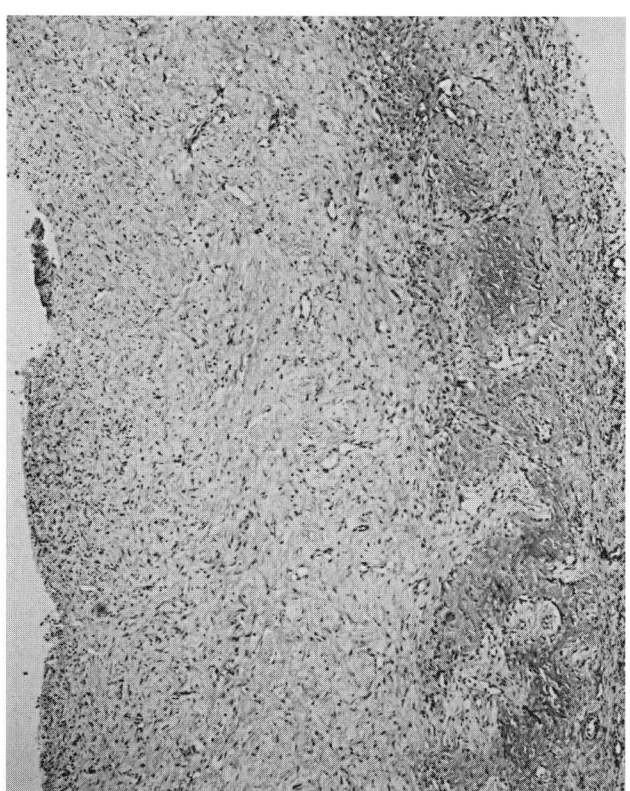

Figure 13-7 ■ The lining of a unicameral bone cyst—bland fibrous tissue with a few spicules of reactive bone.

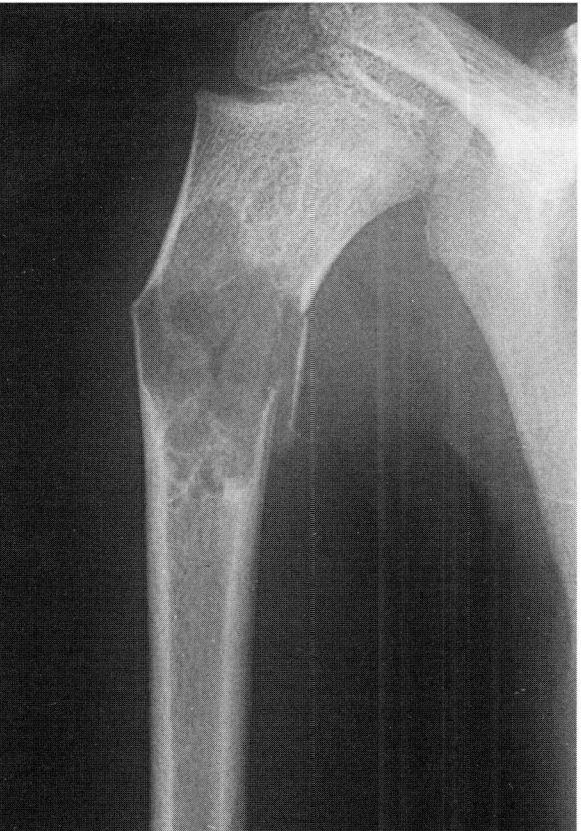

Figure 13-9 ■ A unicameral bone cyst of the proximal humerus with a pathologic fracture. A pathologic fracture is a common presentation of this lesion.

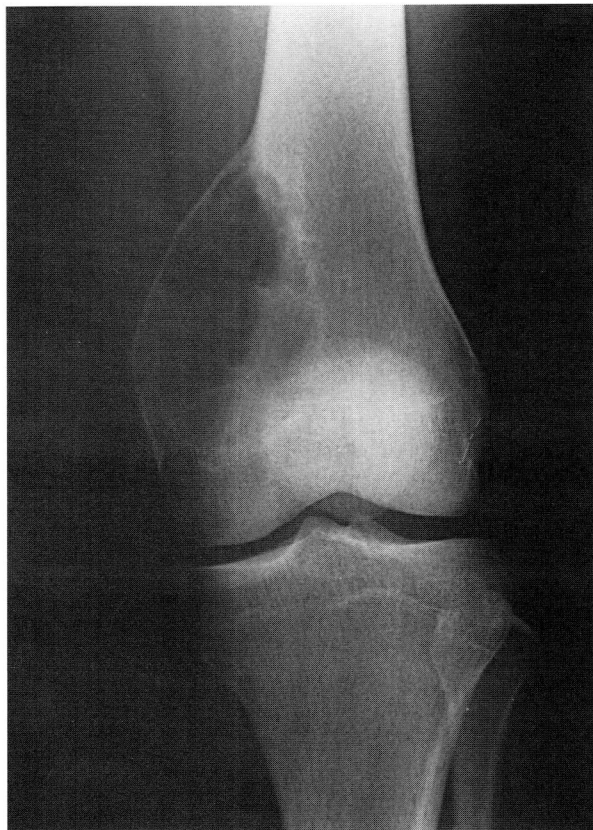

Figure 13-10 ■ Aneurysmal bone cyst of the distal femoral metaphysis. This zone is one of the most common locations for aneurysmal bone cyst.

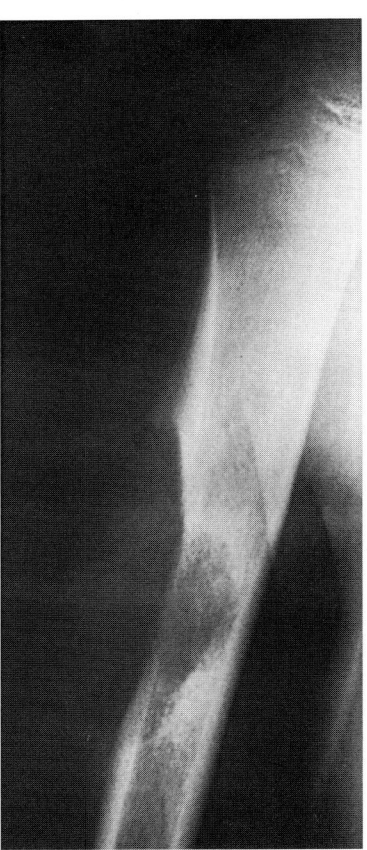

Figure 13-11 ■ An aneurysmal bone cyst of the proximal humerus showing an aggressive permeative pattern with aneurysmal expansion into the adjacent soft tissues.

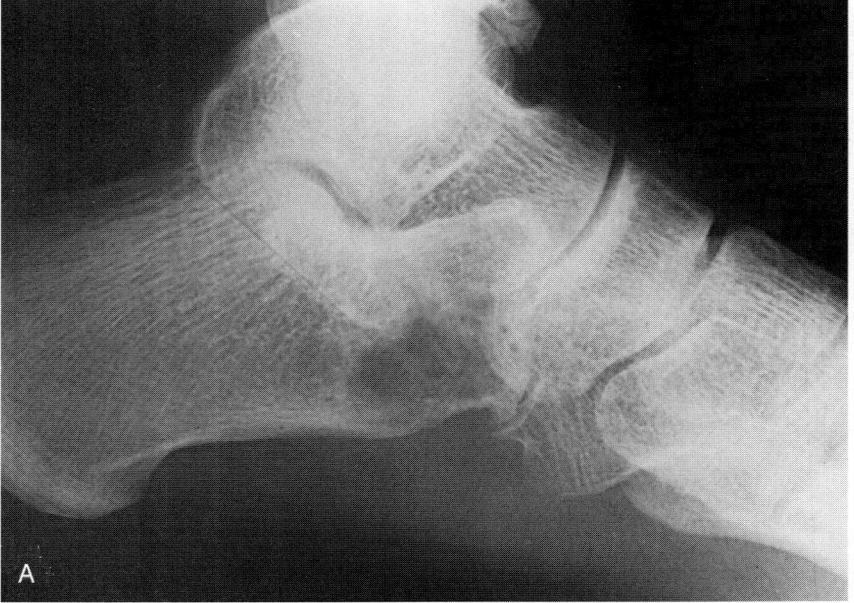
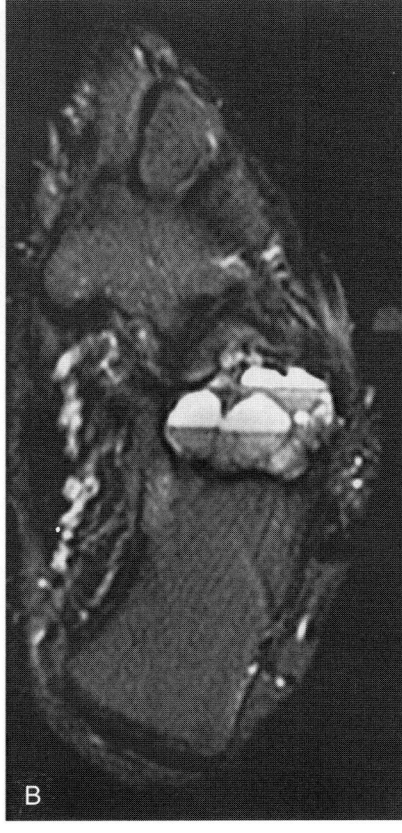

Figure 13-12 ■ Aneurysmal bone cyst of the calcaneus. **A,** A poorly defined radiolytic lesion. **B,** A T_2-weighted MRI showing features diagnostic of an aneurysmal bone cyst. Multiple locules of fluid that demonstrate serum-blood lines are present.

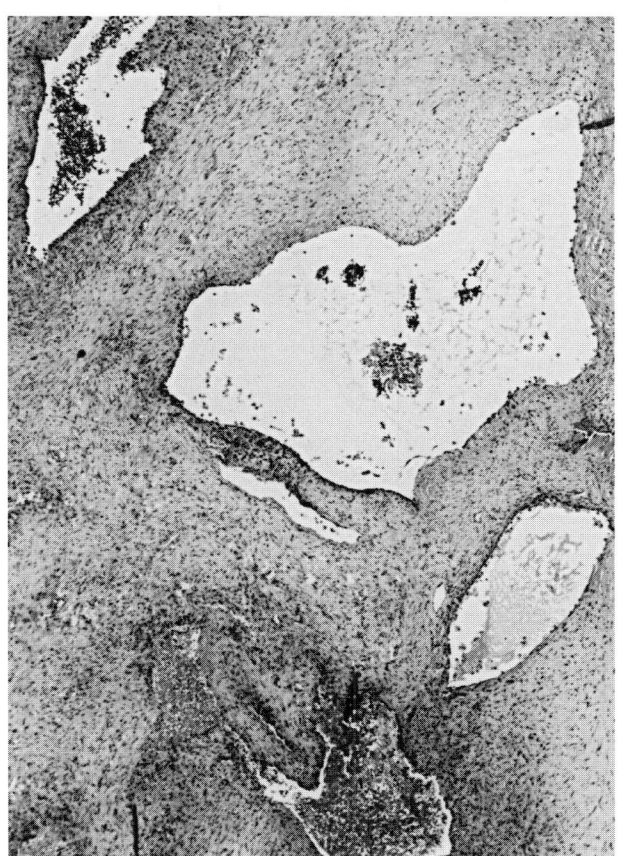

Figure 13-13 ■ Low-power photomicrograph of aneurysmal bone cyst showing multiple blood lakes.

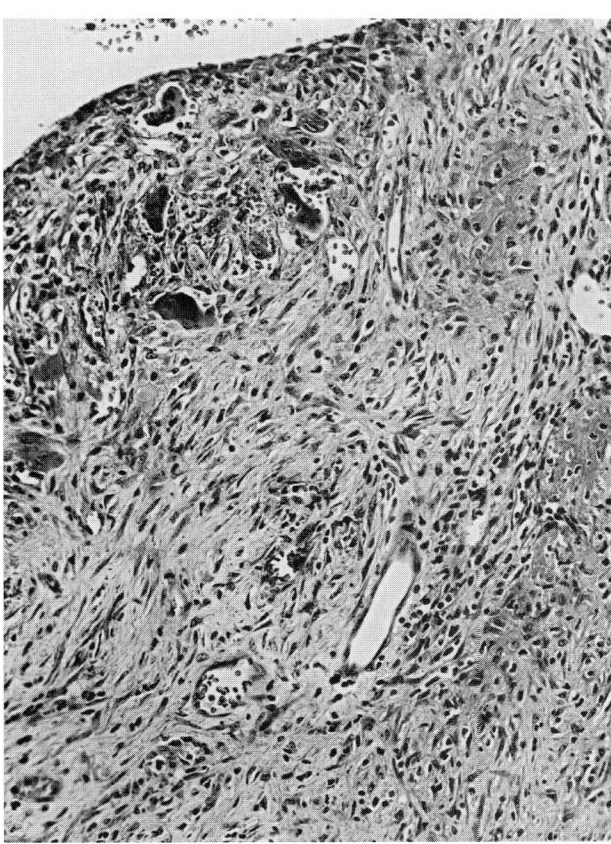

Figure 13-14 ■ Lining of aneurysmal bone cyst showing multinucleated giant cells and a fibroblastic stroma. A few spicules of reactive bone are present.

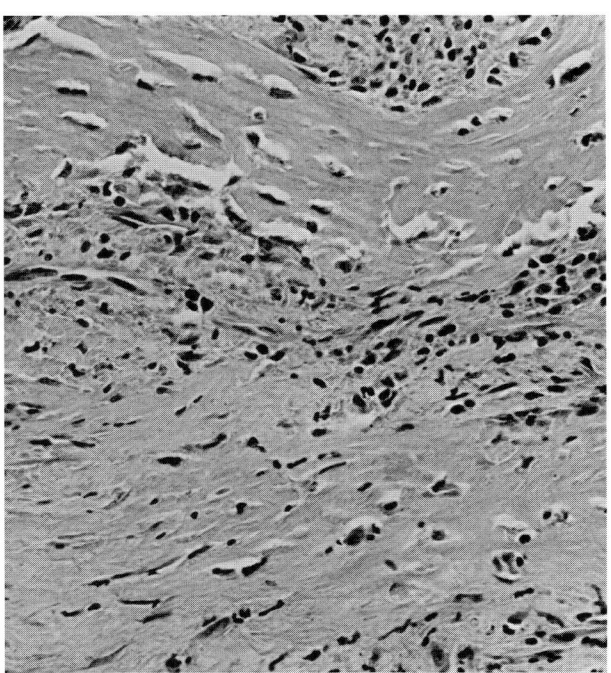

Figure 13-15 ■ The broad bands of reactive new bone in the lining of an aneurysmal bone cyst.

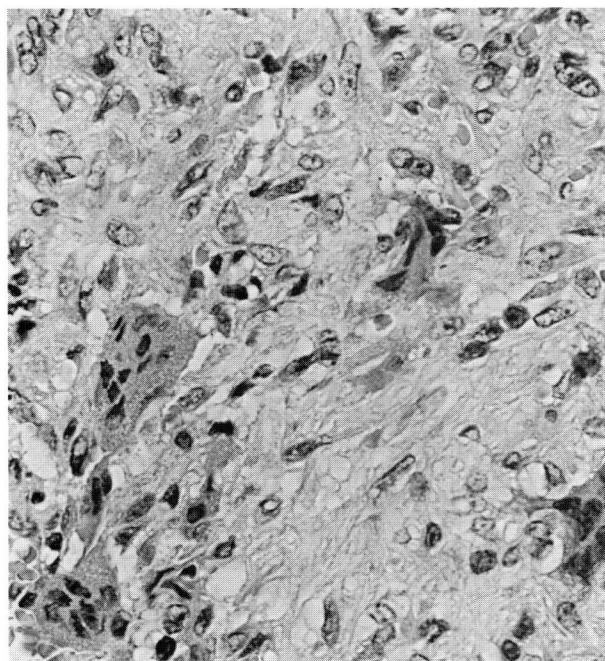

Figure 13-16 ■ The fibroblastic stroma from a septum in an aneurysmal bone cyst. The fibroblasts are bland, and mitotic figures are rare.

The entire surgical specimen of an aneurysmal bone cyst should be studied histologically to identify, if present, a preexisting bone tumor. Features suggestive of a preexisting neoplasm should be interpreted in the light of the patient's clinical presentation and radiographs. For example, to conclude that chondroblastoma is present in an aneurysmal bone cyst, the lesion must involve the epiphyseal end of the bone, the typical location of a chondroblastoma. In addition, the focal presence of a sarcomatous stroma in an otherwise typical aneurysmal bone cyst indicates a telangiectatic osteosarcoma.

Some pathologists recognize a variant called "solid aneurysmal bone cyst."[17] This lesion is histologically identical to giant cell reparative granuloma with small foci of aneurysmal bone cyst change.

Treatment

In rare cases, aneurysmal bone cysts heal spontaneously.[18] Most lesions, however, require curettage with bone grafting. Because of the potential for heavy bleeding, preoperative embolization is often required.[19,20] Although the recurrence rate after curettage is 50% (most recurrences appearing within 6 months), reoperation ultimately results in complete cure for most patients.

SUBCHONDRAL CYSTS

Acquired subchondral bone cysts, known by a variety of names depending on clinical and radiographic features, are probably all caused by trauma to the joint surface. These lesions include osteoarthritic cysts, intraosseous ganglia, and post-traumatic cysts. Injury to the articular cartilage stimulates granulation tissue proliferation in the marrow spaces of the subchondral bone. Then, foci of myxomatous change appear in the granulation tissue. Finally, because of enlargement and coalescence of these foci, a cyst forms and causes local bone resorption. Regardless of the clinical setting, the result of this process is a subchondral radiolytic defect filled with granulation tissue and acellular myxoid material (Fig. 13–17). Therefore, because of identical histologic features, the types of subchondral cysts must be distinguished by clinical and radiographic presentation.

Osteoarthritic Cysts

Osteoarthritic cysts are a component of the degenerative changes of osteoarthritis.[21,22] In addition, large subchondral cysts, occasionally referred to as geodes, often complicate chronic pyrophosphate arthropathy or late rheumatoid arthritis.[23] Patients are in their 50s and 60s, the usual age range for the onset of osteoarthritis. The subchondral cysts usually occur adjacent to areas of maximal joint space narrowing and are often present on both sides of a joint. The hip and knee are the most common joints to develop these cysts because these joints are most frequently involved by osteoar-

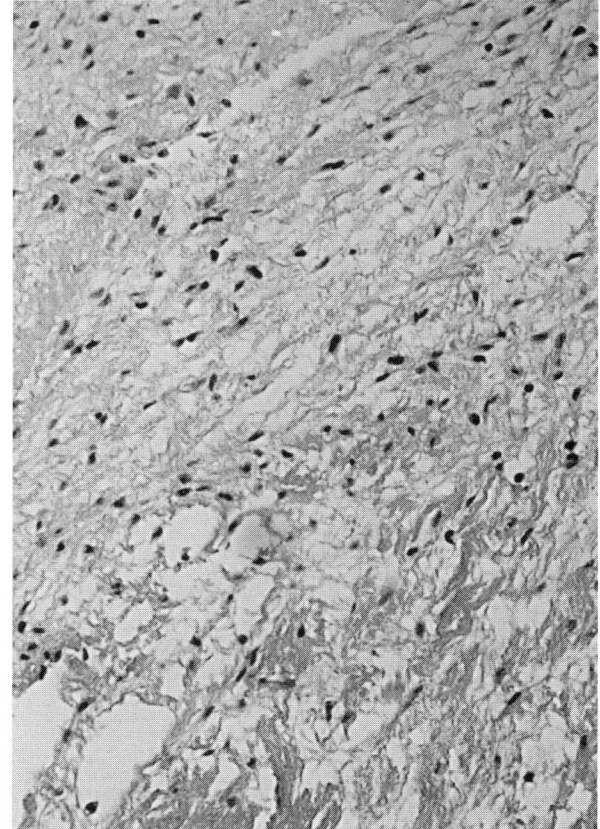

Figure 13-17 ■ The contents of a subarticular cyst. Fibrous tissue is undergoing mucoid degeneration.

thritis. Osteoarthritic cysts vary in size from a few millimeters to several centimeters.

Diagnostic problems occasionally arise because a subchondral cyst may develop when other radiologic features of osteoarthritis are minimal or even absent.[24] In this event, a large cyst may radiographically mimic a bone neoplasm, particularly giant cell tumor (Fig. 13–18). This diagnostic problem is most frequently encountered in osteoarthritic cysts of the proximal tibia.[25] However, careful radiographic study usually demonstrates subtle changes of osteoarthritis. For example, patients may have small osteophytes or joint space narrowing visible only on weight-bearing films. In addition, tiny cysts may be present on the other side of the joint. Finally, the MRI will correctly identify the fluid-filled cystic nature of these subchondral lesions.

Osteoarthritic cysts are most often present in subchondral bone that has been denuded of articular cartilage. The process begins by focal myxoid degeneration of subchondral granulation tissue. Multiple foci of myxomatous degeneration enlarge and coalesce to form cysts (Fig. 13–19). A mature cyst is lined by fibrous tissue and filled with acellular mucoid material, rich in hyaluronic acid. When denuded of cartilage, the overlying cortex often fractures, and portions of bone and degenerated cartilage fall into the cyst. These subchondral fractures have led to the hypothesis that osteoarthritic cysts are caused by inspissation of synovial fluid into the bone through these defects. However, careful study of osteoarthritic joint surfaces usually reveals early subchondral cyst formation in the absence of fractures and often with substantial overlying cartilage (Fig. 13–20).

In the absence of other significant changes of osteoarthritis, osteoarthritic cysts may be treated conservatively. Although some cysts heal spontaneously, most patients eventually develop more severe osteoarthritis. Large cysts associated with end-stage osteoarthritis must be treated by total joint arthroplasty. Occasionally, during this procedure the cyst must be filled with methyl methacrylate cement or bone graft.

Intraosseous Ganglion

Intraosseous ganglia, although sharing histologic features with osteoarthritic cysts, are regarded as a distinct entity because patients lack other clinical and radiographic features of osteoarthritis. For example, trabecular thickening of the subchondral bone and joint space narrowing, characteristic features of osteoarthritis, are not present with intraosseous ganglia. However, most intraosseous ganglia are probably early manifestations of osteoarthritis before clinical and other radiographic features occur.

Intraosseous ganglia occur in middle-aged patients (mean

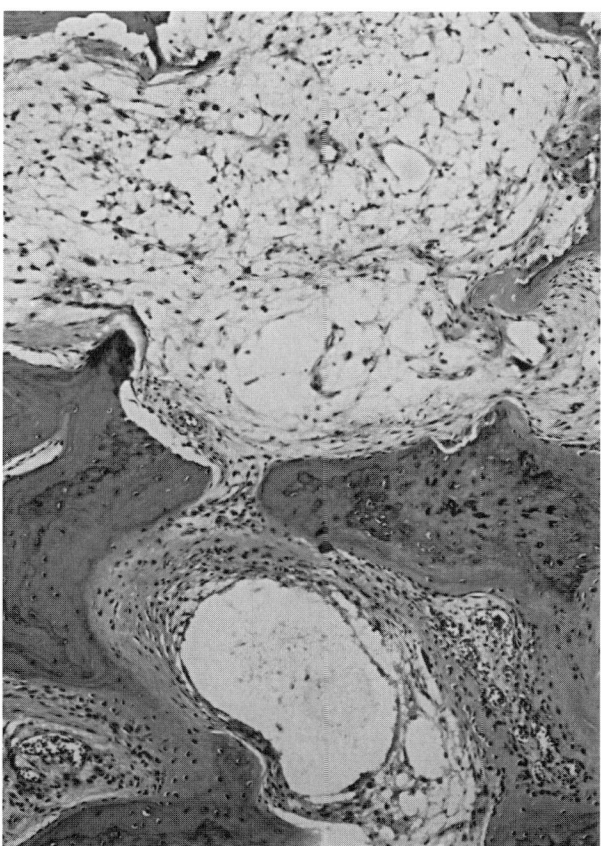

Figure 13-19 ■ Subchondral bone in osteoarthritis showing mucoid degeneration of reparative fibrous tissue.

age, 42 years) and most frequently involve the medial malleolus of the distal tibia, the proximal tibia, the carpal bones, and the acetabulum.[26–29] Radiographically, these lesions are well-defined lytic defects in the epiphysis beneath the subchondral plate (Fig. 13–21). Usually no cortical expansion occurs, and some lesions have a sclerotic rim. In rare cases, intraosseous ganglia occur when soft tissue ganglia erode adjacent bone. Histologically, like osteoarthritic cysts, intraosseous ganglia are filled with acellular mucoid material, and the cyst cavity is lined by a fibrous tissue membrane with focal myxoid degeneration.

Intraosseous ganglia are treated successfully by removal of the myxomatous tissue and curettage of the fibrous lining. Bone grafts are necessary to fill large defects. The incidence of subsequent clinically significant osteoarthritis adjacent to treated intraosseous ganglia is not known.

A lesion histologically similar to an intraosseous ganglion may develop beneath the periosteum. This rare lesion, known as a *periosteal ganglion,* usually occurs in the tibia and causes subtle subperiosteal cortical erosion.[30,31]

Post-Traumatic Cysts

Post-traumatic cysts occur in subchondral bone following severe articular injury. This lesion usually develops within several months of the injury, and it may reach several centi-

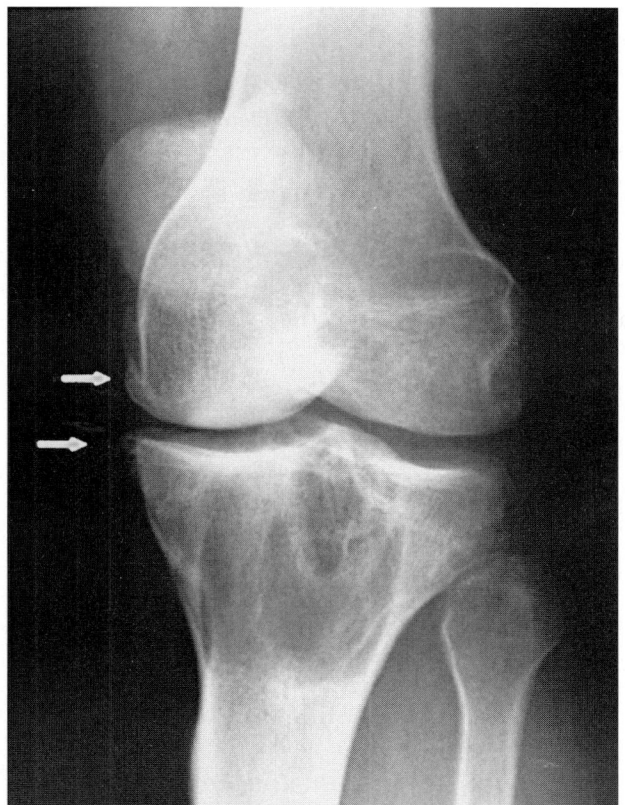

Figure 13-18 ■ A large osteoarthritic cyst of the proximal tibia. This lesion resembles a giant cell tumor of bone. However, small osteophytes on the medial portion of the joint *(arrows)* are the clue that this lesion is probably an osteoarthritic cyst.

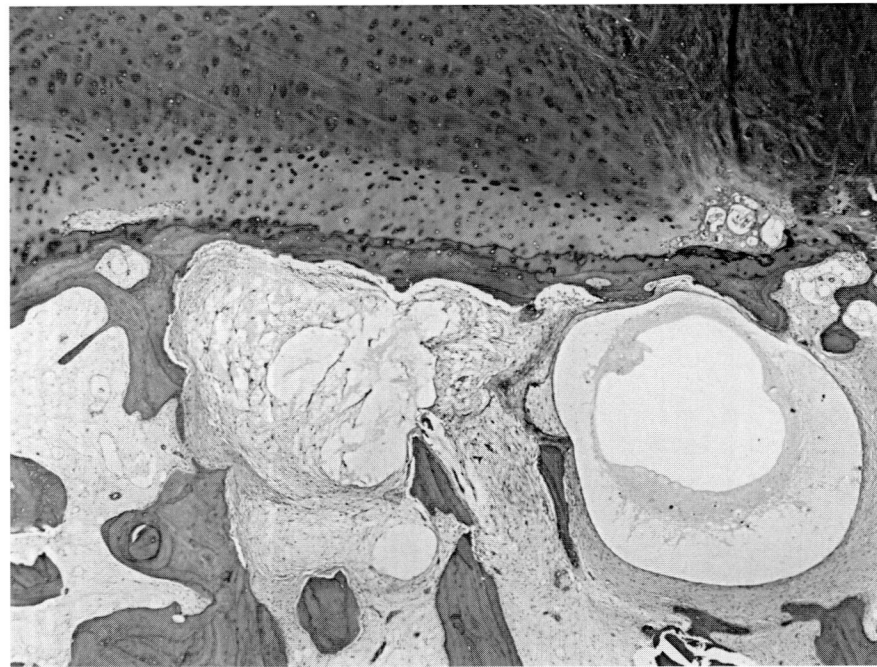

Figure 13-20 ■ Small osteoarthritic cysts beneath an intact subchondral plate with abundant overlying hyaline cartilage.

meters in diameter. Occasionally, the injury to the joint may be severe enough to cause an osteochondral fracture, best visualized with a computed tomography (CT) scan. The proximal tibia and talus are the most common locations of this process (Fig. 13–22).

Like other subchondral cysts, post-traumatic cysts contain acellular material admixed with granulation tissue. In addition, a chondral or osteochondral fragment is occasionally present in the cyst cavity.

Post-traumatic subchondral cysts may be treated with evacuation of the contents and curettage of the lining. Bone grafting is usually necessary to prevent collapse of the articular surface.

INTRAOSSEOUS LIPOMA

Lipomas are very common in soft tissue; they may also occur, although rarely, within the medullary cavity of bone. This lesion, known as an intraosseous lipoma, is characterized by a focus of mature adipose tissue proliferation in the

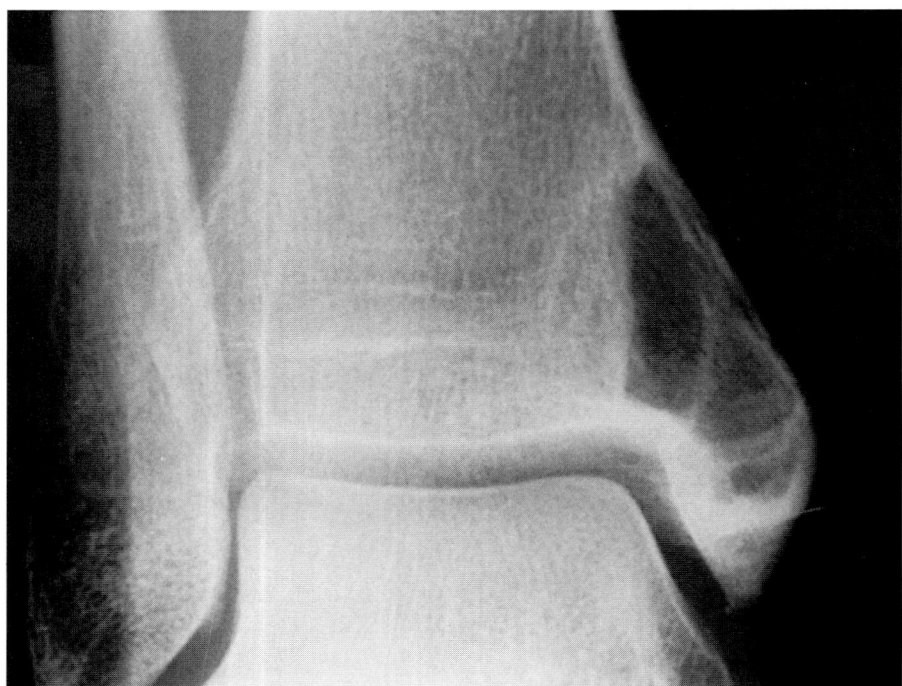

Figure 13-21 ■ An intraosseous ganglion in the medial tibial malleolus. No evidence of osteoarthritis in the ankle joint can be seen. (From McCarthy, E. F.: *Differential Diagnosis in Pathology. Bone and Joint Disorders.* New York and Tokyo, Igaku-Shoin, 1996. With permission from Williams & Wilkins.)

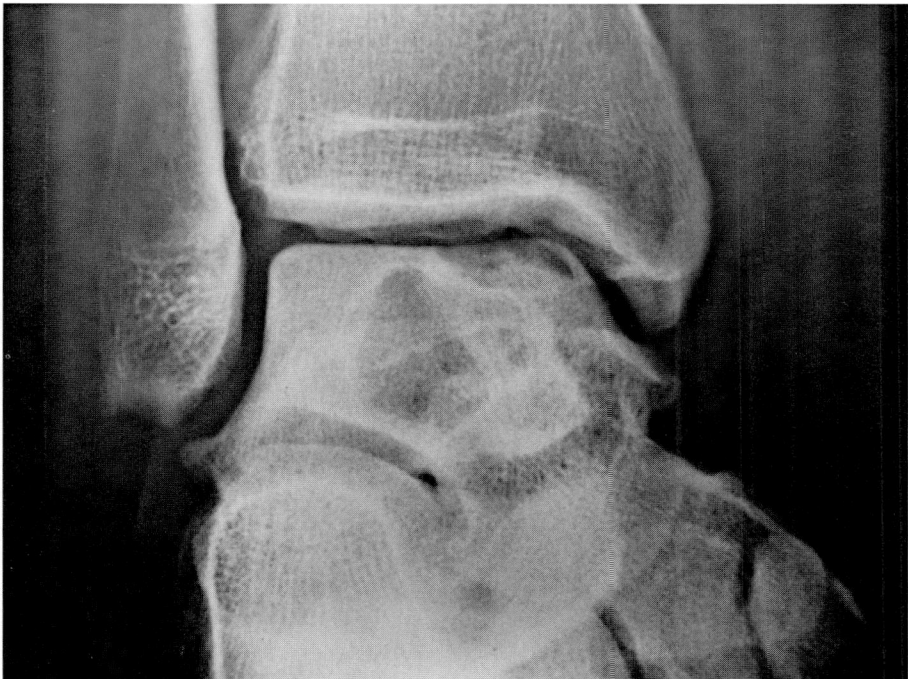

Figure 13–22 ■ A traumatic cyst of the talus. Discontinuity of the articular surface of the talus is present. (From McCarthy, E. F.: *Differential Diagnosis in Pathology. Bone and Joint Disorders*. New York and Tokyo, Igaku-Shoin, 1996. With permission from Williams & Wilkins.)

marrow space. Often the fat undergoes liquefactive necrosis, and the lesion may become a single-chambered cyst. However, unlike unicameral bone cyst, which presents in children and adolescents, intraosseous lipoma usually occurs in middle-aged or older adults. The long bones, particularly the femur and tibia, are the most common sites.[32] Involvement of the calcaneus, ribs, and maxilla is also common. Twenty-nine percent of patients with intraosseous lipoma are asymptomatic; the remainder have vague pain and mild swelling. In contrast to unicameral bone cyst, intraosseous lipoma rarely presents with pathologic fracture.

Radiographically, an intraosseous lipoma is an elongated, well-circumscribed lytic lesion. Located in the center of the medullary canal, it causes uniform cortical thinning, as does unicameral bone cyst. Lesions are usually confined to the metaphysis, but the epiphysis may be involved. Many intraosseous lipomas have focal intralesional radiodensities (Fig. 13–23). These foci are denser and more sharply demar-

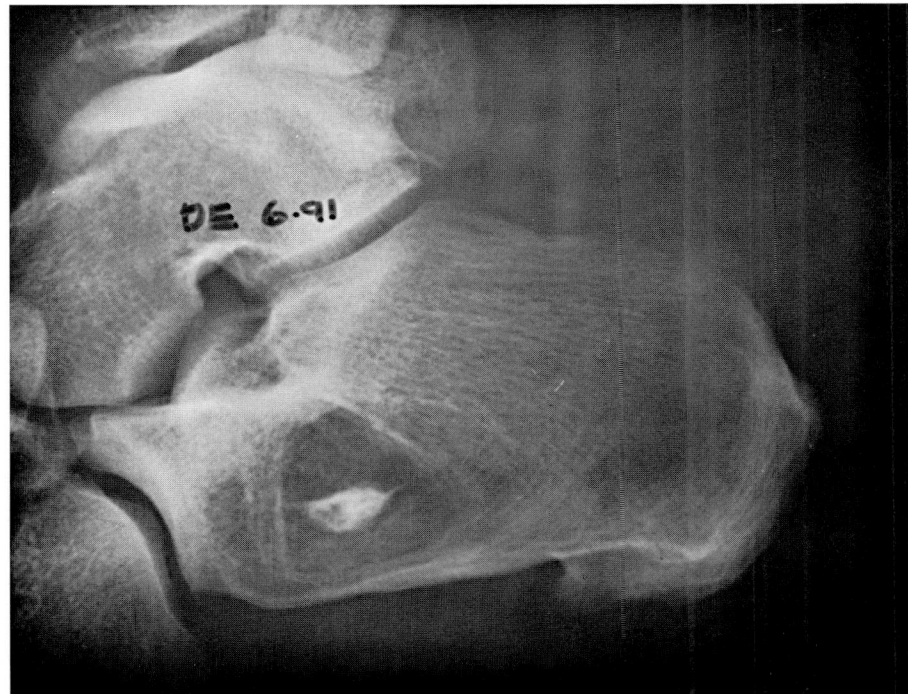

Figure 13–23 ■ An intraosseous lipoma of the calcaneus. An intralesional radiodensity represents focal calcified fat necrosis. (From McCarthy, E. F.: *Differential Diagnosis in Pathology. Bone and Joint Disorders*. New York and Tokyo, Igaku-Shoin, 1996. With permission from Williams & Wilkins.)

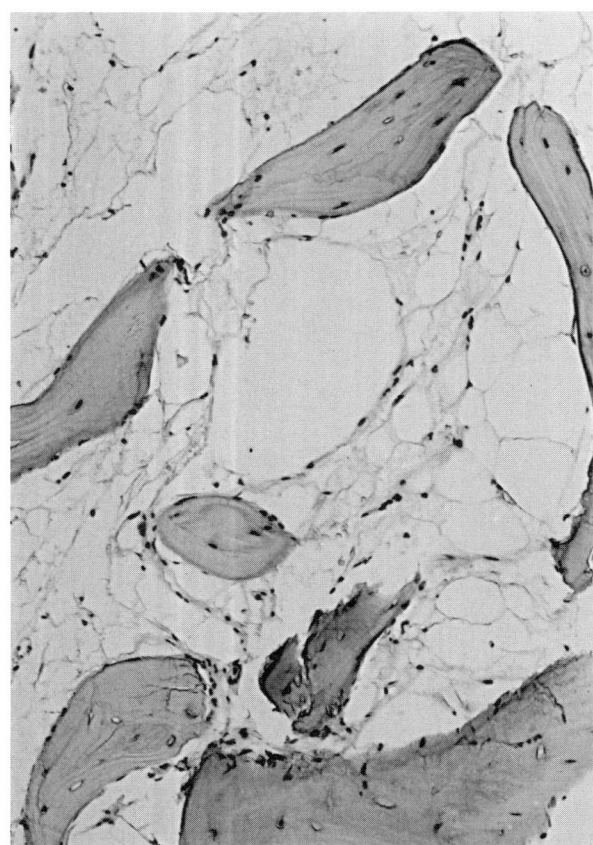

Figure 13-24 ▪ An intraosseous lipoma. Spicules of cancellous bone float in adipose tissue.

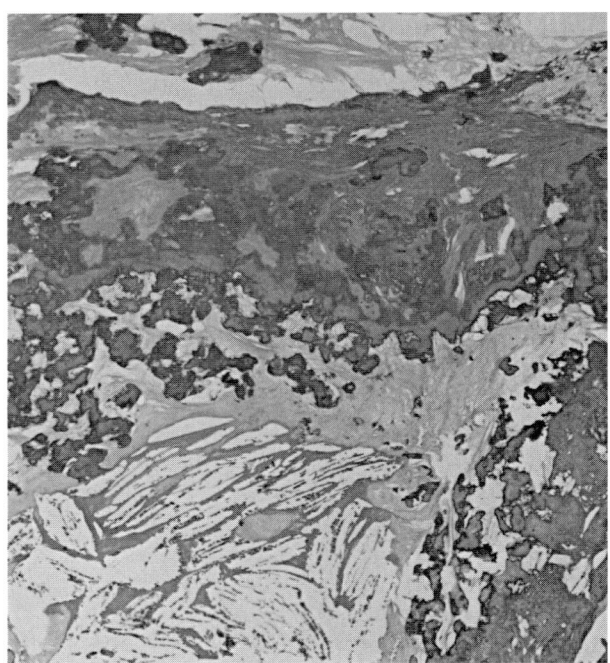

Figure 13-25 ▪ An intraosseous lipoma. Tissue from the interlesional radiodensity showing calcified fat necrosis.

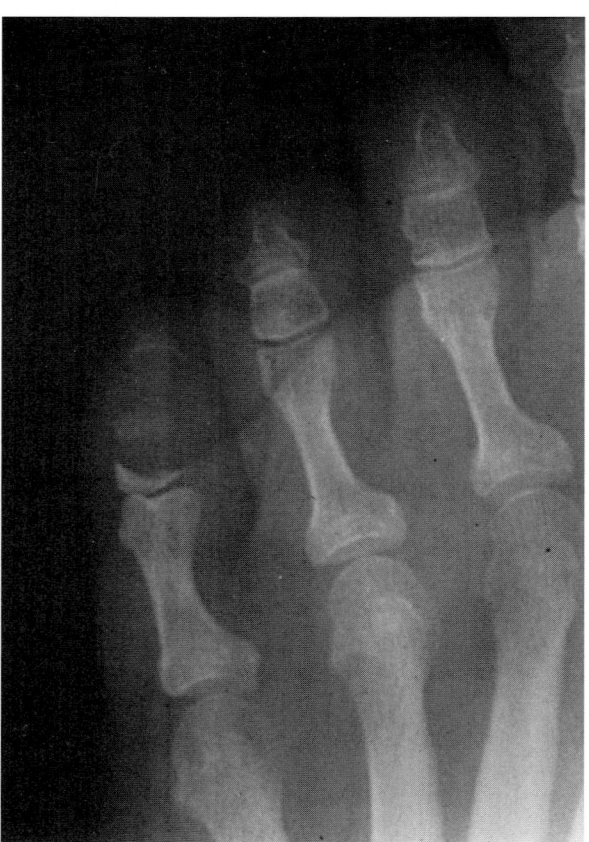

Figure 13-26 ▪ An epidermal inclusion cyst of the distal phalanx of the fifth toe.

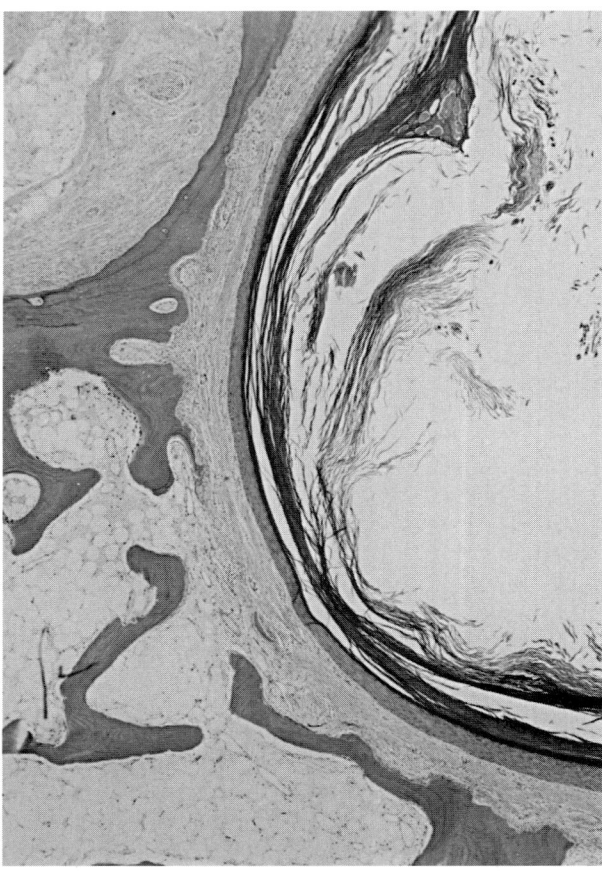

Figure 13-27 ▪ Photomicrograph of an intraosseous epidermal inclusion cyst showing bone containing a squamous-lined cyst with keratin.

cated than those of unicameral bone cyst. The MRI is diagnostic if the intralesional fat has not undergone extensive liquefactive necrosis.[33]

Histologically, intraosseous lipomas replace marrow elements with mature adipose tissue. Often, thin spicules of trabeculae are present in the fat (Fig. 13–24). The thin bone spicules are disconnected and show no orderly trabecular arrangement, features that distinguish intraosseous lipoma from normal trabeculae with surrounding fatty marrow. Most intraosseous lipomas show focal fat necrosis (Fig. 13–25). These foci may become fibrotic and calcify, a feature that causes the intralesional radiodensity. Sometimes the necrotic fat partially repairs and is replaced by a fibromyxoid tissue with varying amounts of reactive bone. Because of these changes, some intraosseous lipomas are misdiagnosed as bone infarcts. In other intraosseous lipomas, the fat necrosis becomes cystic, a change that grossly mimics a unicameral bone cyst. Examination of the curettings of a cystic intraosseous lipoma usually reveals remnants of the characteristic bone spicules dispersed in mature fat.

EPIDERMAL INCLUSION CYST

Epidermal inclusion cyst is a common skin lesion. However, in areas where the skin is tightly adherent to the bone, particularly the distal phalanges, an epidermal inclusion cyst may penetrate the bone cortex.[34] Patients are adults, usually with a history of trauma to the distal phalanx. Presumably, a portion of epidermis is traumatically implanted in the periosteum, where it begins to grow as a cyst. Radiologically, a well-circumscribed lytic lesion is present in the distal phalanx (Fig. 13–26). Curettage of this lesion reveals keratinaceous debris and a lining membrane of squamous epithelium (Fig. 13–27).

REFERENCES

1. Abdelwahab, I. F., Hermann, G., Norton, K. I., Kenan, S., Lewis, M. M., and Klein, M. J.: Simple bone cysts of the pelvis in adolescents. *J Bone Joint Surg* 73A:1091–1094, 1991.
2. Smith, R. W., and Smith, C. F.: Solitary unicameral bone cyst of the calcaneus. *J Bone Joint Surg* 56A:49–56, 1974.
3. Capanna, R., Van Horn, J., Ruggieri, P., and Biagini, R.: Epiphyseal involvement in unicameral bone cysts. *Skeletal Radiol* 15:428–432, 1986.
4. Struhl, S., Edelson, C., Pritzker, H., Seimon, L. P., and Dorfman, H. D.: Solitary (unicameral) bone cyst. The fallen fragment sign revisited. *Skeletal Radiol* 18:261–265, 1989.
5. Mirra, J. M., Bernard, G. W., Bullough, P. G., Johnston, W., and Mink, G.: Cementum-like bone production in solitary bone cysts (so-called "cementoma" of long bones). Report of three cases. Electron microscopic observations supporting a synovial origin to the simple bone cyst. *Clin Orthop* 135:295–307, 1978.
6. Sanerkin, N. G.: Old fibrin coagula and their ossification in simple bone cysts. *J Bone Joint Surg* 61B:194–198, 1979.
7. Capanna, R., Albisinni, U., and Caroli, G. C.: Contrast examination as a prognostic factor in the treatment of solitary bone cyst by cortisone injection. *Skeletal Radiol* 12:97–102, 1984.
8. Scaglietti, O., Marchetti, P. G., and Bartolozzi, P.: The effects of methylprednisolone acetate in the treatment of bone cysts. Results of three years follow-up. *J Bone Joint Surg* 61B:200–204, 1979.
9. Adamsbaum, C., Kalifa, G., Seringe, R., and Dubousset, J.: Direct ethibloc injection in benign bone cysts: Preliminary report on four patients. *Skeletal Radiol* 22:317–320, 1993.
10. Spence, K. F. J., Bright, R. W., Fitzgerald, S. P., and Sell, K. W.: Solitary unicameral bone cyst: Treatment with freeze-dried crushed cortical-bone allograft. A review of one hundred and forty-four cases. *J Bone Joint Surg* 58A:636–641, 1976.
11. Martinez, V., and Sissons, H. A.: Aneurysmal bone cyst. A review of 123 cases including primary lesions and those secondary to other bone pathology. *Cancer* 61:2291–2304, 1988.
12. Burnstein, M. I., De Smet, A. A., Hafez, G. R., and Heiner, J. P.: Case Report 611. *Skeletal Radiol* 19:294–297, 1990.
13. Vergel DeDios, A. M., Bond, J. R., Shives, T. C., McLeod, R. A., and Unni, K. K.: Aneurysmal bone cyst. A clinicopathologic study of 238 cases. *Cancer* 69:2921–2931, 1992.
14. Koskinen, E. V., Visuri, T. I., Holmstrom, T., and Roukkula, M. A.: Aneurysmal bone cyst. Evaluation of resection and of curettage in 20 cases. *Clin Orthop* 118:136–145, 1976.
15. Capanna, R., Springfield, D. S., Biagini, R., Ruggieri, P., and Giunti, A.: Juxtaepiphyseal aneurysmal bone cyst. *Skeletal Radiol* 13:21–25, 1985.
16. Hudson, T. M., Hamlin, D. J., and Fitzsimmons, J. R.: Magnetic resonance imaging of fluid levels. *Skeletal Radiol* 13:267–270, 1985.
17. Sanerkin, N. G., Mott, M. G., and Roylance, J.: An unusual intraosseous lesion with fibroblastic, osteoclastic, osteoblastic, aneurysmal and fibromyxoid elements. "Solid" variant of aneurysmal bone cyst. *Cancer* 51:2278–2286, 1983.
18. McQueen, M. M., Chalmers, J., and Smith, G. D.: Spontaneous healing of aneurysmal bone cysts. *J Bone Joint Surg* 67B:310–312, 1985.
19. Konya, A., and Szendroi, M.: Aneurysmal bone cysts treated by superselective embolization. *Skeletal Radiol* 21:167–172, 1996.
20. DeCristofaro, R., Biagini, R., Boriani, S., Ricci, S., Ruggieri, P., Rossi, G., Fabbri, N., and Roversi, R.: Selective arterial embolization in the treatment of aneurysmal bone cyst and angioma of bone. *Skeletal Radiol* 21:523–527, 1992.
21. Landells, J. W.: The bone cysts of osteoarthritis. *J Bone Joint Surg* 35B:643–649, 1953.
22. Ondrouch, A. S.: Cyst formation in osteoarthritis. *J Bone Joint Surg* 45B:755–760, 1963.
23. Bullough, P. G., and Bansal, M.: The differential diagnosis of geodes. *Radiol Clin North Am* 26:1165–1181, 1988.
24. Eggers, G. W. N., Evans, E. B., Blumel, J., Nowlin, D. H., and Butler, J. K.: Cystic change in the iliac acetabulum. *J Bone Joint Surg* 45A:669–686, 1963.
25. Ostlere, S. J., Seeger, L. L., and Eckardt, J. J.: Subchondral cysts of the tibia secondary to osteoarthritis of the knee. *Skeletal Radiol* 19:287–289, 1990.
26. Helwig, U., Lang, S., Baczynski, M., and Windhager, R.: The intraosseous ganglion. A clinical-pathological report on 42 cases. *Arch Orthop Trauma Surg* 114:14–17, 1994.
27. Bauer, T. W., and Dorfman, H. D.: Intraosseous ganglion. A clinicopathologic study of 11 cases. *Am J Surg Pathol* 6:207–213, 1982.
28. Pope, T. L., Fechner, R. E., and Keats, T. E.: Intra-osseous ganglion. Report of four cases and review of the literature. *Skeletal Radiol* 18:185–187, 1989.
29. Kambolis, C., Bullough, P. G., and Jaffe, H. I.: Ganglionic cystic defects of bone. *J Bone Joint Surg* 55A:496–505, 1973.
30. Okada, K., Unoki, E., Kubota, H., Abe, E., Taniwaki, M., Morita, M., and Sato, K.: Periosteal ganglion: A report of three new cases including MRI findings and a review of the literature. *Skeletal Radiol* 25:153–157, 1996.
31. McCarthy, E. F., Matz, S., Steiner, G. C., and Dorfman, H. D.: Periosteal ganglion: A cause of cortical bone erosion. *Skeletal Radiol* 10:243–246, 1983.
32. Chow, L. T., and Lee, K.: Intraosseous lipoma. A clinicopathologic study of nine cases. *Am J Surg Pathol* 16:401–410, 1992.
33. Blacksin, M. F., Ende, N., and Benevenia, J.: Magnetic resonance imaging of intraosseous lipomas: A radiologic-pathologic correlation. *Skeletal Radiol* 24:37–41, 1995.
34. Byers, P., Mantle, J., and Salm, R.: Epidermal cysts of the phalanges. *J Bone Joint Surg* 48B:577–581, 1966.

CHAPTER 14 | Tumor-Like Lesions

Reactive or degenerative processes in bone or soft tissue occasionally masquerade as neoplasms. Awareness of the clinical, radiologic, and pathologic features of these processes may prevent overdiagnosis. These tumor-like lesions may be grouped in two categories—those in the soft tissue next to bone and those inside bones (Table 14–1). In the soft tissues, tumor-like lesions are often mineralized and radiodense. The mineralization may be in the form of dystrophic calcification, as in tumoral calcinosis, or it may be as heterotopic ossification, as in myositis ossificans.

In contrast to radiodensity produced by some tumor-like lesions of the soft tissues, intraosseous reactive lesions are radiolucent. The most important intraosseous reactive process is giant cell reparative granuloma, a lesion that may be mistaken for a giant cell tumor of bone.

TUMORAL CALCINOSIS

Clinical Presentation

Tumoral calcinosis is the massive deposition of amorphous calcium salts and calcium hydroxyapatite crystals in periarticular soft tissues. This disease occurs in three clinical settings. The first is a sporadic presentation affecting adult patients and usually only involving one joint. In this setting, the calcification is probably initiated by local tissue damage. A small nodule of this process in tendons is known as *calcific tendinitis*. The second setting, accounting for one third of patients with this disease, suggests a familial metabolic abnormality. Several members of a family may be affected in a pattern of autosomal dominant inheritance. These families are usually African-American, and affected members first present in childhood, usually with multiple sites of involvement. Hyperphosphatemia and elevated serum levels of 1,25 $(OH)_2$ vitamin D in many of these patients suggest a metabolic abnormality.[1] In the third setting, tumoral calcinosis may occur in patients on chronic renal dialysis. Multiple joints are usually involved.[2]

Radiographic Features

Plain radiographic images of tumoral calcinosis show multiple, amorphous periarticular radiodensities (Fig. 14–1). The densities are round or oval and are grouped in a mass, sometimes 20 cm or more in diameter. Common sites of involvement are the hips, elbows, and shoulders. The limited form of this disease, calcific tendonitis, occurs most com-

Table 14–1 ■ **TUMOR-LIKE LESIONS OF SOFT TISSUE ADJACENT TO BONE AND TUMOR-LIKE LESIONS OF BONE**

Tumor-Like Lesions of Soft Tissue Adjacent to Bone
Tumoral calcinosis
    Isolated presentation (calcific tendonitis)
    Familial presentation
    Renal dialysis patients
Tumoral calcium pyrophosphate deposition (tophaceous pseudogout)
Heterotopic bone formation
    Myositis ossificans circumscripta
    Heterotopic bone following neurologic injury
    Heterotopic bone following total hip surgery
    Fibrodysplasia ossificans progressiva
Reactive lesions of the hands and feet
    Bizarre parosteal osteochondromatous proliferation
    Florid reactive periostitis
    Subungual exostosis
Infantile cortical hyperostosis

Tumor-Like Lesions of Bone
Giant cell reparative granuloma
    Brown tumor of hyperparathyroidism
    Giant cell reparative granuloma of the jaw, cherubism
    Giant cell reparative granuloma of the hands and feet
    Giant cell reparative granuloma of Paget's disease
Hemophilic pseudotumor

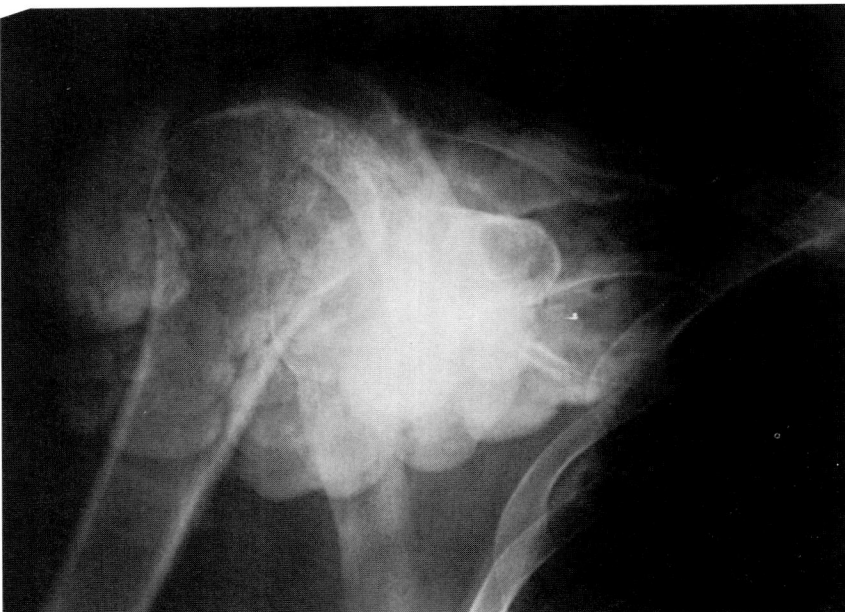

Figure 14-1 ■ Tumoral calcinosis of the shoulder.

monly in the shoulder.[3] A small oval radiodensity is present, usually in the supraspinatus tendon.

Tumoral calcinosis may be mistaken radiographically for a bone- or cartilage-producing neoplasm. However, tumoral calcinosis lacks the stippled and ring-like calcification of cartilage, and it lacks the trabecular pattern of bone (see Chapter 1). Furthermore, two features of tumoral calcinosis are not present in bone or cartilage lesions. First, the radiodensities of tumoral calcinosis are separated by bands of lucency, imparting a "cobblestone" appearance. Second, fluid-calcium levels within the radiodensities are often present on computed tomographic (CT) scans or plain radiographs.[4]

Pathogenesis and Pathologic Features

Tumoral calcinosis is probably initiated by a soft tissue, periarticular hematoma, followed by an infiltrate of histiocytes.[1] Motion of the nearby joint stimulates neobursa formation in the area of hemorrhage. Then, as a result of systemic problems of calcium metabolism, local calcification begins. Fully developed lesions of tumoral calcinosis are characterized histologically by locules of amorphous calcified debris surrounded by a histiocytic and multinucleated giant cell infiltrate (Fig. 14–2). The histiocytes and giant cells show focal degeneration with occasional intracellular calcifications. Extracellular calcification is more prominent, oc-

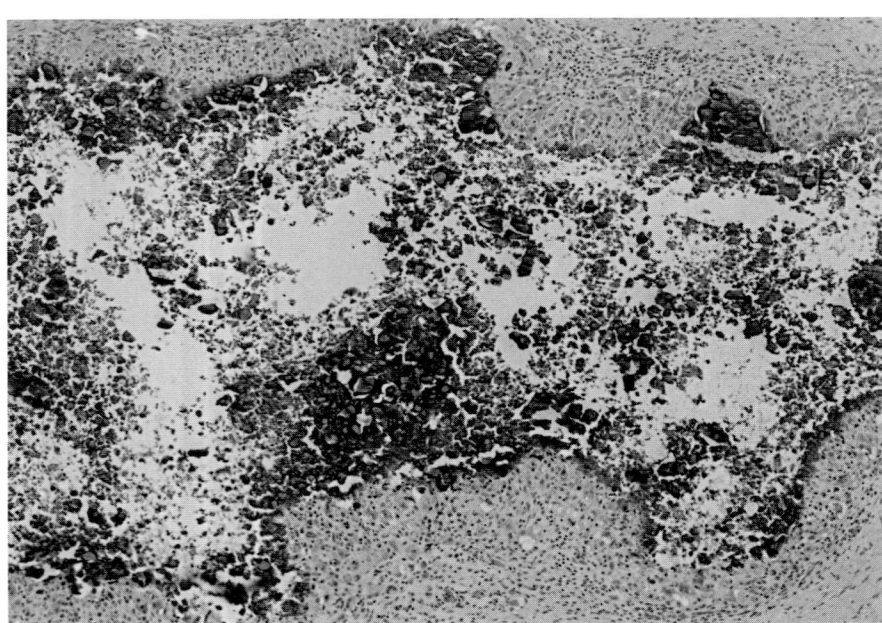

Figure 14-2 ■ Photomicrograph at low power of tumoral calcinosis showing a locule containing calcified debris.

curring as plates or laminated spherules (psammoma bodies) admixed with amorphous debris (Fig. 14–3). The calcifications are deeply basophilic and are not birefringent in polarized light. Calcification may be absent in early lesions, which show only a histiocytic infiltrate. Occasionally, metaplastic bone develops at the periphery of the lesions. Although tumoral calcinosis occurs mainly in the periarticular soft tissues, occasionally the process may erode adjacent bone (Fig. 14–4).

Treatment

Massive lesions of tumoral calcinosis are difficult to eradicate. Large deposits have, in some patients, been reduced by oral administration of phosphate binders, such as aluminum hydroxide.[5] Symptomatic deposits may also be surgically debulked or excised. Smaller lesions may be aspirated or treated symptomatically.

TUMORAL CALCIUM PYROPHOSPHATE DEPOSITION DISEASE

In contrast to the calcium hydroxyapatite deposition characteristic of tumoral calcinosis, calcium pyrophosphate may

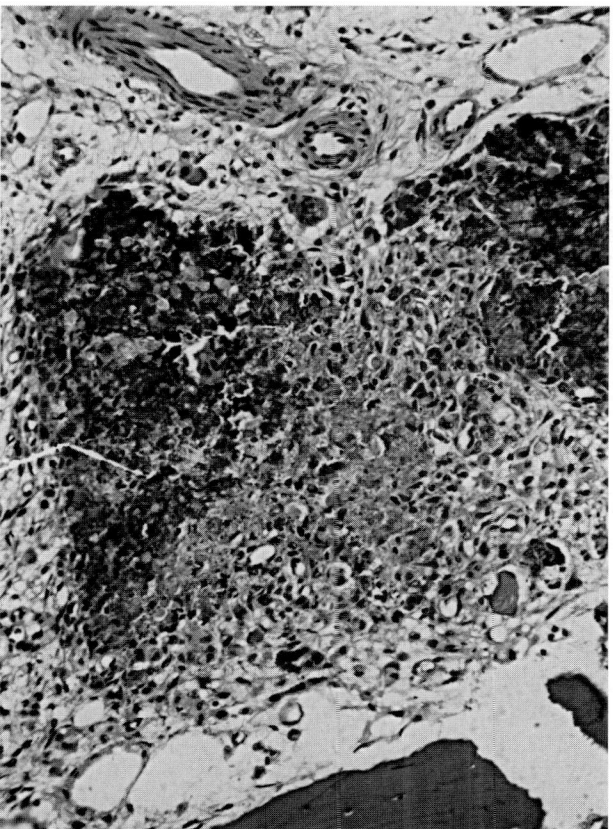

Figure 14-4 ■ Interosseous tumoral calcinosis.

also be deposited as large soft tissue masses. This condition, known as tumoral calcium pyrophosphate deposition disease (also known as tophaceous pseudogout), is a rare manifestation of calcium pyrophosphate deposition disease (see Chapter 16).[6,7] Although radiographically indistinguishable from tumoral calcinosis, certain microscopic features help distinguish these lesions. First, high-power microscopic study of tumoral calcium pyrophosphate deposition disease demonstrates small, uniform, rhomboid calcium pyrophosphate crystals. This contrasts with the plates of calcium hydroxyapatite characteristic of tumoral calcinosis. Second, chondroid metaplasia, not seen in tumoral calcinosis, is common in tissues surrounding deposits of calcium pyrophosphate (Fig. 14–5). This feature, present in most cases, frequently leads to a histologic misdiagnosis of a cartilage neoplasm. However, the demonstration of polarizable pyrophosphate crystals, not present in cartilage lesions, properly identifies tumoral calcium pyrophosphate deposition disease.

Calcium pyrophosphate deposition disease most commonly occurs around the temporomandibular joint or in the fingers (Fig. 14–6). Patients present with pain and swelling and range in age from 31 to 86 years; most are older than 50. Surgical excision is the treatment of choice, although about 20% of patients develop recurrence following this therapy.

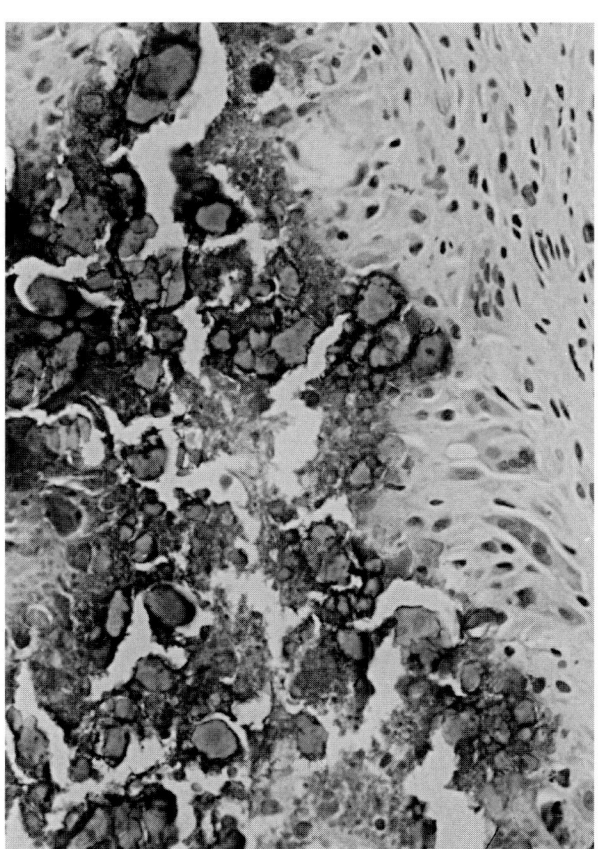

Figure 14-3 ■ Photomicrograph of tumoral calcinosis showing plate-like crystals of calcium hydroxyapatite surrounded by a foreign body giant cell reaction.

CALCIFYING PSEUDOTUMOR OF THE NEURAL AXIS

Calcifying pseudotumor of the neural axis is an unusual lesion that resembles tumoral calcinosis. Histologically, confluent masses of dystrophic calcification are surrounded by histiocytes. However, unlike the paraarticular location of tumoral calcinosis, calcifying pseudotumor of the neural axis occurs adjacent to the spine or at the base of the skull. In the skull, this lesion usually presents as an intracranial nodule adjacent to the foramen magnum and often associated with the dura. Along the spine, the lesion may present at any level, either within the spinal canal or posteriorly, associated with a facet joint. Patients are usually in their 30s, 40s, or 50s and present with pain. Lesions range in size from 1 to 10 cm.[8] Their gray-yellow friable texture, present on gross pathologic examination, has led to an alternative name, "crudoma." The cause of calcifying pseudotumor of the neural axis is not known, although disc degeneration may contribute to some spinal lesions.

HETEROTOPIC BONE

In contrast to amorphous calcification, heterotopic bone formation may also cause a radiodense soft tissue mass. Heterotopic bone occurs in four important clinical presenta-

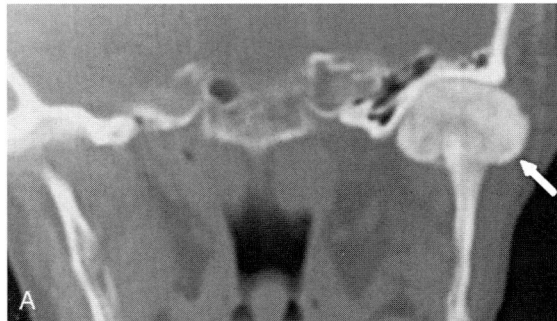
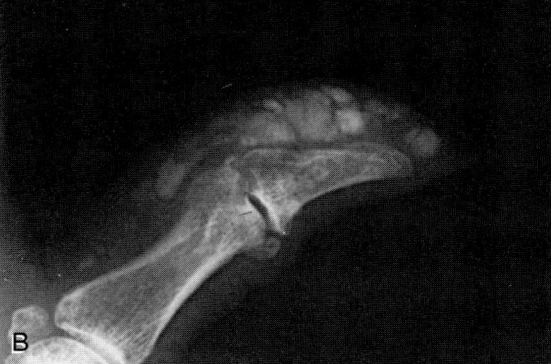

Figure 14-6 ■ The most common locations for tumoral calcium pyrophosphate deposition. **A,** CT scan of the skull showing fluffy mineralization around the temporal mandibular joint *(arrow).* **B,** Fluffy deposits of calcium in the soft tissues adjacent to the distal phalanx of the thumb.

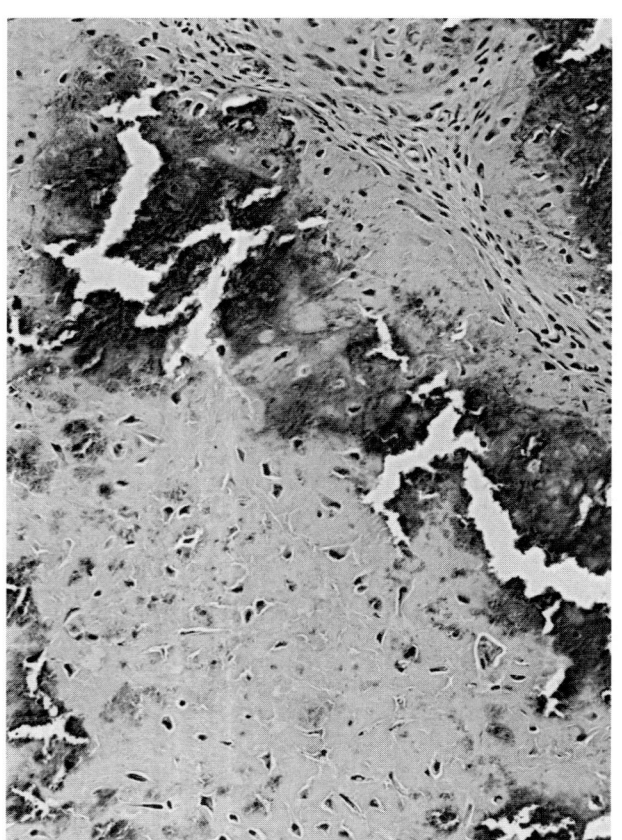

Figure 14-5 ■ Photomicrograph of tumoral calcium pyrophosphate deposition. Extensive chondroid metaplasia is adjacent to the calcified areas.

tions. In the first presentation, known as *myositis ossificans circumscripta,* a localized self-limited proliferation of fibroblasts and heterotopic bone forms in skeletal muscle following trauma. Sometimes patients with this localized presentation have no history of an injury. The second presentation occurs in muscles and periarticular fibrous tissue at multiple sites in patients who have sustained *head trauma or spinal cord injury.* The third clinical presentation is heterotopic bone formation in periarticular soft tissue following *total hip arthroplasty.* In the final presentation, in a rare genetic disorder known as *fibrodysplasia ossificans progressiva,* masses of heterotopic bone progressively accumulate around multiple joints and eventually cause severe disability and early death.

The pathogenesis of the various presentations of heterotopic bone formation has not been clarified. Because lesions of heterotopic bone evolve similar to a fracture callus, bone morphogenetic proteins (BMPs) are probably activated in similar ways in both conditions. However, not all people develop heterotopic bone after muscle trauma. Therefore, patients with this disease probably have a hereditary or acquired tendency to inappropriately activate BMPs in the soft tissues. Patients with fibrodysplasia ossificans progressiva fully express this tendency.

Myositis Ossificans Circumscripta

Myositis ossificans circumscripta is a reactive process characterized by the intramuscular proliferation of fibroblasts, new bone, and, occasionally, cartilage. In this common, self-limited disorder, an osseous mass develops next to bones and joints. Although myositis ossificans may develop spontaneously, the process is initiated by trauma in 60 to 75% of cases. A distinctive feature of myositis ossificans is *lesional maturation,* which is apparent clinically, radiologically, and histologically.

Clinical Presentation

One or two days after trauma to a muscle, a painful mass appears. Sometimes the patient has no history of a single episode of severe trauma. Instead, multiple episodes of minor injury may initiate the process. The lump may even appear spontaneously. The mass grows steadily for a month or two and reaches a size of 4 to 10 cm. Thereafter, the mass becomes hard and ceases to grow. Often, after a year or so, the firm mass becomes smaller, and rarely, it may disappear completely.

Patients with myositis ossificans are usually in their teens and 20s, although patients as old as 84 years and as young as 5 months have been reported.[9] The most common locations are the muscles of the thigh, buttock, or upper arm. These sites correspond to muscles most easily traumatized in young athletic adults, the most common patients to be affected.

Radiologic Features

The radiologic features of myositis ossificans evolve as the lesion matures. For the first few weeks after clinical presentation, a soft tissue mass, best seen on magnetic resonance imaging (MRI), shows no mineralization. On routine MRI, the soft tissue mass is nonspecific.[10] However, after gadolinium administration, the lesion may show rim enhancement, a feature rarely seen in other soft tissue masses.[11] After 3 to 5 weeks, fluffy radiodensities appear in the mass, and a periosteal reaction is often present in the adjacent bone (Fig. 14–7). After about 6 weeks, the mineralization shows a characteristic zonal pattern; mineralization is denser at the periphery of the lesion. This zonal pattern is best visualized with a CT scan (Fig. 14–8). As the lesion ages, orderly lines of mature trabecular bone become very distinct (Fig. 14–9). The mass often attaches to the adjacent bone and, with time, seems to blend with the cortex (Fig. 14–10).

Pathologic Features

The histologic features of myositis ossificans evolve parallel to the radiologic features. The early lesion shows very cellular sheets of plump fibroblasts, and mitotic figures are numerous. These early lesions have the appearance of a tissue culture of fibroblasts. The cells are spindle shaped or stellate and seem to float in a myxoid extracellular matrix (Fig. 14–11). As early as 1 week after the mass becomes clinically palpable, seams of osteoid appear in the peripheral portions (Fig. 14–12). Because of the dense cellularity and osteoid production, lesions at this early stage of evolution

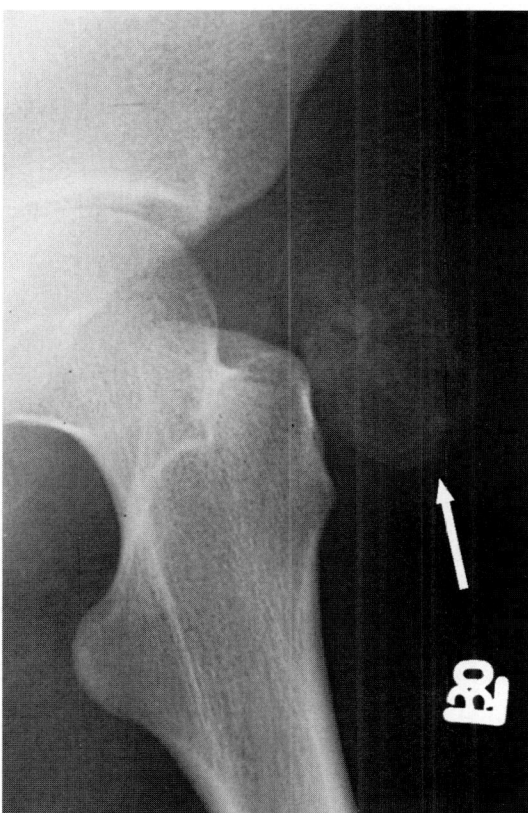

Figure 14–7 ■ Myositis ossificans. This early lesion shows only faint radiodensity in the soft tissues adjacent to the greater trochanter *(arrow)*.

have been called "pseudomalignant osseous tumors of soft tissue."[12,13] However, despite the high degree of cellularity and frequent mitotic figures, cytologic atypia and abnormal mitoses are absent. In some lesions of myositis ossificans, cartilage is present; as the lesion matures, the cartilage undergoes endochondral ossification. A characteristic feature of myositis ossificans is the entrapment of skeletal muscle in the peripheral portions of the mass.

After about 6 weeks, the zonal pattern seen on plain radiographs is also apparent on low-power microscopic study. The outer portion of the mass shows dense lamellar bone arranged as a pseudocortex. Spicules of bone are progressively thinner toward the center of the lesion (Fig. 14–13). After 6 months to 1 year, lesions of myositis ossificans develop an orderly arrangement of thick, mature trabecular bone. In these older lesions, the zonal pattern is no longer apparent, and bone marrow may be present.

Complications

Complications develop as a result of myositis ossificans. Lesions commonly cause mild restriction of movement of the adjacent joints. Sometimes a lesion may impinge on a nearby nerve or blood vessel. Three other complications rarely occur. First, a mature lesion of myositis ossificans may fracture after direct trauma.[14] A painless nonunion usually results. Second, as a result of biopsy, a lesion of myositis

296 ──── TUMOR-LIKE LESIONS

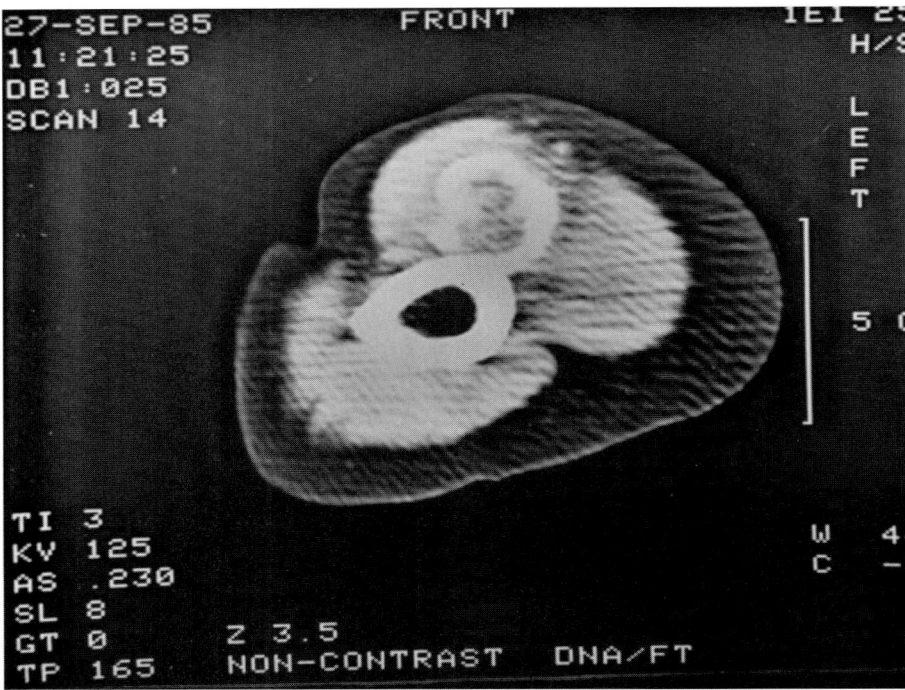

Figure 14-8 ■ Computed tomographic scan of humerus showing zonal pattern of myositis ossificans. The central portion of the lesion is radiolucent. (From McCarthy, E. F.: *Differential Diagnosis in Pathology. Bone and Joint Disorders.* New York and Tokyo, Igaku-Shoin, 1996. With permission from Williams & Wilkins.)

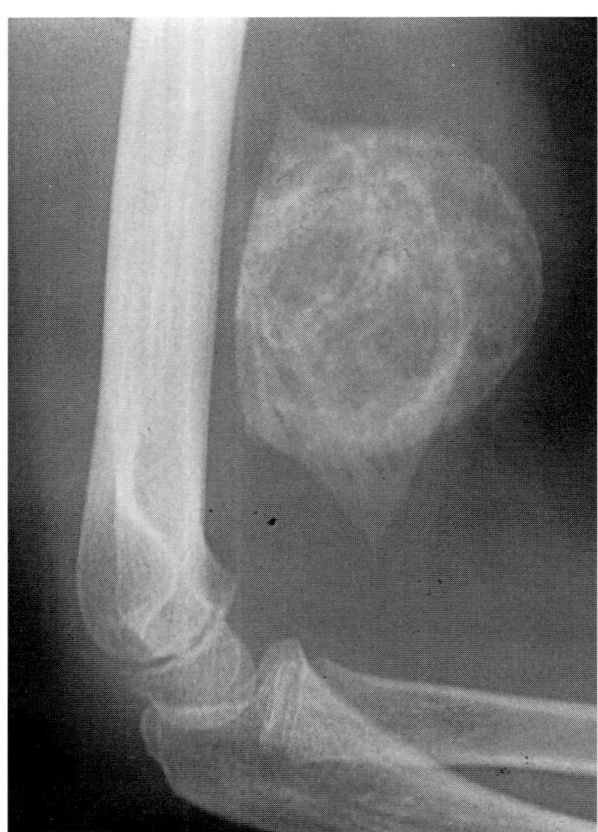

Figure 14-9 ■ A mature lesion of myositis ossificans adjacent to the humerus. Lines of mature trabecular bone are present.

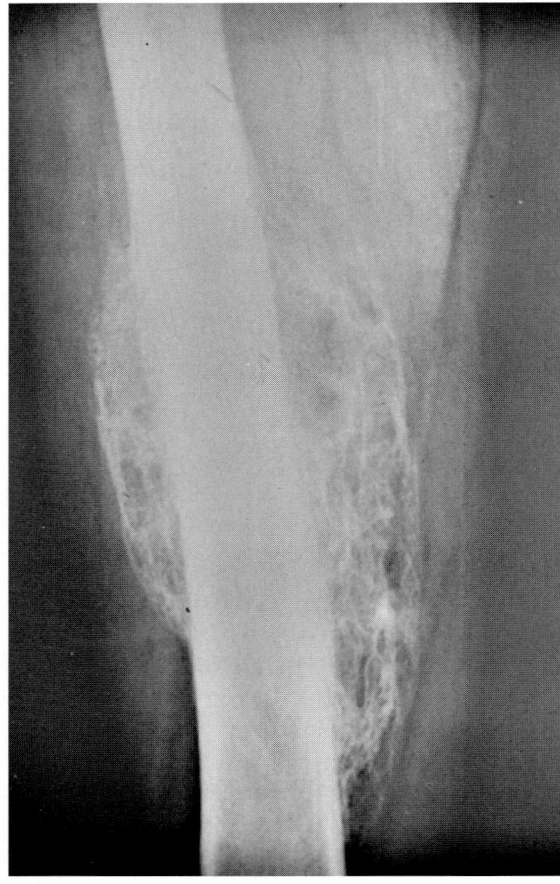

Figure 14-10 ■ Myositis ossificans in the thigh. The ossified mass is attached to the cortex.

ossificans may develop aneurysmal bone cyst change.[15] Finally, myositis ossificans has been reported to undergo malignant transformation to osteosarcoma.[16] However, these reports are rare, and no case is convincing. Most likely, the reported lesions were osteosarcomas from the outset.

Differential Diagnosis

Differential diagnostic problems arise in both early and late lesions of myositis ossificans. An early lesion may be misdiagnosed as a soft tissue osteosarcoma. However, pleomorphic atypical cells with atypical mitotic figures, features characteristic of soft tissue osteosarcoma, are absent in myositis ossificans. A late lesion of myositis ossificans may be confused with a parosteal osteosarcoma. However, parosteal osteosarcoma does not show a zonal pattern of ossification and lacks orderly lines of mature trabecular bone. Also, in parosteal osteosarcoma, cellular atypia, although mild, is always present.

Neurogenic Heterotopic Ossification

Heterotopic bone occasionally develops around joints in patients immobilized after traumatic neurologic lesions.[17] For example, heterotopic bone forms in 20 to 25% of patients paralyzed from a spinal cord injury. In 18 to 35% of these

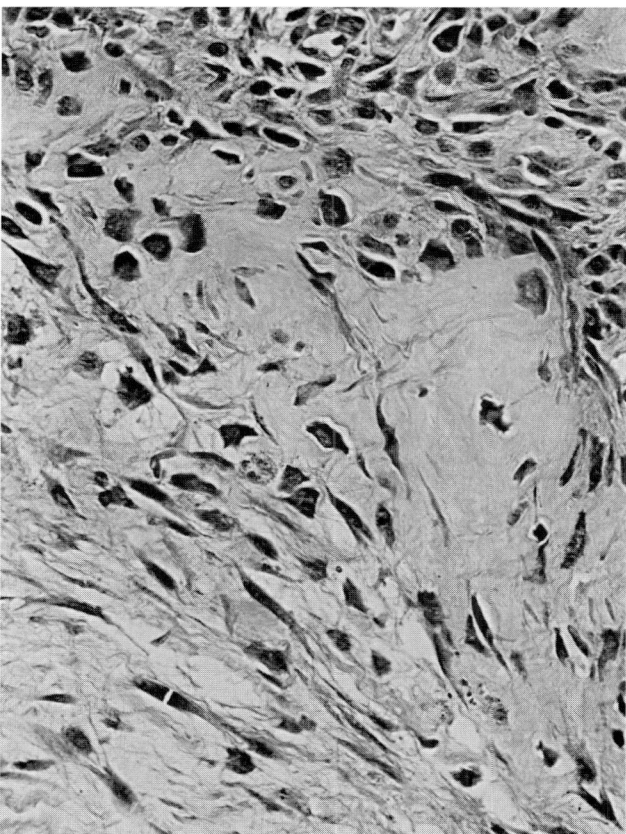

Figure 14-12 ■ Photomicrograph of early lesion of myositis ossificans showing osteoid production in a cellular, fibrous tissue background.

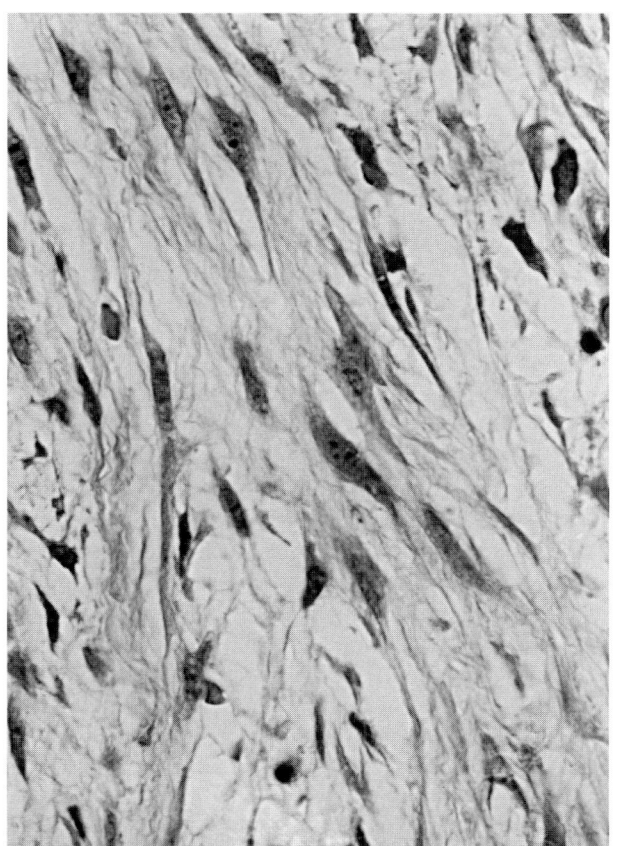

Figure 14-11 ■ Myositis ossificans in the early phases. Spindle-shaped and stellate cells are present in a myxomatous matrix. These areas resemble fibroblasts in tissue culture.

patients, the process is severe enough to cause limitation of joint motion. Patients with low cervical or high thoracic lesions are the most likely to develop this complication. In addition to patients with spinal cord injury, 10 to 20% of patients immobilized due to closed head trauma form heterotopic bone. About 10% of these patients develop severe limitation of joint motion.[18]

Patients with neurogenic heterotopic ossification develop lesions around larger joints. The hip is the most common location, followed by the knees and elbows. A single joint is affected in 40% of patients; in another third, two joints are affected. The heterotopic bone formation begins within 2 months after neurologic injury and is usually fully developed by 2 years. Sometimes the heterotopic bone may be massive and cause complete ankylosis of the affected joint.

The cause of the heterotopic bone formation in these patients is unknown. Vascular stasis, edema, and prolonged swelling are likely contributing factors. In addition, passive manipulation of joints to preserve range of motion may traumatize soft tissue and initiate heterotopic bone formation.[19]

Heterotopic Bone Following Total Hip Surgery

Following total hip surgery, 2 to 7% of patients develop extensive heterotopic bone in periarticular soft tissue.[20] In

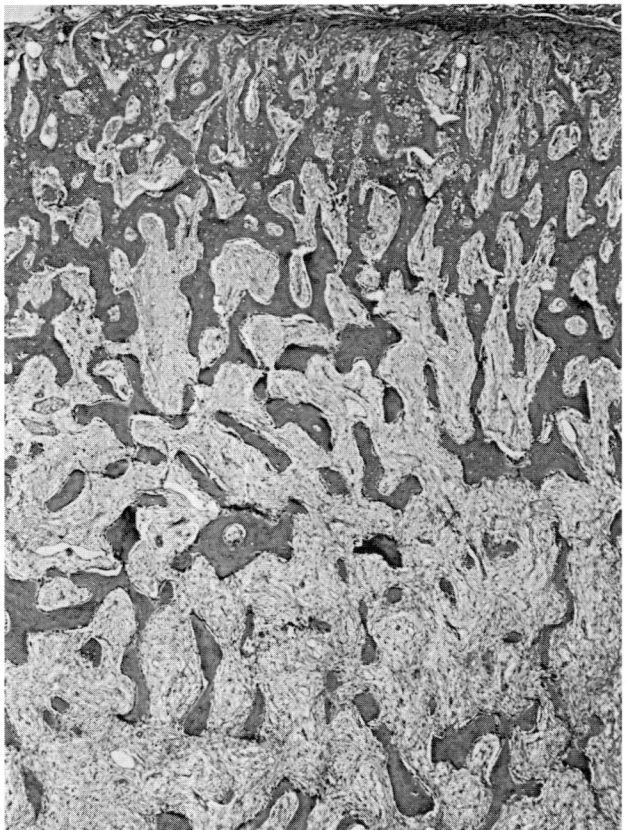

Figure 14-13 ■ A mature lesion of myositis ossificans showing dense bone at the periphery of the lesion and abundant fibrous tissue in the central portion of the lesion.

many of these patients, resulting limitation in motion necessitates a revision arthroplasty. Although the incidence of clinically significant heterotopic ossification is small, asymptomatic heterotopic bone formation occurs frequently; radiographic evidence is present in as many as 56% of patients.[21,22] Patients with ankylosing spondylitis, Paget's disease, and hypertrophic osteoarthritis are at risk to develop this complication.[23] In high-risk patients, as well as those requiring revision arthroplasty for this complication, the incidence of heterotopic bone is reduced by prophylactic low-dose irradiation. Beginning 5 days after surgery, 1000 rads is administered in five divided doses. Postoperative nonsteroidal antiinflammatory drug therapy also reduces the incidence of heterotopic bone.

Fibrodysplasia Ossificans Progressiva

Another manifestation of heterotopic ossification is the severe genetic disorder known as fibrodysplasia ossificans progressiva. In this disorder, extensive heterotopic ossification progressively develops at multiple periarticular sites and eventually causes complete immobilization. Fortunately, this disease is very rare; only about 100 cases are known to exist in the United States.[24] Fibrodysplasia ossificans progressiva almost always arises by a spontaneous mutation, and no gender, racial, or ethnic predilection has been observed. Because the reproductive capacity of most patients is small, familial transmission is rare. However, a few familial cases suggest an autosomal dominant mode of transmission.

Although it is extremely rare, this dramatic syndrome has fascinated physicians for over 200 years. In 1741, Copping described a patient as a "stalactite in the Grotto of Calypso."[25] By 1869, Münchmeyer had collected 12 cases.[26] Because very little has been added to his accurate description, this disorder has been known as Münchmeyer's disease.

Clinical Features

The heterotopic ossification begins in the first decade of life, usually at about age 3 years. The first lesion usually occurs in the back when a soft tissue mass becomes palpable adjacent to the upper spine and shoulder girdle.[27] As the patient ages, other masses appear, usually from cranial to caudal and proximal to distal in the skeleton. Many patients develop a severe scoliosis. Although the disease progresses at different rates in different patients, by the third decade, patients are usually severely crippled with widespread periarticular ossification. Although a few patients survive into middle adulthood (one patient survived to age 70),[28] most die in the third or fourth decade of life due to pneumonia.

In addition to progressive heterotopic ossification, patients have other characteristic congenital skeletal anomalies. For example, almost all patients have short great toes, usually because of synostosis of the phalanges, and some have short thumbs. These phalangeal features are essential to the diagnosis of this disorder.[29] Other congenital bone anomalies are sometimes present. For example, some patients have short and wide femoral necks. Also, small cervical vertebral bodies with large posterior elements are occasionally present.

Pathologic Features

Genetic studies suggest that fibrodysplasia ossificans progressiva is caused by overexpression of a bone morphogenic protein gene. Indeed, bone morphogenic protein 4 mRNA is expressed in circulating lymphoblastoid cells in most patients with this disorder.[30] Most probably, these cells are recruited to sites of soft tissue injury and initiate heterotopic bone. Histologically, lesions of fibrodysplasia ossificans progressiva are similar, but not identical, to those of myositis ossificans circumscripta. The earliest lesions show muscular degeneration and a lymphoid infiltrate. This is followed by the proliferation of highly vascular fibrous tissue. Bone morphogenic proteins 2 and 4 have been demonstrated in this tissue.[31] Then, osteoid forms in this fibroblastic stroma. However, the zonal pattern typical of myositis ossificans circumscripta is not usually present in fibrodysplasia ossificans progressiva. In addition, hyaline cartilage, which is undergoing endochondral ossification, is abundant in fibrodysplasia ossificans progressiva. In fact, endochondral ossification appears to be the principal mechanism of bone formation in this disorder.[32]

HETEROTOPIC BONE IN THE HANDS AND FEET

Myositis ossificans is rare in the muscles of the hands and feet.[33,34] However, other manifestations of heterotopic bone occur in these locations. These manifestations are usually associated with the periosteum or periarticular fibrous tissue and therefore should not be regarded as myositis ossificans.

Reactive lesions in the hands and feet occur in three important clinicoradiologic settings. The first setting, *bizarre parosteal osteochondromatous proliferation* (BPOP), also known as Nora's lesion, is a lobular proliferation of reactive bone and cartilage that forms an exophytic mass adjacent to the bone. Formerly, this process was often regarded as an osteochondroma. The second setting, *florid reactive periostitis*, is a fusiform proliferation of reactive tissue confined beneath the tight periosteum. These first two settings are probably manifestations of the same reactive process in different locations, one being subperiosteal and the other involving the loose alveolar tissues outside the periosteum.[35] When these lesions are mature and firmly attached to the bone surface, they have been referred to as *turret exostoses*.[36] The third reactive lesion of the hands and feet, *subungual exostosis,* is a bony projection from the distal phalanx and is probably a response to trauma.

Like lesions of heterotopic bone in other locations, reactive lesions of the hands and feet may be misdiagnosed as osteosarcoma. Therefore, awareness of their distinctive clinicoradiologic features is necessary to prevent this misdiagnosis.

Bizarre Parosteal Osteochondromatous Proliferation

Bizarre parosteal osteochondromatous proliferation presents as a painless swelling in the soft tissues of the hand or feet. The most common site is adjacent to a proximal phalanx, a metacarpal, or a metatarsal. Similar lesions have been reported in sites other than the hands and feet, such as adjacent to the ulna, femur, and radius. Patients range in age from 8 to 73 years, although most patients are between 20 and 40 years. Approximately 12% of patients have a history of trauma.[37]

On plain radiographs, BPOP is a well-circumscribed radiodense mass that arises from the cortical surface (Fig. 14-14). An additional unmineralized soft tissue mass is absent. The underlying cortex is always intact but occasionally shows slight surface irregularity. The radiodense mass, which shows a trabecular pattern in later stages of development, ranges in size from 0.4 to 3 cm.

Histologically, bizarre parosteal osteochondromatous proliferation consists of irregular aggregates of hyaline cartilage, spindle cells, and new bone (Fig. 14-15). The cartilage, probably formed by chondroid metaplasia of fibrous tissue, often forms a cap at the periphery of the lesion (Fig. 14-16). The cartilage is usually hypercellular with large chondrocytes, some of which are binucleated and show mild atypia. The cartilage lobules are separated by a florid spindle cell proliferation (Fig. 14-17). The spindle cells show mild to moderate mitotic activity, but atypical mitotic figures are not present. Cellular atypia is also absent. In addition, myxoid change is occasionally present. Irregular new bone or osteoid is abundant and is formed in the cartilage lobules by endochondral ossification or by metaplastic ossification in the spindle cell areas. A characteristic histologic feature of BPOP is deep basophilia of the new bone (Fig. 14-18). Older lesions contain mature lamellar bone.

Bizarre parosteal osteochondromatous proliferation should be treated by surgical excision. However, 50% of lesions recur 2 months to 2 years after the first excision. Twenty percent of patients have more than one recurrence. Recurrent lesions should be excised.

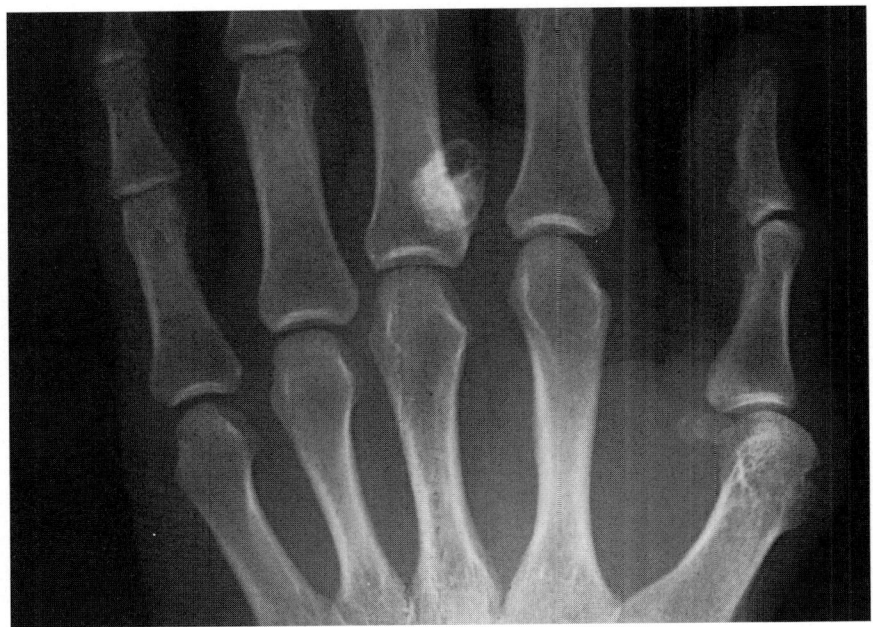

Figure 14-14 ▪ Bizarre parosteal osteochondromatous proliferation of the finger. The lesion is a well-circumscribed radiodensity. (From McCarthy, E. F.: *Differential Diagnosis in Pathology. Bone and Joint Disorders.* New York and Tokyo, Igaku-Shoin, 1996. With permission from Williams & Wilkins.)

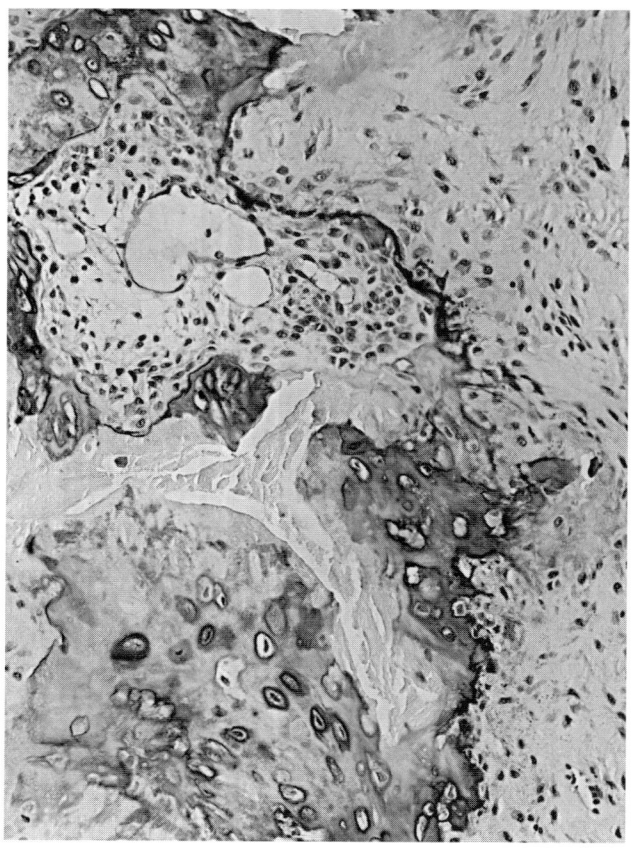

Figure 14-15 ■ Photomicrograph of bizarre parosteal osteochondromatous proliferation. This proliferation shows an admixture of cartilage, fibrous tissue, and osteoid.

Florid Reactive Periostitis

Florid reactive periostitis, like BPOP, affects patients of any age. Also, like BPOP, most patients are between 20 and 40 years of age. However, unlike most patients with BPOP, who have painless swelling, almost all patients with florid reactive periostitis present with pain and a fusiform swelling. A history of trauma is present in 40% of patients. Like BPOP, the proximal phalanges, metacarpals, and metatarsals are the most common sites.[38]

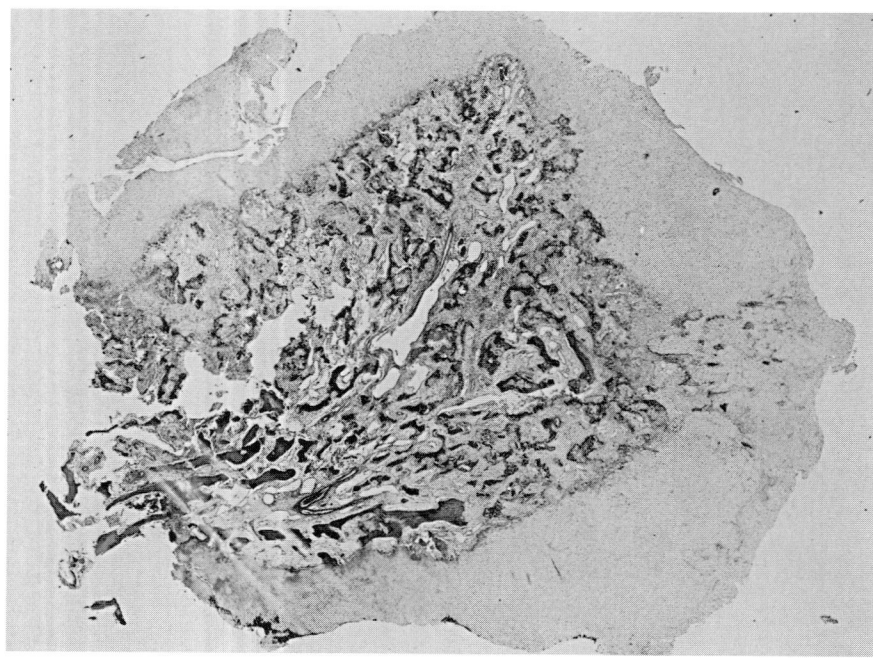

Figure 14-16 ■ Low-power photomicrograph of bizarre parosteal osteochondromatous proliferation showing a cartilaginous cap. (From McCarthy, E. F.: *Differential Diagnosis in Pathology. Bone and Joint Disorders.* New York and Tokyo, Igaku-Shoin, 1996. With permission from Williams & Wilkins.)

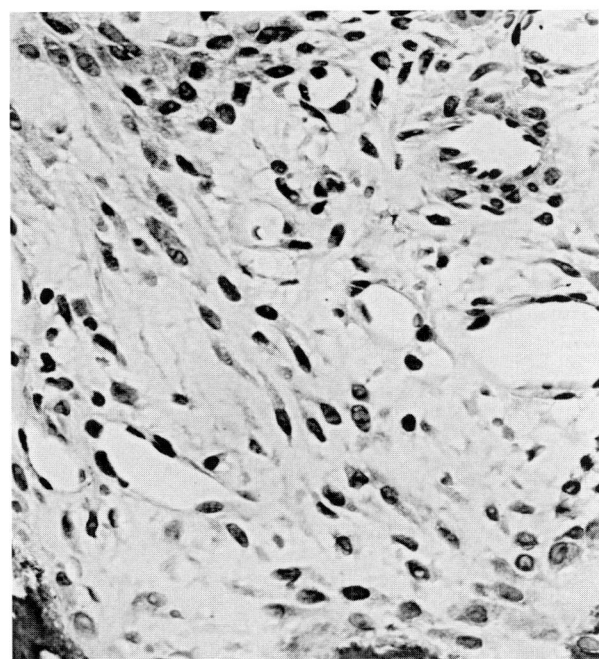

Figure 14-17 ■ High-power photomicrograph of bizarre parosteal osteochondromatous proliferation showing bland spindle cells.

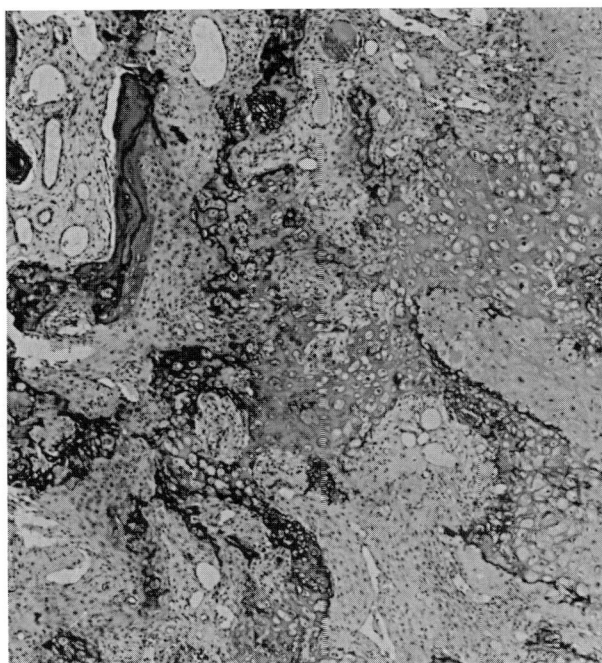

Figure 14-18 ■ Photomicrograph of bizarre parosteal osteochondromatous proliferation showing characteristic deep basophilic osteoid.

Early lesions of florid reactive periostitis show only soft tissue swelling. Later, a smoothly contoured mass of fluffy subperiosteal new bone develops (Fig. 14–19). In the late stages, the new bone matures and becomes incorporated in the cortex. Like BPOP, the underlying bone is unaffected.

Histologically, florid reactive periostitis shows new bone in a fibroblastic proliferation. Although cartilage is occasionally present, it is less conspicuous than in BPOP. In addition, unlike the disorganization of tissue elements in BPOP, florid reactive periostitis tends to have a zonal pattern, with more mature bone in the center of the lesion (Fig. 14–20). The fibroblastic component is usually very cellular, the cells having plump nuclei with a large nucleolus. In addition, mild pleomorphism and numerous typical mitotic figures are present. The osteoid is usually lace-like in early stages and is rimmed by plump uniform osteoblasts (Fig. 14–21). Trabecular bone is present in more mature lesions.

Florid reactive periostitis should also be treated by surgical excision. Unlike BPOP, florid reactive periostitis rarely recurs.

Subungual Exostosis

Subungual exostosis arises on the dorsal surface of the distal phalanx. Lesions range from a few millimeters to 2

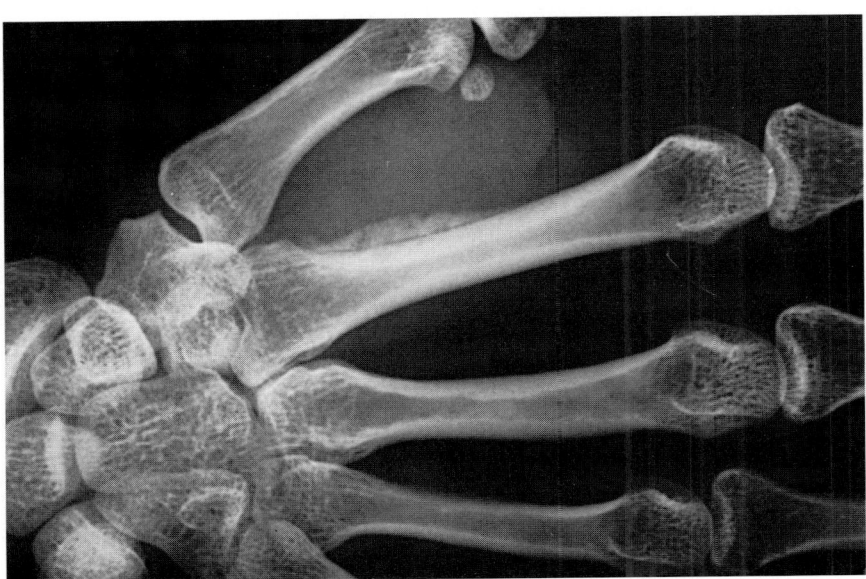

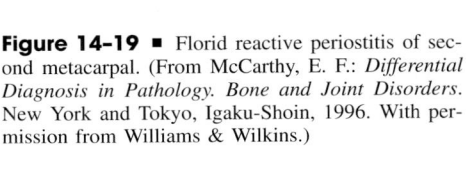

Figure 14-19 ■ Florid reactive periostitis of second metacarpal. (From McCarthy, E. F.: *Differential Diagnosis in Pathology. Bone and Joint Disorders.* New York and Tokyo, Igaku-Shoin, 1996. With permission from Williams & Wilkins.)

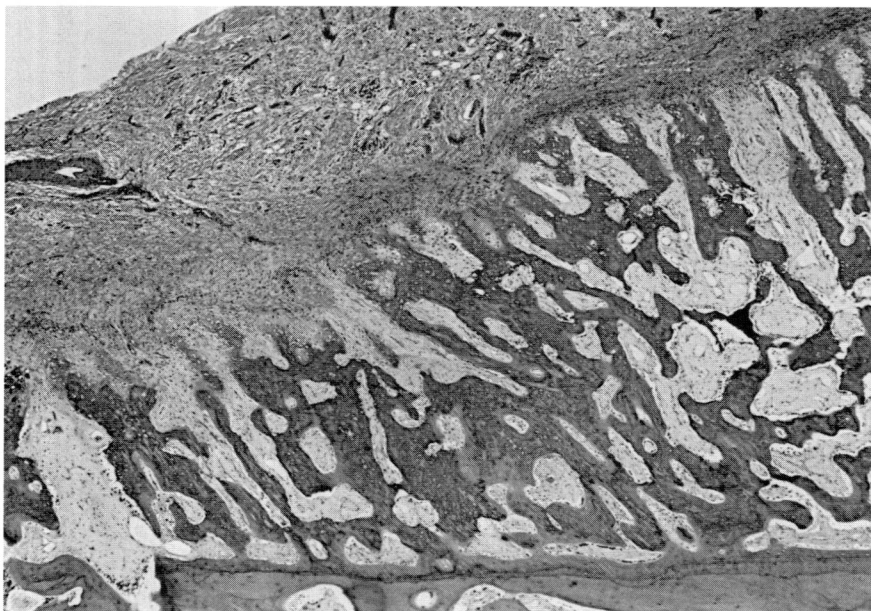

Figure 14-20 ■ Photomicrograph of florid reactive periostitis. Broad bands of woven bone are present adjacent to the cortex, and less mature woven bone is present beneath the periosteum.

cm. Larger lesions elevate the nail and ulcerate the nail bed. Patients, ranging in age from 8 to 55 years (mean, 23.5 years), present with pain. About 75% of subungual exostoses arise in the great toe. The remaining 25% of cases affect the other digits of the hands and feet with equal frequency.[39]

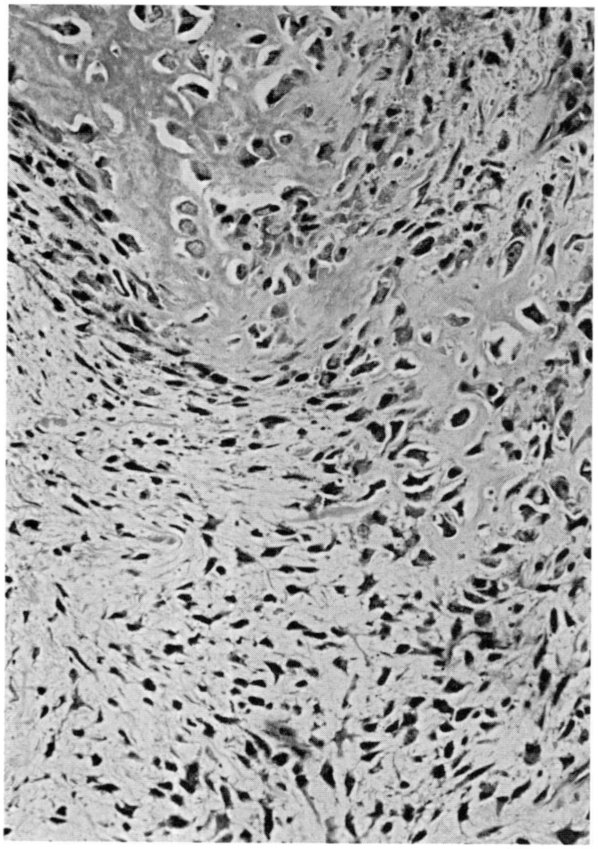

Radiologically, a bony projection from the dorsal portion of the distal phalanx is best seen on a lateral plain radiograph (Fig. 14–22). The underlying bone is unremarkable.

Histologically, a cartilage cap, which arises from chondroid metaplasia of spindle cells beneath the nail, covers the projection of trabecular bone. A zonal arrangement of tissues is apparent (Fig. 14–23). Superficially, spindle cells with chondroid metaplasia are present under the nail, and beneath this tissue, mature cartilage changes to endochondral bone. The deepest portion of the lesion consists of mature trabecular bone, which connects with the cortex of the phalanx.

Subungual exostoses can be cured by simple excision with preservation of the distal phalanx and nail.

INFANTILE CORTICAL HYPEROSTOSIS

Infantile cortical hyperostosis, also known as Caffey's disease, is a very rare pediatric disorder characterized by layers of reactive periosteal new bone (Fig. 14–24). The periosteal new bone may be massive and lead to a misdiag-

Figure 14-21 ■ Florid reactive periostitis showing a zonal pattern. Proliferating fibroblasts are beginning to differentiate into bone-forming cells.

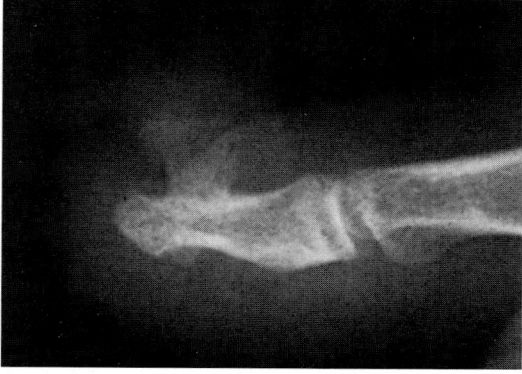

Figure 14-22 ■ Subungual exostosis of the distal phalanx.

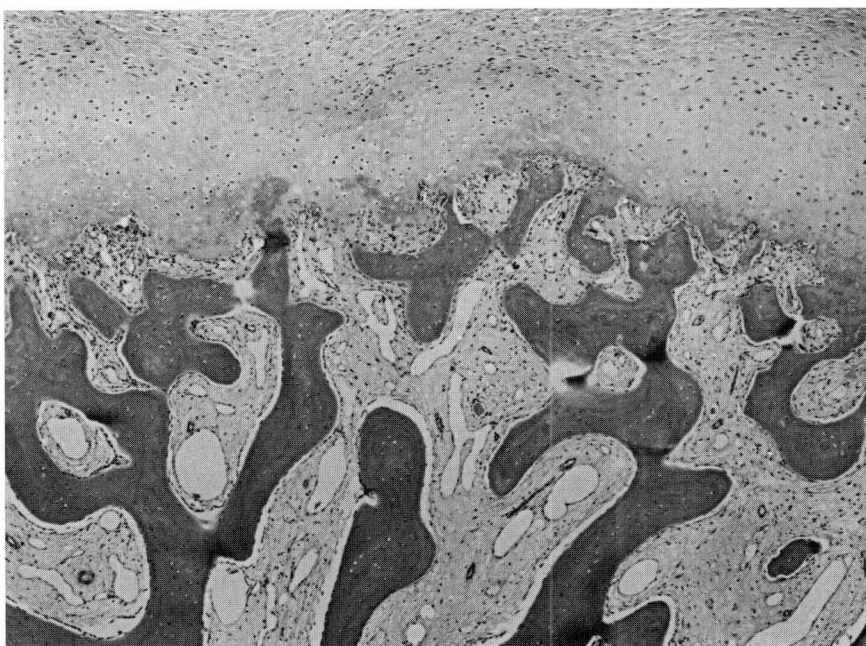

Figure 14-23 ■ Photomicrograph of subungual exostosis. A zonal pattern of fibrous tissue, cartilage, and bone is present.

nosis of a primary bone neoplasm. When the disease affects multiple bones, the battered child syndrome may be suspected.

The clinical features are distinctive. The disease begins in infancy with swelling and tenderness over the affected bone. Almost all patients are younger than 5 months, and some may even develop the disease in utero.[40] Although this disease has not been reported in the phalanges of the hands and feet or the vertebral bodies, any other bone may be involved. Most commonly, the mandible, the clavicle, and the long bones are affected.[41] Frequently, the disease is multicentric.

In addition to swelling and tenderness, other symptoms suggest a systemic component. For example, patients are usually febrile and have a leukocytosis and an elevated erythrocyte sedimentation rate.

Histologically, the periosteum is hypercellular and contains an infiltrate of inflammatory cells, a feature that suggests a microbial etiology. Abundant new bone forms in the periosteum, and the underlying diaphyseal cortex is extensively remodeled and replaced by thick, immature trabecular bone.[42]

Infantile cortical hyperostosis is self-limited and regresses over several years. The periosteal reactive bone matures and is eventually remodeled into a new cortex. Some patients are left with mild skeletal deformity.

GIANT CELL REPARATIVE GRANULOMA

Unlike radiodense reactive processes on the bone surface or in soft tissue, giant cell reparative granuloma, an intraosseous lesion, causes radiolucency. Giant cell reparative gran-

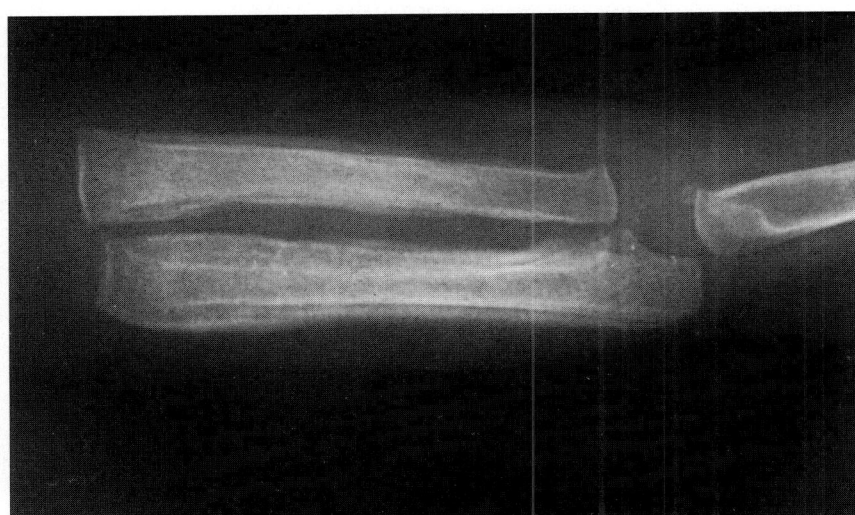

Figure 14-24 ■ Caffey's disease of the forearm. Extensive periosteal bone encases the radius and ulna.

uloma shares many histologic features with conventional giant cell tumor of bone. However, unlike giant cell tumor of bone, giant cell reparative granuloma is not a neoplasm. It is a reactive intraosseous proliferation of connective tissue, probably a result of prior incidents of excessive bone resorption.

Clinical Settings

Giant cell reparative granuloma arises in four clinical settings: in hyperparathyroidism, as a lytic lesion in the jaw, as a lesion in the hands and feet, and in Paget's disease.

Giant Cell Reparative Granuloma of Hyperparathyroidism

Giant cell reparative granuloma occasionally occurs in patients with advanced hyperparathyroidism (see Chapter 4). In this setting, the giant cell reparative granuloma is known as a *brown tumor* due to lesional hemosiderin deposition. Multiple lesions are typical, and the femur and tibia are the most common sites. Because advanced primary hyperparathyroidism is rare today, brown tumors are usually only seen in secondary hyperparathyroidism due to chronic renal failure.

Giant cell reparative granuloma associated with hyperparathyroidism is a well-defined lytic lesion that may involve any portion of the bone. In the long bones, usually the metaphysis or diaphysis is involved. Multiple lesions are often present. Initially, lesions lack a sclerotic rim. However, after parathyroidectomy, lesions show perilesional and intralesional sclerosis, a manifestation of healing.

Giant Cell Reparative Granuloma in the Jaw

The second setting for giant cell reparative granuloma is a lytic lesion in the jaw or face in the absence of hyperparathyroidism. Giant cell reparative granuloma in this setting most commonly (two thirds of cases) affects the anterior portion of the mandible. The maxilla, maxillary sinus, or sphenoid sinus are other sites of involvement.[43] Although patients range in age from 7 to 67 years, most are between 10 and 20 years.[44] The characteristic radiographic pattern is a lytic expansile lesion with a loculated or "soap bubble" pattern. The cause of this lesion is unknown, although trauma has been implicated in some cases. Giant cell reparative granuloma of the jaw is usually cured by simple curettage. Occasionally, this lesion occurs in the gingiva without involving the underlying bone. A lesion in this setting is called a *peripheral giant cell epulis*.

A curious syndrome of multiple giant cell reparative granuloma affecting the mandible in children is known as *cherubism*. In this autosomal dominant disorder, the multiple jaw lesions cause a puffy swelling of the lower face, a feature characteristic of the faces of cherubs in Renaissance paintings. The lesions are symmetric and begin to appear at about age 2 years. They grow until the patients are in their early teens and then begin to regress.[45]

Giant Cell Reparative Granuloma of the Hands and Feet

The third setting for giant cell reparative granuloma is in the bones of the hands and feet, also in the absence of hyperparathyroidism. In this setting, the patient occasionally has a history of trauma, but patients usually have no prior medical problems.[46-48]

Giant cell reparative granuloma of the hands and feet is a lytic lesion that usually affects the metaphysis or diaphysis (Fig. 14–25). The tubular bones of the hands and feet are more commonly involved than the carpal or tarsal bones. These lesions may appear aggressive and occasionally destroy one cortex.

Giant Cell Reparative Granuloma of Paget's Disease

The final clinical setting for giant cell reparative granuloma is as a rare complication of Paget's disease of bone. In these patients, the Paget's disease is usually in the hot phase, and the skull is the most common location.

Radiologically, giant cell reparative granuloma associated with Paget's disease is a well-defined lytic lesion. This contrasts to the highly destructive lytic lesion of a Paget's

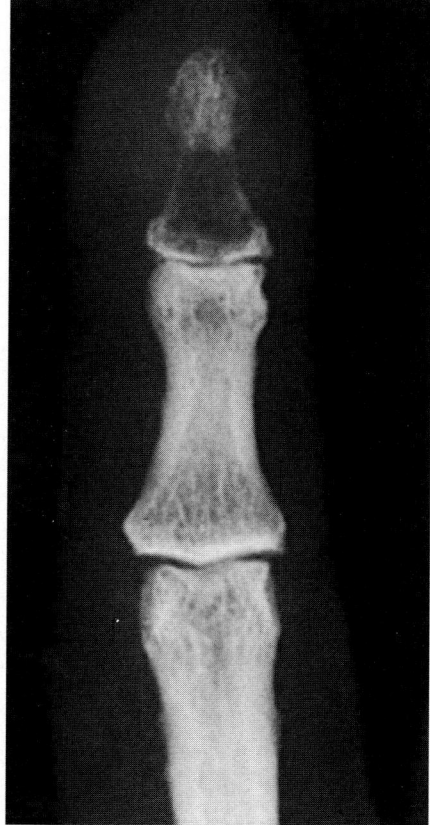

Figure 14-25 ■ Giant cell reparative granuloma of the distal phalanx.

sarcoma. Occasionally, the appearance of a giant cell reparative granuloma may be the initial manifestation of undiagnosed Paget's disease.

Histologic Features

The histologic features of giant cell reparative granuloma are identical in all clinical settings. Stromal cells are admixed with osteoclast-like giant cells. The most important histologic feature of the lesion is a zonal pattern. The clusters of giant cells aggregate around red blood cells (Fig. 14–26). The giant cells are surrounded by a zone of reactive fibrosis, which, in turn, is bounded by reactive bone (Fig. 14–27). This pattern repeats itself numerous times in any low-power field. Giant cell reparative granuloma may also undergo focal aneurysmal bone cyst change. Lesions with focal aneurysmal bone cyst have been called the "solid variant of aneurysmal bone cyst."

Giant Cell Reparative Granuloma Versus Giant Cell Tumor of Bone

Giant cell reparative granuloma presents an important problem of differential diagnosis—it is often confused with giant cell tumor of bone. It is imperative to distinguish these lesions because giant cell tumor of bone is an aggressive neoplasm, whereas giant cell reparative granuloma is an indolent process, often cured by simple curettage.

These two lesions may be distinguished by clinicoradiographic and histologic means. Although giant cell tumor may rarely be multicentric, multiple giant cell lesions are

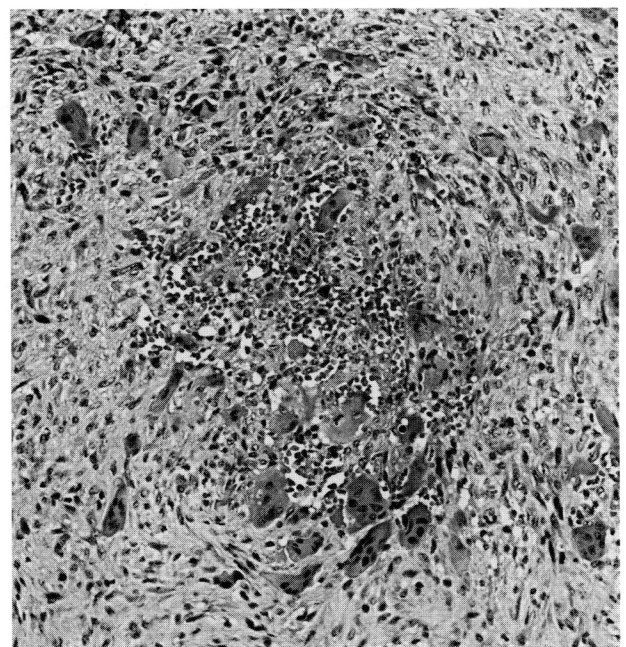

Figure 14–26 ■ Giant cell reparative granuloma showing giant cells aggregated around extravasated red blood cells.

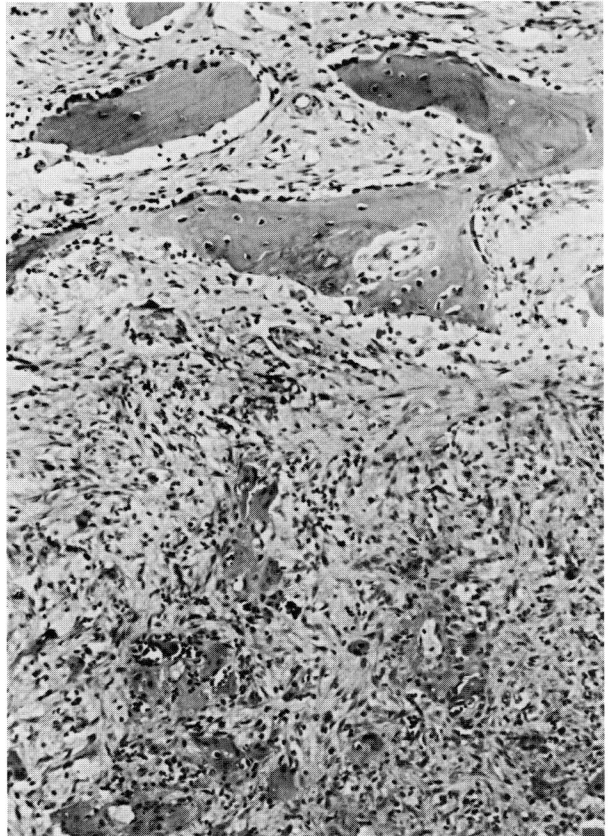

Figure 14–27 ■ Giant cell reparative granuloma showing a zonal pattern. Clusters of giant cells are surrounded by fibrous tissue, which is in turn surrounded by reactive bone.

more likely to be brown tumors of hyperparathyroidism. Serum calcium and parathormone levels should be checked.

Differences in location also aid in distinguishing these lesions. For example, giant cell tumor rarely occurs in the jaw; lesions in this location are probably reparative granulomas. In the long bones, giant cell tumor is centered in the epiphysis and extends into the metaphysis; patients are skeletally mature. By contrast, giant cell reparative granuloma is usually metaphyseal or diaphyseal; patients may be skeletally immature.

Histologic differences are also present. Although both lesions contain giant cells and stromal cells, giant cell tumor lacks the zonal pattern characteristic of giant cell reparative granuloma.

HEMOPHILIC PSEUDOTUMOR

Hemophilic pseudotumor is another lytic bone lesion that may mimic a neoplasm. This rare complication affects only 1% of patients with severe hemophilia. The process begins with subperiosteal bleeding, and the resulting hematoma erodes the underlying bone. With repeated bleeding, the erosion enlarges into a lytic lesion, which may reach 10 cm in diameter. Patients are usually adult hemophiliacs, and the ilium, distal femur, and proximal tibia are the most frequent sites.

The clinical course of hemophilic pseudotumor varies. Some lesions are asymptomatic and do not progress. Other lesions regress. Rarely, a pseudotumor may grow until it perforates, forming a fistula to the skin or into the abdominal cavity.[49]

REFERENCES

1. Slavin, R. E., Wen, J., Kumar, D., and Evans, E. B.: Familial tumoral calcinosis. A clinical, histopathologic, and ultrastructural study with an analysis of its calcifying process and pathogenesis. *Am J Surg Pathol* 17:788–802, 1993.
2. McGregor, D. H., Mowry, M., Cherian, R., McAnaw, M., and Poole, E.: Nonfamilial tumoral calcinosis associated with chronic renal failure and secondary hyperparathyroidism: Report of two cases with clinicopathological, immunohistochemical, and electron microscopic findings. *Hum Pathol* 26:607–613, 1995.
3. Holt, P. D., and Keats, T. E.: Calcific tendonitis: a review of the usual and unusual. *Skeletal Radiol* 22:1–9, 1993.
4. Steinbach, L. S., Johnston, J. O., Tepper, E. F., Honda, G. D., and Martel, W.: Tumoral calcinosis: Radiologic-pathologic correlation. *Skeletal Radiol* 24:573–578, 1995.
5. Gregosiewicz, A., and Warda, E.: Tumoral calcinosis: Successful medical treatment. *J Bone Joint Surg* 71A:1244, 1989.
6. Ishida, T., Dorfman, H. D., and Bullough, P. G.: Tophaceous pseudogout (tumoral calcium pyrophosphate dihydrate crystal deposition disease). *Hum Pathol* 6:587–593, 1995.
7. Sissons, H. A., Steiner, G. C., Bonar, F., May, M., Rosenberg, Z. S., Samuels, H., and Present, D.: Tumoral calcium pyrophosphate deposition disease. *Skeletal Radiol* 18:79–87, 1989.
8. Bertoni, F., Unni, K. K., Dahlin, D. C., Beabout, J. W., and Onofrio, B. M.: Calcifying pseudoneoplasms of the neural axis. *J Neurosurg* 72:42–48, 1990.
9. Heifetz, S. A., Galliani, C. A., and DeRosa, G. P.: Myositis (fasciitis) ossificans in an infant. *Pediatr Pathol* 12:223–229, 1992.
10. DeSmet, A. A., Norris, M., and Fisher, D. R.: Magnetic resonance imaging of myositis ossificans: Analysis of seven cases. *Skeletal Radiol* 21:503–507, 1992.
11. Cvitanic, O., and Sedlak, J.: Acute myositis ossificans. *Skeletal Radiol* 24:139–141, 1995.
12. Ogilvie-Harris, D. J., Hons, C. B., and Fornasier, V. L.: Pseudomalignant myositis ossificans: Heterotopic new bone formation without a history of trauma. *J Bone Joint Surg* 62A:1274–1282, 1980.
13. Lagier, R., and Cox, J. N.: Pseudomalignant myositis ossificans. A pathological study of eight cases. *Hum Pathol* 6:653–665, 1975.
14. Mody, B. S., Patil, S. S., Carty, H., and Klenerman, L.: Fracture through the bone of traumatic myositis ossificans. *J Bone Joint Surg* 76B:607–609, 1994.
15. Amir, G., Mogle, P., and Sucher, E.: Case report 729. *Skeletal Radiol* 21:257–259, 1992.
16. Shanoff, L. B., Spira, M., and Hardy, S. B.: Myositis ossificans: Evolution to osteogenic sarcoma. Report of a histologically verified case. *Am J Surg* 113:537–541, 1967.
17. Damanski, M.: Heterotopic ossification in paraplegia. *J Bone Joint Surg* 43B:286–299, 1961.
18. Garland, D. E.: A clinical perspective on common forms of acquired heterotopic ossification. *Clin Orthop* 263:13–29, 1991.
19. Milgram, J., and Gruhn J. (Eds.): *Radiologic and Histologic Pathology of Nontumorous Diseases of Bones and Joints.* Chicago, IL, Lea & Febiger, 1990, p. 454.
20. Riegler, H. F., and Harris, C. M.: Heterotopic bone formation after total hip arthroplasty. *Clin Orthop* 117:209–216, 1976.
21. Thomas, B. J.: Heterotopic bone formation after total hip arthroplasty. *Orthop Clin North Am* 23:347–358, 1992.
22. Brooker, A. F., Bowerman, J. W., Robinson, R. A., and Riley, L. H.: Ectopic ossification following total hip replacement: Incidence and method of classification. *J Bone Joint Surg* 55A:1629–1632, 1973.
23. Kjaersgaard-Andersen, P., and Ritter, M. A.: Prevention of formation of heterotopic bone after total hip arthroplasty. *J Bone Joint Surg* 73A:942–947, 1991.
24. Kaplan, F. S., Hahn, G. V., and Zasloff, M.: Heterotopic ossification: Two rare forms and what they can teach us. *Am Acad Orthop Surg* 2:288–296, 1994.
25. DeWitt, L. M.: Myositis ossificans. *Am J Med Sci* 120:295–309, 1900.
26. Münchmeyer, E.: Ueber myositis ossificans progressiva. *Zeitschr Rationelle Medizine* 34:9, 1869.
27. Cohen, R. B., Hahn, G. V., Tabas, J. A., Peeper, J., Levitz, C. L., Sando, A., Sando, N., Zasloff, M., and Kaplan, F. S.: The natural history of heterotopic ossification in patients who have fibrodysplasia ossificans progressiva. A study of forty-four patients. *J Bone Joint Surg* 75A:215–219, 1993.
28. Campbell, R. K.: Myositis ossificans progressiva. *Radiological Rev* 55:153, 1933.
29. Smith, R., Russell, R. G., and Woods, C. G.: Myositis ossificans progressiva. Clinical features of eight patients and their response to treatment. *J Bone Joint Surg* 58B:48–57, 1976.
30. Shafritz, A. B., Shore, E. M., Gannon, F. H., Zasloff, M. A., Taub, R., Muenke, M., and Kaplan, F. S.: Overexpression of an osteogenic morphogen in fibrodysplasia ossificans progressiva. *N Engl J Med* 335:555–561, 1996.
31. Gannon, F. H., Kaplan, F. S., Olmsted, E., Finkel, G. C., Zasloff, M. A., and Shore, E.: Bone morphogenetic protein 2/4 in early fibromatous lesions of fibrodysplasia ossificans progressiva. *Hum Pathol* 28:339–343, 1997.
32. Kaplan, F. S., Tabas, J. A., Gannon, F. H., Finkel, G., Hahn, G. V., and Zasloff, M.: The histopathology of fibrodysplasia ossificans progressiva. An endochondral process. *J Bone Joint Surg* 75A:220-230, 1993.
33. Nuovo, M. A., Norman, A., Chumas, J., and Ackerman, L. V.: Myositis ossificans with atypical clinical, radiographic, or pathologic findings: A review of 23 cases. *Skeletal Radiol* 21:87–101, 1992.
34. Johnson, M. K., and Lawrence, J. F.: Metaplastic bone formation (myositis ossificans) in the soft tissues of the hand. *J Bone Joint Surg* 57A:999–1000, 1975.
35. Yuen, M., Friedman, L., Orr, W., and Cockshott, W. P.: Proliferative periosteal processes of phalanges: A unitary hypothesis. *Skeletal Radiol* 21:301–303, 1992.
36. Wissinger, H. A., McClain, E. J., and Boyes, J. H.: Turret exostosis. Ossifying hematoma of the phalanges. *J Bone Joint Surg* 48A:105–110, 1966.
37. Meneses, M. F., Unni, K. K., and Swee, R. G.: Bizarre parosteal osteochondromatous proliferation of bone (Nora's lesion). *Am J Surg Pathol* 17:691–697, 1993.
38. Spjut, H. J., and Dorfman, H. D.: Florid reactive periostitis of the tubular bones of the hands and feet. A benign lesion which may simulate osteosarcoma. *Am J Surg Pathol* 5:423–433, 1981.
39. Landon, G. C., Johnson, K. A., and Dahlin, D. C.: Subungual exostoses. *J Bone Joint Surg* 61A:256–259, 1979.
40. Langer, R., and Kaufmann, H. J.: Case report 363. *Skeletal Radiol* 15:377–382, 1986.
41. Caffey, J.: Infantile cortical hyperostosis. *J Pediatr* 29:541–559, 1946.
42. Pazzaglia, U. E., Byers, P. D., Beluffi, G., Chirico, G., Rondini, G., and Ceciliani, L.: Pathology of infantile cortical hyperostosis (Caffey's disease). *J Bone Joint Surg* 67A:1417–1426, 1985.
43. Rogers, L. F., Mikhael, M., Christ, M., and Wolff, A.: Case report 276. *Skeletal Radiol* 12:48–53, 1984.
44. Waldron, C. A., and Shafer, W. G.: The central giant cell reparative granuloma of the jaws. An analysis of 38 cases. *Am J Clin Pathol* 45:437–447, 1965.
45. Jones, W. A.: Cherubism. A thumbnail sketch of its diagnosis and a conservative method of treatment. *Oral Surg Oral Med Oral Path* 20:648–653, 1965.
46. Lorenzo, J. C., and Dorfman, H. D.: Giant-cell reparative granuloma of short tubular bones of the hands and feet. *Am J Surg Pathol* 4:551–563, 1980.
47. Picci, P., Baldini, N., Sudanese, A., Boriani, S., and Campanacci, M.: Giant cell reparative granuloma and other giant cell lesions of the bones of the hands and feet. *Skeletal Radiol* 15:415–421, 1986.
48. Wold, L. E., Dobyns, J. H., Swee, R. G., and Dahlin, D. C.: Giant cell reaction (giant cell reparative granuloma) of the small bones of the hands and feet. *Am J Surg Pathol* 10:491–496, 1996.
49. Ahlberg, A. K. M.: On the natural history of hemophilic pseudotumor. *J Bone Joint Surg* 57A:1133–1136, 1975.

Diseases of Synovial Membrane

Many joint diseases are caused by systemic factors that target the synovial membrane directly or indirectly. These diseases, such as the inflammatory and crystal-induced arthritides, cause an intense synovitis that can erode adjacent bone. Multiple joints are usually affected. Occasionally, however, synovial membrane is affected by a primary disease. Primary synovial disease can also erode adjacent bone, but unlike systemic disease, usually only one joint is affected. Of the primary diseases of synovial membrane, synovial chondromatosis and pigmented villonodular synovitis cause the most diagnostic problems. Other primary diseases include synovial hemangioma and synovial lipomatosis.

SYNOVIAL CHONDROMATOSIS

Synovial chondromatosis (also known as synovial chondrometaplasia or osteochondromatosis) is characterized by the proliferation of hyaline cartilage nodules in synovial membrane. This disease occurs in two clinical settings. First, patients with preexisting disease, such as osteoarthritis, occasionally develop cartilage nodules in the synovial membrane. This process, known as *secondary synovial chondromatosis,* is initiated by cartilage and bone denuded from the joint surface. In the second setting, patients have no evidence of preexisting joint disease. In this process, known as *primary synovial chondromatosis,* metaplastic cartilage nodules form de novo, and the cause is not known.

Primary Synovial Chondromatosis

Primary synovial chondromatosis is an idiopathic proliferation of metaplastic cartilage nodules in synovial membrane. This process may occur within joints as well as in extraarticular synovial membrane, such as bursae or tendon sheaths. In any of these sites, all or only a portion of the synovial membrane may be involved. Synovial chondromatosis has three stages of evolution.[1] In the first stage, cartilage nodules develop in the synovial membrane by metaplasia of subsynovial fibroblasts. Many of these nodules become calcified and undergo endochondral ossification. In the next phase, some of these nodules detach from the synovial membrane and become loose bodies in the joint space. Finally, osteochondral loose bodies, sometimes hundreds, fill the joint, and the process of chondrometaplasia becomes quiescent in the synovial membrane.

Clinical Features

Synovial chondromatosis usually affects patients 30 to 50 years of age, although a 5-year-old child has been reported with this disease.[2] It is twice as common in men. Invariably, only one joint is affected, usually the knee (involved in two thirds of cases). Other joints often involved are the hip, elbow, wrist, ankle, shoulder, and temporomandibular joint. Patients present with pain, swelling, and stiffness, which may be present years before the diagnosis is made.

Extraarticular synovial chondromatosis, sometimes referred to as *chondroma of soft parts,*[3] most commonly presents as cartilage nodules in the tendon sheaths of the hands and feet.[4] Other extraarticular locations include the biceps tendon bursa, the iliopectineal bursa, and the ischial bursa. Occasionally, synovial chondromatosis occurs in bursae that develop over large osteochondromas, a condition sometimes called "exostosis bursata."[5]

Radiologic Features

Plain radiographic images of synovial chondromatosis show a spectrum of features. The process may be focal in a joint, or it may massively involve all the synovial tissues. Early in the course of the disease, only joint swelling is visible because the cartilage nodules have not yet begun to ossify. In this stage, they are best visualized with magnetic resonance imaging (MRI). Later in the disease process, fine

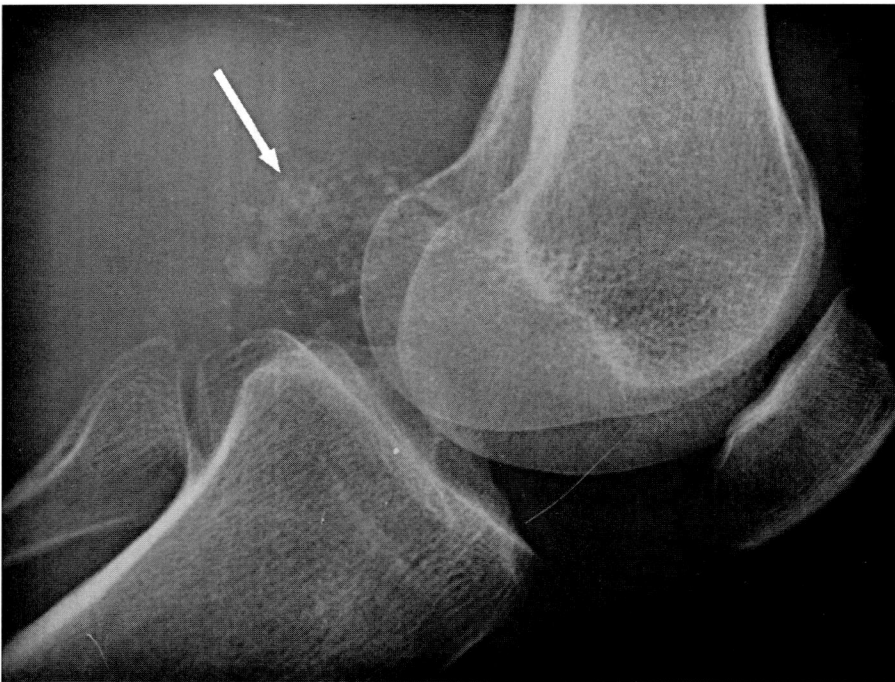

Figure 15-1 ▪ Synovial chondromatosis of the knee. Fine, stippled radiodensities are present in the posterior aspects of the joint *(arrow).* (From McCarthy, E. F.: *Differential Diagnosis in Pathology. Bone and Joint Disorders.* New York and Tokyo, Igaku-Shoin, 1996. With permission from Williams & Wilkins.)

stippled calcifications occur (Fig. 15-1). However, as the cartilage nodules grow, endochondral bone formation causes ring-shaped densities (Fig. 15-2). Occasionally, some of these densities may fuse into one giant osteochondral mass.[6]

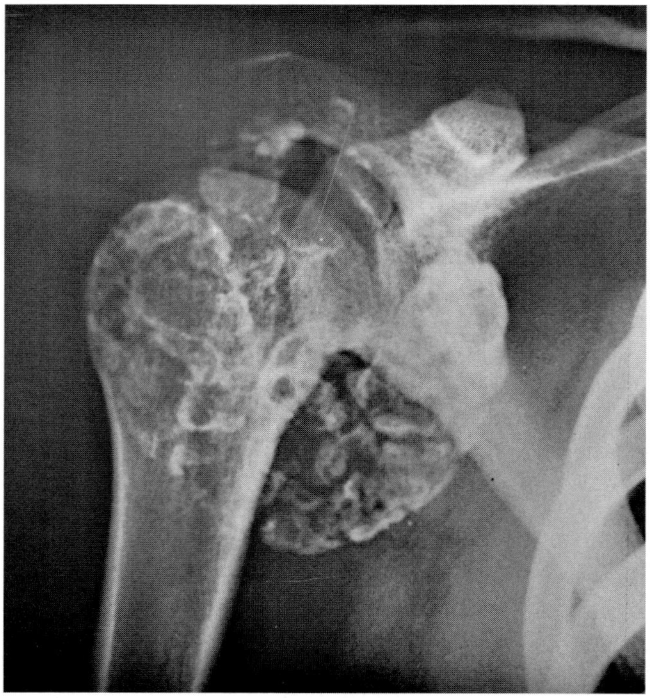

Figure 15-2 ▪ Synovial chondromatosis in the biceps tendon bursa. Ring-shaped radiodensities are present. The radiodensities are marginated by the limits of the bursa. (From McCarthy, E. F.: *Differential Diagnosis in Pathology. Bone and Joint Disorders.* New York and Tokyo, Igaku-Shoin, 1996. With permission from Williams & Wilkins.)

In addition, intraarticular synovial chondromatosis may cause bone erosion or damage the articular cartilage.[7]

Characteristically, the densities are well marginated, corresponding to the limits of the involved bursa or joint. A computed tomography scan may be useful in defining the limits of the lesion.

Pathologic Features

At surgery, a joint involved by primary synovial chondromatosis may be filled with hundreds of osteocartilaginous loose bodies. Histologic examination of the synovial membrane shows multiple discrete nodules of hyaline cartilage, some of which are focally calcified or ossified (Fig. 15-3). Ossification occurs at the periphery of the lobules, a pattern that causes the ring-shaped densities seen on plain radiographs. The chondrocytes within these nodules are arranged in clones or clusters (Fig. 15-4), and they often show mild cytologic atypia. In addition, binucleated chondrocytes and rare mitotic figures may be present. These features would be sufficient to diagnose malignancy in an intraosseous cartilage neoplasm. However, chondrocyte atypia is a characteristic feature of synovial chondromatosis and, in this setting, is not an indication of malignancy.[8]

As the disease evolves, the nodules of cartilage continue to calcify and undergo endochondral ossification. Even after the osteochondral nodules become loose bodies, they may continue to grow, nourished by the synovial fluid.

Prognosis and Treatment

Synovial chondromatosis is a self-limiting disease. However, because the process may damage the joint, removal of

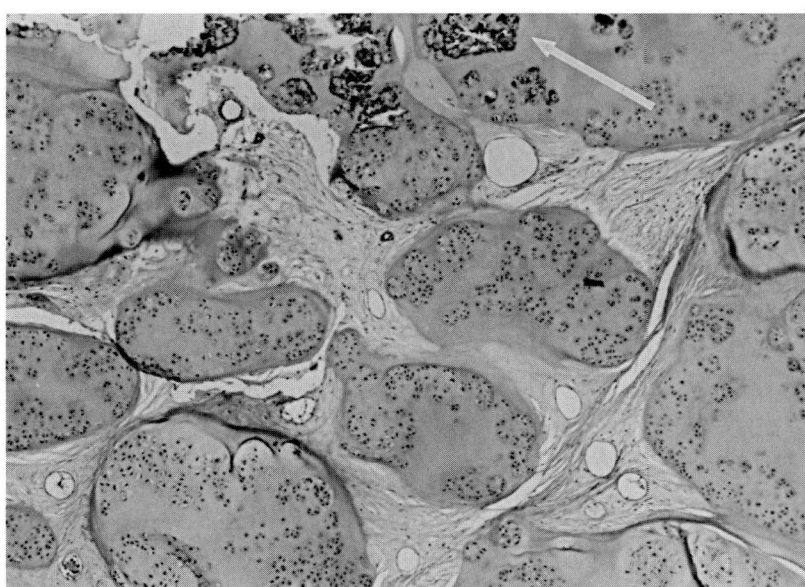

Figure 15–3 ▪ Cartilage nodules of synovial chondromatosis. A few are focally calcified *(arrow)*.

the loose bodies and, in the early phases, a synovectomy are necessary. Incomplete synovectomy in the active phases of the disease usually results in recurrence.

Problems in Diagnosis

Three factors of synovial chondromatosis may lead to overdiagnosis as a chondrosarcoma. First, the chondrocyte atypia, characteristic of primary synovial chondromatosis, may be interpreted as evidence of malignancy. Second, primary synovial chondromatosis may massively involve a joint and cause a huge soft tissue mass. Third, primary synovial chondromatosis often recurs. Awareness of these features and the knowledge that chondrosarcomas almost never occur in synovial membrane are crucial to avoid unnecessary surgery. On very rare occasions, however, a chondrosarcoma does arise in the synovial membrane. The only reliable diagnostic feature of this lesion, known as *synovial chondrosarcoma*, is metastasis. This neoplasm has only been documented in nine published cases.[9] These nine cases have demonstrated characteristic histologic features that may be diagnostic of malignancy before metastasis occurs. The first feature is the arrangement of the chondrocytes in solid sheets instead of clusters typical of synovial chondromatosis. Second, the chondrocytes of synovial chondrosarcoma tend to assume a spindle shape at the periphery of cartilage lobules. Third, chondrocytes of synovial chondrosarcoma are much more atypical and mitotic figures more numerous than in synovial chondromatosis (Fig. 15–5).

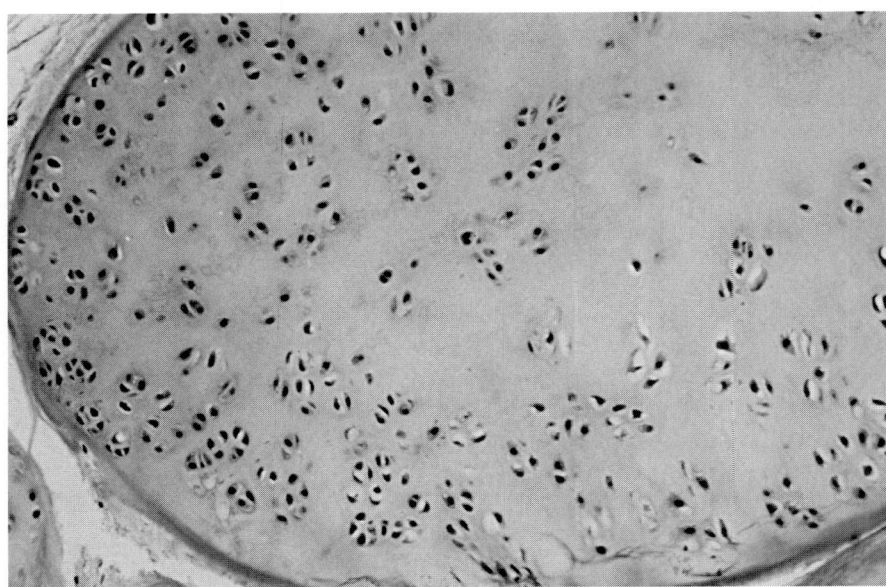

Figure 15–4 ▪ Nodule of synovial chondromatosis showing clones of chondrocytes.

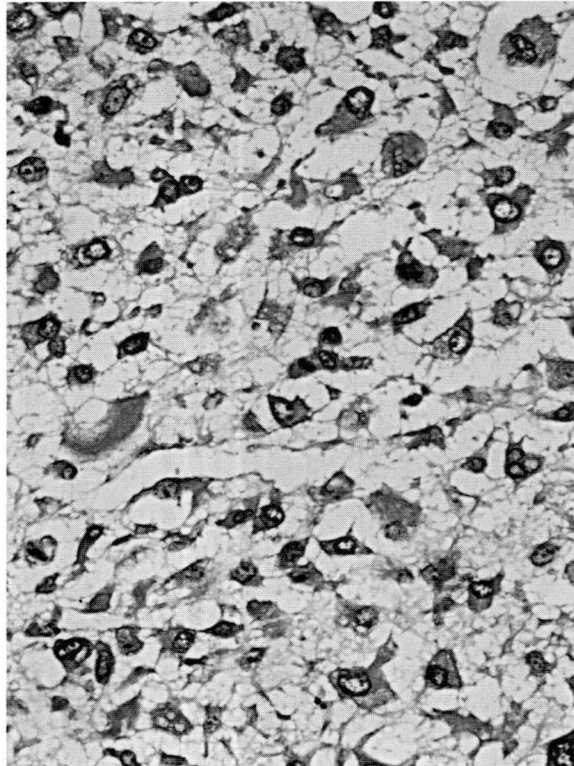

Figure 15-5 ▪ Synovial chondromatosis. The chondrocytes are markedly atypical.

Secondary Synovial Chondromatosis

Secondary synovial chondromatosis is a reactive proliferation of cartilage in the synovial membrane caused by other joint diseases. Fragments of cartilage and bone, called nidi, detach from the articular surface of diseased joints and become embedded in the synovial membrane, where they stimulate cartilage metaplasia. This process occurs in older patients, usually older than 60 years, who have osteoarthritis (Fig. 15–6). It also occurs when patients with osteonecrosis shed fragments of dead bone.[10] The metaplastic cartilage nodules stimulated by these detached fragments undergo ossification to form osteocartilaginous bodies. Unlike primary synovial chondromatosis, the cartilage nodules of secondary chondromatosis often vary in size, a reflection of the variation in size of the denuded fragments and the severity of the primary joint disease. Also, unlike primary synovial chondromatosis, multiple joints are often involved.

Histologically, the diagnostic feature of secondary synovial chondromatosis is the presence of an articular cartilage nidus in the center of the nodule. This nidus has a pale basophilic matrix with rare chondrocytes. Subchondral bone, if detached with the articular cartilage, is necrotic. Another characteristic histologic feature is the arrangement of the metaplastic cartilage in concentric rings around the nidus (Fig. 15–7). These rings are a manifestation of lamellar growth, which may continue when the nodule becomes a loose body.[11]

PIGMENTED VILLONODULAR SYNOVITIS

Pigmented villonodular synovitis (PVNS) is a disease of synovial membrane characterized by a proliferation of mononuclear cells, probably of histiocytic origin, deep to the synovial lining cells. In addition to mononuclear cells, multinucleated giant cells, foam cells, and hemosiderophages are present in varying amounts. As a result of these cells, the synovial membrane is transformed into thickened brownish nodules and greatly elongated villi. Like synovial chondromatosis, PVNS can involve both intraarticular or extraarticular (bursae, tendon sheaths) synovial membrane. In either site, PVNS occurs in one of two growth patterns—a localized nodule or a diffuse villous hyperplasia of large portions of synovial membrane. The localized form, when arising in tenosynovium, is sometimes called *giant cell tumor of tendon sheath*.

The etiology of pigmented villonodular synovitis is uncertain. Because many of the mononuclear cells show trisomy 7, a feature that suggests clonality, a neoplastic origin is possible.[12] A neoplastic origin is further supported by the observation that some cells in this process are aneuploid.[13] Another observation has confirmed the histiocytic differenti-

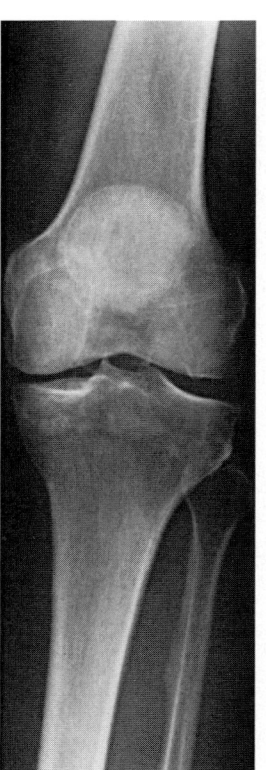
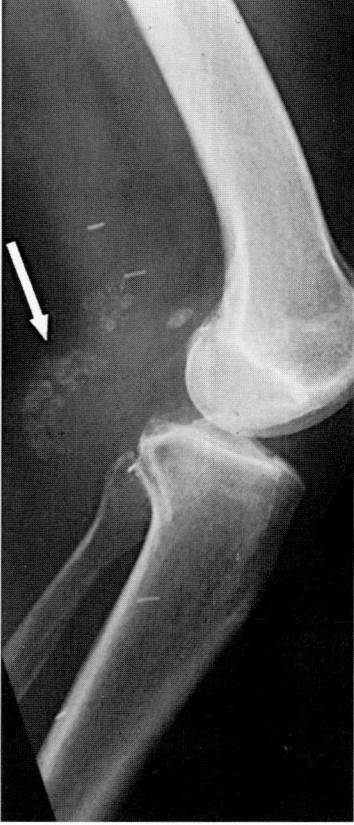

Figure 15-6 ▪ Secondary synovial chondromatosis. Ring-shaped radiodensities are present in the posterior compartment of the knee joint *(arrow)*. Anteroposterior radiograph *(left)* shows early joint space narrowing of the medial compartment consistent with early osteoarthritis. The presence of osteoarthritis excludes the possibility of primary synovial chondromatosis.

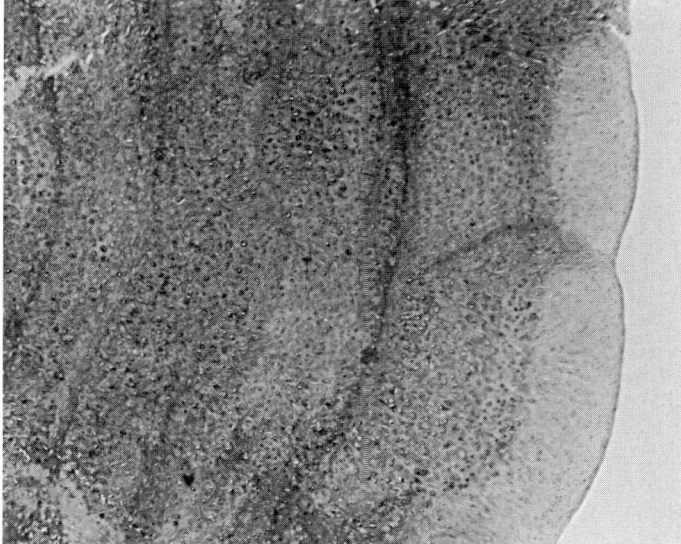

Figure 15-7 ■ Osteocartilaginous loose body from a lesion of secondary synovial chondromatosis. Concentric cartilage rings are present.

ation of the mononuclear cells—most contain the histiocyte markers Leu-M$_3$ and Leu-3.[14]

Clinical Features

Pigmented villonodular synovitis most commonly affects adult patients in the third or fourth decade of life. Patients present with joint pain, swelling, and stiffness. The process rarely affects children, although an 11-year-old with this disease has been reported.[15] Although any joint may be affected by PVNS, the knee is the most common site, involved in 80% of cases. Other joints frequently involved are the hip, shoulder, and ankle. Usually only one joint is affected. Rarely, PVNS may be polyarticular. In these cases, patients are younger, and several members of a family may be affected. Sometimes these family members have additional disorders such as the multiple lentigenes syndrome, fibrous dysplasia, and pectus excavatum. This observation suggests a possible genetic contribution to the development of pigmented villonodular synovitis.[16]

The extraarticular nodular form of PVNS (giant cell tumor of tendon sheath) presents with different features. This condition most commonly affects the hand and wrist. Patients report a slow-growing, painless, well-defined nodule in the subcutaneous tissue.

Radiologic Features

Because pigmented villonodular synovitis is a radiolucent intraarticular process, MRI is the most effective imaging modality. An intraarticular mass that shows signal dropout on a gradient echo or T$_2$-weighted image is highly suspicious for PVNS (Fig. 15-8). The signal dropout, due to the paramagnetic effect of iron, is caused by the hemosiderin present in this lesion.[17] Although PVNS is a primary disease of synovial membrane, its propensity to erode bone occasionally allows diagnosis with plain radiographs (Fig. 15-9). Bone erosion occurs in 15 to 50% of cases and is more common in the so-called "tight joints," such as the hip, elbow, and wrist.[18] In these joints, the capsule is not readily expandable. As a result, the diseased synovial membrane penetrates bone through vascular foramina near the chondroosseous junctions.[19] Plain radiographs show single or multiple well-circumscribed defects, usually on both sides of the joint. These defects, which usually have a sclerotic rim, occasionally penetrate into the metaphysis and mimic primary bone neoplasms such as giant cell tumor of bone.

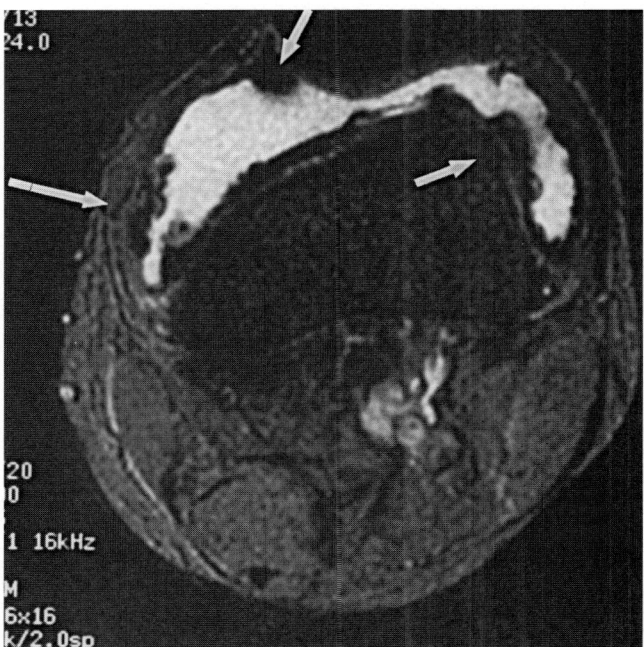

Figure 15-8 ■ Magnetic resonance image of knee showing pigmented villonodular synovitis. This gradient echo sequence shows numerous foci of signal dropout (arrows).

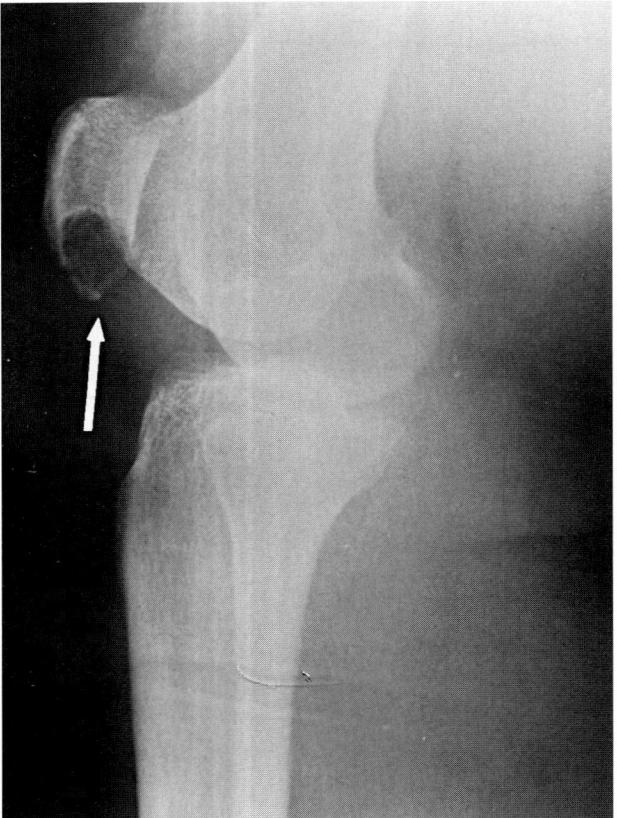

Figure 15-9 ■ Pigmented villonodular synovitis of the knee with erosion of the inferior pole of the patella *(arrow)*.

An additional feature of bone involvement by PVNS is the lack of juxtaarticular osteoporosis.

Histologic Features

The diagnostic feature of pigmented villonodular synovitis is an infiltrate of mononuclear stromal cells in the synovial membrane[20] (Fig. 15–10). These cells are round or oval and have an eosinophilic cytoplasm with a large round nucleus. Mitotic figures are present and average 10 per 20 HPFs. Admixed with these cells are varying numbers of hemosiderin-laden macrophages, which impart the dark brown color to the synovial membrane (Fig. 15–11). Sometimes, however, hemosiderin may be extremely scant. In addition to mononuclear cells and hemosiderin-laden macrophages, multinucleated giant cells and foam cells may be present. However, the stromal cell proliferation by itself is sufficient for the diagnosis. The localized nodular expression of PVNS, whether intraarticular or extraarticular, often shows areas of dense stromal hyalinization in addition to the cellular elements.

Treatment and Prognosis

Diffuse intraarticular pigmented villonodular synovitis must be treated with total synovectomy. Following meticulous total synovectomy, the recurrence rate is as low as 8%. Less than complete synovectomy results in recurrence rates as high as 46%. Therefore, arthroscopic surgery is inadequate to eradicate pigmented villonodular synovitis.[21]

Differential Diagnosis

Pigmented villonodular synovitis presents several problems in differential diagnosis. First, *hemosiderotic synovitis,* a reaction to chronic hemarthrosis, is often misdiagnosed as PVNS. Like PVNS, hemosiderotic synovitis shows brown discoloration of synovial membrane caused by hemosiderin deposition. However, hemosiderin deposition, no matter how extensive, is not diagnostic of PVNS. Only the proliferating mononuclear cell is diagnostic, and this cell is absent in hemosiderotic synovitis (Fig. 15–12). Also, multinucleated giant cells and foam cells are usually absent in hemosiderotic synovitis. Hemosiderotic synovitis commonly occurs in hemophiliacs because more than half of these patients bleed into their joints, usually the knee. It also occurs in patients who have had a traumatic hemarthrosis or in patients receiving anticoagulant therapy.

Another possible diagnostic difficulty arises when PVNS invades bone—it may be misdiagnosed as a bone tumor. With extensive bone involvement, both the epiphysis and metaphysis are involved. This results in a radiographic pattern very similar to that of giant cell tumor.[22] Moreover, like giant cell tumor, PVNS often contains many multinucleated giant cells, posing diagnostic problems histologically. Two features help distinguish giant cell tumor from bone involvement by PVNS. First, PVNS usually involves bone on both sides of a joint, a pattern not seen in giant cell tumor. Careful search for small lesions on the opposite joint surface is required. Second, giant cell tumor lacks the heavy hemosiderin deposition characteristic of PVNS in bone.

SYNOVIAL HEMANGIOMA

A synovial hemangioma is a hamartomatous proliferation of blood vessels in the synovial membrane. This rare disease, which may involve the synovial membrane of joints or bursae, is often mistaken for other synovial lesions such as chronic synovitis or pigmented villonodular synovitis. The clinical symptoms of synovial hemangioma are nonspecific. Affected patients, usually children or young adults, have had an intermittently swollen painful joint for as long as 2 years. The knee is the most commonly involved joint (60% of cases), followed by the elbow and joints of the hand. Aspiration of the involved joint often yields bloody fluid.

The MRI is the most effective way to diagnose a synovial hemangioma preoperatively.[23,24] Characteristically, on T_1-weighted images the signal is similar to that of surrounding muscle. However, the signal on T_2-weighted images is very bright. The lesion is well defined and contains punctate or linear areas of lower signal corresponding to fibrofatty septae. Synovial hemangiomas may have numerous gross and microscopic patterns.[25] Grossly, the lesion may be a single

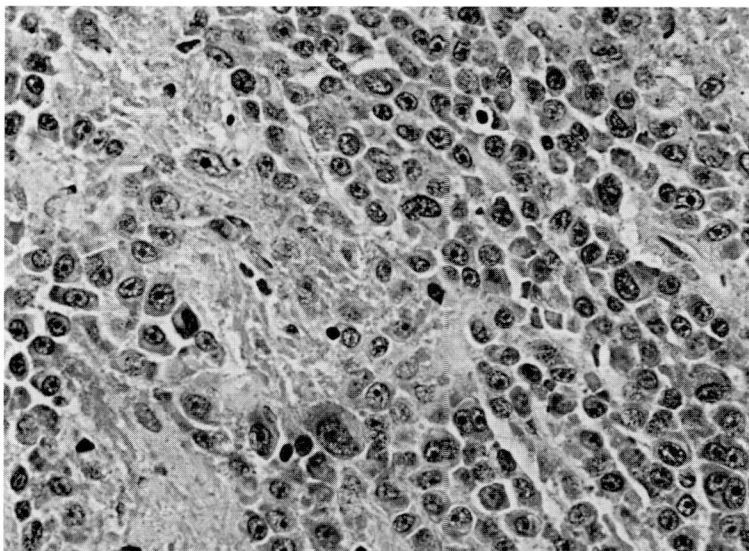

Figure 15-10 ■ Pigmented villonodular synovitis. The synovial membrane is infiltrated by sheets of mononuclear cells.

nodule as large as 6.0 cm in diameter, or it may be a diffuse villous growth involving part or all of the synovial membrane. Microscopically, lesions show the same spectrum of histologic patterns found in hemangiomas in other tissues. Synovial hemangiomas may show a capillary or cavernous pattern, and some may show features of an A-V malformation (Fig. 15–13). Intravascular thrombosis is occasionally present, and hemosiderin deposition is often abundant. These histologic features may cause diagnostic confusion. For example, the numerous vascular spaces may be mistaken for the prominent vascularity of chronic synovitis, and the extensive hemosiderin deposition may lead to the misdiagnosis of pigmented villonodular synovitis.

SYNOVIAL LIPOMATOSIS

Synovial lipomatosis, lipoma arborescens, and *Hoffa's disease* are various names for symptomatic hyperplasia of adi-

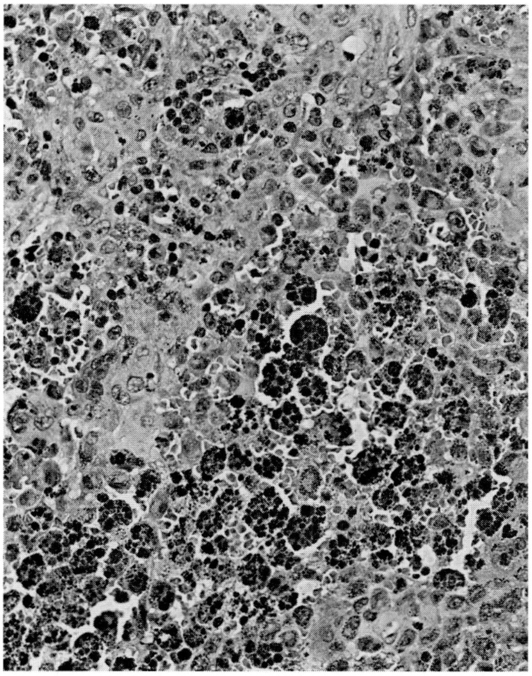

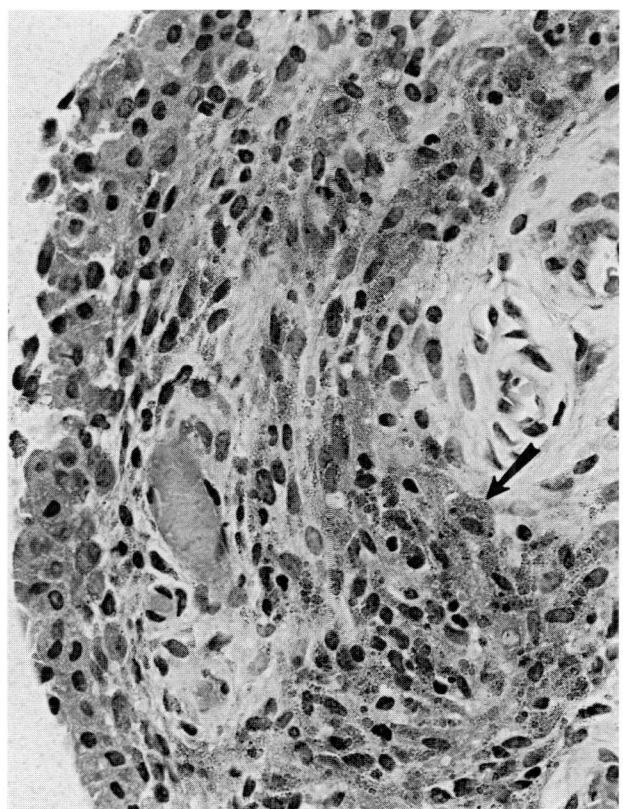

Figure 15-11 ■ Pigmented villonodular synovitis. Mononuclear cells are heavily laden with hemosiderin.

Figure 15-12 ■ Hemosiderotic synovitis. Mononuclear cells are absent, although hemosiderin deposition is present in synovial lining cells *(arrow)*.

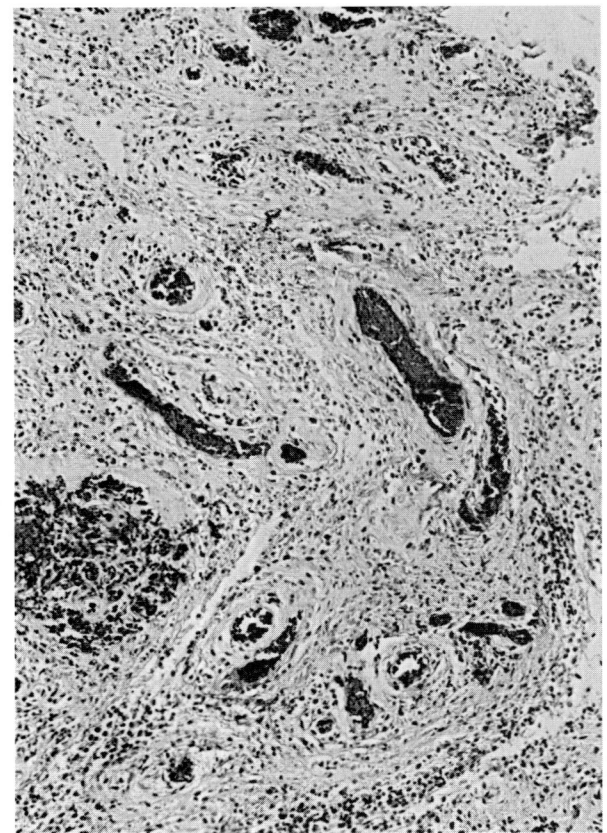

Figure 15-13 ■ Synovial hemangioma. Multiple thick walled blood vessels are present.

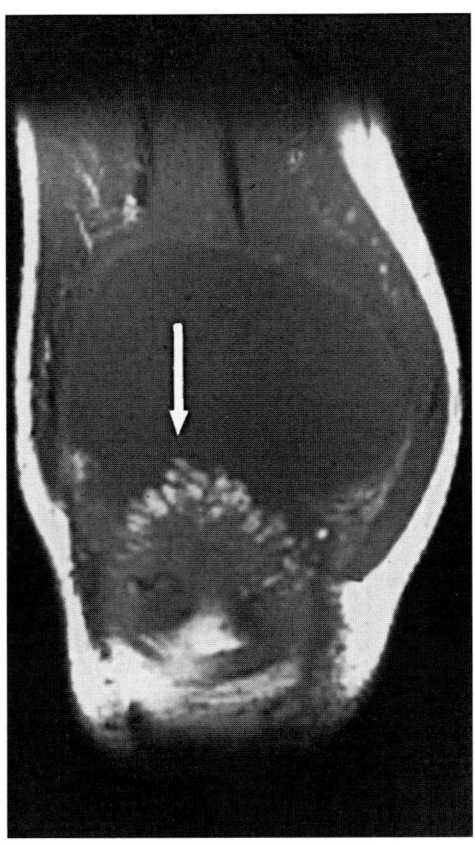

Figure 15-14 ■ Magnetic resonance image of synovial lipomatosis. This T_1-weighted sequence shows increased signal from villus fronds of fat *(arrow)*.

pose tissue in the synovial membrane. Patients with this rare disorder, usually middle-aged men, report a slowly progressive joint swelling over a period of years. Almost always, only one joint is involved, usually the knee, although the wrist or ankle may also be affected. Synovial lipomatosis almost always accompanies an underlying joint disorder, such as a meniscal tear or osteoarthritis. This suggests that the adipose tissue proliferation is reactive rather than neoplastic.[26] Patients may have symptoms of the underlying

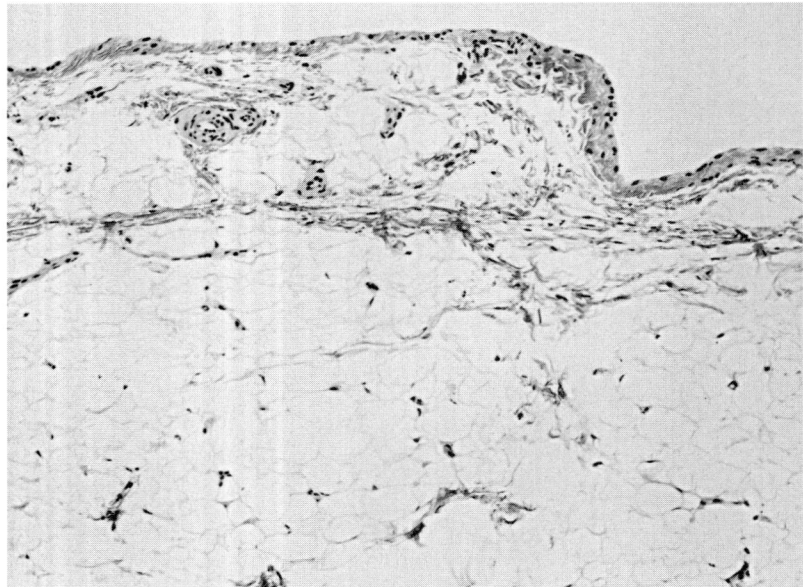

Figure 15-15 ■ Synovial lipomatosis. The synovial membrane is extensively infiltrated by fat.

joint abnormality as well as acute episodes of pain and effusion due to mechanical injury of the enlarged synovial fronds.

The MRI is the most specific imaging modality to diagnose synovial lipomatosis (Fig. 15–14). Sequences demonstrate a villous intraarticular mass with the signal intensity of fat.[27] Unlike other diseases of synovial membrane, such as PVNS or synovial chondromatosis, synovial lipomatosis does not cause bone erosion.

A joint involved by lipomatosis shows a villous proliferation of the synovial membrane caused by extensive fatty infiltration. The process may be focal or diffuse within the joint. Microscopically, the fatty infiltration is deep to the synovial lining cells (Fig. 15–15).

The treatment of synovial lipomatosis is synovectomy. Following this procedure, symptoms of the mass are relieved, and the lesion does not recur. However, the symptoms of the underlying joint abnormality may progress.

REFERENCES

1. Milgram, J. W.: Synovial osteochondromatosis. *J Bone Joint Surg* 59A:792–801, 1977.
2. Milgram, J. W., and Pease, C. N.: Synovial osteochondromatosis in a young child. *J Bone Joint Surg* 62A:1021–1023, 1980.
3. Chung, E. B., and Enzinger, F. M.: Chondroma of soft parts. *Cancer* 41:1414–1424, 1978.
4. Dahlin, D. C., and Salvador, A. H.: Cartilaginous tumors of the soft tissues of the hand and feet. *Mayo Clin Proc* 49:721–726, 1974.
5. Borges, A. M., Huvos, A. G., and Smith, J.: Bursa formation and synovial chondrometaplasia associated with osteochondromas. *Am J Clin Pathol* 75:648–653, 1981.
6. Edeiken, J., Edeiken, B. S., Ayala, A. G., Raymond, A. K., Murray, J. A., and Guo, S.: Giant solitary synovial chondromatosis. *Skeletal Radiol* 23:23–29, 1994.
7. Friedman, B., Nerubay, J., Blankstein, A., Kessker, A., and Horoszowski, H.: Case report 439. *Skeletal Radiol* 16:504–508, 1987.
8. Villacin, A. B., Brigham, L. N., and Bullough, P. G.: Primary and secondary synovial chondrometaplasia: Histopathologic and clinicoradiologic differences. *Hum Pathol* 10:439–451, 1979.
9. Bertoni, F., Unni, K. K., Beabout, J. W., and Sim, F. H.: Chondrosarcomas of the synovium. *Cancer* 67:155–162, 1991.
10. Osburn, A. W., Bassett, L. W., Seeger, L. L., Mirra, J. M., and Eckardt, J. J.: Case report 609. *Skeletal Radiol* 9:237–241, 1990.
11. Milgram, J. W.: The development of loose bodies in human joints. *Clin Orthop* 124:292–303, 1977.
12. Ray, R. A., Morton, C. C., Lipinski, K. K., Corson, J. M., and Fletcher, J. A.: Cytogenetic evidence of clonality in a case of pigmented villonodular synovitis. *Cancer* 67:121–125, 1991.
13. Abdul-Karim, F. W., El-Nagger, A. K., Joyce, M. J., Makley, J. T., and Carter, J. R.: Diffuse and localized tenosynovial giant cell tumor and pigmented villonodular synovitis. *Hum Pathol* 23:729–735, 1992.
14. Wood, G. S., Beckstead, J. H., Medeiros, L. J., Kempson, R. L., and Warnke, R. A.: The cells of giant cell tumor of tendon sheath resemble osteoclasts. *Am J Surg Pathol* 12:444–452, 1988.
15. Soifer, T., Guirguis, S., Vigorita, V. J., and Bryk, E.: Pigmented villonodular synovitis in a child. *J Pediatr Surg* 28:1597–1600, 1993.
16. Wendt, R. G., Wolfe, F., McQueen, D., Murphy, P., Solomon, H., and Housholder, M.: Polyarticular pigmented villonodular synovitis in children: Evidence for a genetic contribution. *Rheumatol* 13:921–926, 1986.
17. Sher, M., Lorigan, J. G., Ayala, A. G., and Libshitz, H. I.: Case report 578. *Skeletal Radiol* 19:131–133, 1990.
18. Zwass, A., Abdelwahab, I. F., and Klein, M. J.: Case report 463. *Skeletal Radiol* 17:81–84, 1988.
19. McMaster, P. E.: Pigmented villonodular synovitis with invasion of bone. Report of six cases. *J Bone Joint Surg* 42A:1170–1183, 1960.
20. Flandry, F., Hughston, J. C., McCann, S. B., and Kurtz, D. M.: Diagnostic features of diffuse pigmented villonodular synovitis of the knee. *Clin Orthop* 298:212–220, 1994.
21. Flandry, F. C., Jacobson, K. E., Hughston, J. C., Barrack, R. L., McCann, S. B., and Kurtz, D. M.: Surgical treatment of diffuse pigmented villonodular synovitis of the knee. *Clin Orthop* 300:183–192, 1994.
22. Jergesen, H. E., Mankin, H. J., and Schiller, A. L.: Diffuse pigmented villonodular synovitis of the knee mimicking primary bone neoplasm. *J Bone Joint Surg* 60A:825–832, 1978.
23. Greenspan, A., Azouz, E. M., Matthews, J. II, and Decarie, J. C.: Synovial hemangioma: Imaging features in eight histologically proven cases, review of the literature, and differential diagnosis. *Skeletal Radiol* 24:583–590, 1995.
24. Llauger, J., Monill, J. M., Palmer, J., and Clotet, M.: Synovial hemangioma of the knee: MRI findings in two cases. *Skeletal Radiol* 24:579–581, 1995.
25. Devaney, K., Vinh, T. N., and Sweet, D. E.: Synovial hemangioma: A report of 20 cases with differential diagnostic considerations. *Hum Pathol* 24:737–745, 1993.
26. Hallel, T., Lew, S., and Bansal, M.: Villous lipomatous proliferation of the synovial membrane (lipoma arborescens). *J Bone Joint Surg* 70A:264–270, 1995.
27. Grieten, M., Buckwalter, K. A., Cardinal, E., and Rougraff, B.: Case report 873. *Skeletal Radiol* 23:652–655, 1994.

CHAPTER 16 | Diseases of Joints

Joint disorders are among the most common of all medical problems. In England, for example, joint disorders account for almost 20% of presenting complaints to general practitioners.[1] Similarly, 20% of the population in the Netherlands has a rheumatologic problem.[2] In the United States, 32% of all adults are currently affected with musculoskeletal signs and symptoms such as joint swelling, limitation of motion, or pain on motion.[3] In some of these cases, the joint symptoms are mild. However, they can also cripple a patient. For example, in the United States, osteoarthritis of the knee is the most common cause of disability after heart disease. In fact, about 100,000 people in the United States are unable to walk independently from the bed to the bathroom because of osteoarthritis of the hip or knee.[4]

More than 100 specific diagnostic entities of joint disease exist, but in this chapter, we discuss only the most common. They can be grouped into three major categories: degenerative, inflammatory, and metabolic (Table 16–1). Degenerative diseases are caused by primary failure of joint structures. In this group, osteoarthritis is the most common. Other frequently seen degenerative disorders include spondylosis deformans, diffuse idiopathic skeletal hyperostosis, and neuropathic joints. The second category, inflammatory joint disease, is characterized by systemic factors that target the synovial membranes. Resulting inflammatory change in the synovial membrane causes secondary destruction of other joint structures. Of these diseases, rheumatoid arthritis is the prototype. We also discuss juvenile rheumatoid arthritis, ankylosing spondylitis, psoriatic arthritis, reactive arthritis, and arthritis associated with systemic lupus erythematosus. In the third category, metabolic joint disease, problems are caused by the deposition of crystals. We discuss the two most important diseases in this category—gout and calcium pyrophosphate deposition disease.

Two other major categories of joint disease exist. One of these, traumatic disorders, is not discussed in this book. The other, infectious arthritis, is discussed in Chapter 8.

HISTORY

The Paleopathologic Record

Joint diseases not only are common in modern times but also have affected humans (and animals) throughout history. In fact, they are among the most frequently observed disorders in fossilized and archeologic bone specimens. For example, the hypertrophic changes of osteoarthritis have been demonstrated in the weight-bearing bones of many species of dinosaur. One example is severe spinal osteoarthritis of a Comanchean dinosaur from 100 million years ago.[5]

Early hominids also suffered from osteoarthritis, as evidenced by hypertrophic changes in the knees and spine of a Neanderthal specimen.[6] Another Neanderthal specimen, dating from 40,000 to 54,000 years ago, showed alterations of the wrist, ankle, and shoulder characteristic of calcium pyrophosphate deposition disease.[7]

Egyptian mummies, because of their excellent preservation, often provide a record of the antiquity of joint disease. A radiographic survey of the mummies from the royal families showed osteoarthritis of the knee, hip, or spine in 3 of 12 specimens.[8] In another mummy, changes consistent with gouty arthritis were present, and urate crystals were identified.[9]

Evidence of osteoarthritis is present in paleopathologic material from all cultures in all historical periods. By contrast, evidence of inflammatory arthritis is very scant. It is possible that ankylosing spondylitis affected early humans. For example, numerous spine specimens show fusion of the vertebral bodies, a feature of ankylosing spondylitis. One of the earliest of these specimens is from a Neolithic grave (3500 BC) in northern France.[10] However, distinguishing ankylosing spondylitis from spondylosis deformans is difficult in archeologic specimens. The absolute diagnosis of ankylosing spondylitis requires sacroiliac joint changes, and these joints are usually poorly preserved.

The scant evidence of inflammatory joint changes has

Table 16-1 ■ **CATEGORIES OF JOINT DISEASES**

Degenerative
    Osteoarthritis
        Generalized osteoarthritis
        Spondylosis deformans
        Neuropathic joint
        Diffuse idiopathic skeletal hyperostosis
Inflammatory
    Rheumatoid arthritis
    Juvenile rheumatoid arthritis
    Seronegative spondyloarthropathies
        Ankylosing spondylitis
        Reactive arthritis
        Psoriatic arthritis
        Reiter's syndrome
        Arthritis associated with inflammatory bowel disease
    Arthritis of systemic lupus erythematosus
Metabolic (crystal induced)
    Gout
    Calcium pyrophosphate deposition disease
        Pseudogout
        Chronic pyrophosphate arthropathy
        Tophaceous pseudogout
Traumatic
Infectious

led to controversy among paleopathologists regarding the antiquity of rheumatoid arthritis. Despite thousands of skeletal specimens showing bone disease, osteologic evidence of rheumatoid arthritis is extremely rare. In fact, unequivocal evidence of rheumatoid arthritis has not been found in any specimens dated before the 18th century. This has prompted scholars to search for visual evidence of rheumatoid arthritis in early paintings. Although numerous possible examples were found, particularly among 15th- and 16th-century Flemish paintings, none is convincing.[11] As a result of this lack of convincing osteologic and visual evidence, it has been suggested that rheumatoid arthritis is a relatively new disease, an almost unique situation in human pathology.

Recently, however, skeletal remains of an ancient (3000–5000 years ago) Native American population in Alabama showed a symmetric, erosive, polyarthritis of the small and large joints of several skeletal specimens.[12] These changes are highly suggestive of rheumatoid arthritis. They raise the possibility that rheumatoid arthritis was present in prehistoric times in the New World and crossed the Atlantic, like syphilis, in 1492.[13]

The Medical Record

Descriptions of joint disease are present in the earliest medical literature. In the *Hippocratic Corpus,* the chapter "On Articulations" contains descriptions of joint pain, swelling, and stiffness. In the works of Galen, the treatise *On the Function of the Parts of the Human Body* contains numerous similar descriptions. Although the Greeks used the term *arthritis,* the Romans preferred the word *gout* to describe joint swelling. This word was based on the Latin word *gutta,* which means a drop. According to the theory of the four humors, joint swelling occurred because phlegm, one of the humors, was distilled by the brain and "dropped" into weakened joints, painfully distending them.[14]

In the 17th and 18th centuries, two major categories of joint disease were described: those that were accompanied by suppuration and those that were chronic but nonsuppurative. Joints in this latter category contained a watery fluid, a characteristic leading to the use of the term *rheumatic* (from the Greek root *rheuma,* meaning "watery"). This term, first used by Guillaume de Baillou in 1570 (republished in Geneva in 1762), was applied to all chronic, nonsuppurative arthritis.[15] Often, the term *rheumatic gout* was used.

In the late 18th century, specific subtypes of the so-called rheumatic diseases were recognized. For example, in 1797, William Wollaston discovered urates in the swollen joints of some patients.[16] By 1848, Alfred Garrod of England recognized that this finding represented a specific disease. He devised the famous "thread test" to identify urates. This test was one of the first bedside tests ever used for diagnostic purposes. It is based on the observation that synovial fluid in inflamed joints has less viscosity and does not form a thread when a drop is pulled apart. Garrod, in 1859, introduced the term *rheumatoid arthritis* to distinguish those chronic joint diseases that were not true gout.[17]

Garrod's son, Archibald, continued his father's studies. By 1890, he had recognized that the arthritides were a group of joint diseases having as their only common characteristic the pain and stiffness of multiple joints: "The realization that we are here dealing with a group of maladies and not with a single disease is in itself a great advance."[18] Garrod used the term *osteoarthritis* to describe those chronic joint diseases characterized by bone hypertrophy. Almost 100 years earlier, Heberden had described "little hard knots" adjacent to the distal interphalangeal joints of the hand. He recognized that these were a manifestation of chronic arthritis and were not related to gout.[19] These nodules, now called Heberden's nodes, are examples of the hypertrophic changes of osteoarthritis.

In 1904, Joel Goldthwaite of Boston proposed another classification. He called one group of joint diseases "hypertrophic" and another "atrophic."[20] Goldthwaite believed that these categories, based on pathologic features, corresponded to Garrod's osteoarthritis and rheumatoid arthritis. Goldthwaite noticed that atrophic arthritis tended to involve multiple joints in younger patients. Hypertrophic arthritis, by contrast, affected fewer joints in older patients.

The subdivision of the arthritides has continued up to the present. In 1927, Mandl recognized a difference between primary and secondary osteoarthritis. The most recently described entity was calcium pyrophosphate deposition disease. In 1962, McCarty and colleagues discovered that a gout-like syndrome was caused by calcium pyrophosphate crystals.[21] Even today, most clinicians believe that both osteoarthritis and rheumatoid arthritis are not single diseases but are in fact groups of separate but similar processes.

Before discussing our current knowledge of the various disease entities, a description of normal joints is necessary.

THE NORMAL JOINT

The human body has 327 joints. They vary greatly in size and complexity. For example, the largest joint, the knee, is many times larger than the tiny joints of the ear. Also, the knee, with its subtle rotational and translational motions, is far more complex than the simple ball-and-socket structure of the hip joint.

In addition to varying size and complexity, joints also allow different degrees of motion. In some joints, called *syndesmoses,* the bones are joined by a thin connective tissue ligament. These joints, which include the cranial sutures, allow almost no movement. In another category of joint called *synchondroses,* the bones are joined by cartilage and allow only slight motion. The joints between the vertebral bodies—the intervertebral discs—are synchondroses. In the final category, *diarthrodial joints,* the bones move freely relative to one another. Most joints in the body are diarthrodial joints.

Diarthrodial Joints

Diarthrodial joints are characterized by having a joint capsule that encloses the bone ends in a joint space. The bone ends are covered by articular cartilage, and the joint space is partially lined by synovial membrane (Fig. 16–1). The fluid secreted by the synovial membrane is a lubricant that allows virtually frictionless motion of one bone end against the other. Although movement is free, supporting tissues of the joint maintain structural stability and limit the joint's range of motion.

The supporting tissues of diarthrodial joints include the joint capsule and various ligaments. The capsule is a dense fibrous tissue sheath that encases the joint and, by its continuity with the periosteum, is tightly bound to the bone. Articular ligaments are specialized condensations of connective tissue that tightly attach one bone to another. These ligaments (the knee has four, for example) stabilize the joint by limiting the range of motion.

A radiograph of a normal diarthrodial joint shows a uniform radiolucent zone between the bone ends. This zone, known as the joint space, is occupied by the articular cartilage (Fig. 16–2).

Fibrocartilage

Some joints have a specialized tissue called *fibrocartilage,* which helps stabilize the joint or facilitates motion. The labra of the glenoid and acetabulum, the menisci of the knee, and the annulus fibrosus of the intervertebral discs are fibrocartilaginous structures. In addition, the terminal portion of a tendon or ligament, at its insertion into bone, is fibrocartilage. Fibrocartilage consists of a dense fibrous extracellular matrix composed mainly of type I collagen. In this respect, fibrocartilage is identical to fibrous connective tissue. However, instead of elongated fibroblasts, the cells of fibrocartilage are round chondrocytes (Fig. 16–3). They are present in lacunae and surrounded by a small amount of bluish, chondroid matrix.

Synovial Membrane

Diarthrodial joints are lined by synovial membrane. This membrane covers much of the inside of the joint capsule, as well as the intraarticular portions of bone not covered by

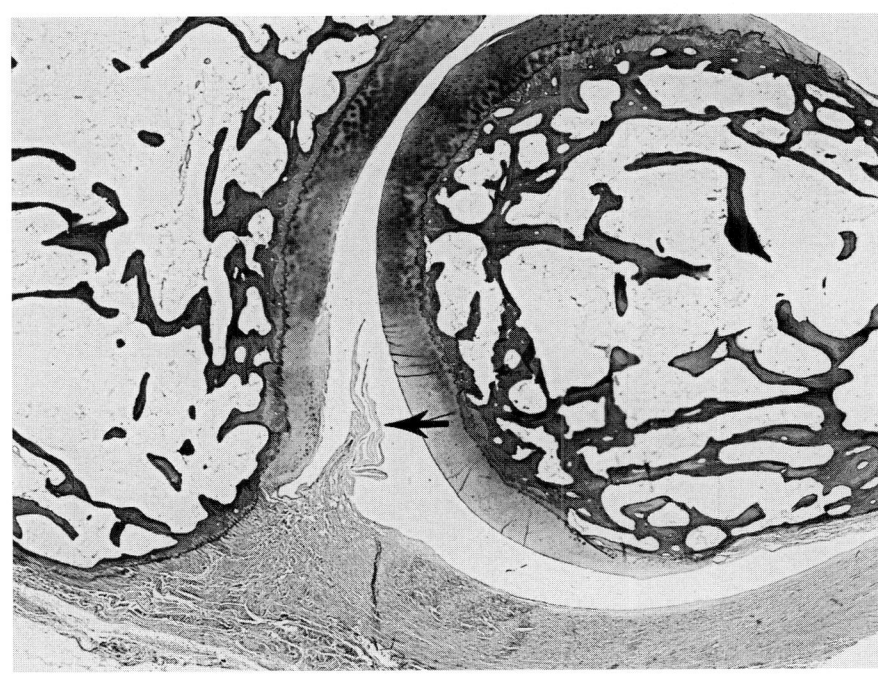

Figure 16-1 ■ Low-power photomicrograph of a diarthrodial joint. The bone ends are covered by articular cartilage and are encased in a fibrous capsule. A portion of synovial membrane *(arrow)* arises from the inner surface of the joint capsule.

320 DISEASES OF JOINTS

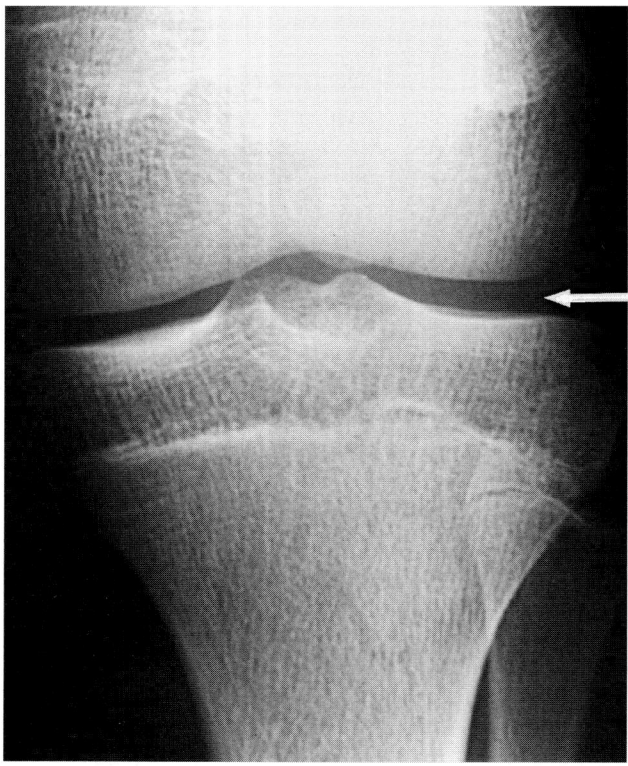

Figure 16-2 ■ Radiograph of diarthrodial joint. The uniform space between the bone ends is occupied by radiolucent hyaline cartilage *(arrow)*.

Synovial Fluid

Each diarthrodial joint contains a small amount of thick, viscous liquid, known as synovial fluid. The knee joint, for example, contains about 4 ml of this fluid. The synovial fluid lubricates the articular cartilage and allows almost frictionless motion of one articular surface on the other.

Most of the synovial fluid is a transudate of water and solutes from the blood. In addition, hyaluronic acid and a glycoprotein, lubricin, are added by the lining cells of the synovial membrane. These molecules provide the lubricating characteristics of the synovial fluid. Another compound found in the synovial fluid (and probably synthesized by the synovial lining cells) is *link protein,* a crucial component of the articular cartilage matrix. This protein is responsible for binding proteoglycans to hyaluronic acid.

Articular Cartilage

Articular cartilage covers the bone ends that are encapsulated in diarthrodial joints (Fig. 16-6). It provides a smooth, slippery surface so the bones glide freely on one another. In addition, articular cartilage absorbs mechanical shock and spreads forces evenly onto the supporting bone underneath. It has no nerve supply and no blood supply, and it receives oxygen and nutrients by diffusion from the synovial fluid.

The cartilage of articular surfaces is known as *hyaline cartilage.* It consists of chondrocytes that are scattered throughout an abundant extracellular matrix. The chondrocytes, which compose less than 10% of the total tissue volume, are located in lacunae in the extracellular matrix. In living tissue, the chondrocytes conform to the round shape of the lacunae. However, in histologic preparations, they are stellate and appear shrunken and retracted from the inner wall. In adults, chondrocytes do not divide. Despite this lack of cell turnover, chondrocytes are extremely active

articular cartilage. The synovial membrane is composed of loose fibrovascular tissue admixed with varying amounts of fat (Fig. 16-4). Characteristically, the surface area of this membrane is increased by numerous villous fronds. On the surface of the villi are one or two layers of cells with features of both macrophages and fibroblasts (Fig. 16-5). These are the synovial lining cells, and they secrete some of the components of the synovial fluid.

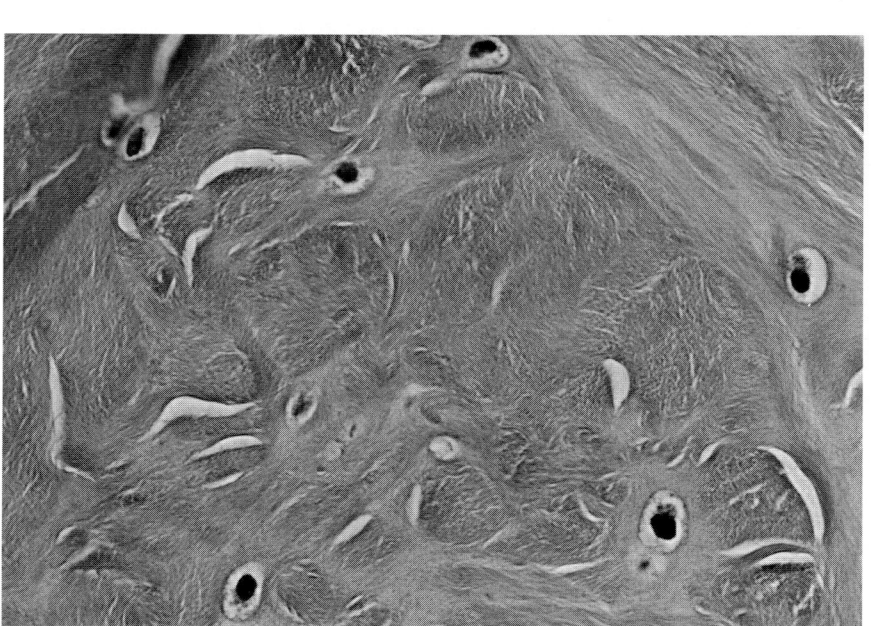

Figure 16-3 ■ High-power photomicrograph of fibrocartilage. The extracellular matrix is dense type I collagen, and the cells are round chondrocytes in lacunae.

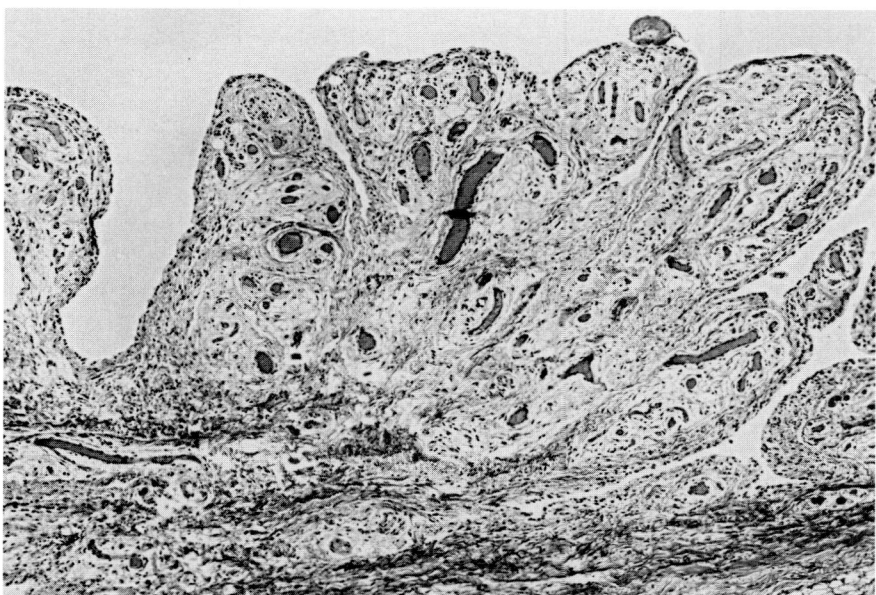

Figure 16-4 ■ Low-power micrograph of normal synovial membrane. The surface area of this membrane is increased by the numerous villi.

metabolically. They are responsible for the synthesis, maintenance, and catabolism of the extracellular matrix, a substance that requires constant turnover.

Extracellular Matrix of Hyaline Cartilage

Water. The extracellular matrix of cartilage consists of three major components: water, a network of type II collagen fibrils, and proteoglycan aggregates. Cartilage has a unique cushioning property because 65 to 80% of the extracellular matrix is water. The water is trapped in the matrix by the hydrophilic proteoglycan aggregates within the interstices of the collagen framework. The compressibility of the cartilage is due to the mobility of the water. Mechanical forces on the cartilage move water within the matrix as well as out of the cartilage into the joint. Because cartilage has no blood supply, movement of water is the mechanism by which nutrients enter from the synovial fluid.

Collagen. Type II collagen is the most abundant organic compound in the extracellular matrix of hyaline cartilage. This type of collagen is also found in elastic cartilage, the intervertebral disc, and in the vitreous of the eye. Unlike the broad type I collagen fibrils, which aggregate into larger fibers, type II fibrils are narrow and are arranged in a delicate three-dimensional lattice uniformly distributed throughout the extracellular space. The arrangement of the fibrils is purposeful. In the superficial zone nearest the joint space, the collagen fibrils are oriented parallel to the surface. Although the collagen fibers are thinner in this superficial zone, they are packed closer together. In the deepest layer of the articular cartilage, adjacent to the bone, the type II collagen fibrils are oriented perpendicular to the subchondral bone. Between the superficial and deep layers, the collagen fibrils gently curve with a trajectory that has been likened to Gothic arches.

In addition to type II collagen, articular cartilage contains other collagens, although in much smaller amounts. About 10% of the total collagen content consists of types V, VI, IX, X, and XI. Unlike type II collagen, which is distributed throughout the articular cartilage, most of the other collagens are located in specific areas. For example, type VI collagen

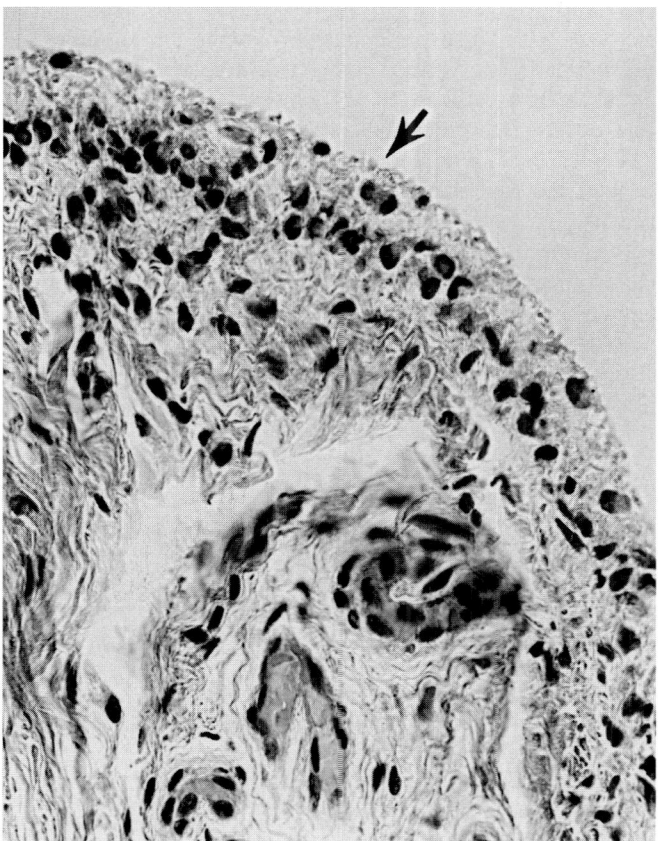

Figure 16-5 ■ High-power photomicrograph of surface of a synovial villus. Each villus is lined by one or two layers of lining cells *(arrow)*.

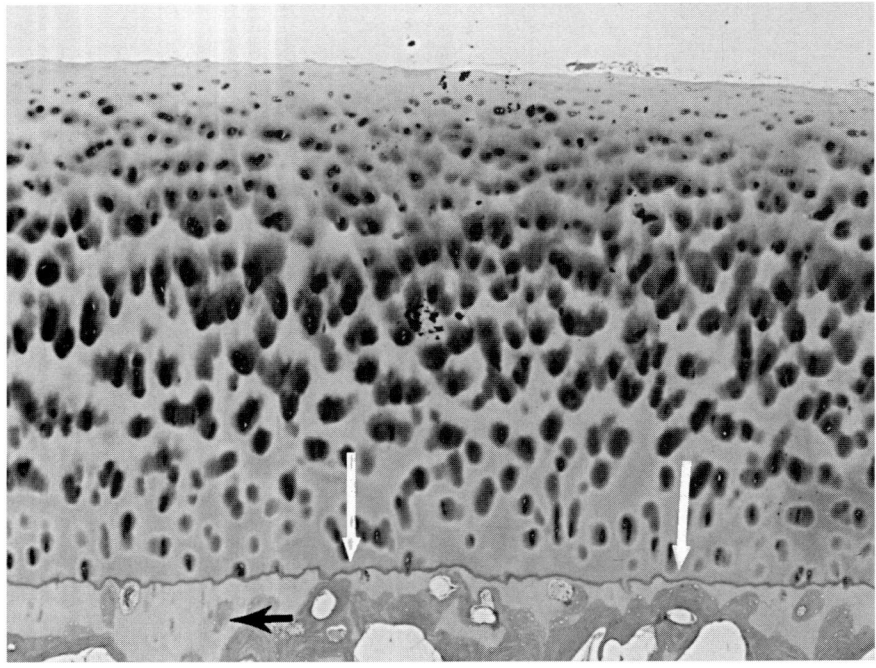

Figure 16-6 ■ Low-power photomicrograph of normal articular cartilage. Tiny chondrocytes are uniformly dispersed in the extracellular matrix. The unmineralized cartilage is separated from the bone by the tidemark *(white arrows)*. Beneath the tidemark is the zone of calcified cartilage *(black arrow)*.

appears to be located in the areas of matrix immediately adjacent to the chondrocytes, and type X collagen is limited to the very deepest layer adjacent to the bone. The function of these additional collagens is not known, although they appear to be stabilizers of the fibrous network of the matrix. Because each chain of a collagen fiber is the product of a distinct gene, the various collagens in the articular cartilage are encoded by at least 10 different genes located on at least four different chromosomes.

Proteoglycans. Proteoglycans are the third major component of the articular cartilage. Whereas the collagen fibers provide tensile strength, proteoglycans function to hold water in the cartilage. Proteoglycans, formerly called mucopolysaccharides, are among the largest molecules produced by cells anywhere in the body. They consist of a protein core to which are attached sulfated glycosaminoglycans. A glycosaminoglycan is a long-chain unbranched molecule made up of repeating disaccharide units. In articular cartilage, the principal glycosaminoglycans are keratan sulfate and chondroitin sulfate. Typically, as many as 100 chondroitin sulfate and 50 keratan sulfate chains radiate from the protein core like the bristles on a bottle brush. In the articular matrix, about 90% of the proteoglycans attach to a long chain of hyaluronic acid. A special protein, known as link protein, binds the proteoglycan to the hyaluronic acid. Proteoglycans that attach themselves to hyaluronic acid (as many as 200 molecules may be attached) are known as aggrecans (Fig. 16–7).

The large size of the proteoglycan aggregates provides a very large array of COO^- and SO_4^{2-} groups. Water, therefore, being trapped and immobilized by these negative charges, creates a gel that is supported by the fine, reticular arrangement of the collagen fibers (Fig. 16–8).

Zones of the Articular Cartilage. Because of variation in the distribution of proteoglycans and collagen, the articular cartilage may be divided into four zones (Fig. 16–9). The

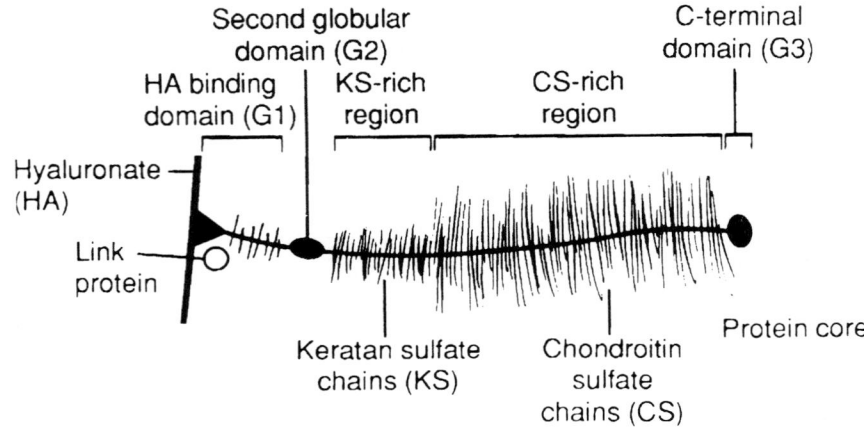

Figure 16-7 ■ Proteoglycan molecule. Many glycosaminoglycan molecules are lined up along the protein core. The protein core is attached to a molecule of hyaluronic acid by link protein. (Reproduced with permission from Mankin, H. J., Maw, V. C., Buckwalter, J. A., Iannotti, J. P., and Ratcliffe, A.: Form and function of articular cartilage. Simon, S. R., Ed. *Orthopaedic Basic Science.* American Academy of Orthopaedic Surgeons, 1994.)

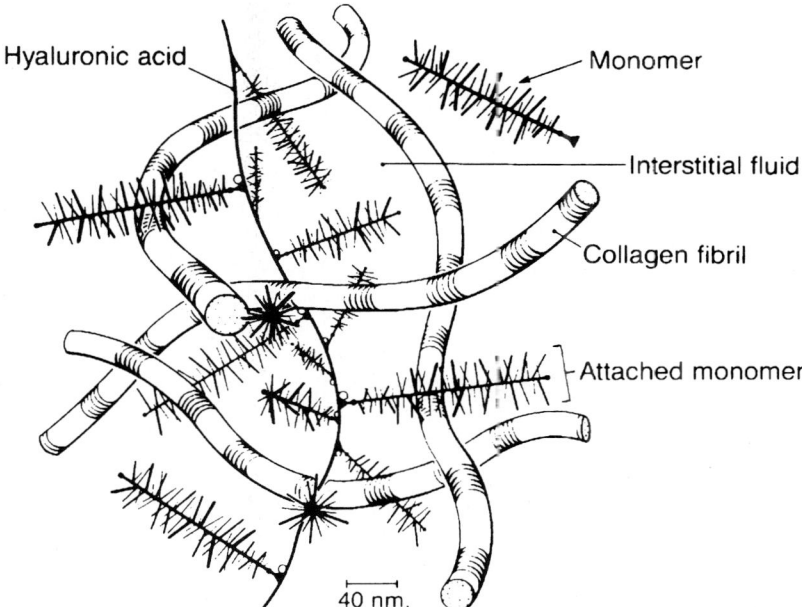

Figure 16-8 ■ The arrangement of proteoglycans and type II collagen fibrils in the hyaline cartilage matrix. (From Maw, V. C., Proctor, C. S., and Kelly, M. A.: Biomechanics of articular cartilage. Nordin, M., Frankel, V. H., Eds. *Basic Biomechanics of the Musculoskeletal System,* 2nd ed. Philadelphia, Lea & Febiger, 1989. With permission from Waverly.)

superficial zone is relatively rich in collagen and poor in proteoglycans. In the second zone, known as the transitional zone, the number of proteoglycans increases, and the molecules are distributed evenly throughout the arching collagen fibers. In the third zone, proteoglycans seem to be concentrated around chondrocytes. This zone has the highest concentration of proteoglycans and the lowest water content. The deepest zone of cartilage, directly adjacent to bone, is calcified. This layer, known as the zone of calcified cartilage, is separated from the uncalcified cartilage by a blue line (with a hematoxylin and eosin stain), known as the *tidemark* (Fig. 16–10).

The matrix components also vary according to proximity to chondrocytes. For example, the thin area immediately surrounding a chondrocyte, known as the pericellular region, contains almost exclusively proteoglycans and almost no collagen fibrils. Outside the pericellular region is the territorial zone. In this zone, collagen fibrils are present, and they form a fibrillar network that is organized around a particular chondrocyte. Between the territorial zones of specific chondrocytes, the interterritorial regions form the largest areas of the extracellular matrix. These interterritorial areas contain the largest collagen fibers and the highest concentrations of proteoglycans.

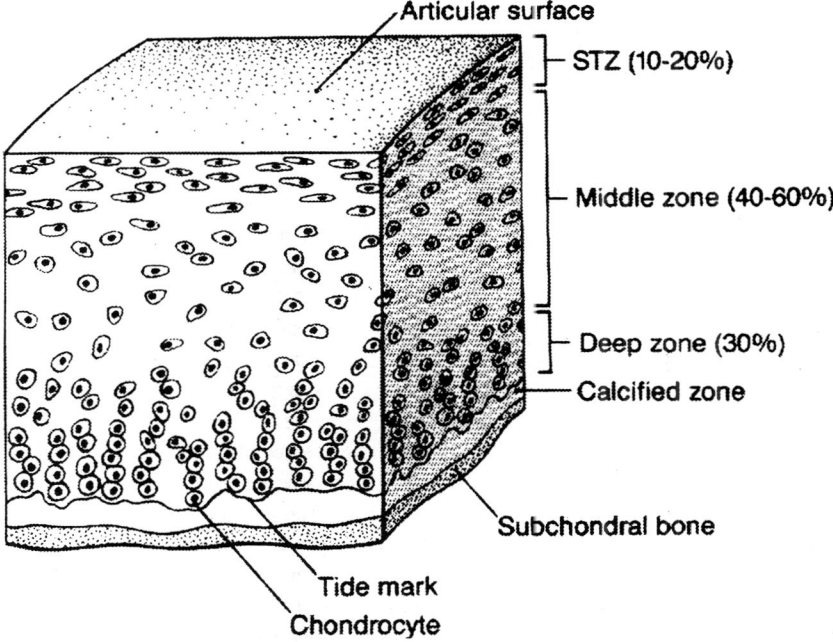

Figure 16-9 ■ The zones of articular cartilage. (From Maw, V. C., Proctor, C. S., and Kelly, M. A.: Biomechanics of articular cartilage. Nordin, M., Frankel, V. H., Eds. *Basic Biomechanics of the Musculoskeletal System,* 2nd ed. Philadelphia, Lea & Febiger, 1989. With permission from Waverly.)

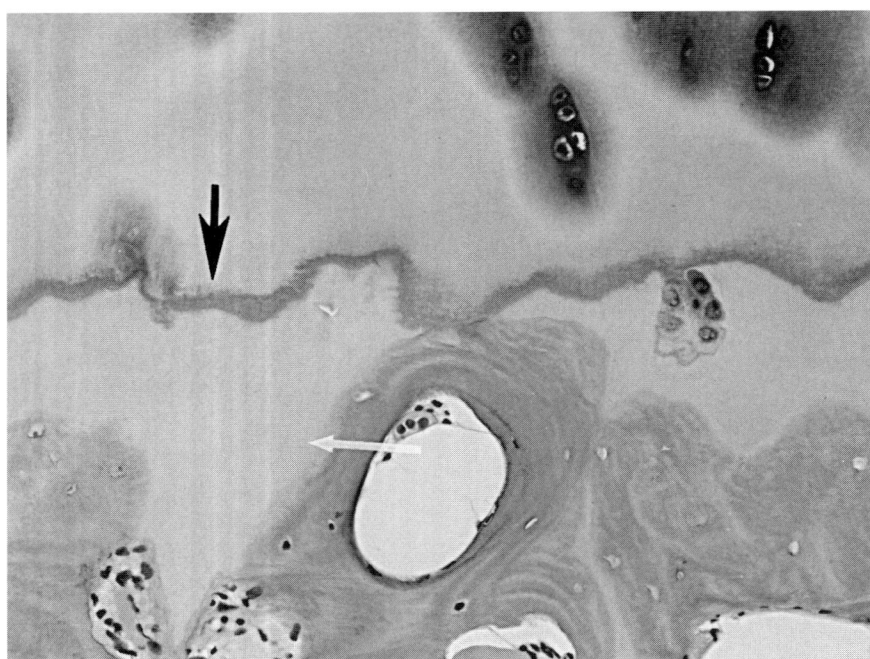

Figure 16–10 ■ High-power photomicrograph of the tidemark *(black arrow)*. Between the tidemark and the lamellar bone is an irregular zone of calcified cartilage *(white arrow)*.

Metabolism of Articular Cartilage. The extracellular matrix of articular cartilage is in a constant state of turnover. The chondrocytes synthesize and assemble the matrix components and direct their distribution within the tissue. By enzymatic secretion, chondrocytes also control the breakdown of matrix components.

Synthesis of the matrix occurs in various stages. For example, gene transcription results in the synthesis of glycosaminoglycans, core proteins, and hyaluronic acid. Then, numerous post-translational changes, such as sulfation of the repeating disaccharide units and their attachment to the protein core, occur in the Golgi apparatus. After secretion, the assembly into the large proteoglycan aggregates occurs in the extracellular matrix.

Breakdown of the proteoglycans occurs by extracellular enzymatic degradation. Various metalloproteinases and cathepsins are secreted by the chondrocytes and cleave the core protein, link protein, and hyaluronate at specific locations. The fragments are small enough to diffuse from the articular cartilage into the synovial fluid. From the joint, the fragments are taken up by lymphatics and moved into the circulating blood. Eventually, proteoglycan fragments are excreted in the urine.

Joint motion and loading are necessary to maintain healthy articular cartilage. Reduced joint loading, in the form of rigid immobilization or casting, leads to atrophy or degeneration of the cartilage. Animal studies have shown that these changes occur within as few as 4 weeks of immobilization. Motion and loading have two positive affects on articular cartilage. Having no blood supply, the cartilage depends on the diffusion of oxygen and nutrients from the synovial fluid. Pressure is necessary to force nutrients into the cartilage and to promote their diffusion into the deepest layers. The second positive effect of loading is that chondrocyte deformation is required to maintain homeostasis of the extracellular matrix. Cartilage contains no nerves and therefore receives no direct regulatory messages from the rest of the body. In addition, the cartilage matrix is impermeable to cellular and humoral immune responses. Therefore, mechanical stresses on chondrocytes are an important factor that regulates the balance between matrix synthesis and breakdown. Absence of the stresses ultimately disrupts the homeostasis of the matrix.

OSTEOARTHRITIS

Osteoarthritis is a disease characterized by loss of the articular cartilage and secondary changes in the subchondral bone (Fig. 16–11). Usually, the bone changes are sclerosis, cyst formation, and the development of osteophytes. Osteoarthritis is also known as degenerative joint disease, hypertrophic arthritis, and osteoarthrosis. Although any joint can be affected, osteoarthritis usually develops in the hips, knees, spine, and small joints of the hand and wrist. Pain and stiffness are the principal symptoms.

Osteoarthritis is a heterogeneous disorder. Many factors lead to loss of the articular cartilage. If the factor is a well-defined, preexisting joint disorder, the disease is called *secondary osteoarthritis*. For example, osteonecrosis, crystal deposition disease, trauma, congenital dysplasias, and inflammatory arthritis all may lead to secondary osteoarthritis. In the absence of preexisting joint disease, loss of articular cartilage is known as *primary osteoarthritis*. However, even in this setting, the cause of the cartilage failure probably varies in different patients.

Incidence

Osteoarthritis is the most common joint disease and affects elderly men and women of all racial and ethnic groups.

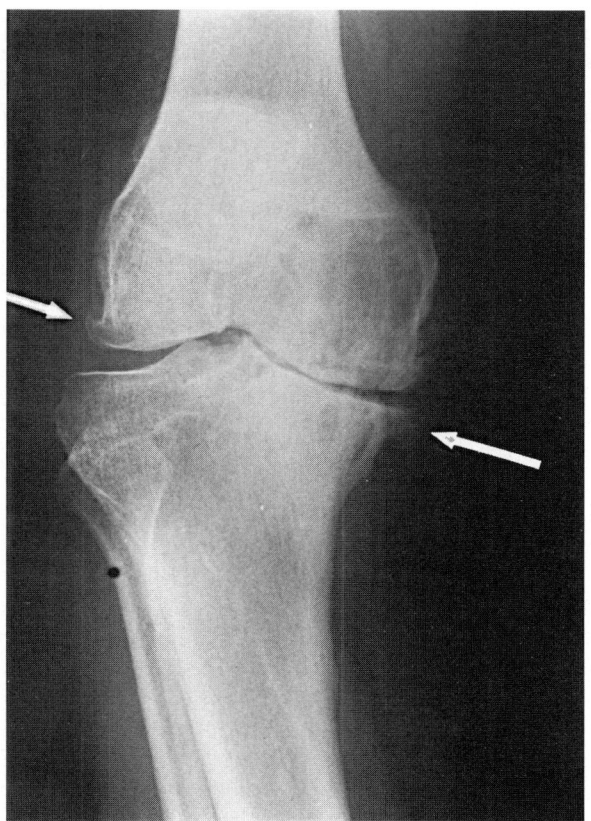

Figure 16-11 ■ Radiograph of the knee with osteoarthritis. The medial joint space is narrowed, and subchondral sclerosis is present in both the femur and tibia. Small osteophytes *(arrows)* are present.

This joint disease is rare in people younger than 40 years and extremely common after age 60. An autopsy study of 1000 patients older than 65 revealed cartilage damage in almost 100%.[22] The radiographic prevalence is a bit lower. About 75% of women older than 60 have radiologic changes of osteoarthritis of the hand. Despite the predilection for the elderly, primary osteoarthritis does occur in younger individuals. By age 40, 10 to 20% of subjects have radiographic osteoarthritis of the hands and feet.

Osteoarthritis more commonly affects women than men, and multiple joints are usually involved, the hands being most frequently affected. Osteoarthritis of the hip is an exception. In this location, men and women are affected equally, and other joint involvement is often not present. These observations have led to the theory that osteoarthritis of the hip has a different pathogenesis. Osteoarthritis of the hip strikes about 5% of the population older than 55 years, and about one half of these patients require hip surgery.[23]

A characteristic feature of osteoarthritis is that clinical symptoms often do not correlate with radiographic severity. Patients with severe radiographic changes may have minimal symptoms. This is often observed in osteoarthritis of the hands. By contrast, patients with little radiographic disease may have very painful joints.

Clinically significant osteoarthritis is not as prevalent as radiologic changes. However, the clinical prevalence is high enough to make osteoarthritis a major cause of disability. In 1974, 2.3% of men and 1.3% of women in the working population of Britain had to retire from employment because of osteoarthritis. As a result, 4.7 million working days were lost that year.[24] In addition, 5% of individuals 55 to 64 years of age are required to leave their employment for three or more months because of osteoarthritis.[25] In the United States, moderate to severe osteoarthritis affects over 14 million people.[26]

Etiology

The etiology of osteoarthritis is not known with certainty. Undoubtedly, many factors contribute to articular cartilage failure. Traditionally, aging and overuse were thought to be two of these factors. However, osteoarthritis is not a direct result of either. Although a strong association with age exists, that association is not causal. For example, many older people have some joint space narrowing and small marginal osteophytes, but most do not have clinically significant symptoms. In addition, osteoarthritis almost never develops in the ankle, a weight-bearing joint, even in old age.[27]

Excessive use of joints also does not inevitably lead to osteoarthritis.[28] Although athletes, dancers, musicians, and heavy laborers may develop symptomatic traction spurs and soft tissue syndromes associated with overuse, they do not develop premature osteoarthritis. In fact, distance runners, ballet dancers, and professional keyboard or string musicians actually have a lower incidence of osteoarthritis of the "overused" joints. However, they may develop secondary osteoarthritis due to severe joint trauma, such as a torn ligament. These joint injuries, common in athletes, cause secondary osteoarthritis because of disrupted joint mechanics. It is likely that many successful musicians and dancers have been "self-selected" by a hereditary protection against osteoarthritis. By contrast, if a person is predisposed to develop osteoarthritis, overuse may accelerate, but not cause, its development.

If aging or overuse does not directly cause osteoarthritis, then what does? Two main theories exist. One theory suggests that a defect in the articular cartilage matrix leads to premature failure. The other theory suggests that the primary abnormality is in the underlying bone, and cartilage failure is secondary. These bone alterations may be either an increased hardness or a change in shape.

In support of the theory of primary matrix failure is the recent discovery of a type II collagen mutation in some families with premature osteoarthritis.[29,30] In these cases, the mutation substitutes a cysteine for an arginine in type II procollagen$_2$ chains. The onset of osteoarthritis in these families is in the fourth decade. Because patients lack the abnormally shaped bone ends that characterize the chondrodysplasias, a few of which are also caused by type II collagen mutations, cartilage failure is most likely due to matrix changes.

Changes in the underlying bone, either in its shape or hardness, are probably important factors in the failure of articular cartilage. These alterations result in biomechanical changes that subject normal articular cartilage to increased trauma, even with normal joint use.

Joint shape, as determined by heredity, may be a factor in the development of osteoarthritis. Joint shape is related to body habitus, and this determines, in part, a person's gait pattern. For example, similar body habitus and gait patterns are observed in multiple generations within families. Perhaps a particular familial gait pattern subjects the articular cartilage to abnormal stresses and accounts for the increased incidence of osteoarthritis in these families. The possibility of abnormally shaped joints being a cause of osteoarthritis may have its root in primate evolution. It has been suggested that many joints have insufficiently adapted to the functional changes necessary for an upright posture.[31]

The ends of bone also change shape with aging. Bone ends are continuously remodeling, a process that results in subtle alterations in joint contour.[32] Histologic evidence for remodeling of the bone ends is present at the tidemark, the line separating uncalcified and calcified cartilage. In aging, gradual replacement of calcified cartilage by endochondral bone formation occurs. The calcified cartilage front then advances into the articular cartilage and causes a duplication of the tidemark (Fig. 16–12). This process, probably a response to joint loading, occurs nonuniformly in the joint. As a result, the joint contour is slightly changed, and some surfaces may be exposed to increased mechanical forces.[33] Minor alterations in the shape of joints have been associated with osteoarthritis of the knee[34] and hip.[35]

In addition to alterations of joint contour, increasing hardness of subchondral bone also predisposes to articular cartilage failure.[36] Aging bone contains less water and is therefore harder. This results in decreased bone compliance, which exposes the articular cartilage to more trauma. Perhaps microfractures through the dense but brittle subchondral bone begin the arthritic process.[37] Two observations support this hypothesis. First, patients with osteoporosis are usually protected against osteoarthritis,[38] a protection that is most prominent in the hip joint. Pathologists rarely see a femoral head from an osteoporotic femoral neck fracture that also has significant osteoarthritis. Second, patients with very hard bones develop accelerated osteoarthritis. Osteopetrosis and juxtaarticular Paget's disease, for example, are almost always complicated by severe osteoarthritis.

Although changes in subchondral bone may be important factors leading to articular cartilage failure, other structural abnormalities are probably also important. Hereditary ligamentous laxity is one such factor. Generalized joint laxity is a feature of some hereditary collagen disorders, such as the Ehlers-Danlos syndrome. However, joint laxity is also present in a significant number of healthy people. In general, women have more ligamentous laxity than men, and Asians more than whites. Undoubtedly, ligamentous laxity leads to increased joint trauma and possibly to osteoarthritis.[39]

A final possible etiologic factor in osteoarthritis is disuse. Because the health of the articular cartilage, like that of bone, depends on it being stressed, underutilization of a joint's range of motion may contribute to the development of osteoarthritis.[40] Once disuse changes are present in the articular cartilage, even normal joint stresses can lead to osteoarthritis.[41]

Biochemical Alterations in Osteoarthritic Cartilage

Two important biochemical alterations in osteoarthritic cartilage are a decrease in the amount of proteoglycans and

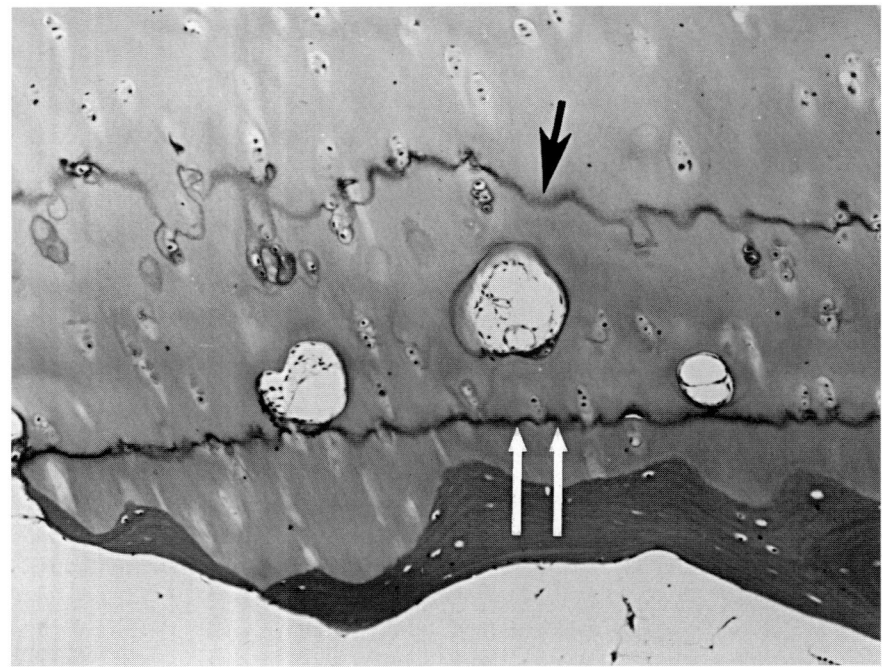

Figure 16-12 ■ Duplication of the tidemark. The original tidemark *(white arrows)* is closest to the lamellar bone. The calcification has advanced into the articular cartilage to form a second tidemark *(black arrow)*.

an increase in the amount of water. Although proteoglycans are decreased overall, their rate of synthesis is increased.[42] This increased proteoglycan synthesis is caused by metabolic hyperactivity of the chondrocytes and is one of the earliest events in arthritic cartilage. However, the increased proteoglycans are structurally abnormal. The proportion of chondroitin sulfate increases relative to keratan sulfate in the proteoglycan molecules, and they aggregate less efficiently with hyaluronic acid cores. Although proteoglycan synthesis is increased, the decrease in their levels in the cartilage matrix results from an even greater increase in their rate of breakdown. This accelerated proteoglycan catabolism is caused by increased activities of normally present active enzymes.

The catabolism of proteoglycans is mediated by interleukin-1. Although this compound usually originates in the monocytes of the synovial membrane, it is also synthesized by chondrocytes.[43] A paracrine effect of interleukin-1 stimulates the activity of various degradative enzymes normally present in the articular cartilage. Most important among these enzymes are the metalloproteinases, which include collagenase, gelatinase, and stromelysin. These degradative enzymes are synthesized within chondrocytes and are activated extracellularly. In the extracellular matrix, they degrade proteoglycans by cleaving the core protein. Then, the proteoglycan fragments pass out of the articular cartilage into the joint space.

The decreased proteoglycan concentration in the cartilage matrix causes an increased water content. As a result, a disruption of the tight interaction between individual collagen fibers as well as between collagen fibers and proteoglycans occurs. Also, collagen fibers are damaged or disrupted. As a result, the swollen cartilage becomes softer and less resistant to forces on the joint, and further damage occurs in a vicious cycle.

Pathology

Changes in the Cartilage

The pathologic changes of osteoarthritis occur first in the articular cartilage and then in the underlying bone. In the cartilage, the initial change is disruption of the *lamina splendens,* the most superficial layer characterized by collagen fibers running parallel to the joint surface. Then, reflecting failure of the matrix, the cartilage becomes fibrillated, eroded, or cracked (Fig. 16–13). These changes worsen until, in certain areas, all the cartilage disappears from the bone surface.

Adjacent to the cracks in the articular cartilage matrix, clones of chondrocytes appear. These clones are evidence of cellular division (Fig. 16–14). The matrix is intensely basophilic around these clones, a feature that is caused by their increased synthesis of proteoglycans. The chondrocyte division and increased matrix synthesis is the cartilage's attempt to repair itself. Unfortunately, the newly synthesized matrix never fills up the defects.

Changes in the Subchondral Bone

Changes in the subchondral bone begin as cartilage damage advances. The principal change is the deposition of new bone on subchondral trabeculae. In some cases, bone deposition is a response to trabecular microfractures. The source of the new bone is reparative granulation tissue, which originates in the marrow and permeates the subchon-

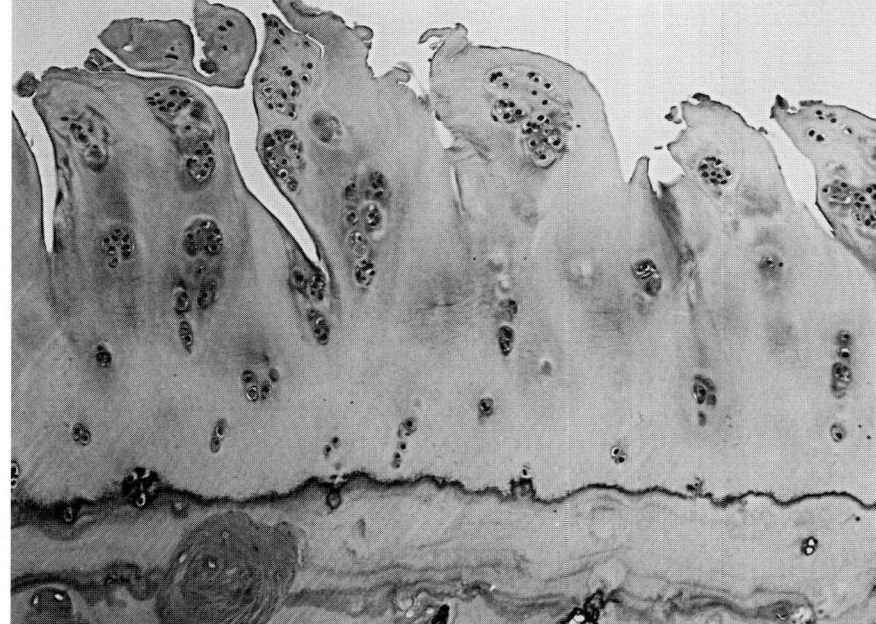

Figure 16-13 ▪ Photomicrograph of articular cartilage with early osteoarthritic change. Superficial erosions and fissuring of the cartilage are present.

328 DISEASES OF JOINTS

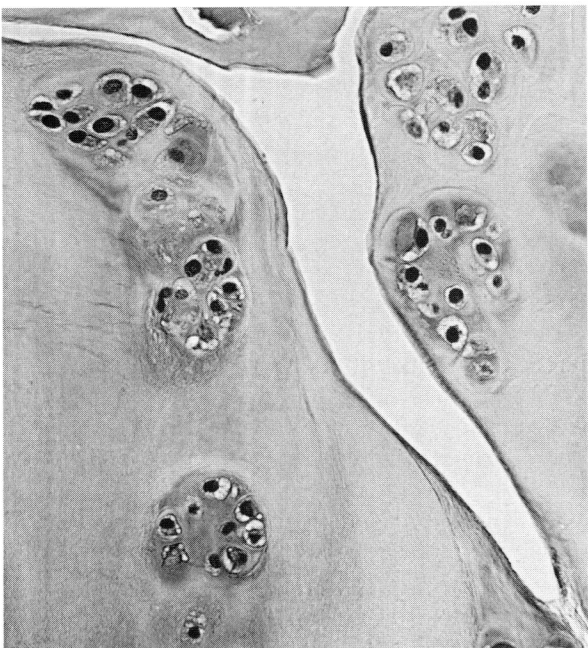

Figure 16-14 ■ Clones of chondrocytes, indicating cellular division, are adjacent to a matrix fissure. Cellular division is an attempt to heal the defect.

dral area of the bone. Perivascular mesenchymal cells in this tissue differentiate into osteoblasts, which progressively thicken the native trabeculae (Fig. 16–15).

In areas of total cartilage erosion, the thickened subchondral bone becomes polished by the opposing denuded joint surface. This process is called *eburnation*, because the shiny, polished bone resembles ivory (Fig. 16–16).

Attempts to resurface the denuded joint also originate in the subchondral granulation tissue. This tissue herniates through defects in the bone and forms buds of fibrocartilage, which protrude from the denuded bone surface (Fig. 16–17). In some cases, the buds of fibrocartilage may coalesce to form a somewhat continuous surface of repair tissue on the previously denuded bone.

The reparative granulation tissue from the marrow frequently undergoes focal myxomatous degeneration. These foci coalesce to form *subchondral cysts,* structures that may reach several centimeters or more (Fig. 16–18). Often, the overlying cortex fractures into a subchondral cyst, an event that has led to the erroneous theory that cysts form by inspissation of synovial fluid into the bone through cracks in the articular cartilage. However, evidence against this theory is that focal myxomatous change and small cysts are often seen even when the overlying articular cartilage and subchondral plate are intact (Fig. 16–19).

Superficial necrosis is another change that occurs in the thickened, exposed bone. These areas of necrosis are caused by trauma or pressure. Unlike osteonecrosis of vascular etiology, the necrosis of osteoarthritis is not segmental.

Another subchondral bone change is the formation of *osteophytes,* bony projections that originate at the margins of an osteoarthritic joint. Osteophytes arise because of abnor-

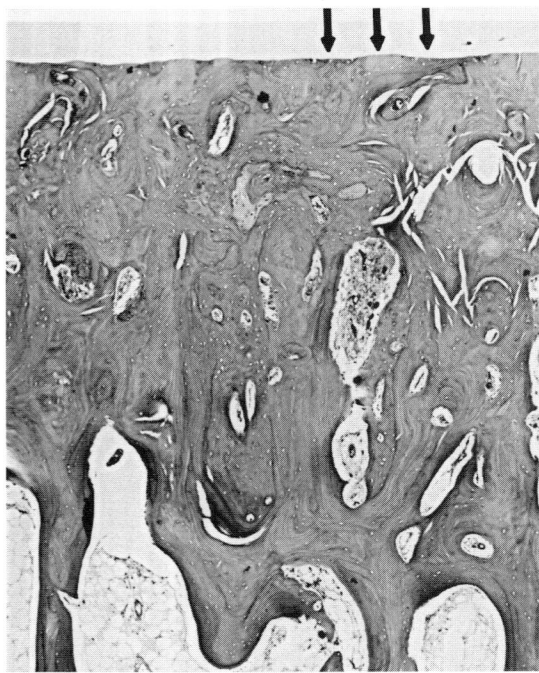

Figure 16-15 ■ Low-power photomicrograph showing advanced osteoarthritis. The articular cartilage is completely denuded. Dense thickening of the subchondral cortex and subchondral trabeculae is present *(arrows).*

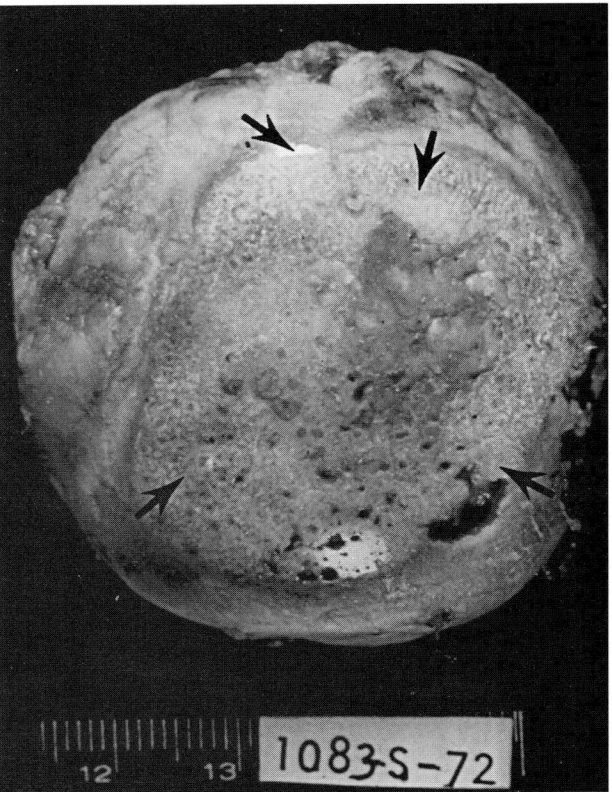

Figure 16-16 ■ Gross photograph of the surface of an osteoarthritic femoral head. The cartilage is denuded and the underlying bone has been polished *(arrows).* This process is known as eburnation.

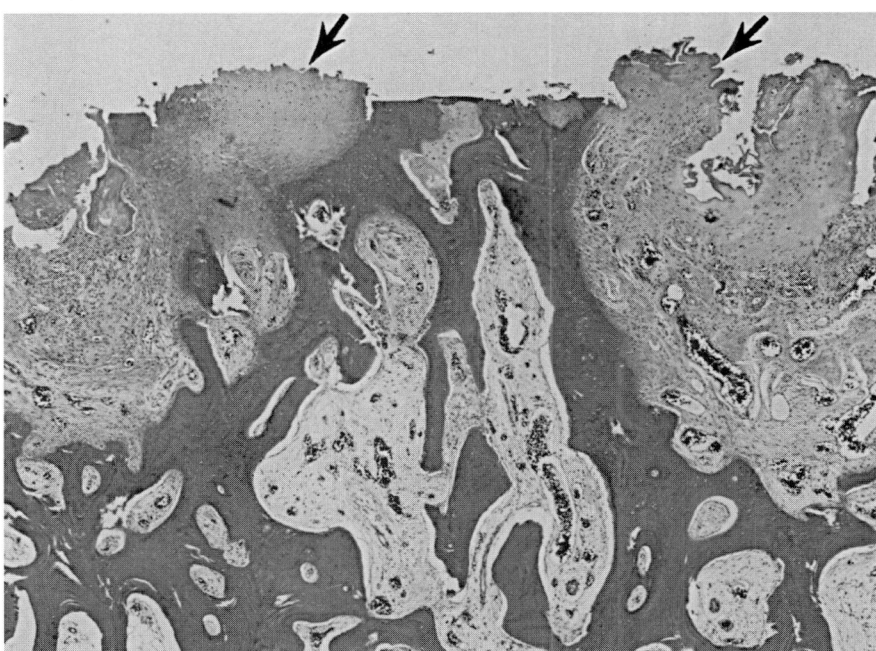

Figure 16-17 ■ Photomicrograph of osteoarthritis. Buds of reparative granulation tissue project from the bone surface in an attempt to resurface the joint *(arrows).*

malities of bone-cartilage interaction, an abnormal interaction that begins early in the development of osteoarthritis. Vascular buds from the subchondral marrow penetrate the tidemark and initiate endochondral ossification in the articular cartilage (Fig. 16–20). At the same time, duplication of the tidemark occurs as the front of calcified cartilage advances toward the joint surface. These changes are normal in the aging process, but they are exaggerated in osteoarthritis. Ultimately, this process leads to the formation of an osteophyte (Fig. 16–21).

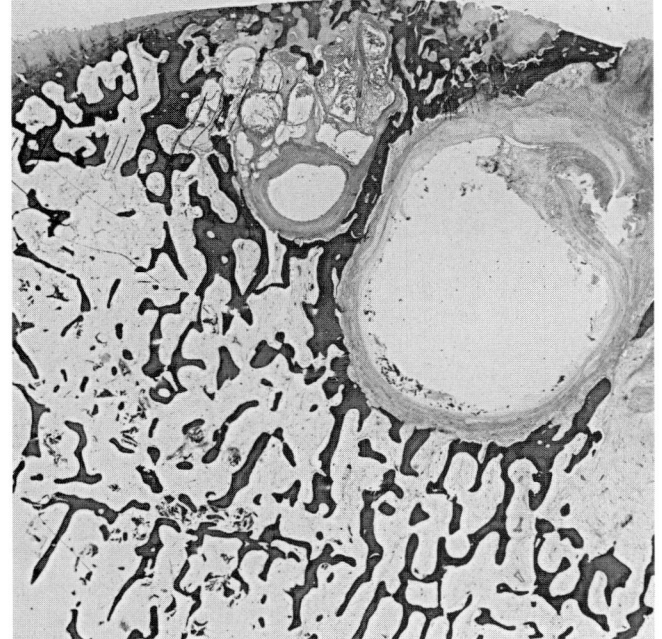

Figure 16-18 ■ Low-power photomicrograph of an osteoarthritic cyst.

Osteophytes form in two different manners. The first is endochondral ossification within the articular cartilage initiated by vascular penetration of the tidemark. As a result, the contour of that region of the bone surface is altered, and frequently, remnants of the original articular cartilage are present at the base of the osteophyte (Fig. 16–22). Osteophytes also form by cartilage metaplasia at the margins of the joint, usually near capsular or ligament insertions. The ossification process in this metaplastic cartilage is similar to that in the epiphyseal plate.

Changes in the Synovial Membrane

The synovial membrane in osteoarthritic joints shows several secondary changes. Edema of the synovial fronds and mild hyperplasia of the synovial lining cells are present. In addition, a mild chronic inflammatory reaction consisting predominantly of lymphocytes usually occurs. A few plasma cells are also present. Frequently, fragments of denuded articular cartilage or subchondral bone become embedded in the synovial membrane. These fragments provoke a more intense inflammatory reaction, a process known as *detritic synovitis* (Fig. 16–23). Occasionally, these fragments lead to secondary synovial chondrometaplasia. Cartilage around these fragments proliferates, and the cartilage nodules detach and become loose bodies. The loose bodies are characterized by concentric rings of hyaline cartilage, often with the original cartilage fragment in the center (see Chapter 15).

Clinical and Radiographic Presentation

Symptoms of primary osteoarthritis usually begin at about age 60. Those of secondary osteoarthritis, accounting for

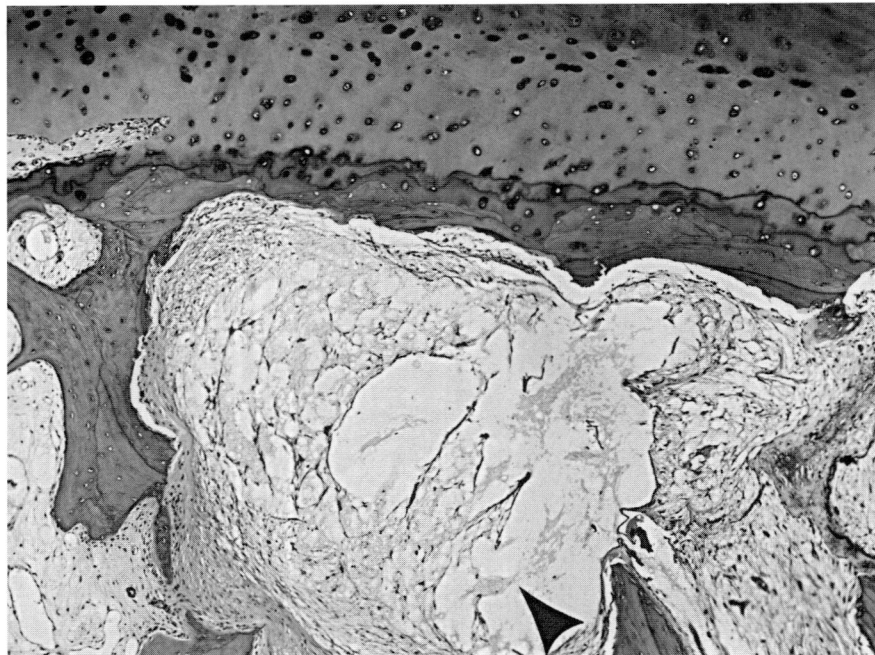

Figure 16-19 ■ An osteoarthritic cyst *(arrowhead)* beneath an intact subchondral plate and thick articular cartilage. The cyst forms by mucoid degeneration of subchondral granulation tissue.

approximately 20% of cases, begin about 10 years earlier. In primary osteoarthritis, an insidious onset of joint pain and stiffness occurs. Pain is typically worse in the morning, but it eases up during the early day. By night, the pain is again severe. In addition to pain, the joints are stiff, and the range of motion is markedly reduced. Usually, symptoms increase over the years, although long plateaus may occur in their progression. Often, other joints become involved.

The earliest radiographic change is narrowing of the joint space (Fig. 16–24). Later, subchondral sclerosis, marginal osteophytes, and subchondral cysts appear (Fig. 16–25). Any one of these changes may predominate. For example, large subchondral cysts, particularly in the acetabulum, may be associated with only minimal joint space narrowing. Osteophytes also may be present with minimal joint space narrowing. Therefore, weight-bearing radiographs are often necessary to demonstrate subtle narrowing of the joint space.

The architecture of the joint may be severely distorted. For example, large medial osteophytes cause a marked lateral displacement of the femoral head (Fig. 16–26). Remodeling

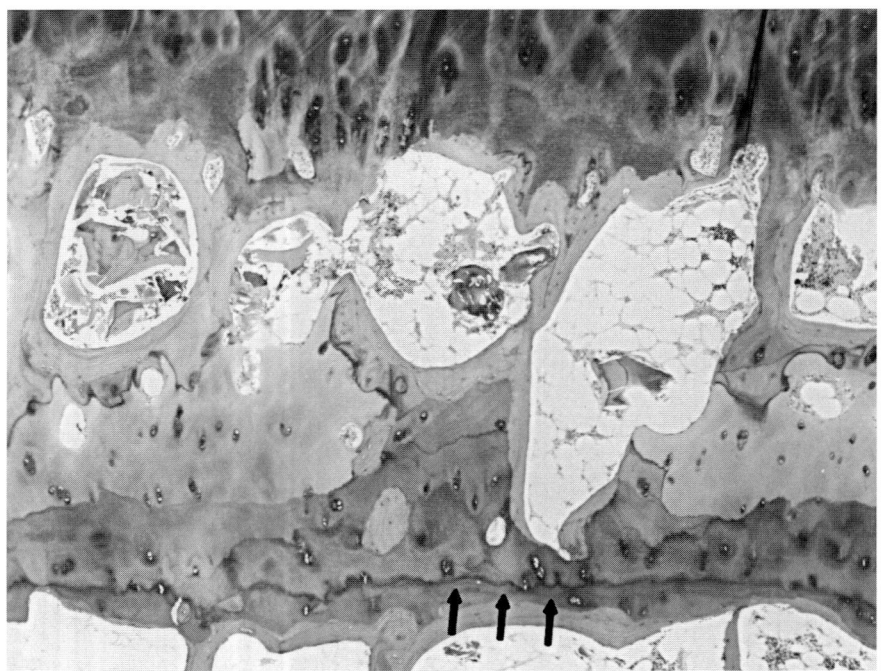

Figure 16-20 ■ Photomicrograph showing an early change in the articular cartilage, which eventually leads to an osteophyte. Endochondral ossification has occurred within the articular cartilage as evidenced by marrow spaces. The original tidemark is marked by *arrows*.

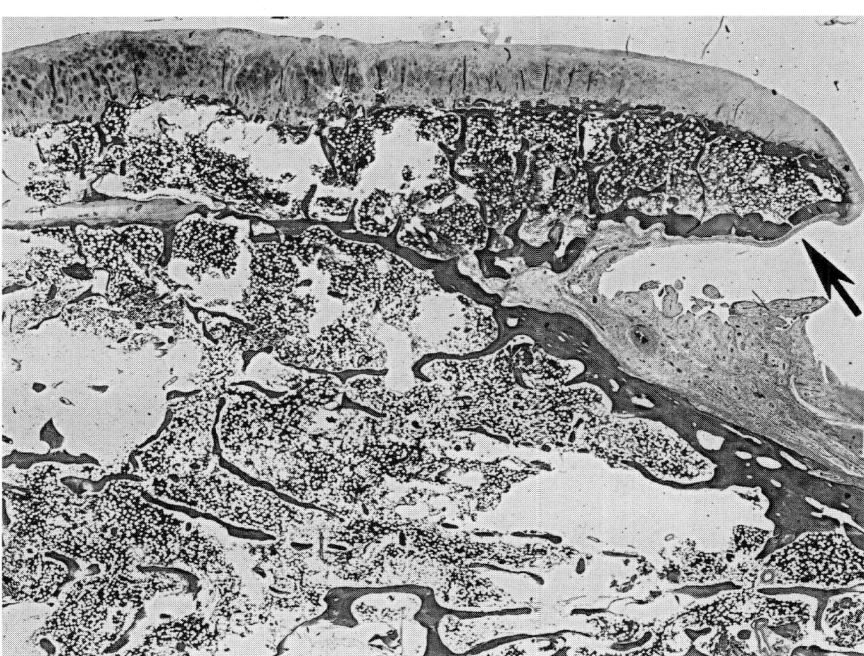

Figure 16-21 ■ Low-power photomicrograph of a marginal osteophyte. The osteophyte is covered by hyaline cartilage *(arrow)*.

of the acetabulum may occur such that the femoral heads migrate medially, a process resulting in *protrusio acetabuli*, the so-called "Otto pelvis" (Fig. 16–27).

The evolution of an arthritic joint is variable. In many cases, the disease progresses to almost complete ankylosis. However, sometimes the disease plateaus and does not worsen during the remainder of a patient's life. In a few patients, osteoarthritis improves both clinically and radiographically. In these fortunate patients, the joint space widens, and subchondral cysts get smaller.

Distribution Patterns

Three major distribution patterns of osteoarthritis exist.[44] The first is osteoarthritis of the hip with little involvement of other joints except the facet joints of the spine. In whites,

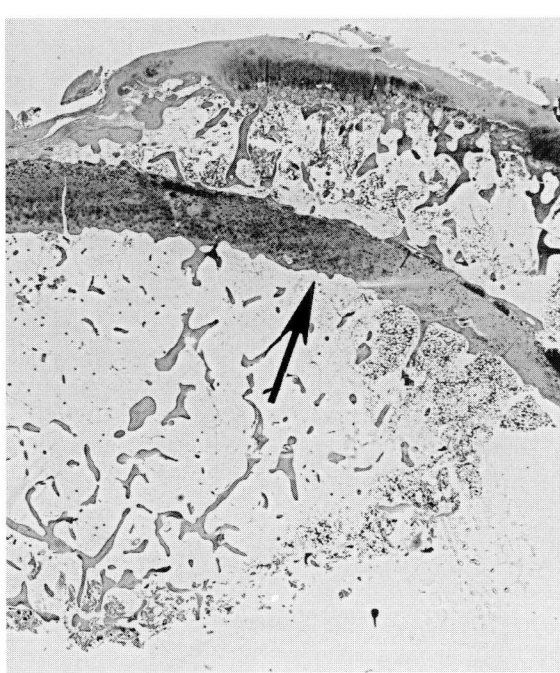

Figure 16-22 ■ Low-power photomicrograph of an osteophyte. Extensive endochondral ossification in the articular cartilage has led to reduplication of the cartilage. The original articular surface is shown with an *arrow*.

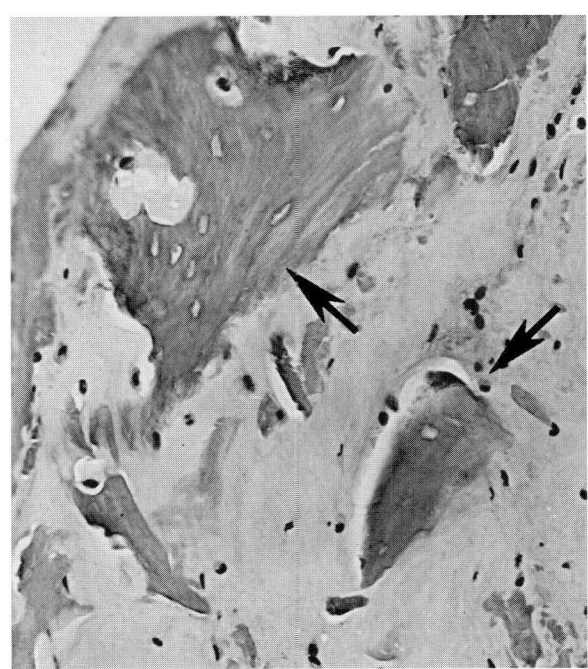

Figure 16-23 ■ Photomicrograph of synovial membrane from an osteoarthritic joint. Fragments of bone are embedded in the synovial membrane producing a detritic synovitis *(arrows)*.

this pattern is more common in men. A second pattern is osteoarthritis of the knee in obese, sometimes hypertensive, women. These women also tend to have osteoarthritis of the hands. A third pattern is known as *generalized osteoarthritis.*

Generalized osteoarthritis, also known as disseminated osteoarthritis of Kellgren, is a pattern characterized by hypertrophic osteoarthritis of the hands, the knee, and, occasionally, the hip.[45] This disorder usually affects middle-aged women and tends to cluster in families. In addition, affected patients have an increased frequency of human leukocyte antigen (HLA)-A1, B8.[46] Characteristically, patients with this syndrome develop Heberden nodes, subcutaneous nodules at the distal interphalangeal joints caused by marginal osteophytes.

Treatment

Total joint arthroplasty has revolutionized the therapy for advanced osteoarthritis. Patients no longer need to spend their older years crippled with the pain and stiffness of severe osteoarthritis. However, the average, uncomplicated total joint arthroplasty lasts from 10 to 15 years. After this interval, many patients require revision because wear of prosthetic material eventually leads to loosening.

Because total joint prostheses have a limited life span, arthroplasty should be postponed as long as possible. There-

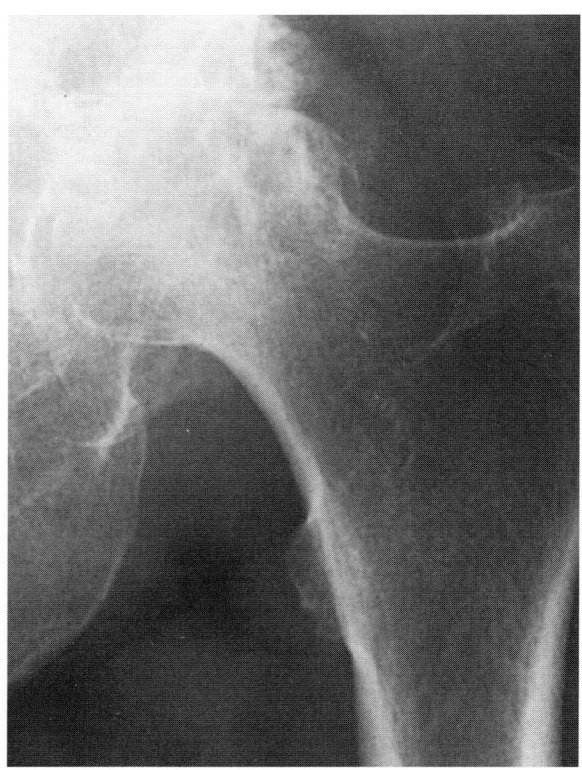

Figure 16-25 ■ Severe osteoarthritis of the hip. The joint space is narrowed, and subchondral sclerosis with marginal osteophytes is present.

fore, patients should be treated conservatively in the early stages of osteoarthritis. Total joint arthroplasty should be reserved for patients who can no longer tolerate the pain. Many aspects of conservative management exist. Muscle strengthening exercises and nonsteroidal antiinflammatory drugs are effective; in addition, walking with a cane may relieve some pain. Obese patients should be encouraged to lose weight.

Recent evidence suggests that estrogen replacement therapy in postmenopausal women protects against osteoarthritis of the hip.[47] In addition to preventing osteoporosis, estrogens appear to have a direct effect on articular cartilage. Also, estrogen may minimize the remodeling of the bone ends, which may have a causal role in articular cartilage failure.

Vitamin D replacement in patients with low serum vitamin D levels may slow the advance of existing osteoarthritis.[48] Presumably, mild osteomalacia exaggerates the progress of osteoarthritis because it induces an exaggerated remodeling reaction. Vitamin D, like estrogen, may also have a protective effect on the articular cartilage.

SPECIAL FORMS OF OSTEOARTHRITIS

Osteoarthritis of the Spine

A form of osteoarthritis, known as *spondylosis deformans,* affects the vertebral bodies and discs of the spine. Although the intervertebral discs are not diarthrodial joints, they de-

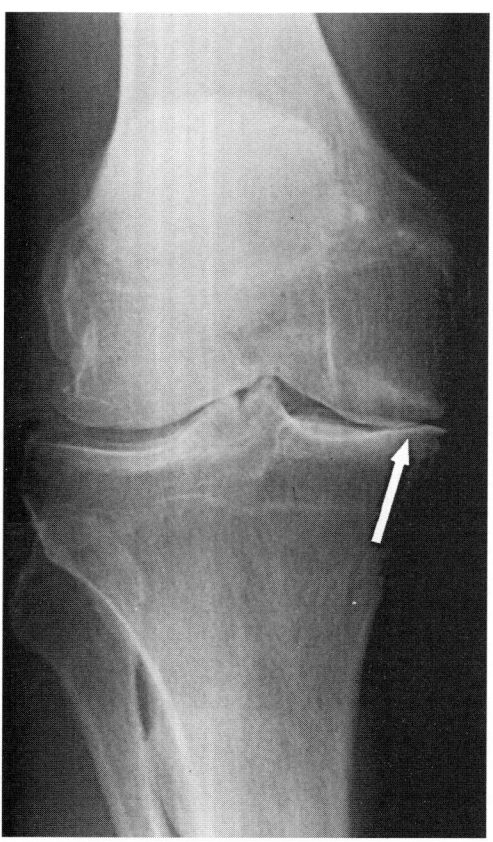

Figure 16-24 ■ Early radiographic features of osteoarthritis. The medial joint compartment is narrowed *(arrow),* but little osteosclerosis is present.

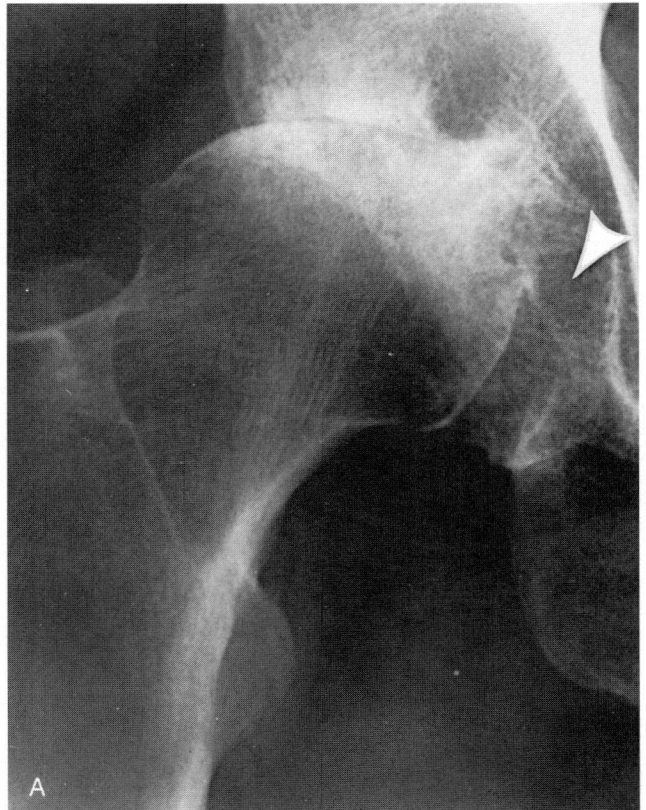
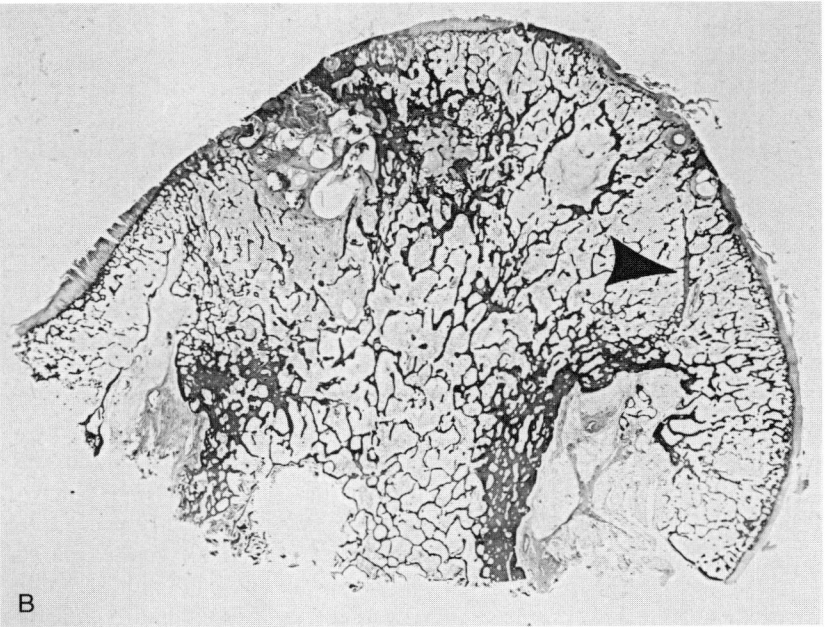

Figure 16-26 ■ **A,** Radiograph showing a large medial osteophyte that displaces the femoral head laterally *(arrowhead).* **B,** Low-power photomicrograph showing the large medial osteophyte. The original joint line is designated by the *arrowhead.*

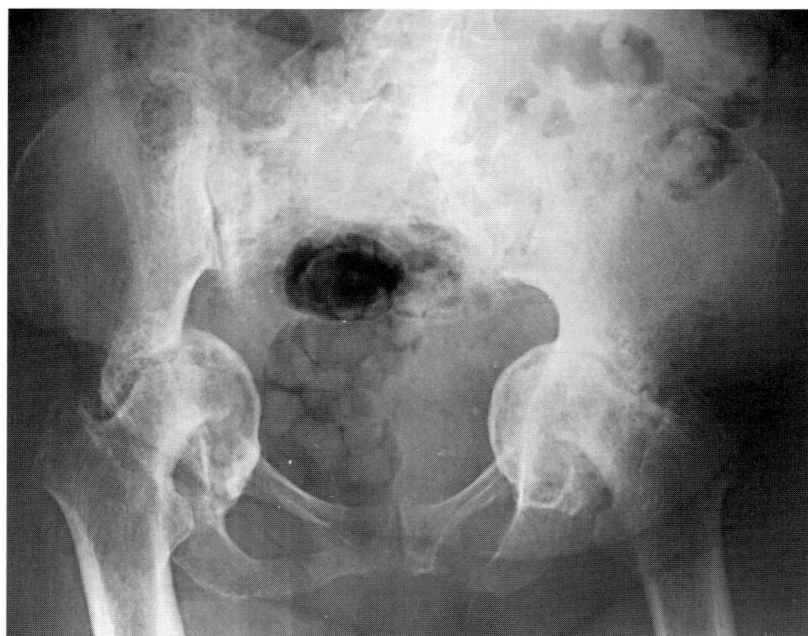

Figure 16-27 ■ Bilateral osteoarthritis of the hips with medial migration of the femoral heads, a condition known as protrusio acetabuli.

velop similar degenerative changes. The process is most severe in the lumbar and cervical spine. This manifestation of osteoarthritis, like that of diarthrodial joints, evolves through a series of pathologic changes. First, the cartilage of the vertebral endplates becomes fibrillated and cracked, and the subchondral bone becomes sclerotic as the disc space narrows (Fig. 16–28). Then, disruption of collagen fibers in the annulus fibrosus leads to disc herniation, usually anteriorly. The bulging annulus fibrosus causes traction of the bony endplates, and the traction results in marginal osteophytes. Further traction at the edges of the vertebral body occurs with the pull of spinal muscles and tendons, and this increases the size of the osteophytes. As this process advances, the traction spurs between adjacent vertebral bodies fuse to form an arched bone bridge between the vertebral bodies (Fig. 16–29). Thus, the characteristic feature of this disorder is the fusion of multiple vertebral bodies by bony prominences covering the narrowed intervertebral disc space.

Another feature of spinal osteoarthritis is the development of Schmorl's nodes. Schmorl's nodes are herniations of intervertebral disc material into the vertebral body (Fig. 16–30). Radiologically, they are lytic defects surrounded by reactive bone. In addition to occurring in spondylosis deformans, Schmorl's nodes are also seen in osteoporotic spines. In this setting, the thin bony endplates easily rupture, allowing intrusion of disc material.

Diffuse Idiopathic Skeletal Hyperostosis

Occasionally, the same process that causes traction spurs in the spine can be generalized throughout the skeleton (Fig. 16–31). This condition, known as diffuse idiopathic skeletal hyperostosis (DISH), is also called Forestier's disease. In this condition, traction spurs develop at ligament and tendon insertions, sites known as *entheses,* throughout the body.

Diffuse idiopathic skeletal hyperostosis is a common disorder. Twenty-five percent of men and 15% of women older than 50 develop this disorder. These figures rise to 44% in men and 20% in women older than 80.[49] The incidence is much higher in certain ethnic groups, such as the Pima tribe of Native Americans, and it is also higher in patients with Paget's disease and gout. The disorder is very uncommon before age 45.

In addition to the spine, new bone is exuberant at the entheses of the hands, feet, elbows, and knees. Despite this widespread involvement, patients are often asymptomatic. Some, however, have stiffness of the back, neck, or peripheral joints.

The cause of DISH is unknown. Most likely, a systemic metabolic factor underlies the tendency to develop bone spurs. Two factors, obesity and adult-onset diabetes, may have causal roles, as suggested by its high prevalence in patients with these conditions.[50] Although the role of obesity is not clear, the insulin intolerance of adult-onset diabetes may have a direct causal role. Insulin levels are significantly higher in DISH patients compared with controls,[51] and perhaps the growth factor–like activity of insulin initiates the new bone formation. Indeed, bone density is generally increased in patients with hyperinsulinemia compared with those with normal or low serum insulin levels.[52]

Patients with vitamin A toxicity develop skeletal changes identical to DISH.[53] Vitamin A toxicity occasionally occurs in individuals who consume large quantities of vitamins or those treated with retinoids for acne or related skin conditions. Affected patients develop arthralgias and new entheseal bone formation.

Bone formation at tendon and ligament insertions (bone

spurs) is the principal pathologic feature of DISH. The earliest change, however, is a fibrovascular connective tissue proliferation at these sites. This is followed by chondroid metaplasia and endochondral bone formation. Then, vascular buds from the normal bone penetrate the tidemark of the ligament insertion and cause union with the new bone.

Neuropathic (Charcot) Joint

Denervation of a joint results in an unusual form of osteoarthritis characterized by either joint destruction with fragmentation of the bone ends or massive osteophyte formation. This condition is known as either a *Charcot joint* or a *neuropathic joint*. Although the condition was originally described as a complication of tabes dorsalis, diabetes is now known to be the leading cause of neuropathic joints. However, peripheral neuropathy due to a wide range of other diseases also produces this form of arthritis. These diseases include syringomyelia, alcoholism, amyloidosis, and demyelinating processes. Depending on the cause, any joint may develop neuropathic changes. In the diabetic, the foot is the most common location, particularly the tarsometatarsal joints or the metatarsophalangeal joints.

Radiologically, two overlapping patterns characterize this

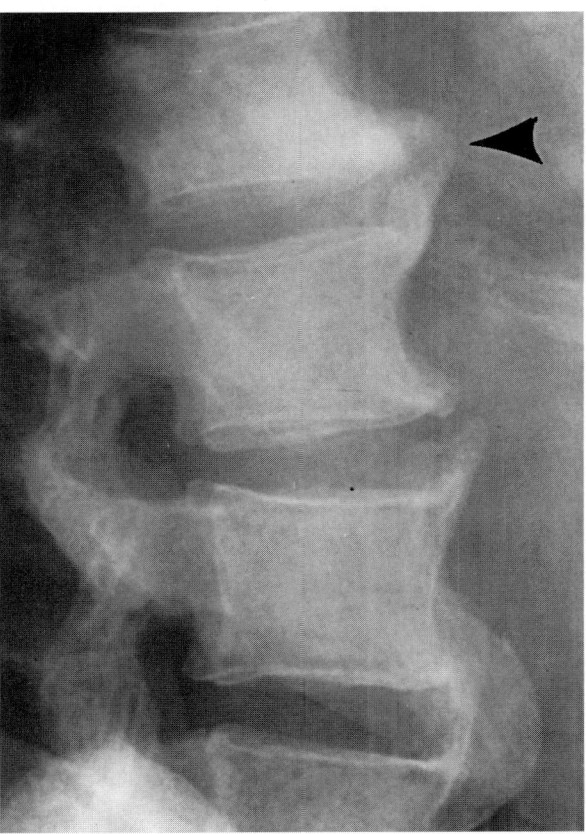

Figure 16-29 ■ Radiograph of spondylosis deformans. Bridging osteophytes are forming to connect the vertebral bodies *(arrowhead).*

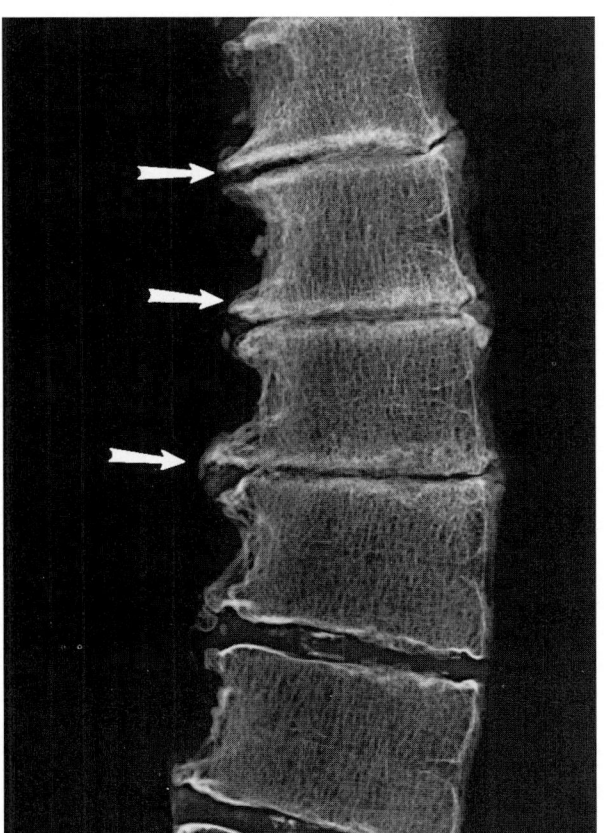

Figure 16-28 ■ Specimen radiograph showing spondylosis deformans. The disc spaces are narrowed. Subchondral sclerosis with marginal osteophytes is present *(arrows).* These osteophytes have not yet fused to form bridges between the vertebrae.

disorder. One pattern shows severe erosive changes. The bone ends are osteopenic and fragmented, and total loss of joint congruity occurs (Fig. 16–32). The other pattern is hypertrophic—the bone ends are enlarged by massive osteophytes.

Two theories have been proposed to explain the exaggerated joint changes.[54] One theory suggests that denervation leads to a loss of the protective function of pain. As a result, repetitive trauma leads to microfractures that ultimately destroy joint continuity. The second theory suggests a neurally mediated vascular reflex causes the bone changes. The vascular reflex leads to increased blood flow to the bones. This, in turn, leads to increased osteoclastic activity and osteopenia. The bones are therefore more susceptible to fractures and destruction of their articular surfaces.

In diabetic patients, a frequently encountered diagnostic problem is distinguishing neuropathic changes in the foot from osteomyelitis (Fig. 16-33). Even more difficult is deciding whether both processes are present, a problem that usually arises in the setting of a stasis ulcer. Making this distinction is sometimes impossible both clinically and pathologically. The neuropathic changes result in bone destruction and a granulation tissue response in the marrow, changes identical to those of osteomyelitis. Microbiologic cultures are usually not diagnostic because patients have usually been on antibiotics. One pathologic feature favors a diagnosis of infection—suppuration in the bone marrow with a heavy neutrophilic infiltrate and necrosis.

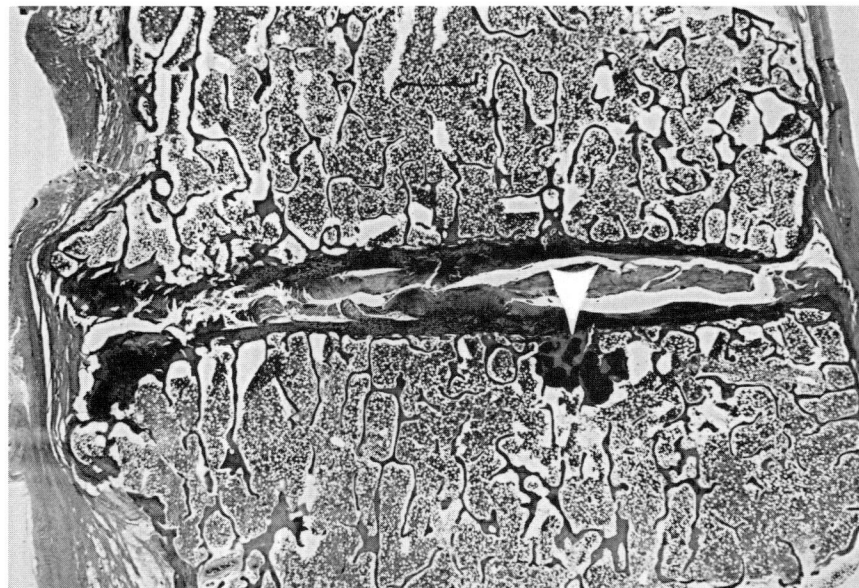

Figure 16-30 ■ Low-power photomicrograph of spondylosis deformans. The disc space is narrowed. Marginal osteophytes and a Schmorl's node *(arrowhead)* are present.

INFLAMMATORY ARTHRITIS

Whereas osteoarthritis is caused by failure of joint structures, inflammatory arthritis is an articular manifestation of a systemic process. Depending on the systemic process, the joints are targeted to varying degrees. For example, in some diseases, like rheumatoid arthritis, the joints are the principal targets of the systemic process. In other diseases, such as psoriasis, joints are less commonly involved.

The inflammatory arthritis syndromes share many patho-

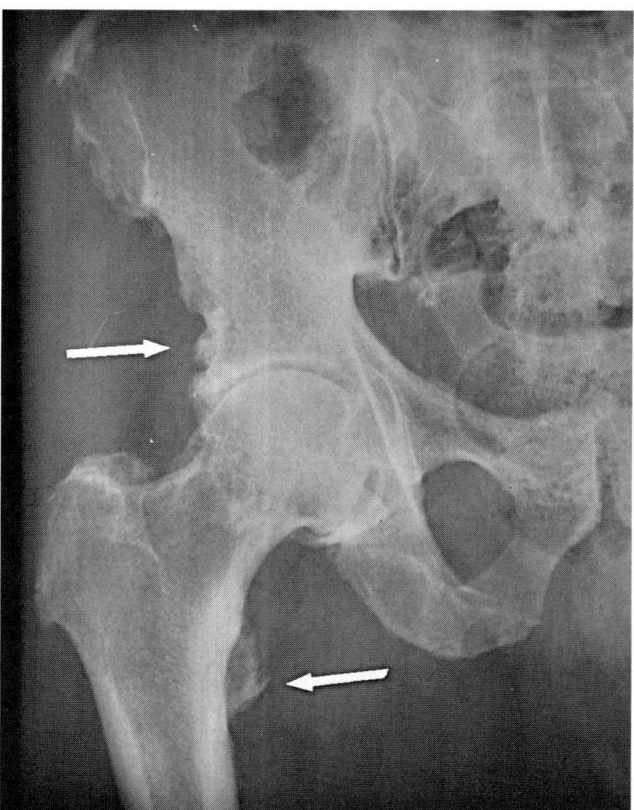

Figure 16-31 ■ Radiograph of the pelvis in diffuse idiopathic skeletal hyperostosis. Multiple osteophytes are present at tendon insertions *(arrows)*.

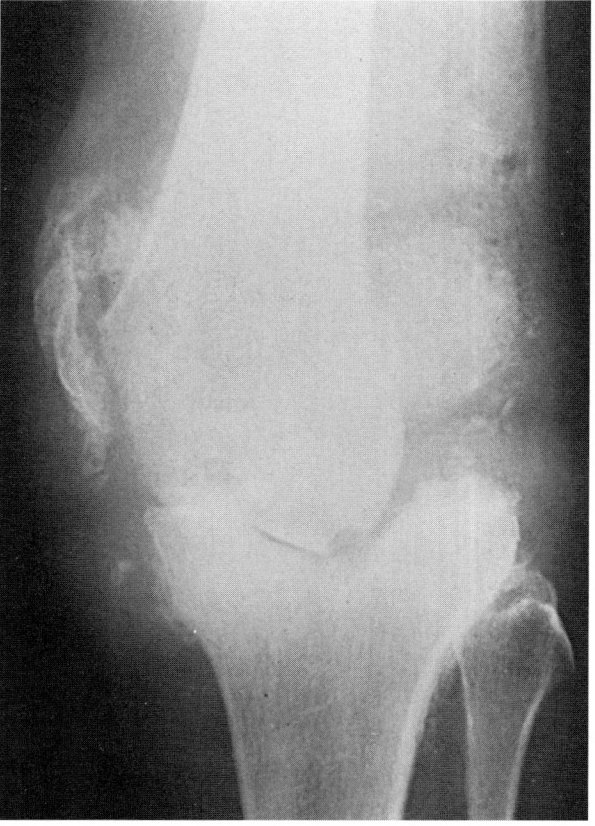

Figure 16-32 ■ Radiograph of a neuropathic knee joint. Extensive bone destruction has occurred.

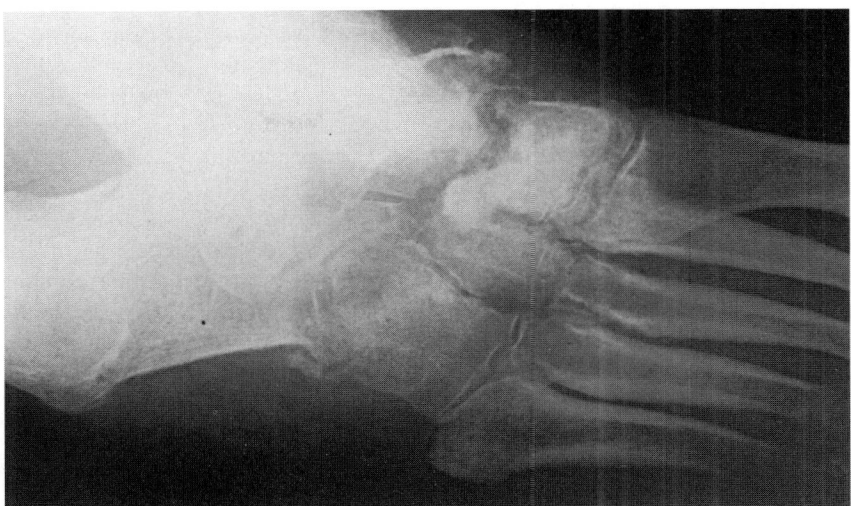

Figure 16-33 ■ Radiograph of a Charcot foot in a patient with diabetes. Marked erosive changes are present in the intertarsal joints.

genetic and histopathologic features. In all syndromes, inflammation of the synovial membrane is the primary disease process, and bone and cartilage destruction is secondary. The histopathologic features of the diseased synovial membrane are similar in all syndromes, and the mechanism of bone destruction is also the same.

The histopathologic similarities in the various syndromes reflect similar etiologies and pathogenetic mechanisms. First, each syndrome requires a genetic predisposition. For example, most patients with ankylosing spondylitis are HLA-B27 positive. In addition to a genetic predisposition, an environmental triggering agent, probably a microorganism, initiates the disease. This agent most likely initiates a cascade of immune events that target the synovial membrane and other tissues. The immune reaction may be autoimmune—antigens to the infective agent cross-react with normal tissues. Alternatively, the immune response may be a hypersensitivity reaction to continuous antigenic presentation.

RHEUMATOID ARTHRITIS

Rheumatoid arthritis is the most common inflammatory arthritis. This disease affects about 1% of whites in the United States, Canada, and most of Europe.[55] This prevalence is somewhat higher in some Native American groups and lower in Asians. Women are affected two to three times more frequently than men. This disease often results in severe disability; therefore, the cost of caring for affected patients is enormous. For example, in 1992, 225,000 adults with rheumatoid arthritis were living in private households in England. An additional 7748 severely handicapped patients were living in communal establishments. The economic impact of rheumatoid arthritis in England that year was £1.256 billion, of which 52% was a result of production loss due to disability.[56] In the United States, an estimated 2.1 million adults suffer from rheumatoid arthritis.[26]

A genetic predisposition for rheumatoid arthritis is clear. In most populations of patients with this disease, the frequency of HLA-DRw4 is about twice that of the general population. In Jewish and Asian patients with rheumatoid arthritis, the association is not with HLA-DRw4 but with HLA-DR1.[57] Concordance in identical twins is variable, but in one study a ninefold increase in the incidence of monozygotic twins was seen.[58]

Clinical Features

The clinical features of rheumatoid arthritis are extremely variable. The onset has ranged from the first few weeks of life to the ninth decade. However, in most patients, the disease begins between the ages of 20 and 60, and distinct peaks occur at ages 35 and 45. The disease is characterized by generalized fatigue and weakness and local symptoms referable to involved joints. All joints in the body can be affected by rheumatoid arthritis. Typically, the joints affected earliest and most frequently are those in the hand, usually the metacarpophalangeal joints and the proximal interphalangeal joints. An affected joint is swollen, red, tender, and stiff. In the late stages, marked ligamentous laxity and, often, subluxation are present. In the hand, dislocation of the metacarpophalangeal joints results in the characteristic ulnar drift. Other joints commonly involved are those in the feet, wrists, elbows, knees, and hips. Some patients develop rheumatoid arthritis of the spine. In the cervical region, resulting subluxations can be life threatening.

Rheumatoid arthritis progresses at variable rates. In some patients, the disease progresses very slowly; involvement of one or two joints for a few months may be followed by a remission lasting a few years. In other patients, the number of involved joints continually increases, resulting in widespread disease. In these patients, most joint destruction occurs within the first 4 to 5 years. About 10% of patients have an acute onset, with the development of polyarticular disease within a few days.

The most helpful (although not diagnostic) laboratory

study in the diagnosis of rheumatoid arthritis is the serum *rheumatoid factor.* Rheumatoid factors are circulating immune complexes formed by an autoantibody, usually an immunoglobulin (Ig) M, to the Fc portion of autologous IgG. Rheumatoid factors are present in 80% of patients with rheumatoid arthritis. However, because they are present in other disease states as well as in healthy individuals, their presence is not diagnostic of rheumatoid arthritis. Other laboratory findings, although nonspecific, are consistently present in this disease. These findings include an elevated erythrocyte sedimentation rate and a leucocytosis.

Pathogenesis

The etiology of rheumatoid arthritis is not known. However, evidence suggests that an infectious agent initiates an immune response.[59] Search for an etiologic microorganism has been long standing. Candidates have included the Epstein-Barr virus, retroviruses, parvoviruses, mycobacteria, and mycoplasma. Hypothetically, an infectious agent could initiate the disease in two manners. First, antibodies formed against the agent may cross-react with normal tissue. Once sensitization occurs, an ongoing autoimmune reaction to the normal tissue occurs. Second, persistence of the causative organism may cause a T-lymphocyte–mediated hypersensitivity reaction. Because no viable organism has ever been cultured from a rheumatoid joint, perhaps persistent microbial antigens located within an affected joint may stimulate the immune reaction.

Whatever the etiologic agent, it most probably acts locally in joints by inciting an inflammatory response. This response injures small blood vessels, and mononuclear cells accumulate in the perivascular areas. Then, macrophages process the pathogenic materials and present them to lymphocytes. Local antibody production ensues, and antigen-antibody complexes activate the complement cascade to induce further inflammation.

Numerous cytokines released from the inflammatory cells, particularly macrophages, incite destruction of the articular cartilage. Important cytokines include several interleukins and tumor necrosis factors.[60] The cytokines stimulate the release of collagenases from the synovial cells as well as from the chondrocytes of the articular cartilage. The result is a breakdown of the cartilage matrix. In addition, locally released prostaglandins activate osteoclasts, which results in osteopenia of the periarticular bone.

Histopathologic Features

All the inflammatory arthritis syndromes share similar histologic features. Although the changes are most pronounced in rheumatoid arthritis, they also occur in the peripheral arthritis of ankylosing spondylitis, psoriasis, lupus erythematosus, Lyme disease, and the various reactive arthritides. Attempts have been made to identify specific patterns of synovial inflammation in these various diseases.[61] However, because most of these syndromes have a similar pathogenesis, histologic features overlap considerably.[62]

Synovial Membrane Changes

Pathologic changes in rheumatoid arthritis initially occur in the synovial membrane. Synovial fronds are edematous, and hyperplasia of the synovial lining cells is present (Fig. 16–34). An infiltrate of inflammatory cells is the most characteristic feature, and the principal inflammatory cell is the small lymphocyte. Most of these cells are CD-4–positive T lymphocytes, and they are most prominent in perivascular

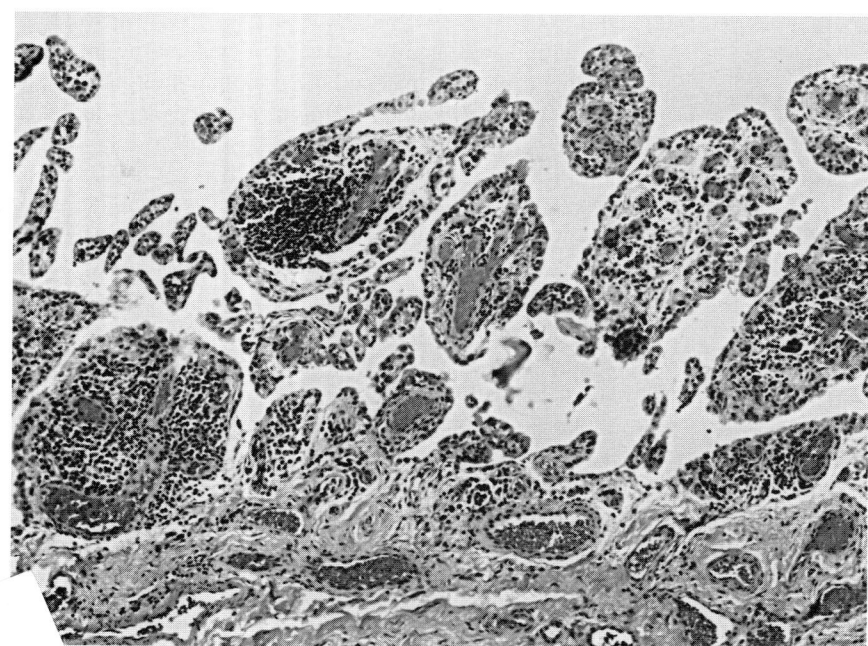

Figure 16–34 ■ Photomicrograph of synovial membrane with early rheumatoid arthritis. The synovial fronds are edematous and filled with chronic inflammatory cells.

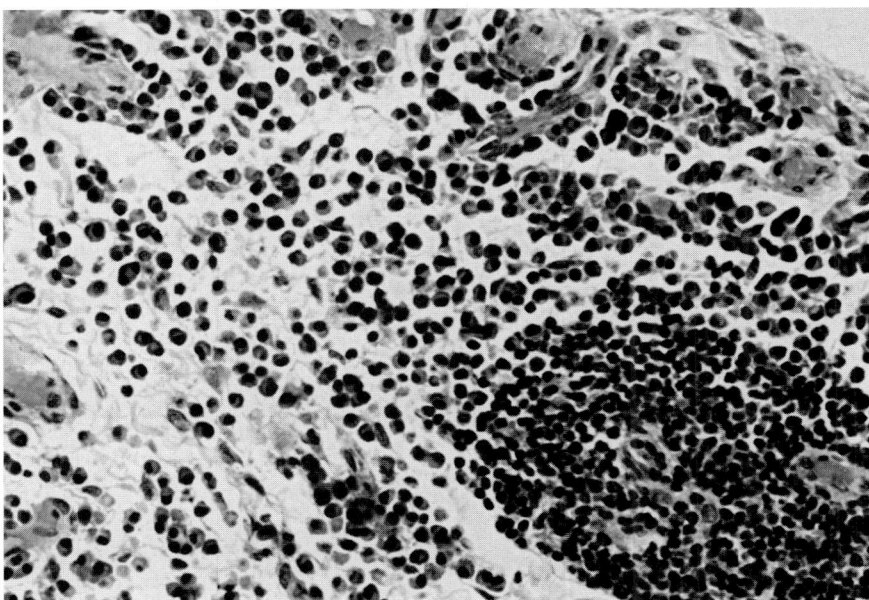

Figure 16-35 ■ High-power photomicrograph of synovial membrane in rheumatoid arthritis. Numerous plasma cells and a lymphoid aggregate are present.

locations. Other lymphocytes, particularly CD-8–positive T cells, are also present diffusely, but these tend to accumulate near the surface of the synovial membrane. In the late stages of the disease, lymphoid follicles consisting of B lymphocytes are also present (Fig. 16–35). In addition, plasma cells and macrophages are usually diffusely present. In active rheumatoid arthritis, neutrophils are also present.

A characteristic feature of rheumatoid synovitis is fibrinoid necrosis of the tips of the synovial fronds (Fig. 16–36). Frequently, these necrotic zones slough into the joint, where they become rice bodies (Fig. 16–37).

Articular Cartilage Changes

The articular cartilage changes are secondary to the inflamed synovial membrane. Granulation tissue originating in the synovial membrane creeps over the surface of the articular cartilage (Fig. 16–38). Cytokines released from this tissue, known as the *pannus,* activate chondrocytes to resorb the matrix. Cartilage is also resorbed directly by action of collagenases released from the pannus. In the late phases of the disease, the granulation tissue of the pannus becomes fibrotic, a change that occasionally causes fibrous ankylosis of the joint. If the cartilage has been completely destroyed, a bony ankylosis sometimes occurs. Eventually, the entire thickness of the cartilage may be destroyed, and the underlying bone begins to be resorbed (Fig. 16–39).

Subchondral Bone Changes

Inflammatory changes also occur in the subchondral bone. Collections of lymphocytes and plasma cells are present in

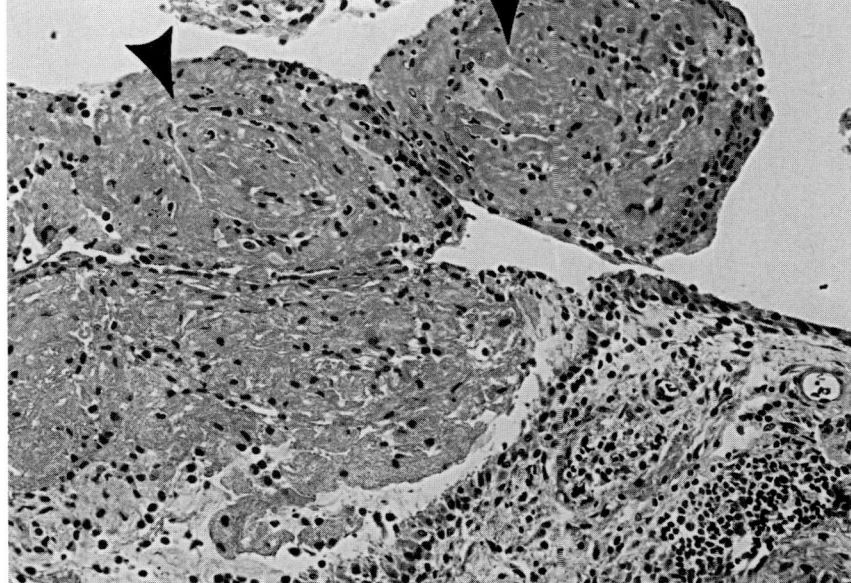

Figure 16-36 ■ Photomicrograph of synovial membrane in rheumatoid arthritis. The tips of a few synovial fronds show fibrinoid necrosis *(arrowheads).*

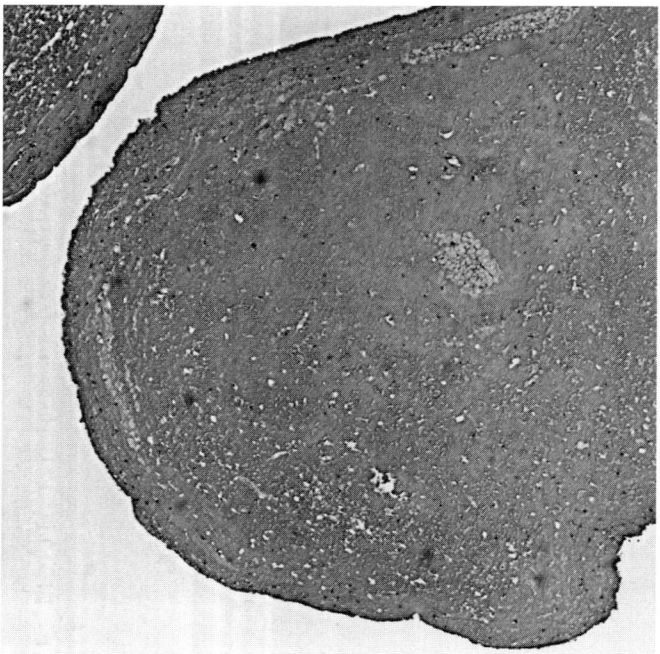

Figure 16-37 ■ Photomicrograph of a rice body from a rheumatoid joint. This tissue forms by fibrinoid necrosis of synovial membrane and is released into the joint space as a loose body.

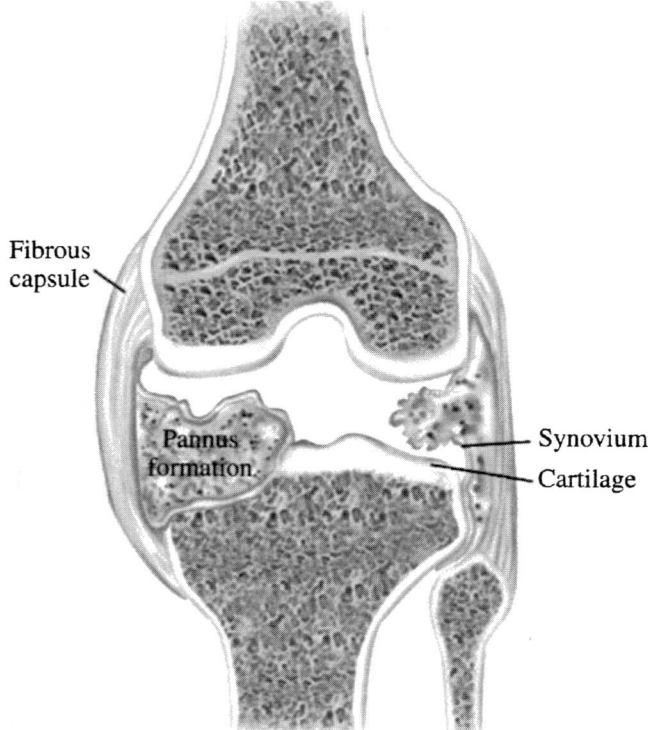

Figure 16-39 ■ Rheumatoid arthritis in the knee. Synovial membrane is hyperplastic and forms a pannus that erodes the bone at the margins of the joint.

a background of loose fibrous tissue (Fig. 16–40). Usually this inflammatory infiltrate is contiguous with the synovial membrane through defects in the cortex or the subchondral plate. These inflammatory marrow changes should not be mistaken for osteomyelitis. In addition to inflammation, the subchondral bone is diffusely osteopenic.

Radiologic Features

Joint space narrowing, marginal erosions, and periarticular osteopenia are the principal radiographic features of rheumatoid arthritis. Unlike the asymmetric joint space narrowing of osteoarthritis, the narrowing in rheumatoid arthritis tends to be concentric (Fig. 16–41). This reflects a uniform amount of cartilage loss over the entire joint surface. Also, osteophytes and subchondral sclerosis are less common than in osteoarthritis.

Marginal erosions are most conspicuous in the small bones of the hands and feet. These erosions are radiolucent cortical

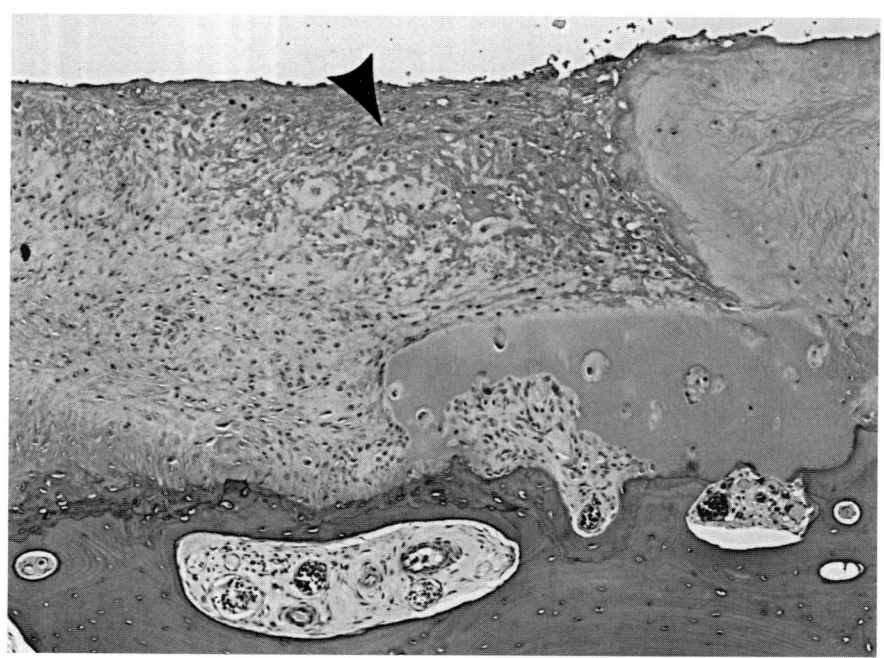

Figure 16-38 ■ Low-power photomicrograph of a joint surface with rheumatoid arthritis. Pannus has eroded the articular cartilage *(arrowhead)*.

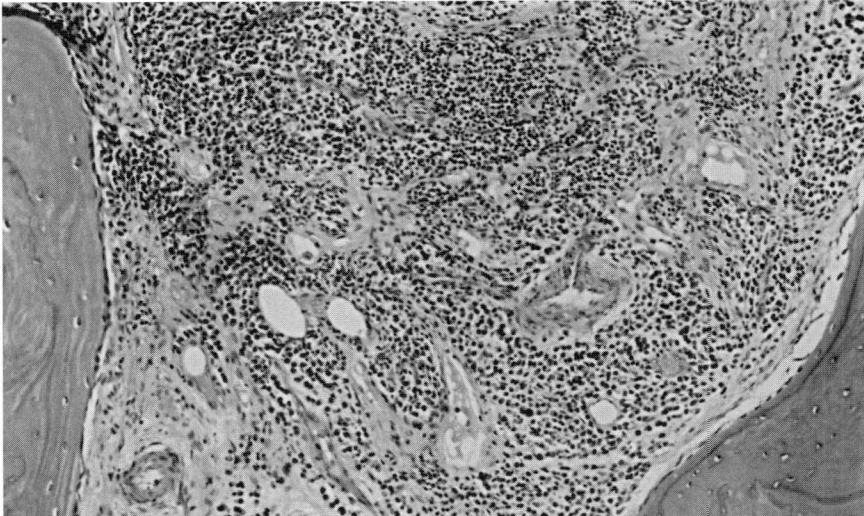

Figure 16-40 ■ Photomicrograph of bone in rheumatoid arthritis. The marrow space has been replaced by fibrous tissue and chronic inflammatory cells. These changes should not be mistaken for chronic osteomyelitis.

defects that usually first occur below the subchondral plate (Fig. 16–42). They are manifestations of bone destruction by the pannus spreading from the margin of the joint. In the carpus and tarsus, the erosions appear as multiple punched-out lesions. Bone destruction at the joint margins frequently disrupts the supporting ligaments of the joint. As a result, joint subluxations and dislocations are common (Fig. 16–43).

Periarticular osteopenia, another radiographic feature of rheumatoid arthritis, has three causes. First, painful joints often lead to disuse atrophy in the adjacent bone. Second, cytokines released from the inflamed synovial membrane act directly on bone to activate osteoclastic resorption. Third, many patients with rheumatoid arthritis are on long-term steroid therapy, drugs that lead to generalized osteoporosis.

Occasionally, in the late stages of the disease, secondary osteoarthritis may become engrafted on the changes of rheumatoid arthritis. In this setting, subchondral bone sclerosis, osteophytes, and subchondral cysts develop. However, these changes are less pronounced than in primary osteoarthritis.

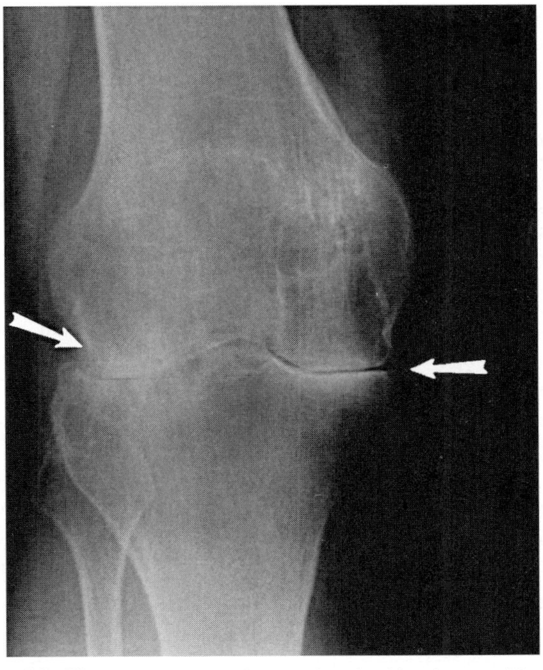

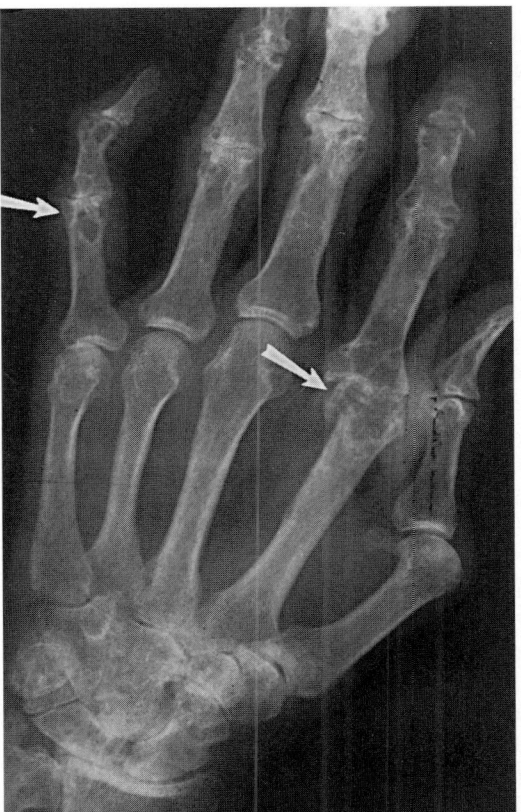

Figure 16-41 ■ Radiograph of a knee involved by rheumatoid arthritis. The loss of joint space is uniform in both compartments *(arrows)*, and subchondral sclerosis is minimal.

Figure 16-42 ■ Rheumatoid arthritis of the hands. Extensive bony erosions *(arrows)* are present along the metacarpophalangeal and interphalangeal joints.

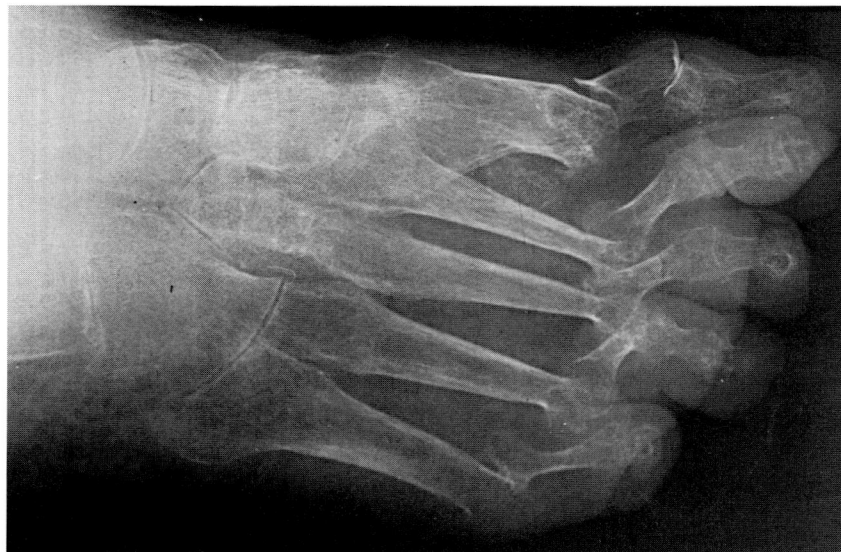

Figure 16-43 ■ Rheumatoid arthritis involving the foot. The ligaments of the metacarpophalangeal joints have been destroyed resulting in subluxation.

Treatment

Most patients with rheumatoid arthritis suffer some disability for the remainder of their lives, and some are severely crippled. In fact, the overall life expectancy is reduced by 3 to 7 years. This reduced life expectancy is often a result of therapeutic complications. Gastrointestinal bleeding from long-term use of aspirin and infections acquired as a result of prolonged steroid therapy are the most common causes of death.

Drug therapy is the mainstay of the management of rheumatoid arthritis. Both steroidal and nonsteroidal antiinflammatory drugs are used in almost all patients. Also, some patients respond to methotrexate, minocycline, or intraarticular gold injections. In addition to drug therapy, patients must continually work to maintain muscle strength and range of motion. Assisted weight bearing and orthotic bracing are also effective.

Surgery is reserved for the intermediate or late stages of the disease. Synovectomy, followed by ligament reconstruction, is often the first surgical procedure indicated. This procedure is particularly effective for rheumatoid synovitis in the hands. Total joint arthroplasty, especially for the hips or knees, is useful in the late stages.

JUVENILE RHEUMATOID ARTHRITIS

Juvenile rheumatoid arthritis, also known as *Still's disease*, is the most common rheumatologic disorder of children. It is an important cause of disability and, occasionally, blindness in children. Children with this disease develop an inflammatory arthritis similar to rheumatoid arthritis in adults (Fig. 16–44). However, about 90% of affected children are seronegative—they lack serum rheumatoid factors. In general, children with juvenile rheumatoid arthritis have more systemic manifestations of the disease than adults with rheumatoid arthritis. Also, unlike adults with rheumatoid arthritis, many children recover completely. Juvenile rheumatoid arthritis is not uncommon. Using prevalence studies, it can be estimated that about 63,000 active and inactive cases exist in the United States.[63]

Three main clinical patterns of juvenile rheumatoid arthritis have been described.[64,65] The largest subtype, accounting for 55 to 75% of cases, is the *pauciarticular* pattern. These patients have involvement of four or fewer joints, and they usually present before age 5 (peak onset, between 1 and 3 years of age). Typically, affected children lack systemic manifestations, and the knee is the most commonly involved joint. Many of these children develop uveitis, which, if severe, can cause blindness. A subtype of this presentation occurs in older children, and the hip is commonly affected.

The second pattern of juvenile rheumatoid arthritis is the *polyarticular* form of the disease. This pattern accounts for about 20% of cases. Some children with this presentation have serum rheumatoid factor. Patients usually present with low-grade fever and hepatosplenomegaly, and five or more joints become involved in the first 6 months of the disease. Joint involvement is usually symmetric, and the knees, wrists, and ankles are most commonly affected. The prognosis for this presentation is excellent. About 30% of patients have a complete remission by 5 years, and many of the remainder suffer only limited disability.

Systemic-onset juvenile rheumatoid arthritis, accounting for 20% of cases, is the third clinical pattern. This is the most serious manifestation of the disease and is associated with significant morbidity and even mortality. Patients present first with fever, a rash, and generalized lymphadenopathy. Hepatosplenomegaly is also usually present. Polyserositis is common, and, on occasion, children develop pericarditis and pleuritis. Approximately 75% of children with this presentation develop polyarthritis within 3 to 12 months of the onset of fever. Although any joint can be affected, the knees, wrists, and ankles are the most commonly involved. The

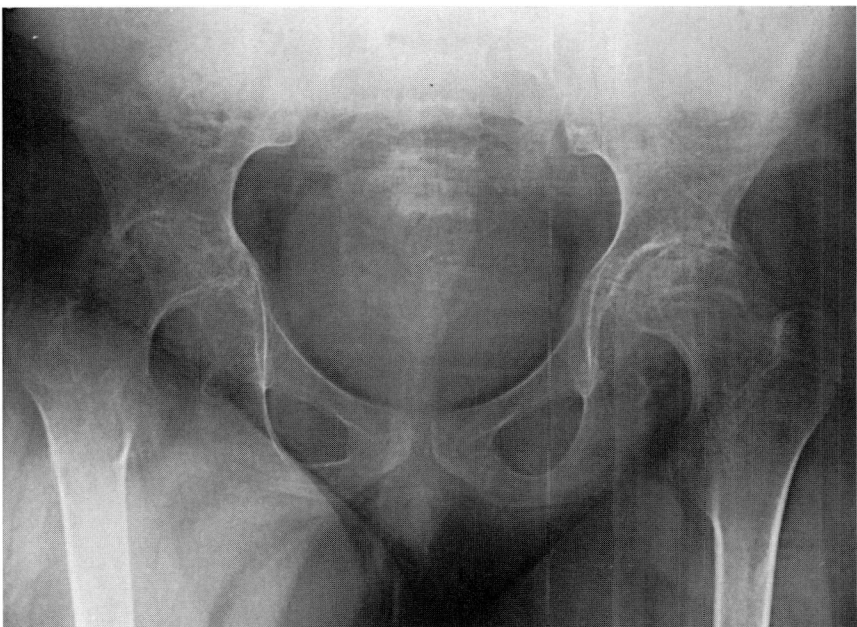

Figure 16-44 ■ Juvenile rheumatoid arthritis involving both hips. Loss of joint space and erosions in both sides of each joint are present.

course of systemic onset juvenile rheumatoid arthritis is variable. At least 50% of patients recover completely, whereas the remainder have progressive polyarthritis. After 2 to 5 years, most of the systemic features usually disappear.

The etiology of juvenile rheumatoid arthritis, like that of adult rheumatoid arthritis, is unknown. Like rheumatoid arthritis, a viral initiation of an autoimmune response has been suggested. The pathogenesis of the joint destruction and histopathologic features are similar to those of adult disease.[66]

ANKYLOSING SPONDYLITIS

Ankylosing spondylitis, also known as *Marie-Strümpell disease,* is an inflammatory arthritis syndrome belonging to the family of disorders known as *seronegative spondyloarthropathy.* Other syndromes in this family are psoriatic arthritis and reactive arthritis. The seronegative spondyloarthropathies have a linking feature—most patients are HLA-B27 positive.[67] This association with HLA-B27, an antigen present in only 8% of the general population, suggests that these disorders share a common pathogenesis.[68,69] One proposed pathogenesis for ankylosing spondylitis is that a triggering microbial infection, with *Yersinia* or *Klebsiella* organisms, for example, elicits an antibacterial immune response that cross-reacts with the HLA-B27 molecule itself.[70] In fact, a striking amino acid sequence homology has been demonstrated between HLA-B27 and proteins produced by *Klebsiella* and *Yersinia* organisms, both known to produce reactive arthritis.

In ankylosing spondylitis, the joint inflammation tends to be localized to the spine, although about one third of patients also develop peripheral joint involvement, particularly of the hips, knees, and shoulder.

Most of the skeletal pathology is explained by changes that take place at tendon or ligament insertions, known as entheses. The pathologic process, called *enthesopathy,* results in ossification of these sites. DISH is also a manifestation of this process. In ankylosing spondylitis, enthesopathy in the spine leads to vertebral body fusion, the characteristic feature of this disease.

Pathologic Features

Histologically, enthesopathy is first characterized by an erosive inflammatory response at ligament insertions.[71] Then, exuberant reactive new bone fills in the defect of the eroded bone, and the eroded end of the ligament becomes ossified. Thus, a new insertion site forms above the original cortical surface. Finally, an irregular bony prominence forms, and sclerosis of the underlying cancellous bone occurs.

In the spine, the erosive lesions occur at the ligament insertions at the outer attachments of the annulus at the edge of the vertebral body. Fusion of the bony prominences of adjoining vertebrae results in an osseous bridge that is level with the vertebral body. This fusion differs from the "Roman-arch" pattern of bony bridges that develops in degenerative spondylosis deformans.

Peripheral joint involvement in ankylosing spondylitis shares many histopathologic features with rheumatoid arthritis.[72] A severe synovitis and the formation of a destructive pannus are present. On occasion, an acute chondrolysis may involve the peripheral joints. In this process, an inflammatory infiltrate originating in the subchondral bone penetrates the tidemark and erodes the articular cartilage from underneath (Fig. 16-45).

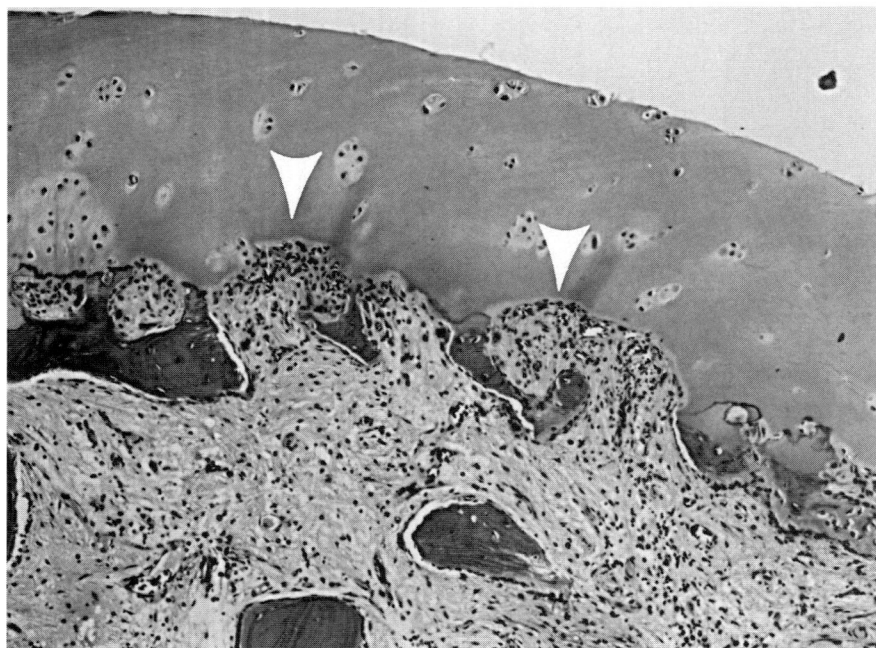

Figure 16-45 ■ Photomicrograph of acute chondrolysis. The articular cartilage is being eroded from below by granulation tissue, which has penetrated the subchondral plate *(arrowheads)*. This pattern of cartilage destruction is often seen in the peripheral joint involvement of ankylosing spondylitis.

Clinical and Radiographic Features

Most patients with ankylosing spondylitis are men. In 1985, an estimated 229,000 men and 89,000 women in the United States were affected with this disorder.[26] These figures are probably underestimated because many patients have mild disease and do not seek medical attention. The disease begins in late or early adulthood, the average age being 26. Onset after age 40 is rare. About 90% of affected individuals are HLA-B27 positive. The process begins in the sacroiliac joints, and patients present with low back pain and stiffness. Sacroiliac joint involvement is best visualized with a computed tomography scan (Fig. 16-46). The initial changes are bony erosions on both sides of the joint. Later, the joint fuses. Because this disorder is not uncommon, any young man presenting with low back pain and sacroiliac joint tenderness should undergo measurement of the erythrocyte sedimentation rate, a laboratory test that shows elevated levels in 75% of ankylosing spondylitis patients.

The course of ankylosing spondylitis is variable. In most patients, the disease is self-limiting and mild, and the majority of patients remain fully employed.[73] In a small number of patients, the disease slowly progresses up the spine over many years. In these patients, the entire spine may become fused into a single bony rod, the so-called "bamboo spine" (Fig. 16-47). Characteristically, severely affected patients are stooped forward, a posture caused by a combination of spinal curvature and flexion deformities of the hip.

Extraskeletal manifestations of ankylosing spondylitis include anterior uveitis, present in 25 to 30% of patients at some time in the course of their disease.[74] Also, on rare occasions, patients develop aortic valve disease.

In most patients, ankylosing spondylitis can be managed conservatively. Often, nonsteroidal antiinflammatory drugs and muscle strengthening and posture exercises are sufficient. Long-term steroid therapy has no role in ankylosing spondylitis. Some severely affected patients respond to methotrexate or cyclophosphamide. In severe cases, surgery may be necessary to stabilize atlantoaxial subluxations of the cervical spine.

REACTIVE ARTHRITIS

Reactive arthritis is a syndrome of nonpurulent arthritis that is secondary to an infection elsewhere in the body.[75]

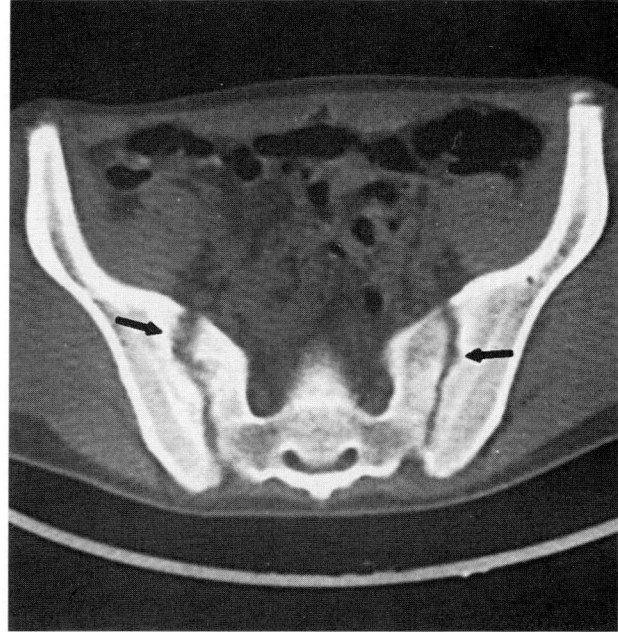

Figure 16-46 ■ Computed tomography scan of sacroilial joints. Irregular erosions *(arrows)* are present on both sides of each sacroilial joint.

DISEASES OF JOINTS   **345**

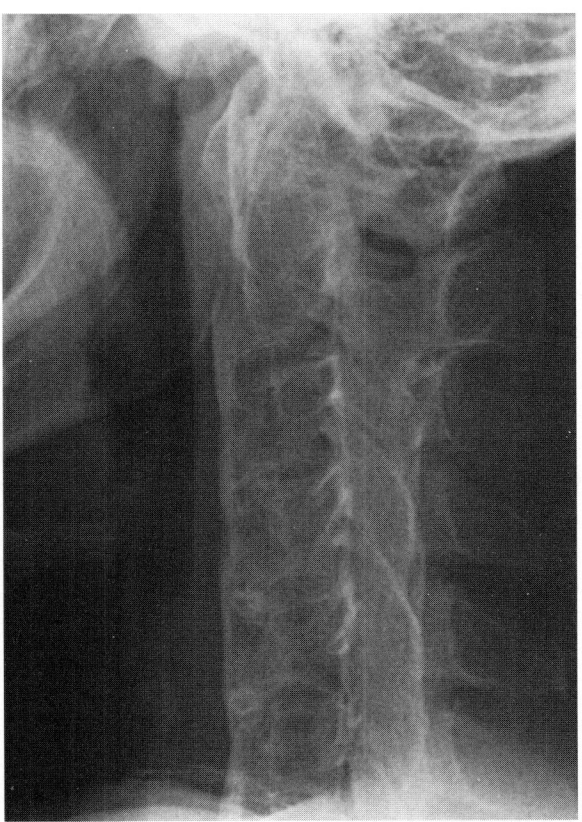

Figure 16–47 ■ Radiograph of ankylosing spondylitis involving the neck. All the vertebrae are fused into a continuous mass, resulting in the so-called bamboo spine.

Patients also occasionally have extraarticular symptoms such as conjunctivitis, erythema nodosum, and painful tendon insertions (enthesopathy). The disease is usually triggered by a urogenital or enteric infection. Reactive arthritis and conjunctivitis following a urogenital infection is known as *Reiter's syndrome*.[76] An important feature of reactive arthritis is HLA-B27 positivity, present in 80% of patients.

Clinical Course

The clinical course of reactive arthritis is similar irrespective of the inciting organism or site of infection. Patients, usually young adults, recover well from the initial infection. However, after a few weeks, they develop an asymmetric oligoarthropathy, usually in the weight-bearing joints. Monoarticular manifestations occur in only 5 to 20% of patients. Joints become swollen, stiff, and painful. Patients often have mild constitutional symptoms, including a low-grade fever. A distinctive symptom of reactive arthritis, a symptom common to all the seronegative spondyloarthropathies, is enthesopathy—inflamed tendon insertions. The inflammatory process at these sites usually leads to the formation of bone spurs. Frequently, this complication occurs at the insertions of the Achilles tendon or plantar fascia (Fig. 16–48). The first episode of arthritis usually resolves within 6 months.

However, symptoms recur in as many as 50% of patients, and in 5 to 30% of patients the arthritis becomes chronic.[77] Some patients with chronic reactive arthritis develop ankylosing spondylitis.

Pathogenesis

The pathogenesis of reactive arthritis is only partially understood. Presumably, bacteria or bacterial products migrate to joints from the site of infection. There they trigger a local synovial immune response. Organisms associated with reactive arthritis are numerous and include *Shigella, Salmonella, Yersinia,* and *Chlamydia,* all of which are known to easily penetrate mucosal membranes. Although none of these organisms has ever been cultured from an inflamed joint, their antigenic products have been identified.[78] Presumably these intraarticular bacterial antigens cause a persistent immune-mediated synovitis. Histologically, the synovial membrane shows features identical to those of other inflammatory joint diseases.

Reactive Arthritis of Inflammatory Bowel Disease

Another manifestation of reactive arthritis occurs in patients with inflammatory bowel disease, that is, ulcerative colitis or Crohn's disease. A total of 10 to 20% of patients with inflammatory bowel disease develop a migratory oligoarthropathy of the large joints and spine. Some develop ankylosing spondylitis. This complication of inflammatory bowel disease is usually limited to patients who are HLA-B27 positive. Symptoms last for several months to years.

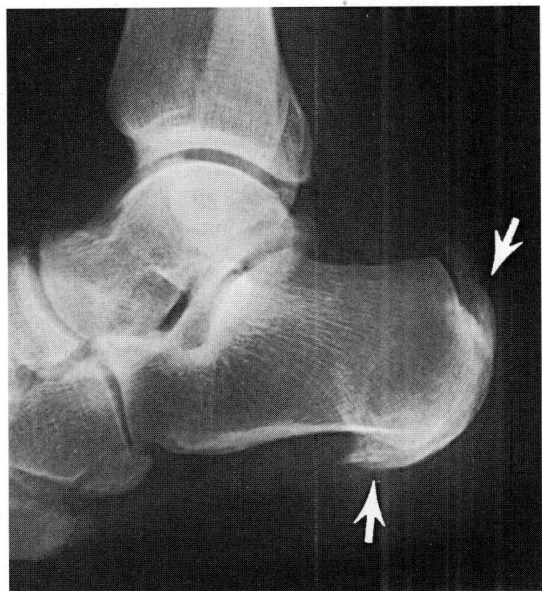

Figure 16–48 ■ Radiograph of the foot in a patient with reactive arthritis. Bone spurs are seen at the insertions of both the Achilles tendon and the plantar fascia *(arrows)*.

The course of the joint disease does not correlate with that of the bowel disease, and only rarely does permanent joint damage occur. A suggested pathogenesis is that mucosal damage caused by the inflammatory bowel disease permits "leakage" of normal bacterial flora into the circulation. The bacteria find their way to the joint, where they initiate an immune reaction.

PSORIATIC ARTHRITIS

Psoriasis is one of the most common skin diseases, affecting 1 to 2% of the population. About 5% of psoriasis patients, representing 160,000 persons in the United States, develop arthritis.[26] Joint symptoms develop slowly but are acute in one third of patients. Occasionally, joint symptoms precede the skin lesions by months or years.

Three clinical patterns of psoriatic arthritis exist.[79] First, about 50% of patients have an asymmetric polyarthritis frequently involving the proximal interphalangeal and distal interphalangeal joints of the hand. Severe involvement at these sites causes the characteristic sausage-shaped digits. Other joints, such as the knee, hips, and ankles, are less often involved.[80] In the second clinical pattern, about one fourth of patients with psoriatic arthritis develop severe erosive lesions in the hands, the so-called *arthritis mutilans*. About 25% of these patients, usually women, develop a symmetric polyarthritis that resembles rheumatoid arthritis. The third clinical pattern of psoriatic arthritis, affecting about 25% of patients, is a sacroiliitis similar to ankylosing spondylitis.

Psoriatic arthritis is probably mediated by the immune system, although the exact mechanism is unknown. The histologic changes in the synovial membrane are similar to those in the other inflammatory arthritis syndromes. However, unlike the other seronegative spondyloarthropathies, there appears to be no strong association with any particular histocompatibility antigen.

ARTHRITIS OF SYSTEMIC LUPUS ERYTHEMATOSUS

Arthralgias and arthritis are the most common presenting symptoms of systemic lupus erythematosus.[81] Circulating immune complexes are a characteristic feature of lupus, and presumably, joint disease is caused by the deposition of these immune complexes in synovial membrane. An acute arthritis may involve any joint. However, the small joints of the hands, wrist, and knees are most commonly affected, and in most cases, joint involvement is symmetric. Unlike rheumatoid arthritis, the arthritis of lupus is not erosive. Although bone destruction does not usually occur, joint deformity, due to weakening or rupture of tendons and ligaments, is common. Patients develop ulnar deviation, flexion contractures, and swan neck deformities of the fingers. This pattern of nonerosive but deforming disease has been called Jaccoud's arthritis.[82] Histologically, the synovial membrane shows changes similar to but less severe than rheumatoid arthritis. A pannus is not usually present.

GOUT

Gout and calcium pyrophosphate deposition disease are the two principle metabolic joint diseases. Both are characterized by the deposition of crystals. Gout is the tissue deposition of monosodium urate crystals, most prominently around joints. It is the clinical manifestation of the various systemic processes that cause hyperuricemia. About one million Americans suffer from this disease.

Hyperuricemia

Uric acid is the final breakdown product of purine, one of the building blocks of nucleic acids. Urates, the ionized form of uric acid, are normally found in plasma, extracellular fluid, and synovial fluid. Almost all urates exist as monosodium urate at normal pH and body temperature. A normal serum urate level is 6.8 mg/dl or lower.

About 10% of all people are hyperuricemic, defined by serum urate concentrations greater than 7.0 mg/dl. Most of these people, however, never develop gout, although their risk for the disease is increased, depending on the severity of hyperuricemia. Ultimately, less than 10% of hyperuricemic people begin to deposit urate crystals.

Hyperuricemia has multiple causes. In some situations, known as *secondary hyperuricemia,* preexisting disease leads to increased serum urate levels. For example, in chronic renal failure, urate excretion is decreased, and in neoplastic disorders, urates are increased because of high nucleic acid turnover. Secondary hyperuricemia accounts for 10% of all cases; the rest are primary. Some of these primary hyperuricemic patients overproduce urates, presumably from failure of feedback inhibition in purine catabolism. However, most patients with hyperuricemia have decreased renal excretion. They have likely inherited an isolated renal abnormality in urate clearance.[83] Patients with this defect who challenge themselves with high protein or alcohol consumption are most likely to develop gout.

Clinical Features

Acute gout is characterized by sudden pain, redness, and swelling of the affected joint. Ninety percent of the initial attacks are monoarticular.[84] In over 50% of cases, the first attack affects the metatarsophalangeal joints, usually of the great toe. Other sites, such as the instep, heel, ankle, or knee may also be involved. Mild attacks resolve within 1 or 2 days, whereas more severe attacks may last several weeks. Most patients develop another attack within a year or two.

Repeated attacks over several years, especially if untreated, result in chronic gout. *Tophi,* soft tissue masses of urate, begin to appear, usually after at least 10 years of intermittent attacks. Tophi are usually associated with overlying soft tissue inflammation, and sometimes they ulcerate the skin. Although tophi usually develop adjacent to joints, they also form in tendons and bursae, especially the Achilles tendon and olecranon bursa.

Pathogenesis

Gout begins with the formation of crystals in solutions that are hypersaturated with monosodium urate. The joints are locations that favor crystal formation because the synovial fluid is a poorer solvent than plasma, and in the peripheral joints, such as in the feet, lower temperatures facilitate crystallization. The precipitated crystals are chemotactic, and they activate compliment. Then, incoming neutrophils phagocytose the crystals and release potent lysosomal enzymes. In addition, macrophages also release interleukins and tumor necrosis factors, which intensify the inflammatory reaction.

Radiographic Features

The diagnosis of gout usually has been established before significant radiologic changes occur because bone erosions require multiple attacks over many years.[85] During the early stages, the only radiographic finding is the soft tissue swelling of edema and inflammation. Later, paraarticular soft tissue densities, corresponding to tophi, may be present. Occasionally, focal calcification develops in the soft tissue densities. In the late stages of gout, almost all patients develop characteristic bone erosions, most prominent in the hands and feet (Fig. 16–49), but the elbows, knees, wrists,

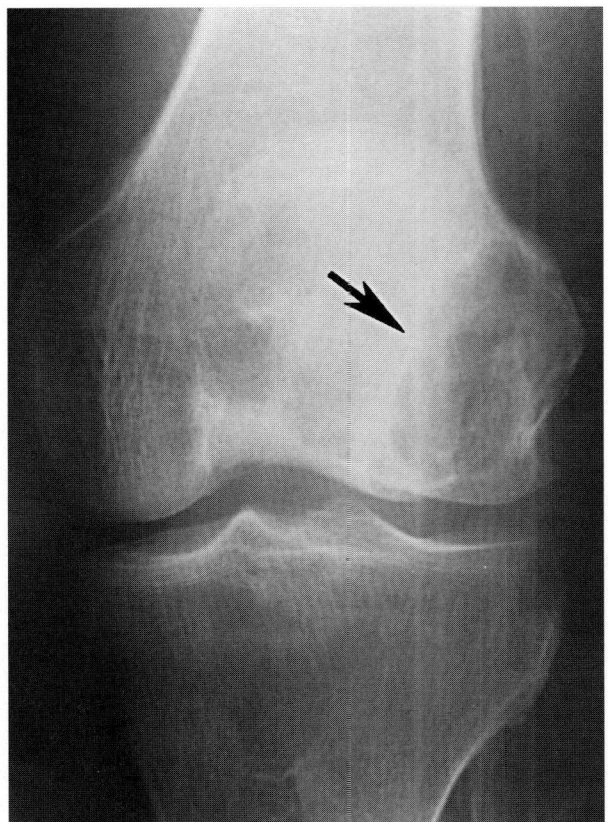

Figure 16-50 ■ A knee radiograph showing an intraosseous gouty tophus involving the medial condyle of the femur (arrow).

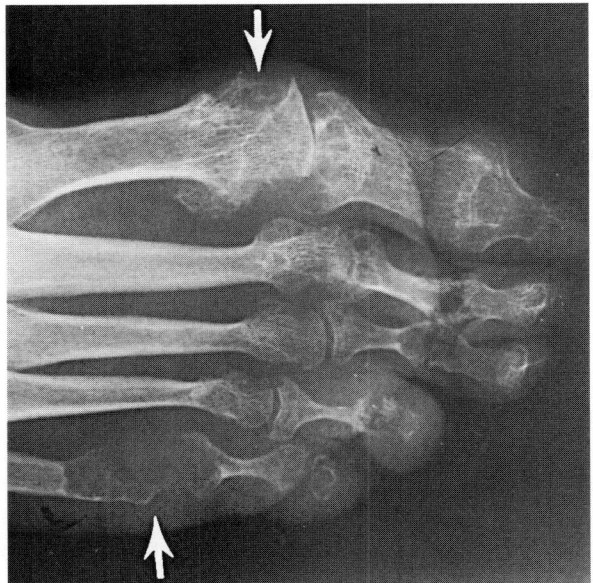

Figure 16-49 ■ Radiograph of a foot in a patient with gout. Bony erosions are present at the joint margins (arrows), particularly at the metatarsophalangeal joints. This foot does not show significant osteoporosis, a feature that helps distinguish these changes from those of rheumatoid arthritis.

and ankles may also be involved. The erosions are paraarticular or intraarticular punched-out lesions, often with a sclerotic rim. Frequently, a lip of subchondral bone overhangs the lytic defect. Occasionally, a gouty tophus may present as a large intraosseous lytic defect resembling a bone tumor (Fig. 16–50).

These radiologic changes are similar to those of rheumatoid arthritis. However, two features help distinguish these diseases. First, gout lacks the periarticular osteoporosis that is characteristic of rheumatoid arthritis. In fact, increased bone density sometimes occurs in gout because of the calcification of intraosseous tophi.[86] Second, the joint space is maintained in gout, a feature that contrasts to the early joint space narrowing seen in rheumatoid arthritis. However, on occasion, joint space narrowing does occur in gout, but it is the result of secondary osteoarthritis.

Pathologic Features

The histologic features of gout are the result of the deposition of sodium urate crystals in the synovial membrane and periarticular tissues (Fig. 16–51). In the early stages, a heavy infiltrate of polymorphonuclear lymphocytes exists in the synovial membrane. Lymphocytes and macrophages are also present. Crystals, sometimes difficult to demonstrate in tissue

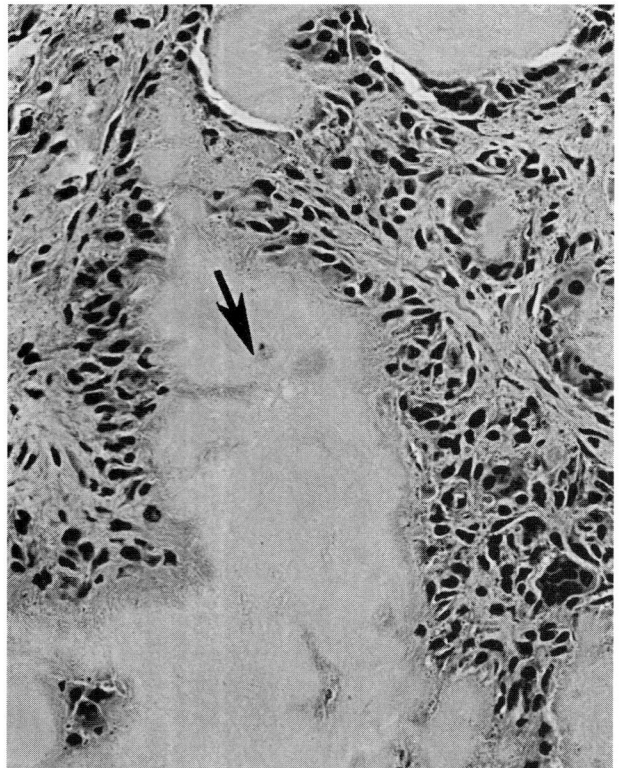

Figure 16-51 ■ Photomicrograph of a tophus *(arrow)*. Amorphous acellular material is surrounded by an inflammatory reaction of macrophages and foreign body giant cells.

in early stages of gout, are usually found in the cytoplasm of the acute inflammatory cells.

Although crystals are difficult to demonstrate in tissue at this stage, they are easily found in the synovial fluid. Wet mount preparations of synovial fluid aspirates demonstrate many needle-shaped crystals, 5 to 25 μm long. These crystals are birefringent in polarized light, and they show a strong negative birefringence with compensated polarized microscopy.

After multiple attacks of gout, tophi begin to form. A tophus, the principle pathologic feature of chronic gout, is a mass of sodium urate surrounded by fibroinflammatory tissue. Each tophus is a white, chalky mass that may reach several centimeters in diameter. Although tophi usually develop adjacent to joints, they also occur in tendons, bursae, subcutaneous tissue, and bone.

Initially, only microtophi are evident in tissues. They appear as small foci of pale, acellular amorphous material surrounded by an infiltrate of macrophages and foreign body giant cells. The acellular amorphous material represents dissolved urate crystals. Sodium urate crystals are soluble in water; therefore, they dissolve in aqueous formalin and are not usually evident in routine histologic sections. In cases of suspected gout, the surgeon or pathologist should fix a small portion of diseased tissue in 100% ethanol, a fixative that preserves the crystals. Microtophi are sometimes mistaken for small caseating granulomas. Because negative stains for microorganisms do not necessarily rule out an infection, clinical and radiographic correlation is usually necessary.

In addition to microtophi, the synovial membrane shows other changes. A diffuse synovitis and fibrosis can be seen. The hyperplastic synovial membrane, loaded with sodium urate, erodes the adjacent bone and often undermines the articular cartilage. The bone erosions are continuous with the soft tissue component of the tophus.

Treatment

Although surgery is occasionally required to reconstruct bone lesions produced by tophi, drug therapy is the mainstay in treating patients with gout. Therapy of gout is directed to the management of acute attacks and the prevention of further attacks.[87] In managing the acute affects, the nonsteroidal antiinflammatory drugs, such as indomethacin, are effective. With these drugs, pain begins to ease within a few hours after administration. In those patients in whom nonsteroidal antiinflammatory drugs are contraindicated, colchicine, a drug that inhibits crystal phagocytosis, offers relief of acute attacks. However, the therapeutic and toxic levels of colchicine are very close, and patients usually experience nausea and vomiting. Steroids may be useful in severe attacks.

Managing hyperuricemia is necessary to prevent future attacks. No advantage is seen in treating asymptomatic hyperuricemia. However, once an attack of gout has occurred, lowering serum uric acid reduces the number and severity of future attacks. Dietary management is crucial. Low-protein diets and abstinence from alcohol can reduce serum urate levels. In addition, allopurinol, a xanthine oxidase inhibitor, promotes renal excretion of urates. In fact, this drug often reduces serum urate levels to normal.

CALCIUM PYROPHOSPHATE DEPOSITION DISEASE

Calcium pyrophosphate deposition disease (CPPD) is the other important metabolic arthritis characterized by crystal deposition in joints. In this disorder, calcium pyrophosphate crystals are deposited in hyaline cartilage or fibrocartilage, a process that results in several overlapping clinical syndromes.

Pathogenesis

Calcium pyrophosphate deposition disease is most probably caused by an inherited metabolic defect that results in the failure of chondrocytes to properly maintain the extracellular matrix. As a result of the matrix alteration, calcium pyrophosphate crystals form adjacent to the chondrocytes.[88] Then, crystals are shed from the cartilage into the joint, where they seed other tissues, such as synovial membrane, ligaments, and the joint capsule.

The metabolic defect resulting in crystal formation is expressed in various settings. First, it may occur spontaneously in numerous members of certain families and show an autosomal dominant pattern of inheritance. Second, the defect may be unmasked in some patients following joint trauma (including meniscectomy) or following a major illness such as a stroke or a myocardial infarction. Third, a tendency to form crystals may be stimulated by other metabolic or endocrine diseases, such as hyperparathyroidism, hypercalcemia, gout, or hemochromatosis. Finally and most commonly, crystals may form as patients grow old. Six percent of adults older than 70 years have calcium pyrophosphate deposits in their joints.

Clinical Manifestations

Calcium pyrophosphate deposition is associated with several clinical manifestations.[89] Many patients are asymptomatic, and joint calcifications are noted incidentally on radiographs taken for other reasons. Symptomatic patients can be classified as having one of two principal overlapping syndromes. The first, known as *pseudogout*, is an acute synovitis due to the showering of the joint with calcium pyrophosphate crystals released from the articular cartilage. Pseudogout is the most common cause of an acute arthritis in the elderly. One or more joints may be involved, the knee being the most common site. Twenty-five percent of patients with calcium pyrophosphate deposition disease present with the syndrome.

The other major syndrome, *chronic pyrophosphate arthropathy*, mimics primary osteoarthritis. Chronic pyrophosphate arthropathy commonly affects the knees, hips, wrists, and metacarpophalangeal joints of the hand. Whether calcium pyrophosphate crystals actually cause this form of osteoarthritis or if they just modify an existing arthritic process has not been determined. A less common syndrome of CPPD mimics rheumatoid arthritis. Finally, an unusual manifestation of CPPD is the tumoral deposition of crystals in periarticular soft tissue. Patients with tumoral deposition of calcium pyrophosphate, known as *tophaceous pseudogout*, may be misdiagnosed as having a bone or cartilage neoplasm (see Chapter 14).

The radiologic term for the deposition of calcium pyrophosphate in joints is *chondrocalcinosis*. Punctate or linear intraarticular calcifications are present with the menisci, intervertebral discs, or articular cartilage or in tendon insertions. The knee is most commonly involved, but other sites include the hip, the symphysis pubis, the spine, and the wrist (Fig. 16–52).

Radiographs in chronic pyrophosphate arthropathy show joint space narrowing and subchondral sclerosis, the same changes seen in osteoarthritis. However, additional radiologic features may suggest that calcium pyrophosphate deposition is contributing to (or causing) the process. First, large subchondral cysts are suggestive of chronic pyrophosphate arthropathy, and second, unusual hook-shaped osteophytes are also characteristic features. In the knee, the patellofemoral compartment is usually involved, a rare finding in primary osteoarthritis that is uncomplicated by calcium pyrophosphate deposits.

Pathologists encounter calcium pyrophosphate crystals in three types of specimens. First, they may be found in intervertebral disc material removed for degenerative disc disease. Second, they are sometimes found in total joint arthroplasty specimens. In these specimens, the crystals may

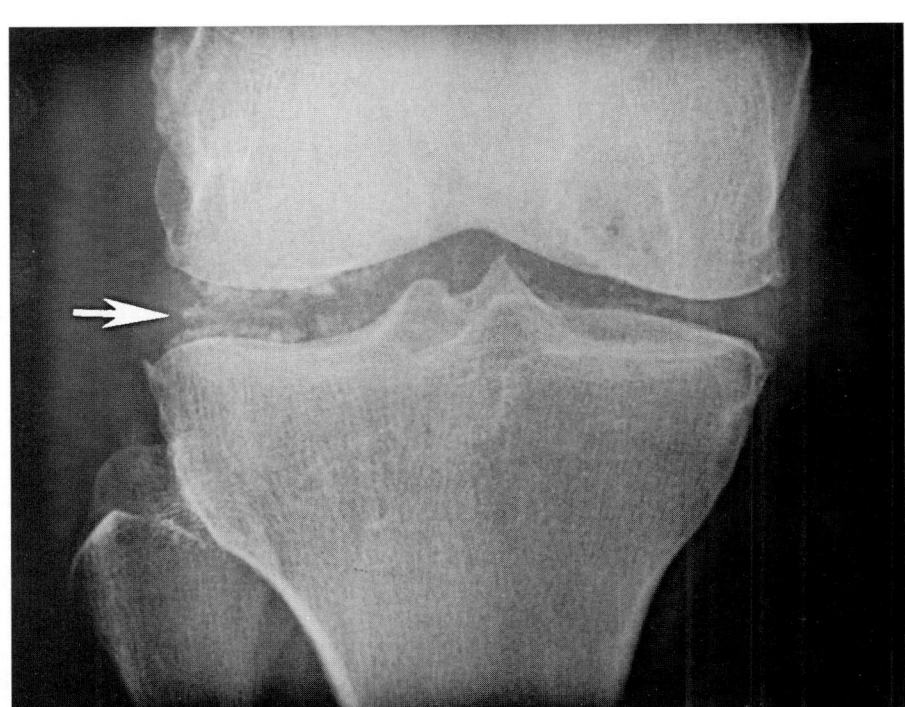

Figure 16–52 ■ Chondrocalcinosis of the knee. Calcifications are present in the articular cartilage of both the femur and tibia as well as in the intervening meniscus *(arrow)*. (From McCarthy, E. F.: *Differential Diagnosis in Pathology. Bone and Joint Disorders.* New York and Tokyo, Igaku-Shoin, 1996. With permission from Williams & Wilkins.)

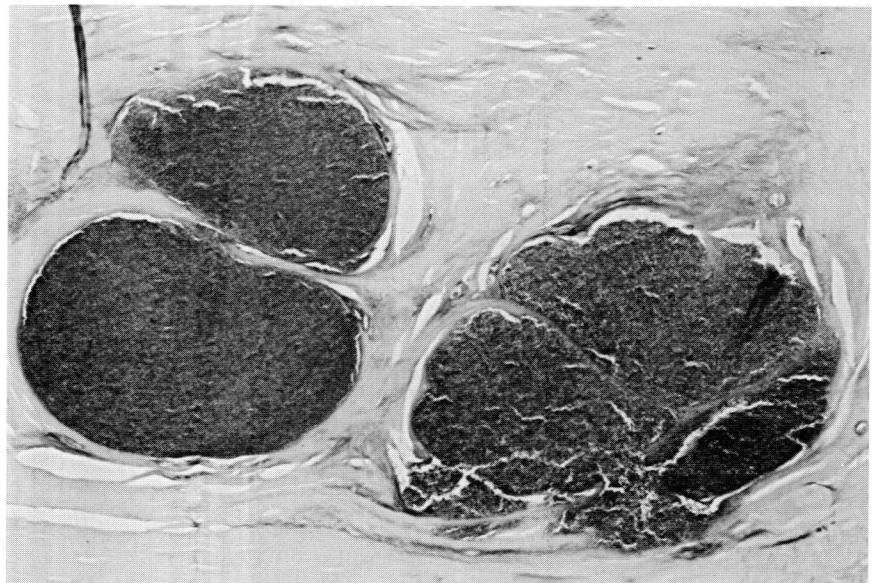

Figure 16-53 ■ Low-power photomicrograph of calcium pyrophosphate deposition disease. The calcium crystals are well-defined clusters of deeply basophilic material.

be present in the articular cartilage, the synovial membrane, the menisci, or the joint capsule. Third, they may be found in small fragments of joint tissue removed during arthroscopy. In this event, the crystals may have prognostic significance.

Histologically, discrete foci of deeply basophilic calcifications are present in the tissues (Fig. 16–53). The calcium pyrophosphate crystals have a uniform rhomboid configuration (1–5 μm long) and show a weak positive birefringence in polarized light (Fig. 16–54). In the articular cartilage and in fibrocartilage, the calcifications characteristically lack an inflammatory or foreign body reaction. By contrast, calcium pyrophosphate crystals in synovial membrane are associated with inflammation. Even when calcium pyrophosphate crystals are inapparent, changes in the cartilage indicate the presence of the disorder. These changes include focal mucoid degeneration and loss of basophilia of the extracellular matrix. In addition, adjacent chondrocytes are usually hypertrophic. These changes precede the deposition of crystals and are diagnostic of CPPD.

The treatment of CPPD is symptomatic. Although the tendency to form crystals cannot be reduced, symptoms can be lessened with nonsteroidal antiinflammatory drugs. Advanced disease, however, such as chronic pyrophosphate arthropathy, usually requires total joint arthroplasty.

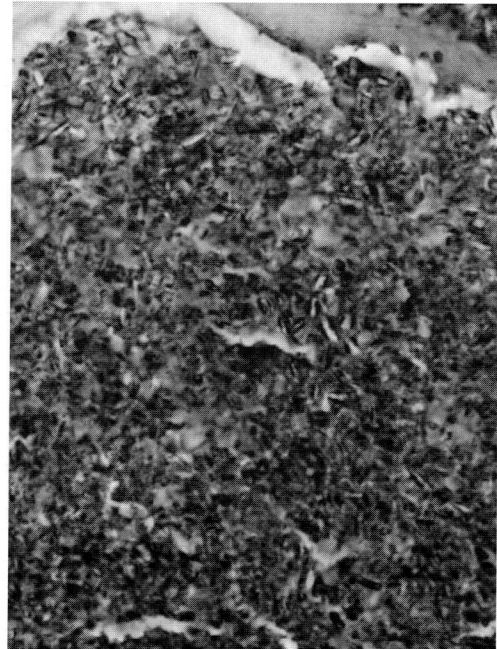

Figure 16-54 ■ High-power photomicrograph of calcium pyrophosphate deposition disease. Small rhomboid crystals are visible in the deeply basophilic material.

REFERENCES

1. Dieppe, P., and Paine, T.: Referral guidelines for general practitioners—which patients with limb joint arthritis should be sent to a rheumatologist. *ARC Report Rheum Dis* 1, 1994.
2. Miedema, H. S.: *Reuma Onderzoek Meedere Echelons (ROME): basisrapport.* Leiden, 1994.
3. Cunningham, L. S., and Kelsey, J. L.: Epidemiology of musculoskeletal impairments and associated disability. *Am J Public Health* 74:574–579, 1984.
4. Brandt, K. D.: Osteoarthritis. Brandt, K. D., Ed. *Harrison's Principles of Internal Medicine.* New York, McGraw-Hill, 1995, p. 1692.
5. Karsh, R. S., and McCarthy, J. D.: Archeology and arthritis. *Arch Intern Med* 105:640–644, 1960.
6. Wells, C.: The palaeopathology of bone disease. *Practitioner* 210:384–391, 1973.
7. Rothschild, B. M., and Thillaud, P. L.: Oldest bone disease. *Nature* 349:288, 1991.
8. Braunstein, E. M., White, S. J., Russel, W., and Harris, J. E.: Paleoradiologic evaluation of the Egyptian royal mummies. *Skeletal Radiol* 17:348–352, 1988.
9. Elliot-Smith, G., and Dawson, W. R.: *Egyptian Mummies.* New York, The Dial Press, 1924.
10. Dastugue, J.: Les maladies de nos ancetres. *La Recherche* 13:980–988, 1982.

11. Dequeker, J.: Rheumatic diseases in visual arts. General review. Appelboom, T., Ed. *Art, History and Antiquity of Rheumatic Diseases.* Brussels, Elsevier, 1987, p. 84.
12. Rothschild, B. M., Turner, K. R., and Deluca, M. A.: Symmetrical erosive peripheral polyarthritis in the late archaic period of Alabama. *Science* 241:1498–1501, 1988.
13. Rothschild, B. M., and Woods, R. J.: Symmetrical erosive disease in archaic Indians: The origin of rheumatoid arthritis in the New World. *Semin Arthritis Rheum* 19:278–284, 1990.
14. Copeman, W. S.: Historical aspects of gout. *Clin Orthop* 71:14–22, 1970.
15. Baillou, G.: Liber de rheumatismo. *Oopera Medica Omnia.* Geneva, 1762.
16. Wollaston, W. H.: On gouty and urinary concretions. *Philos Trans R Soc Lond* 87:386–400, 1797.
17. Garrod, A. B.: *A Treatise on Gout and Rheumatic Gout.* London, Longmans, Green, 1859.
18. Garrod, A. E.: *Treatise on Rheumatism and Rheumatoid Arthritis.* London, Griffin, 1890.
19. Heberden, W.: *Commentaries on the History and Cure of Diseases,* 2nd ed. London, T. Payne, 1803.
20. Goldthwaite, J. E.: The differential diagnosis and treatment of the so-called rheumatoid disease. *Boston Med Surg J* 151:529–534, 1904.
21. Kohn, N. N., Hughes, R. E., McCarty, D. J., and Faires, J. S.: The significance of calcium pyrophosphate crystals in the synovial fluid of arthritic patients: The "pseudogout syndrome." II. Identification of crystals. *Ann Intern Med* 56:738–745, 1962.
22. Heine, J.: Uber die arthritis deformans. *Arch Pathol Anat* 260:521, 1926.
23. Wilcock, G. K.: The prevalence of osteoarthritis of the hip requiring total hip replacement in the elderly. *Int J Epidemiol* 8:247–250, 1979.
24. Wood, P. H., and McLeish, C. L.: Statistical appendix. Digest of data on the rheumatic diseases, 5: Morbidity in industry and rheumatism in general practice. *Ann Rheum Dis* 33:93–105, 1974.
25. Lawrence, J. S., Bremner, J. M., and Bier, F.: Osteoarthrosis. Prevalence in the population and relationship between symptoms and x-ray changes. *Ann Rheum Dis* 25:1–24, 1966.
26. Lawrence, R. C., Hochberg, M. C., Kelsey, J. L., McDuffie, F. C., Medsger, T. A. Jr., Felts, W. R., and Shulman, L. E.: Estimates of the prevalence of selected arthritic and musculoskeletal diseases in the United States. *J Rheumatol* 16:427–441, 1989.
27. Peyron, J. G.: The epidemiology of osteoarthritis. Moskowitz, R. W., Howell, D. S., Goldberg, V. M., Mankin, H. J., Eds. *Osteoarthritis.* Philadelphia, W. B. Saunders, 1984, p. 16.
28. Alexander, C. J.: Osteoarthritis: A review of old myths and current concepts. *Skeletal Radiol* 19:327–333, 1990.
29. Palotie, A., Ott, J., Elima, K. E., et al.: Predisposition to familial osteoarthrosis linked to type II collagen gene. *Lancet* 1:924–927, 1989.
30. Eyre, D. R., Weis, M. A., and Moskowitz, R. W.: Cartilage expression of a type II collagen mutation in an inherited form of osteoarthritis associated with a mild chondrodysplasia. *J Clin Invest* 87:357–361, 1991.
31. Hutton, C. W.: Generalised osteoarthritis: An evolutionary problem. *Lancet* 1:1463–1465, 1987.
32. Johnson, L. C.: Morphologic analysis in pathology: The kinetics of disease and general biology of bone. Frost, H. M., Ed. *Bone Biodynamics.* Boston, Little, Brown & Company, 1964, pp. 543–654.
33. Bullough, P. G.: The geometry of diarthrodial joints, its physiologic maintenance and the possible significance of age-related changes in geometry-to-load distribution and the development of osteoarthritis. *Clin Orthop Rel Res* 156:61–66, 1981.
34. Cooke, T. D. V.: Pathogenic mechanisms in polyarticular osteoarthritis. *Clin Rheum Dis* 11:203–238, 1985.
35. Murray, R. O.: The aetiology of primary osteoarthritis of the hip. *Br J Radiol* 38:810, 1965.
36. Sokoloff, L.: Osteoarthritis as a remodeling process. *J Rheumatol* 14(Suppl 14):7–10, 1987.
37. Radin, E. L., et al.: Response of joints to impact loading: III. Relationship between trabecular microfractures and cartilage degeneration. *J Biomech* 6:51–57, 1973.
38. Dequeker, J., Goris, P., and Utterhoeven, R.: Osteoporosis and osteoarthritis (osteoarthrosis): Anthropometric distinctions. *JAMA* 249:1448–1451, 1983.
39. Bird, H. A., Tribe, C. R., and Bacon, P. A.: Joint hypermobility leading to osteoarthrosis and chondrocalcinosis. *Ann Rheum Dis* 37:203–211, 1978.
40. Alexander, C.: Relationship between the utilisation profile of individual joints and their susceptibility to primary osteoarthritis. *Skeletal Radiol* 18:199–205, 1989.
41. Bullough, P. G., Goodfellow, J. W., and O'Conner, J. J.: The relationship between degenerative changes and load bearing in the human hip. *J Bone Joint Surg* 55B:746–758, 1973.
42. Hamerman, D.: The biology of osteoarthritis. *N Engl J Med* 320:1322–1329, 1989.
43. Verschure, P. J., and Van Noorden, C. J. F.: The effects of interleukin-1 on articular cartilage destruction as observed in arthritic diseases, and its therapeutic control. *Clin Exp Rheumatol* 8:303–313, 1990.
44. Watt, I., and Dieppe, P.: Osteoarthritis revisited. *Skeletal Radiol* 19:1–3, 1990.
45. Ehrlich, G. E.: Pathogenesis and treatment of osteoarthritis. *Compr Ther* 5:36–40, 1979.
46. Pattrick, M., Manhire, A., and Ward, A. M., et al.: HLA-A, B antigens and α 1-antitrypsin phenotypes in nodal generalized osteoarthritis and erosive osteoarthritis. *Ann Rheum Dis* 48:470–475, 1989.
47. Nevitt, M. C., Cummings, S. R., Lane, N. E., Hochberg, M. C., Scott, J. C., Pressman, A. R., Genant, H. K., and Cauley, J. A.: Association of estrogen replacement therapy with the risk of osteoarthritis of the hip in elderly white women. *Arch Intern Med* 156:2073–2080, 1996.
48. McAlindon, T. E., Felson, D. T., Zhang, Y., Hannan, M. T., Aliabadi, P., Weissman, B., Rush, D., Wilson, P. W. F., and Jacques, P.: Relation of dietary intake and serum levels of vitamin D to progression of osteoarthritis of the knee among participants in the Framingham study. *Ann Intern Med* 125:353–359, 1996.
49. Weinfeld, R. M., Olson, P. N., Maki, D. D., and Griffiths, H. J.: The prevalence of diffuse idiopathic skeletal hyperostosis (DISH) in two large American Midwest metropolitan hospital populations. *Skeletal Radiol* 26:222–225, 1997.
50. Forgacs, S. S.: Diabetes mellitus and rheumatic disease. *Clin Rheum Dis* 12:729–753, 1986.
51. Littlejohn, G. O., and Smythe, H. A.: Marked hyperinsulinemia after glucose challenge in patients with diffuse idiopathic skeletal hyperostosis. *J Rheumatol* 8:965–968, 1981.
52. Smythe, H. A.: Osteoarthritis, insulin and bone density. *J Rheumatol* 14(Suppl 14):91–93, 1987.
53. Seawright, A., English, P., and Gartner, R.: Hypervitaminosis A and hyperostosis of the cat. *Nature* 206:1171–1172, 1965.
54. Meyer, S.: The pathogenesis of diabetic charcot joints. *Iowa Orthop J* 12:63–70, 1996.
55. Hochberg, M. C.: Adult and juvenile rheumatoid arthritis, current epidemiologic concepts. *Epidemiol Rev* 3:27–44, 1981.
56. McIntosh, E.: The cost of rheumatoid arthritis. *Br J Rheumatol* 35:781–790, 1996.
57. Grennan, D. M., Dyer, P. A., Clague, R., et al.: Family studies in rheumatoid arthritis—the importance of HLA-DR4 and of genes for autoimmune thyroid disease. *J Rheumatol* 10:584–589, 1983.
58. Aho, K., Kosekenvuo, M., Tuominen, J., and Kaprio, J.: Occurrence of rheumatoid arthritis in a nationwide series of twins. *J Rheumatol* 13:899–906, 1986.
59. Harris, E. D. Jr.: Rheumatoid arthritis: Pathophysiology and implications for therapy. *N Engl J Med* 322:1277–1289, 1990.
60. Brennan, F. M., Maini, R. V., and Feldmann, M.: Tumor necrosis factor-alpha—a pivotal role in rheumatoid arthritis. *Br J Rheumatol* 31:293–298, 1992.
61. Cooper, N. S., Soren, A., McEwen, C., and Rosenberger, J. L.: Diagnostic specificity of synovial lesions. *Hum Pathol* 12:314–328, 1981.
62. Goldenberg, D. L., and Cohen, A. S.: Synovial membrane histopathology in the differential diagnosis of rheumatoid arthritis, gout, pseudogout, systemic lupus erythematosus, infectious arthritis and degenerative joint disease. *Medicine* 57:239–252, 1978.
63. Singsen, B. H.: Rheumatic diseases of childhood. *Rheum Dis Clin North Am* 16:581–599, 1990.
64. Cassidy, J. T., Levinson, J. E., Bass, J. C., et al.: A study of classification criteria for a diagnosis of juvenile arthritis. *Arthritis Rheum* 29:274–287, 1986.
65. Ansell, B. M.: Joint manifestations in children with juvenile chronic arthritis. *Arthritis Rheum* 20:204–206, 1977.
66. Lang, B. A., and Shore, A.: A review of current concepts on the pathogenesis of juvenile rheumatoid arthritis. *J Rheumatol* 21(Suppl 21):1–15, 1990.
67. Khan, M. A., and van der Linden, S. M.: A wider spectrum of spondyloarthropathies. *Semin Arthritis Rheum* 20:107–113, 1990.

68. Burmeister, G. R., Daser, A., Kamsadt, T., et al.: Immunology of reactive arthritides. *Annu Rev Immunol* 13:229–250, 1995.
69. Sieper, J., and Braun, J.: Pathogenesis of spondyloarthropathies: Persistent bacterial antigen, autoimmunity, or both. *Arthritis Rheum* 38:1547–1554, 1995.
70. Yu, D. T., Choo, S. Y., and Schaack, T.: Molecular mimicry in HLA-B27 related arthritis. *Ann Intern Med* 111:581–591, 1989.
71. Ball, J.: Enthesopathy of rheumatoid and ankylosing spondylitis. *J Pathol Bact* 71:73–84, 1956.
72. Revell, P. A., and Mayston, V.: Histopathology of the synovial membrane of peripheral joints in ankylosing spondylitis. *Ann Rheum Dis* 41:579–586, 1982.
73. Carette, S., Graham, D. C., and Little, H., et al.: The natural disease course of ankylosing spondylitis. *Arthritis Rheum* 26:186–190, 1983.
74. Rosenbaum, J. T.: Acute anterior uveitis and spondyloarthropathies. *Rheum Dis Clin North Am* 18:143–151, 1992.
75. Nordstrom, D. C. E.: Reactive arthritis, diagnosis and treatment. A review. *Acta Orthop Scand* 67:196–201, 1996.
76. Hughes, R. A., and Keat, A. C.: Reiter's syndrome and reactive arthritis: A current view. *Semin Arthritis Rheum* 24:190–210, 1994.
77. Keat, A.: ABC of rheumatology: Spondyloarthropathies. *Br Med J* 310:1321–1324, 1995.
78. Phillips, P. E.: The role of infectious agents in the spondyloarthropathies. *Scand J Rheumatol* 17:435–443, 1988.
79. Kantor, S. M., Hsu, S. H., Bias, W. B., and Arnett, F. C.: Clinical and immunogenetic subsets of psoriatic arthritis. *Clin Exp Rheumatol* 2:105–109, 1984.
80. Helliwell, P., Marchesoni, A., Peters, M., et al.: A re-evaluation of the osteoarticular manifestations of psoriasis. *Br J Rheumatol* 30:339–345, 1991.
81. Cronin, M. E.: Musculoskeletal manifestations of systemic lupus erythematosus. *Rheum Dis Clin North Am* 14:99–116, 1988.
82. Bywaters, E. G. L.: Jaccoud's syndrome: A sequel to the joint involvement of systemic lupus. *Clin Rheum Dis* 1:125–148, 1975.
83. Scott, J. T., and Pollard, A. C.: Uric acid excretion in the relatives of patients with gout. *Ann Rheum Dis* 29:397–400, 1970.
84. Lawry, G. V., Fan, P. T., and Bluestone, R.: Polyarticular versus monoarticular gout: A prospective comparative analysis of clinical features. *Medicine* 67:335–343, 1988.
85. Barthelemy, C. R., Nakayama, D. A., Carrera, G. F., Lightfoot, R. W. Jr., and Wortmann, R. L.: Gouty arthritis: A prospective radiographic evaluation of sixty patients. *Skeletal Radiol* 11:1–8, 1984.
86. Resnick, D., and Broderick, T. W.: Intraosseous calcifications in tophaceous gout. *Am J Roentgenol* 137:1157–1161, 1981.
87. Emmerson, B. T.: The management of gout. *Drug Therapy* 334:445–451, 1996.
88. Pritzker, K. P. H.: Calcium pyrophosphate crystal arthropathy: A biomineralization disorder. *Hum Pathol* 17:543–545, 1986.
89. Fam, A. G.: Calcium pyrophosphate crystal deposition disease and other crystal deposition disease. *Curr Opin Rheumatol* 7:364–368, 1995.

CHAPTER 17
The Pathology of Failed Total Joint Arthroplasty

An *arthroplasty* is a surgical procedure to relieve pain and restore motion or stability to a diseased joint. Many kinds of arthroplasties exist. Some are simple and involve only excision of diseased synovial membrane, removal of osteophytes, or repair of damaged ligaments. Other procedures, known as mold arthroplasties, are more complex and involve resurfacing a joint with foreign material to create smooth articulating surfaces. For example, joints may be resurfaced by interposing molds of glass, ceramic, acrylic, or metal. An even more complex arthroplasty is the replacement of one entire joint surface by a prosthesis, a procedure called a hemiarthroplasty.

Mold arthroplasties and hemiarthroplasties have been only moderately successful in the long-term restoration of joint function. However, total joint arthroplasty, popular only in the past 40 years, is a much more successful operation. In this procedure, both sides of a diseased joint are replaced with prostheses designed to allow normal and stable range of motion. Surgeons, working with specialists in biomechanics and biomaterials, have designed prostheses for almost every joint in the body. However, most total joint arthroplasties are performed for diseases of the hip and knee. Each year in the United States, about 170,000 total hip arthroplasties are performed. Almost 300,000 are done worldwide.[1] About the same number of total knee replacements are performed.

Years of clinical and laboratory experimentation have influenced the evolution in the design and materials of these prostheses. Today, prostheses for the larger joints are combinations of two materials designed to articulate with each other. One side of the joint is metal, usually titanium or a chrome-cobalt alloy, and the other side is polyethylene of ultra high molecular weight. In certain clinical situations, one or both components may be secured to the bone with methyl methacrylate, an acrylic cement (Fig. 17–1). Unlike prostheses for the larger joints, those for the smaller joints, as in the hands and wrist, are usually made from Silastic, a flexible long-chained polymer of silicone.

Total joint arthroplasty is one of the miracles of modern medicine. The results are excellent. As people grow older, many are uncomfortable, disabled, or even crippled by joint diseases, especially osteoarthritis. The total joint arthroplasty allows them to resume pain-free lives. However, despite the major clinical success of this surgical procedure, some total joint prostheses fail. Although a failed prostheses can be replaced, a procedure known as *revision arthroplasty,* the results are not as good the second time around. The tissues are scarred, and less bone is available with which to work. For this reason, prosthetic failure has been the subject of extensive medical research. Studying the failed prostheses and the associated bone and soft tissues provides insight into the causes of failure.

Although on rare occasions failures are caused by infection, most are the result of structural limitations of the prosthetic materials. Material failure may be sudden, such as a fatigue fracture of a metal prosthetic stem or the rapid crumbling of a polyethylene cup. These catastrophic failures are rare and are not discussed in this chapter. A much more common cause of a failed total joint arthroplasty is gradual aseptic loosening of the prostheses. For example, following total hip arthroplasty, almost one third of patients develop some radiographic signs of loosening.[2] However, most of these patients do not have enough pain to require revision arthroplasty. Painful aseptic loosening, which usually requires a new prostheses, occurs at a rate of 1% per year.

Aseptic loosening is caused by both mechanical and biological factors. The mechanical factor is the gradual loss of material from the components of the prosthesis. This loss of material, known as *wear,* results from forces on the joint. For example, normal walking places 3 times the body weight on a hip joint, and running may place 12 times the body weight on this joint. The loss of prosthetic material due to these extreme forces causes the prosthesis to fit less snugly.

The biological factor contributing to loosening is osteoclastic resorption of the bone adjacent to the prosthesis. Two

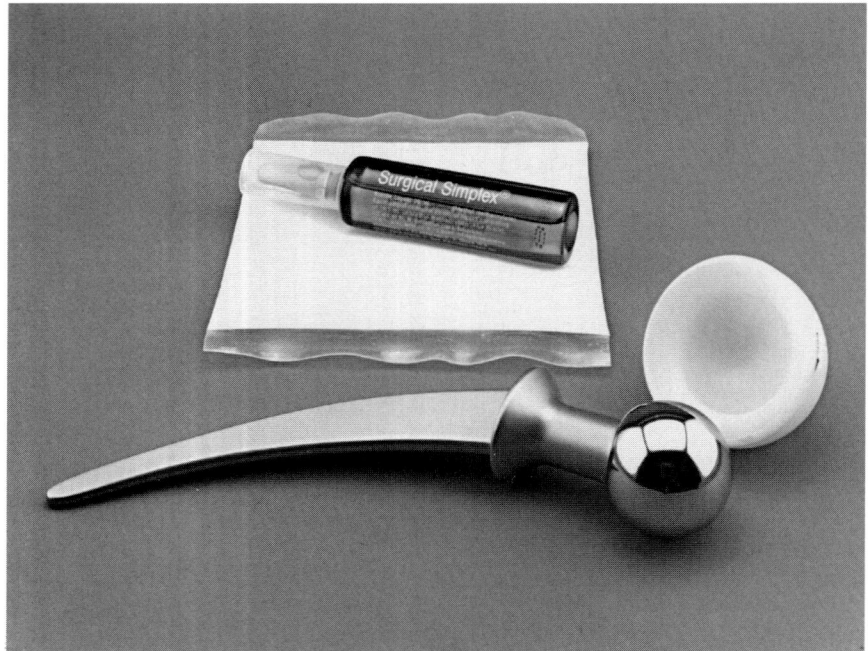

Figure 17-1 ▪ The components of a total hip prosthesis. The prosthesis consists of a metal femoral component, a polyethylene cup for the acetabulum, and the two ingredients for the methyl methacrylate cement.

processes stimulate osteoclastic resorption. First, the stress of the prosthesis on the bone causes increased remodeling, which results in osteopenia. Second, a histiocytic reaction to debris shed from the prosthesis stimulates osteoclasts, a process occasionally called *particle disease*.

These mechanical and biological factors, which eventually cause loosening, are active in all patients. Therefore, the success of a total joint prosthesis depends on the rate with which they occur. The life of any prosthesis is limited, and prostheses in younger, heavier, and more active patients are likely to loosen more quickly. As Sir John Charnley, a pioneer in total joint arthroplasty, put it, "Neither surgeons nor engineers will ever make an artificial hip joint which will last thirty years and at some time in that period enable the patient to play football (p. 1131)."[3]

HISTORY

Three medical advances in the mid- to late 19th century expanded the possibilities for surgical procedures. These advances were the discovery of general anesthesia in 1846; the use of antiseptic surgical techniques, first used by Joseph Lister in the 1860s; and the use of the Esmarck bandage, a technique developed in 1873 that reduced blood loss. These advances allowed orthopedic surgeons to perform extensive painless surgery with much less risk of infection and, in some cases, with minimal blood loss. Surgeons began operating inside joints, and some began to use implants. One such surgeon was Themistocles Gluck, a Romanian working in Germany. In 1890, Gluck published a paper about the implantation of foreign objects to replace diseased joints.[4] He designed numerous machined ivory joint prostheses, especially for the hip and knee, and tried them in war-wounded patients.

At about the same time, Jules Péan, one of the most prominent surgeons in France, was also exploring the idea that diseased tissues could be excised and replaced by implants. One operation that Péan performed in 1893 was the excision of a tuberculous shoulder followed by reconstruction with a total joint prosthesis. Although the prosthesis restored stability and good motion, recurrence of the infection required its removal 2 years later. The prosthesis, made of hard rubber and platinum, may be seen today in the Smithsonian Institute.[5] Even in these early years of experimentation with prostheses, Péan was aware of two principles of implant surgery that are still crucial today: first, the need for sterility, and second, the need for nonresorbable materials.[6]

The development of implants continued in the early decades of the 1900s. Various prosthetic designs and materials were tried for hemiarthroplasties and interposition arthroplasties. For example, in 1937, after experimenting with ceramic, plastic, and glass cups, Smith-Peterson of the Massachusetts General Hospital began to have success with Vitallium, a metal alloy of chrome and cobalt. This alloy is still used today in joint arthroplasty.

The English surgeon Philip Wiles began the first regular experimentation with total joint arthroplasty in 1938. He performed eight total hip operations using a metal acetabular cup and a metal femoral head, which he fixed to the femoral neck with a hip fracture nail. Both components were held in place with metal screws. The results of these early total hip arthroplasties were very poor—they were complicated by metal failure, bone resorption, or heterotopic bone.[7]

In 1951, John McKee of Norwich, England, began to

perform total hip arthroplasties on a regular basis. Like Wiles, he used metal components. However, the McKee femoral component was press-fitted into the medullary canal, similar to the Thompson or the Moore prostheses that had been used for hemiarthroplasties. Although McKee's results were only 54% satisfactory, he remained an advocate of total hip arthroplasty, and his design was adopted in the United States beginning in 1966.

The low plateau of success achieved by McKee was surpassed in the 1960s by Sir John Charnley, also of England. As a result of systematic research on design, materials, and operative procedures, Charnley made three major advances. First, to reduce the problem of friction-induced wear debris when metal rubbed on metal, he diminished the size of the femoral head and replaced the metal acetabulum with a polyethylene cup. Second, Charnley began to use an acrylic cement, polymethyl methacrylate, to tightly hold the implants in the bone.[8] Finally, he developed the use of clean air operating theaters to reduce postoperative infection. This and other innovations of surgical technique brought infection rates down from 10% to about 1%.

Charnley's use of cement was not without precedent in medical fields. Acrylic cement had been used for a long time to construct dental prostheses and to fill calvarial defects created by neurosurgeons. In the early 1950s, Wilse and others began experimenting with cements for possible uses in orthopedic surgery. After experimenting with animals, they suggested that this material could be used to fill defects of bone, to glue fractures, or to anchor prostheses. Although Charnley was the first to use it routinely in total hip surgery, Haboush of New York City had experimented with cement to anchor total hip prostheses in 1953.

Prostheses for the knee joint underwent a similar evolution. In about 1940, prostheses for hemiarthroplasty, including femoral molds and tibial plateaus, were developed. In 1951, Waldius tried the first total knee prosthesis, a hinged joint made from acrylic cement. By 1958, chrome-cobalt was being used to make the hinged prosthesis. Although occasionally used today, hinged prostheses often loosened because they do not allow the normal rotary motion of the knee. Therefore, in 1969, a cemented, metal-polyethylene, polycentric prosthesis was developed at the Charnley Hip Center in England.

In the past 30 years, prostheses have been designed for almost every joint. Each prosthesis has undergone changes in design based on new biomechanical and materials research. For example, many prostheses are now coated with metal beads to allow the growth of reparative tissue into the pores between the beads. Also, some prostheses are coated with apatite compounds to stimulate bone formation. In addition to a gradual evolution of prosthetic design, each manufacturer has its own model. For example, there are at least 30 designs of total hip prostheses used today.

FEATURES OF ASYMPTOMATIC, WELL-FUNCTIONING PROSTHESES

Asymptomatic total hip prostheses retrieved at autopsy often demonstrate an important feature associated with firm fixation—a zone of reactive bone surrounding the prosthesis. This zone, called a neocortex, is a manifestation of the body's acceptance of the prosthesis. Although it is especially prominent in porous coated prostheses, the neocortex is, in most cases, not visible radiologically.[9]

In addition to the neocortex, two other features, one radiologic and one histologic, may also be seen in asymptomatic patients, but these forecast future problems. First, in as many as 50% of patients, a thin radiolucent line develops around the femoral component of a total hip prosthesis[10] (Fig. 17–2). Less frequently, similar lines develop around components of other prostheses.[11] In most cases, these lines, 1 to 2 mm wide, are not associated with symptoms. Two processes contribute to the formation of these radiolucent lines. In the first process, a thin fibrous tissue membrane forms between the bone and the implant.[11] The surface of this membrane that lines the prosthesis develops a layer of plump cells resembling synoviocytes (Fig. 17–3). Thus, the membrane forms a neobursa around the implant. In the second process, bone resorption around the implant causes the radiolucent line. In this process, the radiolucent line and, occasionally, other areas of osteopenia[12] are caused by thinning of trabecular bone and cancellization of endosteal cortex.[13,14]

In addition to the radiolucent line surrounding the prosthesis, another histologic change seen in asymptomatic patients

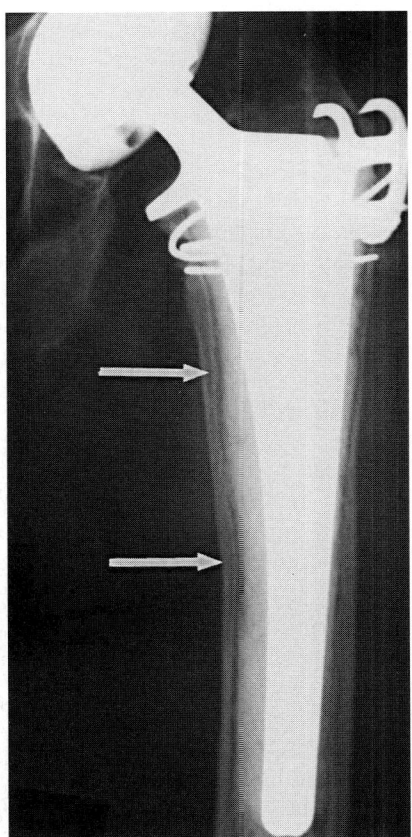

Figure 17–2 ■ An asymptomatic total hip prosthesis. Along the medial border of the proximal femur is a thin radiolucent line separating the radiodense methyl methacrylate from the bone (arrows). Barium is added to methyl methacrylate to make it radiopaque.

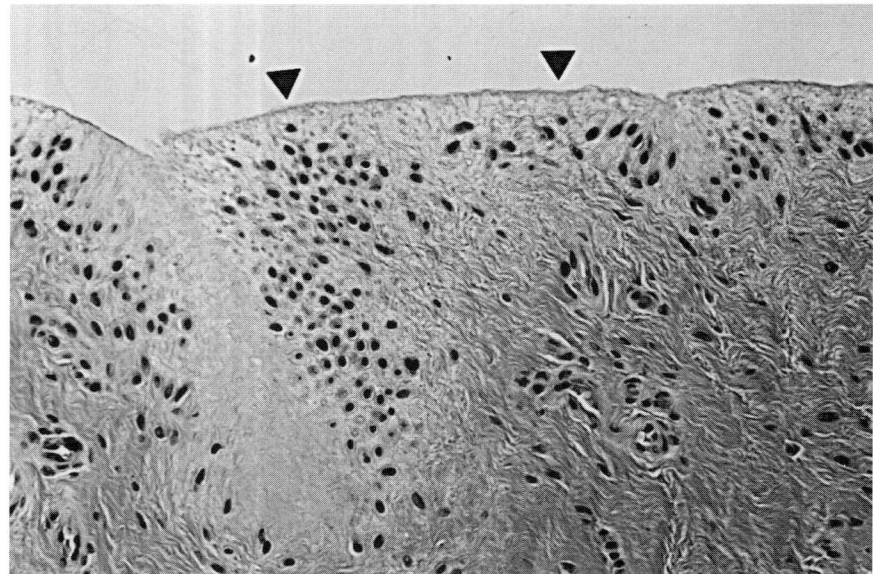

Figure 17-3 ■ Photomicrograph of the membrane removed from between the femoral component of a total hip prosthesis and the bone. One surface of the membrane (arrowheads) shows synovial metaplasia. This membrane forms a bursa around the component.

is the presence of particulate debris in the periprosthetic soft tissues and an associated histiocytic reaction. Particles are also seen in the joint cavity. Because all prostheses lose material from mechanical wear, this change is visible even in well-fixed prostheses.

The radiolucent line and the presence of wear particles do not necessarily mean that a prosthesis is loose. However, the processes that cause these changes in asymptomatic patients, when exaggerated, lead to aseptic loosening.

ASEPTIC LOOSENING

Continuous loss of prosthetic material through wear ultimately leads to loosening. Particles are shed into the surrounding tissue from each of the components of the prosthesis—polyethylene, methyl methacrylate, and metal.

Polyethylene Failure

Polyethylene wear is the primary cause of loosening. Particles are lost where the polyethylene articulates with the metal component. In hip prostheses, loss of material from inside the acetabular cup causes a gradual superior migration of the metal femoral head.[15] The rate of migration averages between only 0.1 and 0.2 mm per year. However, the amount of polyethylene debris shed from this seemingly slow wear rate is staggering—7 billion particles per year, or 20 million particles per day!

Most of the polyethylene debris is shed into the joint cavity. However, some particles migrate far from the joint cavity into spaces between the prosthesis and bone.[16] Polyethylene particles, ranging in size from 1 to 200 μm, provoke a tissue reaction. Smaller particles are phagocytized by histiocytes. Sheets of these cells, with glassy cytoplasm, accumulate in the soft tissues of the joint and in the membrane adjacent to the prostheses (Fig. 17–4). The histiocytes may also accumulate in the marrow spaces. Larger polyethylene fragments are surrounded by foreign body giant cells (Fig. 17–5). These fragments, resembling glass shards, are strongly birefringent in polarized light.

Polyethylene debris from total hips or knees also enters the lymphatic drainage of the leg. This material, accumulating in regional lymph nodes, stimulates a heavy histiocytic infiltrate. This histiocytic reaction is frequently discovered in the lymph nodes of patients with asymptomatic prostheses

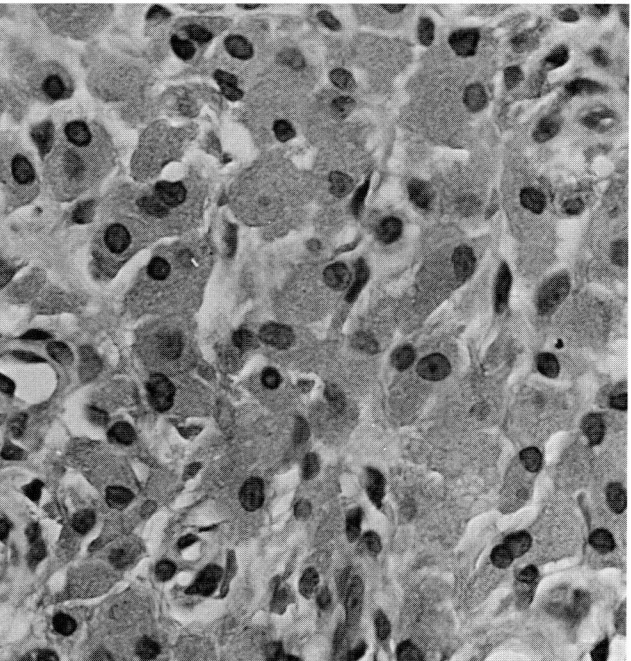

Figure 17-4 ■ Photomicrograph of the histiocytic reaction to polyethylene debris. The cytoplasm of each histiocyte is loaded with polyethylene particles.

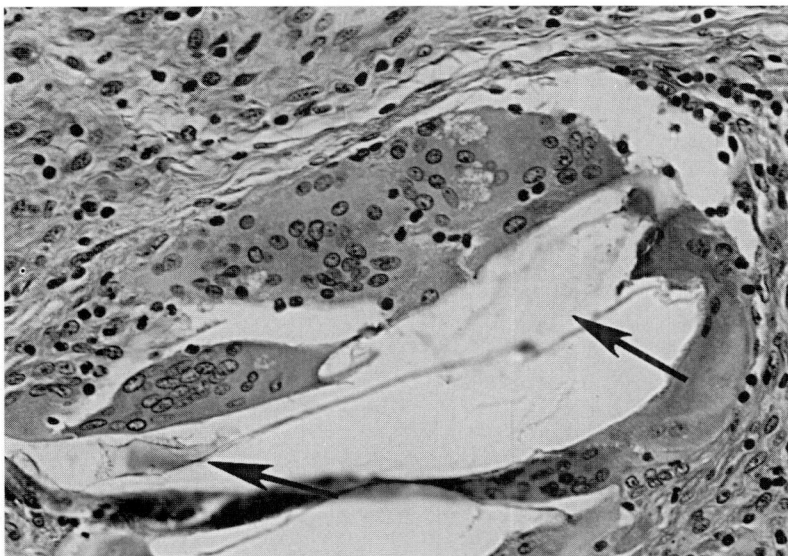

Figure 17-5 ▪ Shards of polyethylene *(arrows)* surrounded by multinucleated, foreign-body giant cells.

who undergo inguinal lymphadenectomy for prostate carcinoma[17,18] (Fig. 17–6).

Cement Failure

In addition to polyethylene failure, fragmentation of methyl methacrylate cement is also a source of particulate debris. Although having no bonding capability, this acrylic serves as a grouting agent to tightly encase the prosthesis. The cement anchors the bone by squeezing into small intertrabecular spaces in the 10 minutes before it hardens.

Methyl methacrylate cement is more brittle than bone. Therefore, stress at the bone-cement interface causes abrasion and fracture of the cement intrusions into trabecular spaces. Like polyethylene debris, the fractured cement particles become embedded in the periprosthetic soft tissue. These particles, 30 to 100 μm in size, are usually dissolved in xylene during processing for routine histologic study.[19] Their presence can be deduced, however, by empty spaces in the soft tissue, spaces often bordered by foreign body giant cells (Fig. 17–7).

Metal Failure

Metal debris may also contribute to aseptic loosening. The metal components, when embedded in human tissue, are in an electrolyte solution. Therefore, oxide layers form on the surface of the chrome-cobalt or titanium, and stresses on the surface of the metal shear the oxides into the surrounding tissues. Titanium oxide is more susceptible to this shear force than chromium oxide. The oxides cause a black pigmentation of the tissues surrounding the implant. Histologi-

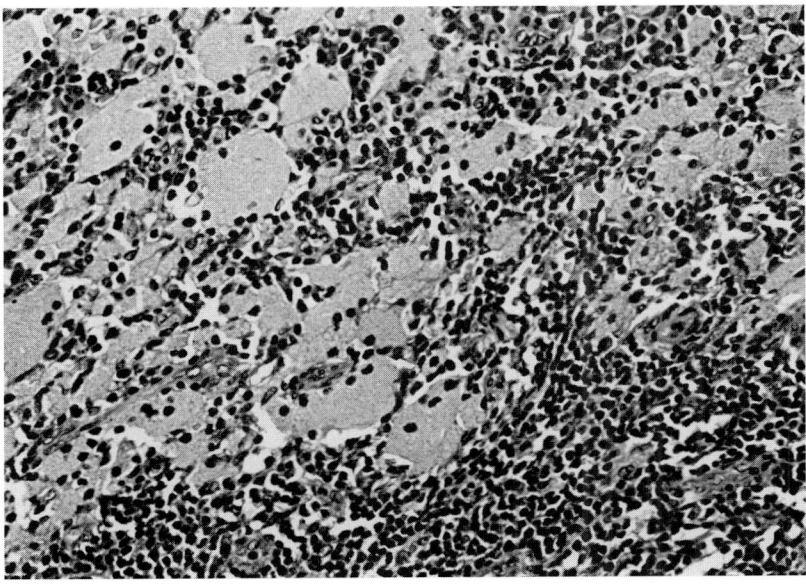

Figure 17-6 ▪ Photomicrograph of a portion of an inguinal lymph node. This lymph node shows an infiltrate of histiocytes containing polyethylene particles.

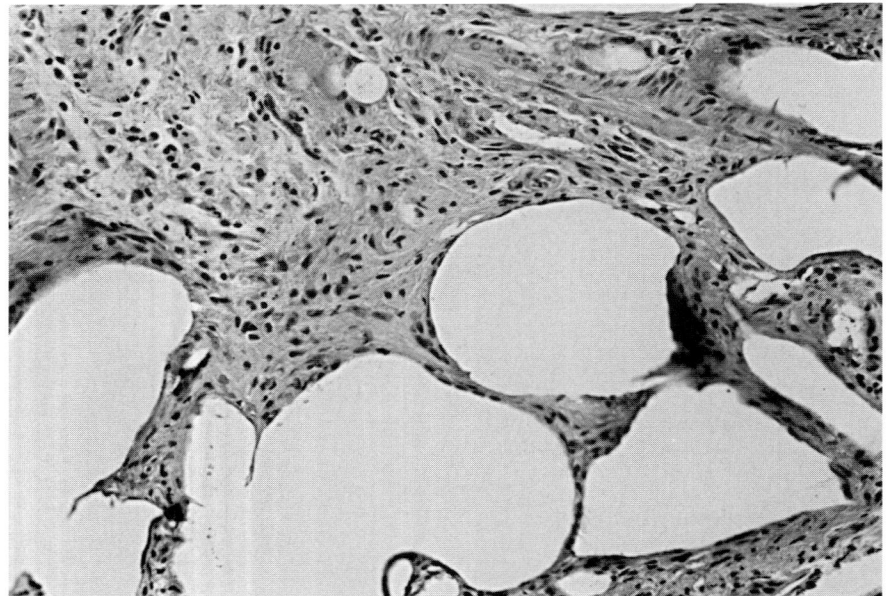

Figure 17-7 ■ Photomicrograph from tissue around the acetabular portion of a total hip prosthesis. The empty spaces were formerly occupied by fragments of methyl methacrylate cement that have been dissolved in tissue processing.

cally, the black deposits of oxidized metal are seen extracellularly as well as in the cytoplasm of histiocytes (Fig. 17–8).

The metal debris may cause symptoms in the absence of loosening. For example, following total hip or total knee replacement, metal debris can cause an intense synovitis with a painful effusion.[20]

In addition to oxidation, the metal components undergo corrosion. As a result of this process, metal is gradually lost, and metallic ions enter the soft tissues and the bloodstream. The systemic effects of the metal ions are not known, but they may inhibit osteoblast function or mineralization.

Silastic Failure

Silastic, a firm but flexible long-chained polymer of silicone, has been used since the 1960s as a prosthetic material for small joints, particularly the interphalangeal and metacarpophalangeal joints of the hands. In addition, Silastic implants are also used to replace diseased carpal bones. Like other prosthetic materials, Silastic fractures and undergoes wear. Silastic particles, usually between 10 and 100 μm, become embedded in the synovial membrane and periarticular soft tissue, where they occasionally cause a painful synovitis known as silicone synovitis (Fig. 17–9). Particles may also enter regional lymphatics. Also, some patients develop multiple subchondral osseous defects filled with fibrous tissue, histiocytes, and Silastic particles[21,22] (Fig. 17–10). The Silastic particles, visible both intracellularly and extracellularly, are not birefringent in polarized light. Although this complication may appear as early as 3 months after insertion of the implant,[21] most patients become symptomatic between 1 and 9 years after surgery (mean, 5.5 years).

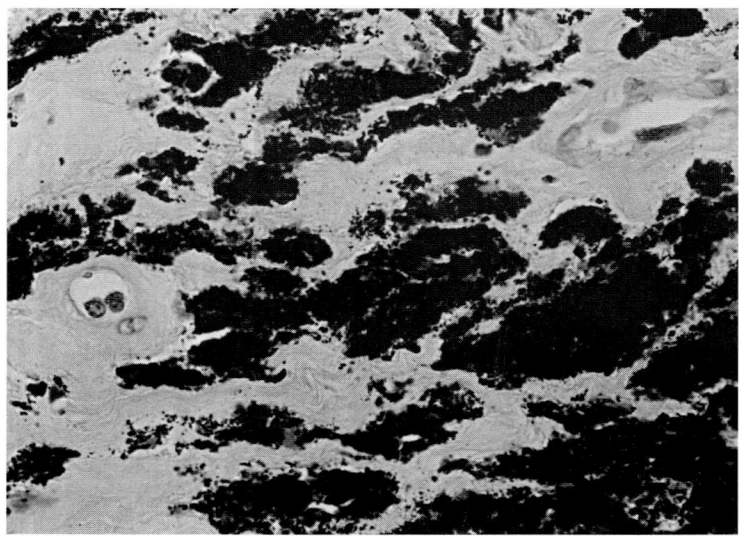

Figure 17-8 ■ Photomicrograph showing extensive black metal deposits. In this case, the metal is titanium, a product that accumulates more oxides than does chrome-cobalt.

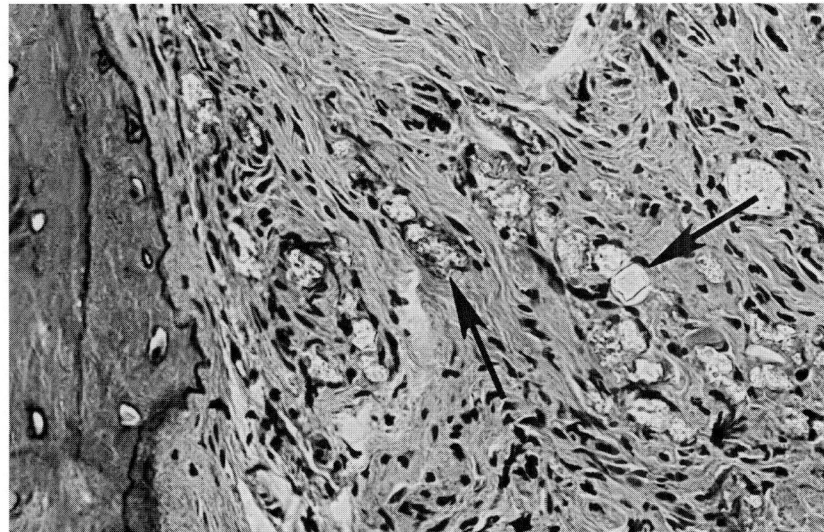

Figure 17-9 ■ Photomicrograph showing marrow fibrosis and refractile Silastic particles (arrows). This tissue was removed from a lytic lesion adjacent to a Silastic finger joint prosthesis.

THE BIOLOGICAL RESPONSE TO TOTAL JOINT PROSTHESES

The biological response to implants is the most important cause of prosthetic loosening. This response is mediated by histiocytes recruited by the vast number of particles, particularly polyethylene particles, shed from the prosthesis. One researcher postulated that during walking, 337,000 polyethylene particles are generated per step! Since a histiocyte can hold about 200 particles of polyethylene, about 1690 histiocytes are recruited per step (Bauer, T., Personal communication, 1996). These cells accumulate in the tissues surrounding the prosthesis. Although areas of necrosis are also present, neutrophils are characteristically absent in aseptic loosening. Lymphocytes and plasma cells, mediators of an immune response, are also usually absent, although they may occasionally be present in patients with rheumatoid arthritis.

The histiocytes initiate the bone resorption.[23] These cells release various factors, particularly prostaglandin E, interleukin-1, and tumor necrosis factor alpha, which stimulate the production of fibrous tissue and the activation of osteoclasts. Therefore, the tissues that accumulate around prosthetic components are potent stimulators of osteolysis. Osteolysis occurs in various regions around total joint prostheses (Fig. 17–11). For example, after total hip replacement, osteolysis is most prominent in the region of the calcar.

GRANULOMATOUS PSEUDOTUMORS

Osteolysis associated with prosthetic implants may be massive and simulate a neoplasm or a focus of infection, a process known as a *granulomatous pseudotumor*[24,25] (Fig. 17–12). This process may occur even in patients with well-functioning prostheses. Lesions are characterized histologically by sheets of histiocytes and foreign body giant cells containing particulate debris. Pseudotumors (or pseudoabscesses) may also present as soft tissue masses adjacent to prostheses,[26] and some of these lesions spontaneously drain fluid (Fig. 17–13). Particulate debris in the fluid draws attention to the relationship with the nearby prosthesis.

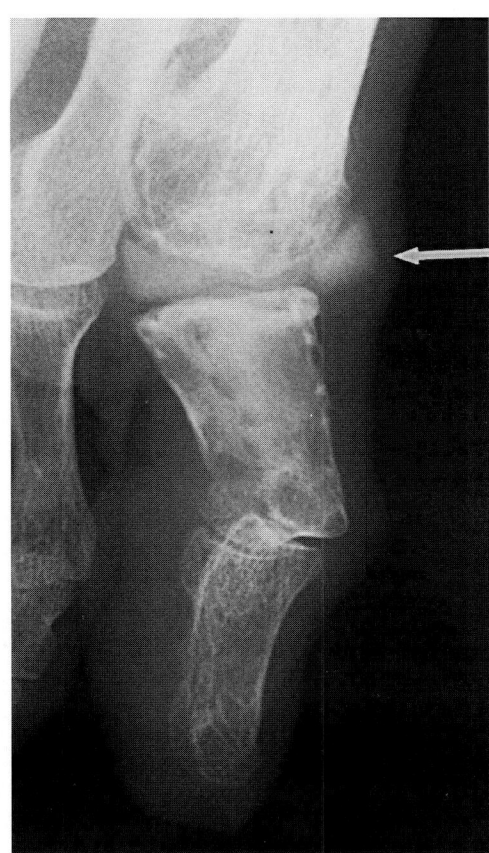

Figure 17-10 ■ A fractured Silastic implant at the metatarsophalangeal joint of the great toe (arrow). Lytic lesions are present in the proximal phalanx.

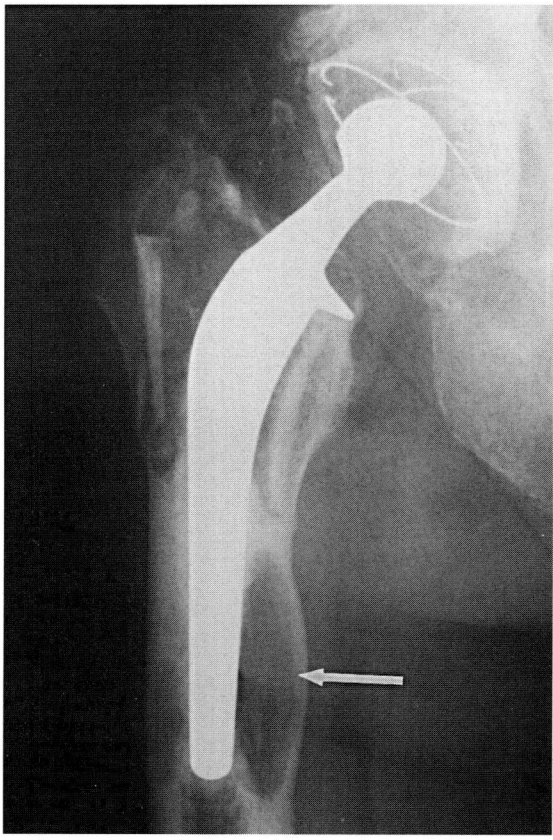

Figure 17-11 ■ A total hip prosthesis with extensive radiolytic changes around the femoral component *(arrow)* secondary to particle disease.

SEPTIC LOOSENING

Although prosthetic loosening is usually caused by gradual material failure, infection around a prosthesis also causes loosening. However, loosening due to infection is more serious and requires more extensive revision surgery. Whereas a noninfected loose prosthesis may be replaced by a single surgical procedure, an infected prosthesis requires complete removal of all cement and débridement of all infected tissue. Usually the implantation of a new prosthesis must be delayed until antibiotics have healed the infection. Sometimes a prosthesis can never be reimplanted, and the patient must have a joint fusion or a pseudarthrosis. In the early days of total joint arthroplasty, almost 10% of total hip prostheses became infected.[27] Today, the infection rate is only about 1.5%, although some centers using clean air systems have reported infection rates as low as 0.5%.[28] Even with very low infection rates, the huge number of total joint arthroplasties performed each year result in a few thousand new cases of prosthetic infection each year.

Pathogenesis

Total joint prostheses become infected by two mechanisms—wound contamination at the time of surgery and hematogenous spread of organisms from a distant site. The first mechanism, wound contamination, is the most common. Bacteria-carrying desquamated skin of operating room personnel may fall directly into the wound. Also, the patient's skin or the surgeon's hand (through a punctured glove) may be a source of organisms. Infections acquired intraoperatively are usually caused by *Staphylococcus epidermidis* or *Staphylococcus aureus*.

The second mechanism of infection, hematogenous spread of organisms, usually occurs late in the postoperative period. Important sources of organisms are infections of skin, soft tissues, respiratory tract, urinary tract, and teeth. Although staphylococcal species are important causes of a hematoge-

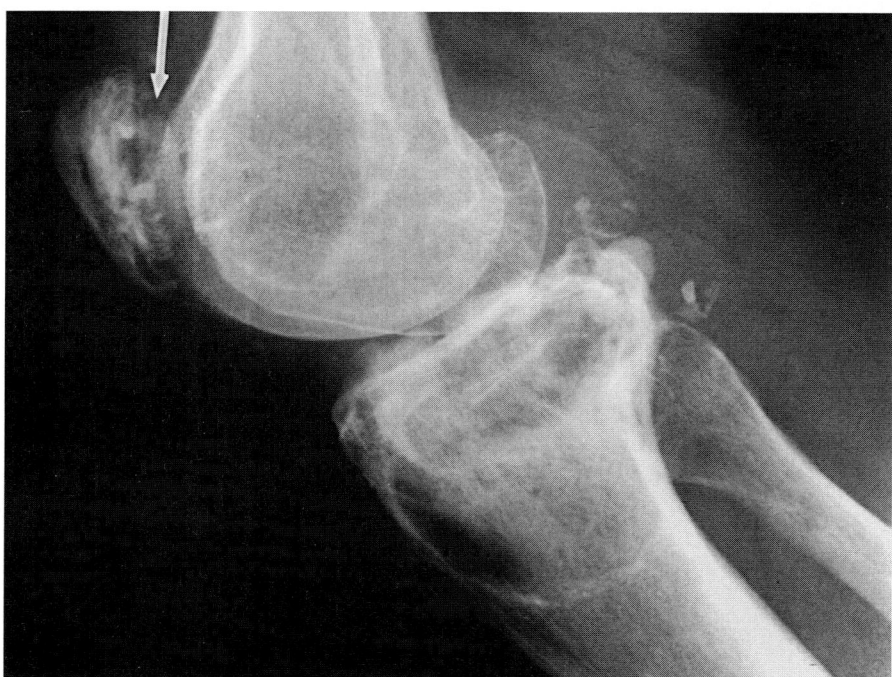

Figure 17-12 ■ A granulomatous pseudotumor of the proximal tibia. A radiolytic lesion is surrounded by a sclerotic rim. This reaction is secondary to polyethylene debris shed from a patellar implant *(arrow)*. (From McCarthy, E. F.: *Differential Diagnosis in Pathology. Bone and Joint Disorders.* New York and Tokyo, Igaku-Shoin, 1996. With permission from Williams & Wilkins.)

This thick protective extracellular coat walls off the bacteria against antibiotics and phagocytosis. Third, certain metals used in implants, such as nickel or cobalt, may depress macrophage function.[30]

Clinical Features

Infection of a total joint prosthesis is sometimes clinically difficult to differentiate from aseptic loosening because of overlapping signs and symptoms. For example, pain is a feature of both noninfected and infected prostheses.[31] However, the character of the pain may help to differentiate between the two. Pain of an infected prosthesis is constant and gradually increases in severity, whereas in a noninfected prosthesis, pain is present only during use of the joint. Other symptoms, such as fever or tenderness, are less constant features of infection and are therefore less helpful in the diagnosis. Also, laboratory studies may be equivocal. With an infected prosthesis, the white blood cell count rarely exceeds 15,000/mm^3, but in some patients it may not even be elevated. The erythrocyte sedimentation rate, if significantly elevated, may indicate infection. However, some patients with an infected prosthesis have a normal erythrocyte sedimentation rate. The level of C-reactive protein has a more predictive value. Levels of more than 220 mg/L are suggestive of infection.

Imaging studies are also of limited value in diagnosing infection. A strongly positive technetium-99 bone scan that shows uniform tracer uptake suggests infection, whereas focal weak positivity is more common with aseptic loosening. Unfortunately, most cases fall into a gray zone between these extremes.

Fine needle aspiration with bacterial cultures may assist in distinguishing septic and aseptic loosening. However, a wide range of sensitivity and specificity for this procedure has been reported.[32-34] Therefore, because of false negatives and false positives, preoperative needle aspiration is not always reliable.

In about 25% of cases, the diagnosis of an infected prosthesis can be made on the basis of clinical history and physical examination.[35] In an additional 50%, the correct diagnosis requires extensive radiographic and laboratory investigations. However, in the remaining 25%, an unequivocal distinction between aseptic and septic loosening cannot be made preoperatively. Therefore, because of the radical difference in surgical management, the correct diagnosis must be made intraoperatively by frozen section. During surgery, the surgeon must work closely with the pathologist. The distinguishing histologic feature of an infected prosthesis, not present in an aseptic loose prosthesis, is an acute inflammatory reaction. The pathologist must carefully search many high-power fields for neutrophils. A finding of five neutrophils per high-power field is presumptive of infection.[36] In addition, large numbers of lymphocytes (more than 50 per high-power field) are highly suspicious for infection. At least three tissue samples from the interface between the

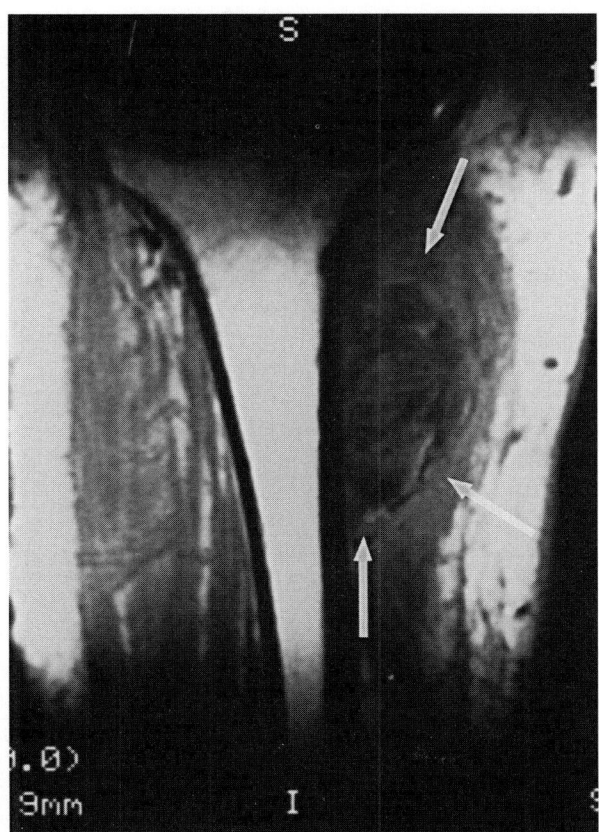

Figure 17-13 ■ A T$_2$-weighted magnetic resonance image showing a soft tissue pseudotumor adjacent to the tibia (arrows). This mass was filled with polyethylene debris and an extensive granulomatous reaction.

nously acquired infection, gram-negative enteric bacteria, such as *Escherichia coli,* commonly play a causative role.

Depending on which of these two mechanisms is at work, infection of prostheses becomes evident at varying time intervals following surgery. Twenty-three percent of infections occur in the first 3 months after surgery.[29] These infections, usually quite virulent, are almost always acquired during the surgical procedure by wound contamination. An additional 27% occur between 3 months and 2 years following surgery. The infection in these patients is often subclinical, and symptoms are very difficult to differentiate from aseptic loosening. Most likely, these infections are also acquired in the operating room. The remaining 50% of infections develop 1 year to as long as 15 to 20 years postoperatively. Most of these patients have a long pain-free postoperative interval and probably acquire their infection by hematogenous spread of organisms.

Once organisms have reached the prosthesis by either of the two mechanisms, three factors facilitate their growth. First, a small amount of bone adjacent to the implant dies as a result of reaming and sawing. In addition, heat generated by the hardening of the cement may also cause osteonecrosis. The dead bone results in a nonvascularized area that permits bacteria to grow, safe from circulating host defenses. Second, when bacteria contact an implant, they secrete a glycocalix.

prosthesis and bone should be studied before acute inflammation is ruled out. Gram staining is not useful in the diagnosis of prosthesis-related infection.[34] Unfortunately, because some low-grade infections fail to stimulate an acute inflammatory reaction, they go undiagnosed until the postoperative period when microbacterial culture results are available.

MALIGNANT NEOPLASMS ARISING IN ASSOCIATION WITH TOTAL JOINT PROSTHESES

On very rare occasions, malignant neoplasms arise in the bone or soft tissues adjacent to total joint prostheses. Neoplasms have also developed at the sites of other kinds of implants, such as metal plates or screws. The neoplasms, numbering only about 20 in the literature,[37] have usually been malignant fibrous histiocytomas or osteosarcomas.[38,39] Most have arisen 5 years or more after implantation.

Implant-associated neoplasms, although rare, raise speculation that the materials are carcinogenic. Some epidemiologic and experimental evidence supports this idea. For example, workers with chromium and nickel, the same materials used in prostheses, have an increased risk of lung cancer.[40] Also, polyethylene has been shown to induce sarcomas in rats.[41]

Malignant degeneration in the long-standing reparative tissues around the implant is an alternative theory to implant carcinogenicity. This suggestion is supported by the observation that malignant neoplasms occasionally arise in association with other conditions characterized by chronic repair, such as a chronic draining sinus tract or around a bone infarct or an ancient enchondroma.

Although clinically interesting, the rarity of prosthesis-associated sarcomas among the millions of patients with total joint prostheses indicates that this complication is probably clinically insignificant.

THE ROLE OF THE PATHOLOGIST IN TOTAL JOINT FAILURE

The pathologist must carefully document the condition of the prosthesis and soft tissue removed during revision arthroplasty. A gross description of the implant should be included in the pathology report. For example, cuts, chips, cracks, or abrasions in the polyethylene and the metal should be described. Ideally, close-up color photographs of the implant components should be taken with the lighting arranged to eliminate distracting highlights. When possible, the implants should be saved indefinitely. In addition to describing the polyethylene and metal, the pathologist should document the amount of methyl methacrylate cement. Care must be taken not to mistake chips of this acrylic cement for bone. This material never softens in decalcification solution! The soft tissues must also be described. Metallic pigmentation is best documented by a color photograph. In addition, purulent material must also be noted. At least three or four blocks of soft tissue should be processed for microscopic study. The amount of wear debris should be noted, as well as the amount of the histiocytic reaction. Finally, the presence of neutrophils should be documented.

In addition to documenting the condition of failed prosthetic implants in the surgical pathology laboratory, efforts should be made to retrieve total joint prostheses at autopsy. An entire joint can be removed en bloc with the prosthesis still in place.[42] Many of these prostheses will have been successful, and by studying them we can learn why some work and others fail.

REFERENCES

1. Pearcy, M. J.: A new generation of artificial hip joints. *Eng Med* 17:199–201, 1988.
2. Stauffer, R. N.: Ten-year follow-up study of total hip replacement with particular reference to roentgenographic loosening of the components. *J Bone Joint Surg* 64A:983–990, 1982.
3. Charnley, J.: Arthroplasty of the hip: A new operation. *Lancet* 1:1129–1132, 1961, p. 1131.
4. Gluck, T. H.: Autoplastik-Transplantation-Implantation von Fremdkorpern. *Berl klin Wsch* 27:421–427, 1890.
5. Lugli, T.: Artificial shoulder joint by Péan (1893). The facts of an exceptional intervention and the prosthetic method. *Clin Orthop* 133:215–218, 1978.
6. Péan, J.: Des moyens prosthetiques destines a obtenir la rearation des parties osseuses. *Clin Orthop* 94:4–7, 1973.
7. Wiles, P.: The surgery of the osteo-arthritic hip. *Br J Surg* 45:488–497, 1958.
8. Charnley, J.: Anchorage of the femoral head prosthesis to the shaft of the femur. *J Bone Joint Surg* 42B:28–30, 1960.
9. Collier, J. P., Bauer, T. W., Bloebaum, R. D., Bobyn, J. D., Cook, S. D., Galante, J. O., Harris, W. H., Head, W. C., Jasty, M. J., Mayer, M. B., Sumner, D. R., and Whiteside, L. A.: Results of implant retrieval from postmortem specimens in patients with well-functioning, long-term total hip replacement. *Clin Orthop* 274:97–112, 1992.
10. Fornasier, V. L., and Cameron, H. U.: The femoral stem/cement interface in total hip replacement. *Clin Orthop* 116:248–252, 1976.
11. Tibrewal, S. B., Grant, K. A., and Goodfellow, J. W.: The radiolucent line beneath the tibial components of the Oxford meniscal knee. *J Bone Joint Surg* 66B:523–528, 1984.
12. Maloney, W. J., Jasty, M., Rosenberg, A., and Harris, W. H.: Bone lysis in well-fixed cemented femoral components. *J Bone Joint Surg* 72B:966–970, 1990.
13. Kwong, L. M., Jasty, M., Mulroy, R. D., Maloney, W. J., Bragdon, C., and Harris, W. H.: The histology of the radiolucent line. *J Bone Joint Surg* 74B:67–73, 1992.
14. Anthony, P. P., Gie, G. A., Howie, C. R., and Ling, R. S.: Localised endosteal bone lysis in relation to the femoral components of cemented total hip arthroplasties. *J Bone Joint Surg* 72B:971–979, 1990.
15. Wroblewski, B. M.: Direction and rate of socket wear in Charnley low-friction arthroplasty. *J Bone Joint Surg* 67B:757–761, 1985.
16. Schmalzried, T. P., Jasty, M., and Harris, W. H.: Periprosthetic bone loss in total hip arthroplasty. *J Bone Joint Surg* 74A:849–862, 1992.
17. Bauer, T. W., Saltarelli, M., McMahon, J. T., and Wilde, A. H.: Regional dissemination of wear debris from a total knee prostheses. *J Bone Joint Surg* 75A:105–110, 1993.
18. O'Connell, J. X., and Rosenberg, A. E.: Histiocytic lymphadenitis associated with a large joint prosthesis. *Am J Clin Pathol* 99:314–316, 1993.
19. Johanson, N. A., Bullough, P. G., Wilson, P. D. Jr., Salvati, E. A., and Ranawat, C. S.: The microscopic anatomy of the bone-cement interface in failed total hip arthroplasties. *Clin Orthop* 218:123–135, 1987.
20. Weissman, B. N., Scot, R. D., Brick, G. W., and Corson, J. M.: Radiographic detection of metal-induced synovitis as a complication of arthroplasty of the knee. *J Bone Joint Surg* 73A:1002–1007, 1991.
21. Yamashina, M., and Moatamed, F.: Peri-articular reactions to microscopic erosion of silicone-polymer implants. Light- and scanning elec-

tron-microscopic studies with energy-dispersive x-ray analysis. *Am J Surg Pathol* 9:215–219, 1985.
22. Telaranta, T., Solonen, K. A., Tallroth, K., and Nickels, J.: Bone cysts containing silicone particles in bones adjacent to a carpal Silastic implant. *Skeletal Radiol* 10:247–249, 1983.
23. Murray, D. W., and Rushton, N.: Macrophages stimulate bone resorption when they phagocytose particles. *J Bone Joint Surg* 72B:988–992, 1990.
24. Griffiths, H. J., Burke, J., and Bonfiglio, T. A.: Granulomatous pseudotumors in total joint replacement. *Skeletal Radiol* 16:146–152, 1987.
25. Santavirta, S., Konttinen, Y. T., Bergroth, V., Eskola, A., Tallroth, K., and Lindholm, T. S.: Aggressive granulomatous lesions associated with hip arthroplasty. *J Bone Joint Surg* 72A:252–258, 1990.
26. Howie, D. W., Cain, C. M. J., and Cornish, B. L.: Pseudo-abscess of the psoas bursa in failed double-cup arthroplasty of the hip. *J Bone Joint Surg* 73B:29–32, 1991.
27. Charnley, J.: Postoperative infection after total hip replacement with special reference to air contamination in the operating room. *Clin Orthop* 87:167–187, 1972.
28. Fitzgerald, R. H.: Infections of hip prostheses and artificial joints. *Infect Dis Clin North Am* 3:329–338, 1989.
29. Bullough, P. G.: Bullough and Vigorita's Orthopedic Pathology. London, Mosby-Wolfe, 1997, pp. 308–321.
30. Rae, T.: A study on the effects of particulate metals of orthopedic interest on murine macrophages in vitro. *J Bone Joint Surg* 57B:444–451, 1975.
31. Fitzgerald, R. H. J.: Problems associated with the infected total hip arthroplasty. *Clin Rheum Dis* 12:537–554, 1986.
32. Roberts, P., Walters, A. J., and McMinn, D. J.: Diagnosing infection in hip replacements. The use of fine-needle aspiration and radiometric culture. *J Bone Joint Surg* 74B:265–259, 1992.
33. Phillips, W. C., and Kattapuram, S. V.: Efficacy of preoperative hip aspiration performed in the radiology department. *Clin Orthop* 179:141–146, 1983.
34. Barrack, R. L., and Harris, W. H.: The value of aspiration of the hip joint before revision total hip arthroplasty. *J Bone Joint Surg* 75A:66–76, 1993.
35. Fitzgerald, R. H. Jr.: Infected total hip arthroplasty: Diagnosis and treatment. *J Am Acad Orthop Surg* 3:249–262, 1995.
36. Fehring, T. K., and McAlister, J. A.: Frozen histologic section as a guide to sepsis in revision joint arthroplasty. *Clin Orthop* 304:229–237, 1994.
37. Galante, J. O., Lemons, J., Spector, M., Wilson, P. D. Jr., and Wright, T. M.: The biologic effects of implant materials. *J Orthop Res* 9:760–775, 1991.
38. Brien, W. W., Salvati, E. A., Healey, J. H., Bansal, M., Ghelman, B., and Betts, F.: Osteogenic sarcoma arising in the area of a total hip replacement. *J Bone Joint Surg* 72A:1097–1099, 1990.
39. Penman, H. G., and Ring, P. A.: Osteosarcoma in association with total hip replacement. *J Bone Joint Surg* 66B:632–634, 1984.
40. Doll, R.: Cancer of the lung and nose in nickel workers. *Br J Ind Med* 15:217–223, 1958.
41. Carter, R. L., and Roe, F. J. C.: Induction of sarcomas in rats by solid and fragmented polyethylene: Experimental observations and clinical implications. *Br J Cancer* 23:401–407, 1969.
42. Wright, T. M., Hughes, P. W., Torzilli, P. A., and Wilson, P. D. Jr.: A method for the postmortem evaluation of an in situ total hip replacement. *J Bone Joint Surg* 61A:661–663, 1979.

CHAPTER 18

Management of Orthopedic Pathology Specimens from the Operating Room to the Microscope

THE CONFERENCE

We have emphasized throughout this book the need for teamwork among the orthopedist, radiologist, and pathologist. This collaboration requires a forum so that individual cases can be discussed before therapeutic decisions are made. We have found that the ideal setting is in the clinic where new patients are being examined. In this setting, decisions can be made before the patient is admitted or leaves for the day. First, based on plain radiographs and clinical examination, a preliminary diagnosis should be established. Then, the orthopedist and radiologist decide which ancillary imaging modalities are needed. Next, the orthopedist, in consultation with the pathologist, decides if a biopsy is required and which type is most efficient and accurate.

If a conference in the new patient clinic is not possible, the orthopedist should review the radiographs with the pathologist before the biopsy is performed. At this time, these two specialists can discuss biopsy alternatives.

Another forum for interdisciplinary dialogue is a weekly conference attended by radiologists, pathologists, radiation therapists, and surgeons. Such a conference, based on individual case presentations, is ideal for teaching residents and medical students.

THE BIOPSY

The biopsy of bone lesion must be carefully planned so that diagnostic tissue is obtained and to ensure that proper ancillary studies are performed. The first question to be addressed is whether an open biopsy or a percutaneous needle biopsy should be performed.[1] In either case, the biopsy site must be chosen such that, if necessary, it can be excised en bloc with the underlying bone lesion.

The Needle Biopsy

Closed needle biopsies offer many advantages over open biopsy. An incision is not required, anesthesia is minimal, and complications are very rare. With computed tomographic guidance, a needle can be placed in any location. Options include fine needle aspiration or various types of cutting needles that yield a core of tissue. With the use of these needle biopsy techniques, diagnostic accuracy rates as high as 90% have been reported.[2]

Despite the advantages of the closed needle biopsy, we have found that this procedure fails to produce diagnostic tissue in all but a few cases. The limiting factor is the small amount of tissue that is obtained. Moreover, the tissue is often crushed and distorted. Radiodense lesions are most apt to be affected by these factors; therefore, needle biopsies in these lesions are rarely diagnostic.

Similarly, closed needle biopsy is seldom helpful in diagnosing primary bone tumors. Because these neoplasms undergo a wide variety of secondary changes, including necrosis, fibrosis, and reactive bone formation, the diagnostic tissue is often obscured. Therefore, for children and young adults with bone tumors, we limit this procedure to those cases in which the radiograph is almost diagnostic and only a few cells are needed. For example, many osteosarcomas and giant cell tumors can be diagnosed with needle biopsies.

Closed needle biopsies are most accurate in lytic lesions in adult patients that are suspicious for metastatic carcinoma. Patients with lesions in the spine or pelvis are also candidates for this technique because open biopsies at these sites require major surgery. In addition, lesions where an open biopsy may cause a pathologic fracture are better biopsied with the closed needle technique.

The Frozen Section

The primary objective of a frozen section of a bone lesion is to determine if diagnostic tissue is present in the biopsy specimen. Because lesional tissue is sometimes obscured by secondary changes such as necrosis or cyst formation, the pathologist may have to send the surgeon back for another specimen. A frozen section cannot be performed on a heavily ossified lesion. However, if soft tissue is present, it can be teased away from the bone and frozen. A small amount of cancellous bone can be included in the frozen section.

Although some institutions claim that 90% of all lesions can be definitively diagnosed by frozen section,[3] we are very conservative in our use of this technique. We feel that definitive surgery should rarely be performed on the basis of a frozen section because of sampling error and obscured cellular detail caused by freezing. Despite these problems, frozen section can be confirmative in cases in which the diagnosis is already strongly indicated by clinical and radiographic features. For example, in high-grade chondrosarcoma or giant cell tumor, only a few cells are needed to confirm the radiographic diagnosis. By contrast, certain lesions, such as low-grade cartilage or osseous tumors, can never be definitively diagnosed by frozen section. In these lesions, the correct diagnosis usually depends on the careful study of many permanent tissue sections in which cellular detail is clearer than in frozen sections.

If a frozen section is performed, the surgeon should always submit an additional sample specifically designated for permanent section. If there is not enough tissue for both, the frozen section should be eliminated. Ideally, the biopsy should be big enough to do ancillary studies in addition to permanent sections. If a malignant lesion is suspected, tissue should be frozen for flow cytometry, and some should be placed in tissue culture media for chromosomal studies. This is particularly important in lesions that will be treated with neoadjuvant chemotherapy. Following this therapy, the entire lesion may be necrotic, and ancillary studies cannot be performed on tissue from the resected specimen.

Frozen sections may also be performed on closed needle biopsy specimens to ensure that diagnostic tissue is present. This is feasible only if it is possible to obtain multiple cores. Soft tissue can be dissected from the needle fragment, and a frozen section performed. If diagnostic tissue is not present, additional cores can be obtained.

HANDLING ORTHOPEDIC SPECIMENS

When preparing biopsy tissue for permanent section, we recommend dividing the tissue into portions that require varying degrees of decalcification. Large bone fragments, such as portions of cortex or sclerotic lesions, require routine decalcification. Cancellous bone requires only light decalcification. Very thin spicules of cancellous bone and soft tissue can be processed without decalcification. We always try to submit some tissue that can be processed without decalcification. Although immunohistochemical stains are not adversely affected by decalcification, we find these stains to be more reliable in nondecalcified tissue. Also, the diagnostic feature of osteoid—mineralization—is not erased.

Cutting Bone Specimens

The quality of the final histologic sections depends on the care with which bone specimens are prepared at the surgical pathology cutting bench. Cutting the bone specimens with a minimum of distortion and bone dust is the first step in preparing good sections. Specimens should be cut to a uniform thickness of 0.4 cm, and they should be small enough to fit in a tissue cassette. Small specimens consisting primarily of cancellous bone may be cut by tapping a single-edge razor blade through the tissue with a hammer. This method makes clean cuts with little distortion and no bone dust.

Motorized saws may be employed for larger specimens.

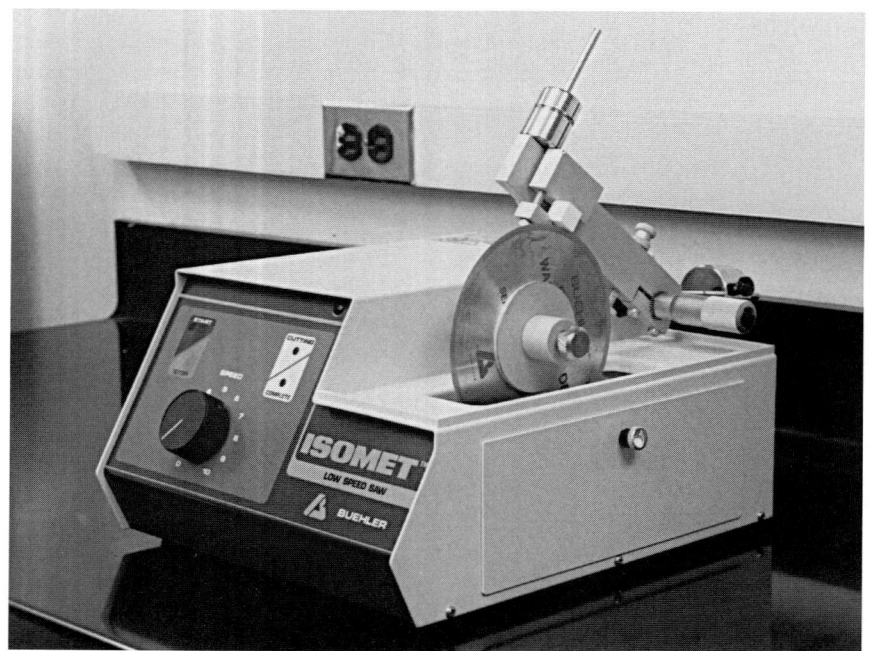

Figure 18-1 ■ A rotary diamond-coated saw. This saw is useful for delicate specimens. It produces almost no artifact.

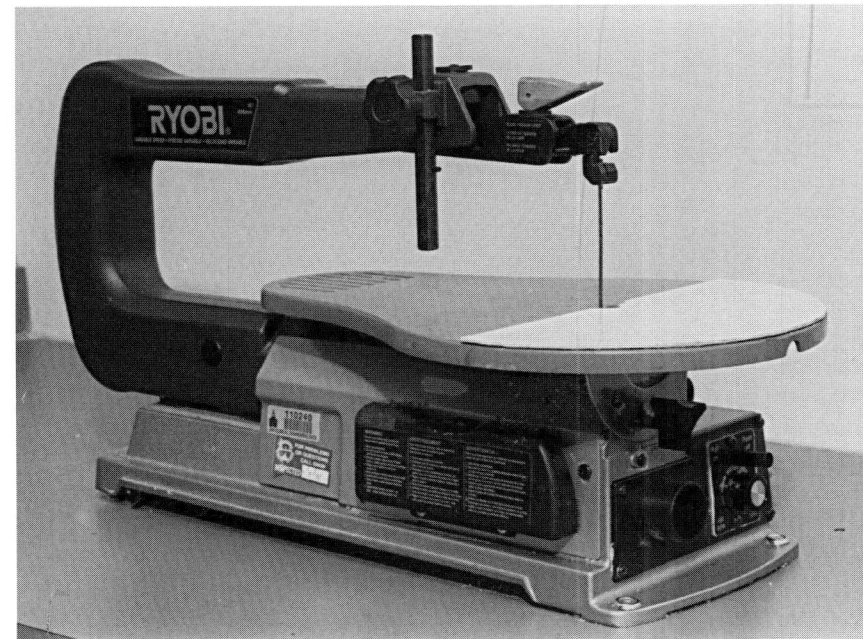

Figure 18-2 ■ A vibrating table saw. Most bone specimens can be cut with this saw.

A rotary diamond-edged saw produces the best results with almost no bone dust (Fig. 18–1). Unfortunately, this saw demands considerable care and is a bit cumbersome and slow. Therefore, we use it only in delicate specimens in which various tissue textures must be preserved in their proper relationship. For routine bone specimens, a small vibrating table saw is ideal (Fig. 18–2). This saw is quick, safe, and easy to use. The small amount of bone dust produced can be gently brushed away under running water with a soft-bristle toothbrush. For large bone specimens, those obtained in amputations and segmental resection for neoplasms, the large band saw is most efficient (Fig. 18–3). Using this saw, however, requires skill and extreme safety precautions. Beginners require close supervision.

Arthroplasty Specimens

The vibrating table saw is ideal for cutting specimens obtained from arthroplasty procedures. These specimens include femoral and humoral heads, as well as articular surfaces removed from total knee arthroplasties.

Some institutions do not process total joint arthroplasty specimens for microscopic study. They justify this practice by retrospective studies in their hospitals that demonstrate high correlation between preoperative clinical diagnosis and postoperative microscopic diagnosis. Because the final diagnosis almost never differs from the clinical diagnosis, the cost of the pathologic examination is, these hospitals argue, not justified.

In our opinion, it is a mistake not to do careful microscopic study of total joint specimens. We believe that the histologic findings are proportional to the quality of the tissue sections and the skill and interest of the pathologist. Many important processes are missed when a microscopic examination is not performed.[4] For example, we often find that cases presumed to be primary osteoarthritis are in fact secondary osteoarthritis. Careful microscopic scrutiny frequently reveals underlying aseptic necrosis, calcium pyro-

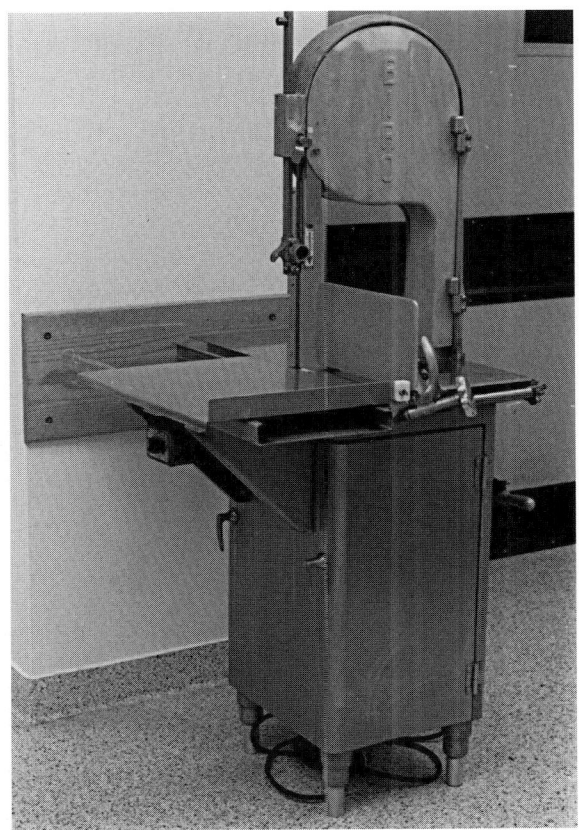

Figure 18-3 ■ A large band saw. This saw is necessary to cut large amputation or resection specimens.

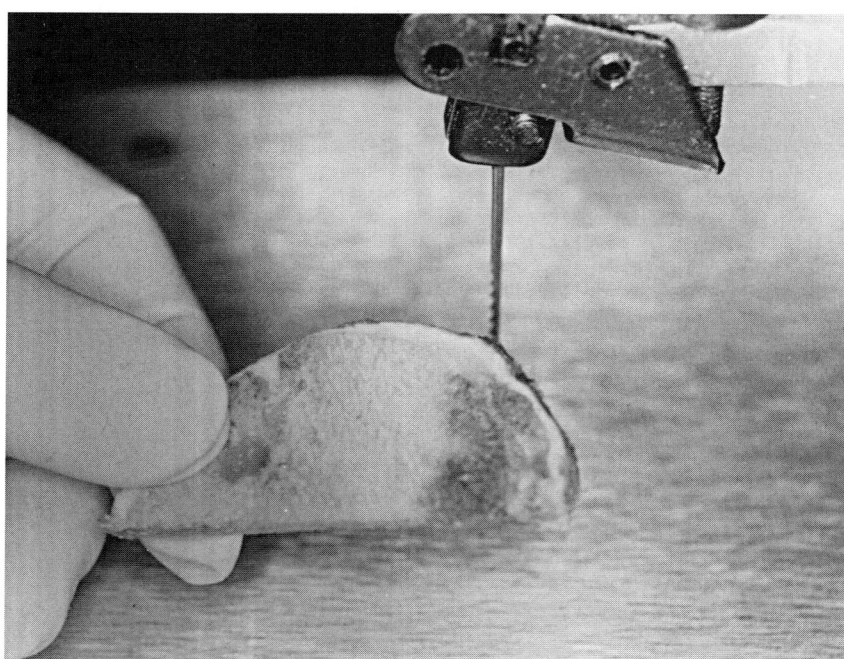

Figure 18-4 ■ A slab section of an osteoarthritic femoral head cut on the table saw. This specimen must be trimmed to fit in a cassette.

phosphate deposition disease, or an inflammatory arthritis. In addition, primary occult synovial diseases, such as pigmented villonodular synovitis, may be factors contributing to joint symptoms. Although these findings may not alter the prognosis, they offer insight into the disease process in that particular patient.

In addition to incidental findings in arthroplasty specimens, prognostically significant changes may also be discovered. For example, we have found unsuspected multiple myeloma, small lymphocytic lymphoma, and metastatic carcinoma. On one occasion, we discovered an undiagnosed chondrosarcoma in a total knee arthroplasty specimen.

Our microscopic study is preceded by a detailed gross examination of the specimen. First, the status of the articular cartilage should be noted. Is it softened, frayed, or eroded? Is the exposed bone eburnated (see Chapter 16)? Are osteophytes present? The cut surface of the bone should also be described. Is it sclerotic or osteoporotic? Are well-demarcated pale areas suggestive of osteonecrosis present?

In addition to articular bone, soft tissue, representing joint capsule and synovial membrane, is frequently a component of these specimens. The character of the soft tissue should also be described. Is it discolored or hemorrhagic? Is detritic bone or cartilage present?

After the gross examination, tissue must be selected for histologic study. Samples from at least two areas of the articular surface should be selected. These samples must include the underlying bone. In addition, one or two samples of periarticular soft tissue should be studied microscopically.

Depending on the specimen, articular surfaces may be cut in any direction that maximizes the exposed bone surface and articular cartilage. Femoral heads, however, are cut according to a standard protocol. First, the neck of the femoral head should be removed, a procedure that exposes a flat bone surface for the table saw. Then, with the vibrating table saw, the specimen is bivalved in a coronal plane. Next, 0.4-cm sections are taken from each half of the bivalved specimen (Fig. 18–4). In femoral heads removed following hip fractures, at least two additional specimens from the fracture site must be studied to rule out an underlying neoplasm.

Specimen Radiography

We frequently radiograph bone specimens with a table x-ray machine (Fig. 18–5). For this procedure, the specimen

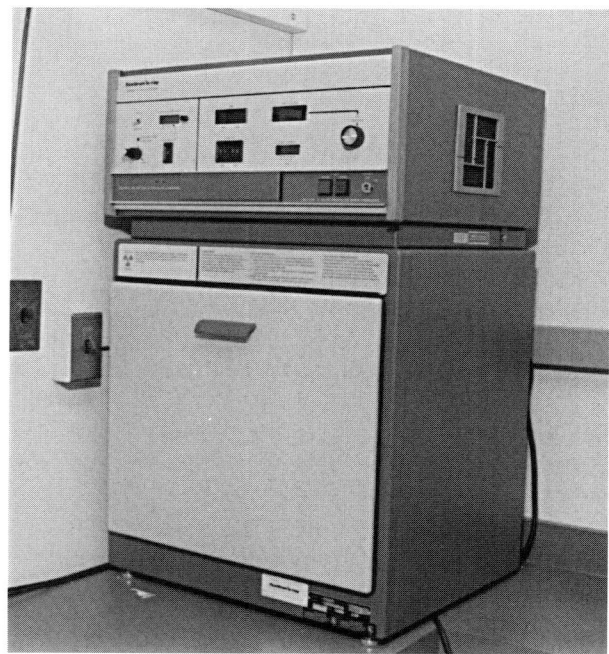

Figure 18-5 ■ A table radiograph machine.

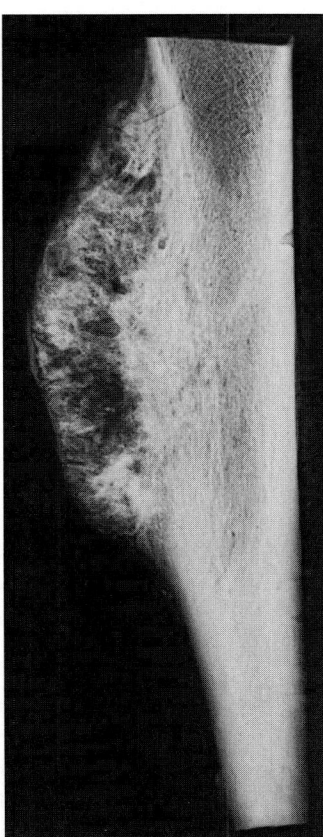

Figure 18-6 ■ A radiograph of a slab section from a periosteal osteosarcoma of the tibia.

(3) to calculate the amount of tumor necrosis. The first of these, evaluating the resection margins, should be completed while the patient is still in the operating room. First, the pathologist inspects the cuff of soft tissue to determine if soft tissue spread of tumor has occurred and if tumor is present at the margin. Suspicious areas may be examined by frozen section. Then, the pathologist incises the soft tissue cuff to the bone on either side of the specimen in the plane that the bone will be sawed. This is followed by bivalving the specimen with the band saw. At this point, the resection margin of the bone marrow can be inspected for the presence of neoplasm. If all margins are clear, the surgeon, delayed by only 15 minutes, may begin the reconstruction process.

The second objective in examining resection specimens is evaluating the extent of bone involvement by tumor. The growth characteristics of the tumor must be documented in the gross description and by photographs (Fig. 18–7 and Table 18–1). First, the location of the tumor, either on the bone surface or in the medullary canal, should be recorded. Its size, in three dimensions, should be documented, as well as its location in the bone (metaphyseal, diaphyseal, epiphyseal). If the epiphyseal plate is present, the amount of tumor penetration should be described. For intramedullary lesions, the presence and degree of cortical invasion should be noted and the amount of extraosseous tumor growth measured.

must be prepared in special ways. First, the initial bivalve through a specimen should be made so that the cut surface exposes the largest area of the disease process. Therefore, specimens should be cut with the guidance of the plain radiograph. When possible, we prefer to cut specimens in the coronal plane. This creates a surface that corresponds to the anteroposterior radiograph. Next, slabs 0.5 to 0.7 cm thick are cut from each portion of the bivalved specimen. The slabs may then be radiographed. Although radiographs taken with this apparatus are of no diagnostic importance, the fine detail of the images creates excellent teaching material (Fig. 18–6). Specimen radiographs may be compared with routine plain radiographs and with histologic sections. Another use of the specimen radiograph machine is to monitor the decalcification process.

Tumor Resection Specimens

Although amputation was formerly the treatment of choice for most primary malignant bone tumors, today many are treated with neoadjuvant chemotherapy and limb-sparing surgical resection. Rather than being an entire limb, the specimen is a segment of bone with a cuff of soft tissue.

The purpose of examining specimens from limb salvage tumor resections is threefold: (1) to evaluate the resection margins, (2) to describe the extent of bone involvement, and

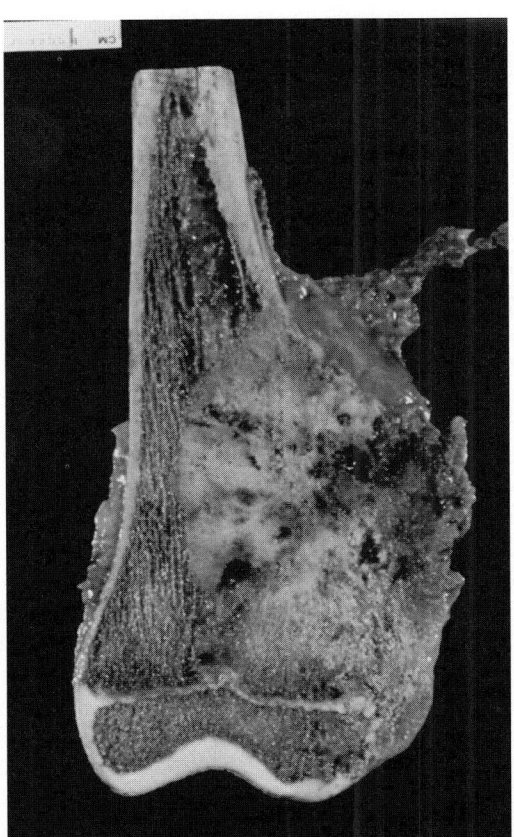

Figure 18-7 ■ Gross photograph of a slab section of a conventional osteosarcoma.

Table 18-1 ■ **EXAMINATION OF RESECTION SPECIMENS FOR PRIMARY MALIGNANT BONE TUMORS**

Resection margins
    Soft tissue cuff margin
    Intramedullary marrow margin
Location of tumor
    Bone involved
    Intramedullary or surface
    Segment involved: epiphyseal, metaphyseal, diaphyseal
Extent of tumor
    Size
    Presence of cortical erosion
    Extent of soft tissue mass
    Extension through epiphyseal plate
Gross features of tumor
    Bony, cartilaginous, or fibrous
    Cystic change
    Necrosis
Histologic features
    Percent of necrotic neoplasm
    Tumor type
    Histologic grade

In addition to the size and location of the tumor, the characteristics of the neoplastic tissue should be described. Is the lesion fleshy, bony, or cartilaginous? Are cystic regions or areas of hemorrhage present? Is grossly necrotic tissue present?

The third objective, quantitation of tumor necrosis, is described in Chapter 12. This procedure is necessary for prognostication in patients who have had neoadjuvant chemotherapy. Neoplasms that have not been treated by chemotherapy should also be studied microscopically. Areas of different gross textures should be examined and the histologic grade established. Well-differentiated lesions should be carefully studied for areas of dedifferentiation.

PROCESSING BONE SPECIMENS

Decalcification

Almost all bone specimens need to be decalcified before processing for microtomy. However, before the process begins, the bone tissue must be completely fixed, preferably in neutral buffered formalin. The decalcification solutions are almost always a mixture of an acid and a buffer. They should be strong enough to ensure timely and adequate decalcification, yet they should not be so strong that the tissue is damaged. Numerous commercial decalcification solutions are available. However, we prefer a 10% formic acid solution with equal parts of a 5% sodium citrate buffer.

There are several important steps in the decalcification process. First, to ensure even decalcification, specimens should always be uniformly trimmed to size before the process begins. Ideally, specimens are no thicker than 0.4 cm. Then, the formalin-fixed bone sections are rinsed in running cold tap water and then suspended in the decalcification solution at room temperature. A motorized agitator decreases the length of time needed in the solution (Fig. 18–8). Depending on the thickness of a specimen, the decalcification process lasts 1 to 4 days. Small fragments of cancellous bone, however, may decalcify in 4 to 6 hours. Typically, a routine section of an osteoarthritic femoral head requires 2 days.

Bone sections should be examined each day to prevent overdecalcification. Determining the endpoint of the process may be done by two methods. The first is manual. An experienced technician can gently probe the tissue with a pin or test its pliability by bending. The second method is to radiograph the tissue samples in a specimen x-ray machine. This method is the more accurate but is time consuming.

If, due to error, an incompletely decalcified specimen is embedded in a paraffin block, surface decalcification may be done. The paraffin block is immersed in a shallow plate filled with the decalcification solution. After about 6 hours, the exposed surface of the block is decalcified for a depth of a few millimeters. This allows cutting of one or two tissue sections.

Cutting and Staining Bone Specimens

After proper decalcification, bone specimens may be processed in the routine manner. Tissue is embedded in paraffin and cut with a rotary microtome. Serial sections should be made of small biopsy specimens. Large bone specimens are prone to tears, wrinkles, or folds. This problem often can be minimized by soaking the face of the block in a 10% glycerin solution for 30 minutes. Adding celloidin to the embedding medium also minimizes these artifacts. Another

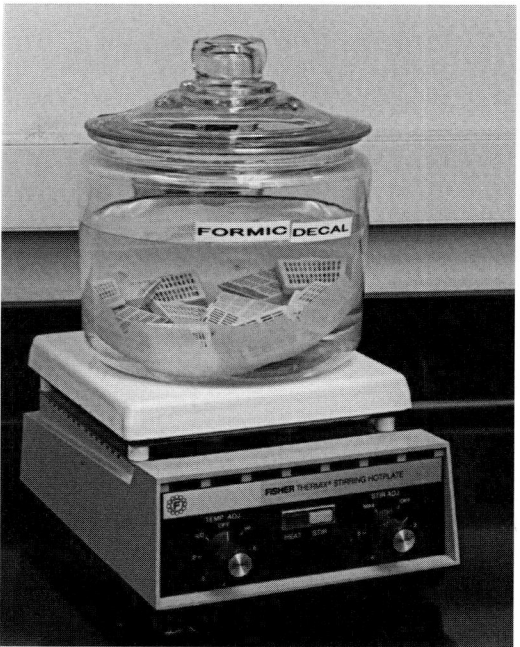

Figure 18–8 ■ A decalcification apparatus. Motorized agitation reduces the time required to decalcify the bone specimens.

artifact, bone dust impacted into the intertrabecular spaces, can be minimized by facing deep into the tissue blocks.

The tissue specimens may then be stained with routine hematoxylin and eosin. Modifications of the staining procedure must occasionally be made to enhance tissue contrast. Because of the acid mucopolysaccharides, hyaline cartilage is basophilic. With routine hematoxylin and eosin staining, it should be blue. However, acid decalcification often weakens this staining characteristic; therefore, we often increase the time in hematoxylin. Eight minutes (instead of the usual three) enhances the basophilia of the hyaline cartilage.

The pathologist should work closely with the histotechnologist to ensure a high quality of bone slides. Tissue prepared with care leads to beautiful histologic sections. With these, the pathologist may accurately correlate microscopic features with radiographs and begin the diagnostic process. The pathologist may then assign the changes to one of the five major disease categories outlined in Chapter 1.

REFERENCES

1. Simon, M. A., and Biermann, J. S.: Biopsy of bone and soft-tissue lesions. *J Bone Joint Surg* 75A:616–620, 1993.
2. DeSantos, L. A., Murray, J. A., and Ayala, A. G.: The value of percutaneous needle biopsy in the management of primary bone tumors. *Cancer* 43:735–744, 1979.
3. Weatherby, R. P., and Unni, K. K.: Practical aspects of handling orthopedic specimens in the surgical pathology laboratory. *Pathol Annu* 17(2):1–31, 1982.
4. DiCarlo, E. F., Bullough, P. G., Steiner, G., Bansal, M., and Kambolis, C.: Pathological examination of the femoral head (FH) [abstract]. *Lab Invest* 70:6A, 1994.

Index

Note: Page numbers in *italics* refer to illustrations; page numbers followed by t refer to tables.

Abscess, in osteomyelitis, *157*
    Brodie's, 155, *156–157*
    intracortical, 155, *155*
    paravertebral, 158, 161, *162*
    subperiosteal, 154, 161
Abuse, alcohol. See *Alcohol abuse.*
    drug, osteomyelitis and, 160
Achondrogenesis type II, 67
Achondroplasia, 65–67, *66–67*
Acid phosphatase, in metastatic carcinoma, 178, 180
    in osteopetrosis, 63
    tartrate-resistant, 8, 30, 33
Aclasis, diaphyseal. See *Exostosis(es), multiple hereditary.*
Acquired immunodeficiency syndrome (AIDS), bone and joint infections in, 159
Acral metastases, 176–177
Acroosteosclerosis, 123
Adamantinoma, 263–264, *263–265*
    differentiated, 264, *265*
    vs. osteofibrous dysplasia, 262–263, 264
Adenocarcinoma, of unknown primary source, 176
    vs. chordoma, 269
Aggrecans, 322
Aging, bone remodeling and, 36, 37
    osteomalacia and, 81
    osteopenia associated with, 3
    vitamin D synthesis and, 45, 81
AIDS (acquired immunodeficiency syndrome), bone and joint infections in, 159
AL amyloid, 190, *191*
Alcohol abuse, neuropathic joint and, 335
    osteonecrosis and, 4, 137–138, 144
    osteoporosis and, 93
Alendronate (Fosamax), for osteoporosis, 95
    for Paget's disease, 172
Alkaline phosphatase, in metastatic carcinoma, 178
    in osteomalacia, 82
    in Paget's disease, 168–169
    in rickets, 79, 80
    mineralization and, 8, 29, 35
Alkaptonuria, 57–58, *58*
Aluminum bone disease, 87–88
    histological diagnosis of, 24, 88, *following page 98*
Amenorrhea, secondary, 93
Amorphous calcification, 9, *9–10*
Amorphous calcium salts, 35, 44, 47
Amputation, 198, *199*
Amyloidoma of bone, 191, *191*
Amyloidosis, 190
    in amyloidoma of bone, 191, *191*
    in chronic renal failure, 88
    in multiple myeloma, 191
    neuropathic joint in, 335
Anemia, bone changes in, 6, 128
    sickle cell anemia and, 128–130, *130*
    thalassemia and, 128, *129*

Anemia *(Continued)*
    bone disorder(s) causing, 8
    multiple myeloma as, 187, 187t
    myelofibrosis as, 131
    osteopetrosis as, 63
Aneurysmal bone cyst, 277, 277t, 279–280, *282–283*, 284
    in giant cell reparative granuloma, 284, 305
    in myositis ossificans, 297
    neoplasm(s) associated with, 279, 284
        chondroblastoma as, 221, 284
        chondromyxoid fibroma as, 225
        fibrous dysplasia as, 246
        giant cell tumor as, 254
        osteoblastoma as, 203
        osteosarcoma as, 208–209
        telangiectatic osteosarcoma as, 284
    solid variant of, 284, 305
    vs. fractured unicameral cyst, 279
    vs. telangiectatic osteosarcoma, 215–215, *218*
Angiomatosis, bacillary, 159
    cystic, 265–267, *266*
Angiosarcoma of bone, 264–265, 268, *268–269*
    in dedifferentiated chondrosarcoma, 243
Ankylosing spondylitis, 343–344, *344–345*
    CT image of, 3-dimensional, *21*
    heterotopic ossification in, 298
    reactive arthritis causing, 345
Ankylosis, in rheumatoid arthritis, 339
Anlage, cartilage, *40–41*
Anorexia nervosa, osteoporosis in, 93
Anticonvulsants, mineralization and, 81
Antiresorptive agents, 95. See also *specific agents.*
Aortic valve disease, ankylosing spondylitis causing, 344
Apatite, 25, 35, 44
Appositional reactive bone, 11, *13–14*
Arthralgias, in acute lymphoblastic leukemia, 127
Arthritis. See also *Ankylosing spondylitis; Osteoarthritis; Rheumatoid arthritis; Synovitis.*
    CPPD as, 348–350, *349–350*
        subchondral cysts in, 284
        tumoral, 293, *294*, 349
    history of, 317–318
    in multicentric reticulohistiocytosis, 125
    in sarcoidosis of bone, 123, *124*
    in systemic lupus erythematosus, 346
    Jaccoud's, 346
    psoriatic, 343, 346
    reactive, 343, 344–346, *345*
        genetic predisposition to, 51
        gonorrheal, 162
    septic, 153, 161–162
    tuberculous, 162
Arthritis mutilans, 346
Arthroplasty, total joint, biological response to, 353–354, 359, *360*
    failure of, aseptic, 353–354, 356–358, *356–359*
        pathologist and, 362

Arthroplasty *(Continued)*
    revision for, 298, 353, 360, 362
    septic, 360–362
  for femoral head osteonecrosis, 141, 144
  for osteoarthritis, 285, 332
  for pyrophosphate arthropathy, 350
  for rheumatoid arthritis, 342
  heterotopic ossification following, 297–298
  history of, 354–355
  in metastatic carcinoma, 180, *182*
  in Paget's disease, 172
  malignancies associated with, 362
  pathology specimens from, 362, 367–368, *368*
  prostheses for, 353, *354,* 355
  tuberculosis reactivated by, 162
  well-functioning, 355–356, *355–356*
  types of, 353
Aseptic necrosis, 136
Athletes, osteoporosis in, 93
Atrophic nonunion, 112, *112*
Atrophy, disuse, 3, 96–97, *96–97*
Autoimmune disease(s), reactive arthritis as, 345
  rheumatoid arthritis as, 337, 338, 343
  sarcoidosis of bone as, 123
  spondyloarthropathies as, 343, 344
Autopsy, in skeletal dysplasias, 72
  total joint prosthesis in, 362
Autosomal dominant disorders, 51–52
Autosomal recessive disorders, 51, 52
Avascular necrosis, 136
Avulsion injury, 4, 114, 116–117, *116–117*
Azzopardi phenomenon, 259–260

Bacillary angiomatosis of bone, 159
Balloon cells, 55
Bamboo spine, 344, *345*
Batson's plexus, 176, *176*
Bence Jones proteins, 185
  in MGUS, 185
  in multiple myeloma, 187
  in solitary myeloma of bone, 190
Benign tumors, 6, 195, 197. See also specific tumors.
  staging of, 198, 198t
Beta$_2$-microglobulin, 88
Biglycan, 34
Biopsy, 365–366
  for histomorphometry, 24
Bisphosphonates, for metastatic carcinoma, 180
  for osteoporosis, 95
    juvenile, 94
  for Paget's disease, 172
Bizarre parosteal osteochondromatous proliferation, 299, *299–301*
Blastic metastases, 5
Blood vessels, in bone, 26, 27, *30*
Blue cell tumors, small round, 258–259
  Ewing sarcoma/PNET as, 258–259, 260
  small cell osteosarcoma as, 216, *219*
BMPs (bone morphogenetic proteins), 35
  in heterotopic ossification, 294, 298
  in osteoblast development, 29
Bone, blood vessels in, 26, 27, *30*
  development of, 37–38, *37–43,* 40–42
  functions of, 25
  mechanical properties of, 105–108, *106–108*
  mineralization of, 35, 37, *38*
  modeling of, 42
    calcitonin and, 48
    in Gaucher disease, 55
  organic matrix of. See *Osteoid.*
  organization of, 25–29, *25–31*
  physiology of, 42–49, *44–45, 48*
  reactive. See *Reactive bone.*
  remodeling of, 35–37, *36*
    calcitonin and, 48

Bone *(Continued)*
    electrical activity in, 30, 37
    resorption of. See *Resorption of bone.*
Bone cyst(s). See *Cyst(s).*
Bone diseases. See also specific disease, e.g., *Osteomyelitis.*
  categories of, 1–7, 1t
  diagnosis of, 7–24
    clinical presentation in, 7–8
    histomorphometry in, 23, 23–24
    immunohistochemistry in, 22
    laboratory studies in, 8
    multidisciplinary, 7, 9, 75, 197, 365
    radiography in, 8–9, 16–22, *19–22*
    radiologic-histologic correlation in, 8–9, *9–18,* 11, 15
Bone grafts, for chronic osteomyelitis, 161
  for nonunion of fracture, 112
Bone island(s), 198–199, *200*
  in osteopoikilosis, 64–65, *66*
Bone marrow, 25, 26. See also *Fat necrosis; Plasma cell dyscrasias.*
  development of, 40
  edema of, in osteomyelitis, 159
    in osteonecrosis, 137, 144
    in transient osteoporosis, 97, 98–99, *98–99*
  expansion of, in hematologic disorders, 6, 127, 128
  fibrosis of, in mastocytosis, 127
    in metastatic carcinoma, 180, *182*
    in myelofibrosis, 130
    in osteomyelitis, 156, 158, *160,* 163
    in renal osteodystrophy, 86, *87, following page 98*
  in leukemias, 127–128
  in mastocytosis, 126–127, *127*
  in osteonecrosis, 138–139, *139*
  inflammation of, 156
  metastatic carcinoma in, 177
Bone mass, definition of, 88
  peak, 88–89, 94–95
Bone morphogenetic proteins (BMPs), 35
  in heterotopic ossification, 294, 298
  in osteoblast development, 29
Bone scan, 16–17, *19*
Bone spurs. See also *Osteophytes.*
  in reactive arthritis, 345, *345*
  traction spurs, in DISH, 334–335, *336*
  in spinal osteoarthritis, 334
Bone turnover, 3. See also *Remodeling of bone.*
  calcium exchange in, 44
  high, bone scan and, 17
    in primary hyperparathyroidism, 76–77
  histomorphometry and, 23, 24
  indices of, 8
  osteocalcin and, 34
Breast carcinoma, metastatic, 175, *176,* 177, 178, 180
Brodie's abscess, 155, *156–157*
Bronchioalveolar tumor, intravascular, 267
Bronchogenic carcinoma, hypertrophic osteoarthropathy in, 131
Brown tumor(s), 304, 305
  in primary hyperparathyroidism, 76, 304
  in renal osteodystrophy, 84, *86,* 304
Brushite, 35, 44, 47
Buckle fractures, 108
Butterfly fractures, *107–108,* 108

Caffey's disease, 302–303, *303*
Calcific tendinitis, 291–292
Calcification. See also *Mineralization.*
  amorphous, 9, *9–10*
  of hyaline cartilage, 9, 11, *11–12*
  radiodensity and, 9
Calcifying pseudotumor, of neural axis, 294
Calcinosis, tumoral, 9, *9,* 291–293, *292–293*
Calcipenic disorders, 78
Calcitonin, 47–48
  for osteoporosis, 95
  for Paget's disease, 172

Calcitonin *(Continued)*
  osteoclast receptors for, 33
Calcitriol, 46. See also *Vitamin D.*
  for osteopetrosis, 64
  for osteoporosis, 95
  in hereditary rickets, 80
Calcium, amorphous salts of, 35, 44, 47
  dietary, 44
    adult requirement for, 95
    deficiency of, 48, 78, 79
    peak bone mass and, 89
  distribution of, in body, 43–44
  exchangeable, 25, 35, 44, 47
    bone remodeling and, 26, 36
    osteocytes and, 29–30
  excretion of, 44, *44,* 47, 48, 49
  intestinal absorption of, 44, *44*
    in osteomalacia, 82
    in rickets, 78, 79
    phytates and, 81
    vitamin D and, 45, 46, 48, 49
  serum levels of, 42–43
    parathyroid hormone and, 46–47, *48,* 48–49
Calcium brushite, 35, 44, 47
Calcium hydroxyapatite, 25, 35, 44
Calcium pyrophosphate deposition disease (CPPD), 348–350, *349–350*
  history of, 318
  subchondral cysts in, 284
  tumoral, 293, *294,* 349
Callus, fracture, 109, *110–111,* 111
  in delayed union, 112
  in nonunion, 112, *113*
  in stress fracture, 114, *116*
Camurati-Engelmann disease, 64, *65*
Canaliculi, 27, 29, *32*
Cancellous bone, 25–26, *25–27*
  microscopic organization of, 27, *30*
  remodeling of, 36, *37*
Cancer. See *Metastatic disease in bone; Tumor(s);* specific neoplasm, e.g., *Osteosarcoma.*
Carbonic anhydrase II deficiency, 64
Carcinoma, breast, metastatic, 175, *176,* 177–178, 180
  bronchogenic, hypertrophic osteoarthropathy in, 131
  lung metastatic, 175–176, 178, *179,* 181
  prostate. See *Prostate cancer.*
Carpal tunnel syndrome, amyloidosis causing, 88
Cartilage. See also *Epiphyseal plate.*
  articular, 26, *27,* 319, *320,* 320–324, *322–324*
    development of, 41
    in osteoarthritis, 326–327, *327–328*
    in rheumatoid arthritis, 339, *340*
    mechanical stresses on, 324, 326
    metabolism of, 324, 326–327
    zones of, 322–323, *323*
  chondrodysplasias of, 65–70, *66–70*
  fibrocartilage as, 319
    CPPD in, 348
    in osteoarthritis repair, 328, *329*
  hyaline, *320,* 320–324, *322–324*
    calcification of, 9, 11, *11–12*
  neoplasms of, 220–221, *222.* See also specific neoplasms.
  ossification of, 37, 38, *39–41,* 40–42
Cartilage-hair hypoplasia, 70
Cat-scratch bacillus, angiomatosis and, 159
Causalgia, 99–100
Cement lines, 27, *31–32*
Cementoma, fibrous, 246, *248*
Cementoossifying fibroma, 246, *248*
Charcot joint, 335, *336–337*
Chemotherapy, for metastatic carcinoma, 180
  neoadjuvant, 219
    biopsy prior to, 366
    tumor necrosis with, 219–220, *220–221*
Cherubism, 304
Cholecalciferol, 45
Chondroblastoma, 220, 221, *223–224*

Chondroblastoma *(Continued)*
  vs. clear cell chondrosarcoma, 240–241
Chondrocalcinosis, 349, *349*
Chondrocytes, defective, in CPPD, 348
    in metaphyseal chondrodysplasia, 70
    in pseudoachondroplasia, 68, *69*
  in endochondral ossification, 38, *39,* 40, 41–42, *42*
    matrix vesicles and, 35
  of cartilage, 11
  of fibrocartilage, 319, *320*
  of hyaline cartilage, 320–321, 323, 324
    in osteoarthritis, 327
Chondrodysplasias, 65–70, *66–70*
  metaphyseal, 69–70, *70*
Chondroid chordoma, 269
Chondroitin sulfate, 55, 322, *322*
  in osteoarthritis, 327
  in Sly syndrome, 57
Chondrolysis, acute, 343, *344*
Chondroma, of soft parts, 307
  periosteal, *222,* 234–235, *235–237*
Chondromatosis, synovial, 220, *222*
  primary, 307–310, *308–310*
  secondary, 307, 310, *310–311*
  vs. chondrosarcoma, 232, 236, 309
  with osteochondroma, *20,* 232, 307
Chondromyxoid fibroma, 220, 221, 225–227, *225–227*
Chondrosarcoma, 235–244
  central, *222,* 235, 236, 239–240, *239–241*
  clear cell, 235, 240–241, *242–243*
  dedifferentiated, 235, 243–244, *243–244*
  enchondromatosis prior to, 230
  histologic grading of, 236, *237–238*
  juxtacortical, 235, 240
  Maffucci's syndrome prior to, 231
  medullary, *222*
  mesenchymal, 235, 241–243, 244
  osteochondroma prior to, 231, 234
  periosteal, 235, 240
  peripheral, *222,* 240, *242*
  secondary, 235
  subtypes of, 235–236, 236t
  surface, *222,* 240, *242*
  synovial, 309
  treatment of, 244
  vs. chondromyxoid fibroma, 226–227
  vs. chordoma, 269
  vs. periosteal osteosarcoma, 212
  vs. synovial chondromatosis, 232, 236, 309
Chordoma, 268–269, *269–271*
  chondroid, 269
  dedifferentiated, 269
Clear cell chondrosarcoma, 235, 240–241, *242–243*
Closed fractures, 108
Closure of physis, 42
Clubbing, in hypertrophic osteoarthropathy, 131–132, *131–132,* 132t
Coagulation, intravascular, in osteonecrosis, 136–137, 137t, 144
Coccidioidomycosis, of spine, 162
Codman's triangle, in osteosarcoma, 208, *209*
Colitis, reactive arthritis of, 345–346
Collagen, breakdown of, markers for, 8, 54
  fibrils of, 33, *34*
    mineralization in, 35
  in bone, 27, 33–34
    woven, 38
  in fibrocartilage, 319, *320*
  in hyaline cartilage, 321–323, *323*
  type I, 33, *34*
    in fibrocartilage, 319, *320*
    in osteogenesis imperfecta, 59, 60–61
  type II, 41, 321, *323*
    defective, 67, 68, 325
  type VI, 321–322
  type X, 41, 322
  type XI, 321
    defective, 67

Collagenases, in osteoarthritis, 327
  in rheumatoid arthritis, 338, 339
Comminution, of fractures, 107, *107,* 108
Compact bone, 25, 26. See also *Cortex.*
  formation of, 38
  microscopic organization of, 25, *27, 28–30, 29*
Complete blood count, 8
Complete fractures, 108
Compliance, of bone, 105
Compressed air, osteonecrosis and, 138, 142–143
Computerized tomography (CT), 16, 17–18, *20–21*
Congenital diseases. See *Genetic disease(s); Skeletal dysplasia(s).*
Cortex, of bone, 25, *25,* 26, *27.* See also *Compact bone.*
  intramembranous ossification of, 37
  modeling of, 42
  remodeling of, 36, 37
Cortical defects, fibrous, 244, *245*
Coupling, of osteoblasts, 37
  uncoupling and, 3
CPPD (calcium pyrophosphate deposition disease), 348–350, *349–350*
  history of, 318
  subchondral cysts in, 284
  tumoral, 293, *294,* 349
Creeping substitution, 140, *140*
Crohn's disease, reactive arthritis of, 345–346
Crudoma, 294
CT (computerized tomography), 16, 17–18, *20–21*
Cutting cone(s), 30, 37
Cyst(s), bone, 277–289
  aneurysmal. See *Aneurysmal bone cyst.*
  intraosseous lipoma as, 277, 277t, 286–287, *287–288,* 289
  unicameral, 117, 277–279, 277t, *278–281*
  diagnosis of, 277, 277t
  epidermal inclusion, 277, 277t, *288,* 289
  subchondral, 277, 284, *284*
    amyloidosis causing, 88
    in CPPD, 349
    intraosseous ganglion as, 277t, 285, *286*
    osteoarthritic. See *Osteoarthritic cyst(s).*
    post-traumatic, 277t, 285–286, *287*
  subperiosteal, in neurofibromatosis, 53
Cystic angiomatosis, 265–267, *266*
Cytokeratin staining, 22
  of chordoma, 269
  of metastatic carcinoma, 180
Cytokines. See also *Growth factor(s); Interleukin(s).*
  in multiple myeloma, 187
  in osteomyelitis, 154
  in osteopetrosis, deficiency of, 63
    interferon-γ for, 64
  in rheumatoid arthritis, 338, 339, 341

Dactylitis, sickle cell, 129, *130*
Decalcification of specimens, 366, 370, *370*
Decorin, 34
Dedifferentiated chondrosarcoma, 235, 243–244, *243–244*
Dedifferentiation, 195
  of giant cell tumors, 255
Degenerative joint disease. See *Osteoarthritis.*
7-Dehydrocholesterol, 45
Delayed union, 112
  strain intolerance causing, 111
Densitometry. See *DEXA (dual energy x-ray absorptiometry) scan.*
Dentinogenesis imperfecta, 60
Dermatan sulfate, 55, 56, 57
Dermatofibrosis lenticularis disseminata, 65
Desferoxamine, for aluminum bone disease, 88
Desmoid, periosteal, 116–117, *117*
Desmoplastic fibroma, 248–249, *249*
  vs. fibrosarcoma, 249–250, *250*
Detritic synovitis, 329, *331*
DEXA (dual energy x-ray absorptiometry) scan, 19, 22, 88, 95
Diabetes, fracture healing and, 112
  idiopathic hyperostosis and, 334

Diabetes *(Continued)*
  neuropathic joint caused by, 335
  osteoporosis in, 93
Diaphyseal aclasis. See *Exostosis(es), multiple hereditary.*
Diaphyseal dysplasia, progressive, 64, *65*
Diaphysis, 26, *27*
Diarthrodial joints, 319, *319*
DIC (disseminated intravascular coagulation), 136
Diffuse idiopathic skeletal hyperostosis (DISH), 334–335, *336,* 343
Dilantin, mineralization and, 81
Discitis, 159
DISH (diffuse idiopathic skeletal hyperostosis), 334–335, *336,* 343
Disseminated intravascular coagulation (DIC), 136
Disseminated osteoarthritis of Kellgren, 332
Disuse osteoporosis, 3, 96–97, *96–97*
  vs. multiple myeloma, 188, *188*
Divers, osteonecrosis in, 138, 142–143
Dominant negative mutations, 61
Drug abuse, osteomyelitis and, 160
Dual energy x-ray absorptiometry (DEXA) scan, 19, 22, 88, 95
Dwarfs, 58
Dysbaric osteonecrosis, 138, 142–143
Dysostosis multiplex, 56, *56,* 57
Dysplasia epiphysealis hemimelica, 51, 70, *71*
Dysplasia(s), skeletal, 1–2, 51, 58–59, 59t. See also specific dysplasias.
  osteochondromatosis as, 232, 234, *235*
  pathologist's role in, 71–72

Eburnation, 328, *328*
Electric currents, disuse atrophy and, 3, 96
  for fracture healing, 112
  osteocytic membrane system and, 30
Embolism, fat, osteonecrosis and, 137, 138, 144
Emperipolesis, 124, *126*
Enchondroma, *222,* 227–228, *227–230*
  dedifferentiated chondrosarcoma with, 243
  MRI of, *21*
  vs. chondrosarcoma, 236, 239–240, *240–241*
Enchondroma protuberans, 228, *229*
Enchondromatosis, 229–230, *230–231*
Endochondral ossification, 11, *12,* 37, 38, *39*
  centers of, 38, 40–42, *40–43*
Endocrine disorders, 2, 75. See also *Hyperparathyroidism.*
Endocrinologists, laboratory studies by, 8, 75
Endosteum, 25, 26
Enneking system, 198, 198t
Enostosis(es), 198–199, *200*
  in osteopoikilosis, 64–65, *66*
Enthesopathy, in ankylosing spondylitis, 343
  in DISH, 334–335, *336*
  in reactive arthritis, 345
Eosinophilic granuloma, 119, 120–121, *120–121*
  vs. chronic osteomyelitis, 22
  vs. Hodgkin's disease, 258
  vs. sinus histiocytosis, 124
Epidermal inclusion cyst, 277, 277t, *288,* 289
Epiphyseal dysplasia, multiple, 68–69, *69*
Epiphyseal plate, 26, *27,* 41–42, *41–43*
  abnormal, in enchondromatosis, 229
    in Legg-Calvé-Perthes disease, 145–146, *146*
    in metaphyseal chondrodysplasia, 69–70, *70*
    in osteogenesis imperfecta, 62, *62*
    in rickets, 79, *80*
  closure of, 42
  matrix vesicles in, 35
Epiphysis(es), 26, *27*
  fusion of, to metaphysis(es), 42
  ossification centers of, *40,* 40–41
Epithelioid hemangioendothelioma, 264–265, 267, *267–268*
Epulis, peripheral giant cell, 304
Erdheim-Chester disease, 124
Erythrocyte sedimentation rate, 8
  in ankylosing spondylitis, 344
  in multiple myeloma, 187, 187t

Erythrocyte sedimentation rate *(Continued)*
   in vertebral osteomyelitis, 158
Estrogen, deficiency of, 91, 93
  for osteoporosis, 95
    osteoarthritis and, 332
Etidronate, for osteoporosis, 95
  juvenile, 94
Ewing sarcoma, 258–261, *259–261*
  immunohistochemistry of, 260–261
  large cell variant of, 259
  pathologic fracture in, 117
  radiographic features of, *18, 259, 259–260*
  vs. acute osteomyelitis, 8
  vs. small cell osteosarcoma, 216
Exostosis(es), multiple hereditary, 232, 234, *235,* 240
  subungual, 299, 301–302, *302–303*
  turret, 299
Exostosis bursata, 307
  vs. chondrosarcoma, 232, 240
Extracellular matrix. See also *Osteoid.*
  of bone, 27, *28*
  of fibrocartilage, 319, *320*
  of hyaline cartilage, 320–324, *322–324*

Fallen leaf sign, 278, *279*
Fat embolism, osteonecrosis and, 137, 138, 144
Fat necrosis, calcification of, 9, *10*
  in intraosseous lipoma, 287, *288,* 289
  in osteonecrosis, 138–139, *139*
  vs. osteosarcoma, 208, *210*
Fatigue fractures, 108, 113, 113t
Femoral cortical irregularity syndrome, distal, 116–117, *117*
Femoral head, osteonecrosis of, in childhood, 145–146, *146*
  intravascular occlusion causing, 4, 137, 141–144
  radiation causing, 150
  staging of, 141–142, 141t, *142–144*
  trauma causing, 135
Fever, bone lesions causing, 8
Fibroblast growth factor receptor 3, 65
Fibrocartilage, 319
  CPPD in, 348
  in osteoarthritis repair, 328, *329*
Fibrocartilaginous mesenchymoma, 247
Fibrodysplasia ossificans progressiva, 294, 298
Fibroma, cementoossifying, 246, *248*
  chondromyxoid, 220, 221, 225–227, *225–227*
  nonossifying, 244–245, *245*
Fibrosarcoma of bone, 249–250, *249–250*
  radiation causing, 249, 271
  treatment of, 252
Fibrous cementoma, 246, *248*
Fibrous cortical defects, 244, 245
Fibrous dysplasia, 245–247, *246–248*
  osteomalacia caused by, 82
  vs. intraosseous well-differentiated osteosarcoma, 213, 215, 247
  vs. Paget's disease, 172
Fibrous dysplasia protuberans, 246
Fibroxanthoma, 245
Fluoride, for idiopathic juvenile osteoporosis, 94
  in apatite crystals, 35
  osteoporosis and, 95
Forces on bone, 105–108, *106–108*
Forestier's disease, 334–335, *336*
C-fos, fibrous dysplasia and, 246
Fosamax. See *Alendronate (Fosamax).*
Fracture(s), 3–4, 105–118
  avulsion injury as, 114, 116–117, *116–117*
  classifications of, *107,* 107–108, 107t, 108t
  healing of, 3–4
    bleeding and, 109, *109*
    delayed union in, 111, 112
    in stress fracture, 114, *116*
    nonunion in, 3–4, 111, 112, *112–113,* 112t
    phases of, 109, *109–110,* 111

Fracture(s) *(Continued)*
   rate of, 108–109
   reduction and, 111–112
  infection of, 5
  mechanics of, 105–108, *106–108*
  osteonecrosis associated with, 4, 135
  pathologic, 4, 108, 117–118, *118*
  reduction of, 111–112
  stress. See *Stress fractures.*
  susceptibility to, 95–96, 95t
    from osteoporosis, 89, 89t, 90, *90,* 96
Freiberg's disease, *146,* 146–147
Frozen section, 365–366, 369
Fungal infections, of bone, 162

Gadolinium contrast, 19
Gammopathies. See *Plasma cell dyscrasias.*
Ganglion, intraosseous, 277, 277t, 285, *286*
  periosteal, 285
Gaucher disease, 54–55, *54–55*
Genetic disease(s), 1–2, 51–52. See also specific diseases.
  fibrodysplasia ossificans progressiva as, 294, 298
  McCune-Albright syndrome as, 245–246, *247*
  rickets as, 78–79, *80,* 80–81, 82, *following page 98*
Geodes, 284
Giant cell epulis, peripheral, 304
Giant cell reparative granuloma, 303–305, *304–305*. See also *Brown tumor(s).*
  in Paget's disease, 171, 304–305
Giant cell tumor of bone, 6, 252–256, *252–256*
  benign metastasizing, 255
  in dedifferentiated chondrosarcoma, 243
  in Paget's disease, 171
  malignant, 255, *256*
  radiologic-histologic correlations in, 15, *17*
  treatment of, 255–256
  vs. giant cell reparative granuloma, 305
  vs. osteoarthritic cyst, 284, *285*
  vs. pigmented villonodular synovitis, 312
Giant cell tumor of tendon sheath, 310, 311
Gigantism, local, in neurofibromatosis, 53
Gla-protein. See *Osteocalcin.*
Glucocerebrosides, in Gaucher disease, 54
Glucocorticoids. See *Steroid therapy.*
β-Glucosonidase, 57
Glycocalyx, 154
Glycosaminoglycans, 55, 322, *322,* 324
Gonorrhea, septic arthritis in, 161–162
Gout, 346–348, *347–348*
Granulomatosis, Langerhans' cell, 119–122, *120–122,* 123t
  lipid, 124
Granulomatous pseudotumor, 359, *360–361*
Greenstick fractures, 108
Growth factor(s), 35. See also *Cytokines.*
  in bone formation, 41, 42
  in bone remodeling, 35, 37
  in metastatic carcinoma, 177
  in myelofibrosis, 130
  TGF-β as, in giant cell tumors, 254
  osteoblasts and, 29, 35
Growth hormone, bone formation and, 41, 42
Growth plate. See *Epiphyseal plate.*
Gunshot wounds, 106

Hamartomas, 195
Harrison grooves, 79
Haversian canals, 25, 27, *29–31*
  enlarged, in disuse atrophy, 97, *97*
  in remodeled bone, 37
Haversian systems, 27, *29–32*
Head trauma, heterotopic ossification caused by, 297
Heberden's nodes, 318, 332

Hemangioendothelioma, epithelioid, 264–265, 267, *267–268*
Hemangioma(s), in Maffucci's syndrome, 230–231, *231*
　skeletal, 264–267, *266*
　synovial, 307, 312–313, *314*
Hemangiopericytoma, 265
　vs. malignant fibrous histiocytoma, 251
Hematologic disorders, 119. See also specific disorders.
Hematoma, aneurysmal bone cyst caused by, 280
　tumoral calcinosis caused by, 292
Hemophilic pseudotumor, 305–306
Hemosiderotic synovitis, 312, *313*
Heparan sulfate, 55, 56, 57
Heterotopic bone, 294–302
　fibrodysplasia ossificans progressiva as, 294, 298
　in hands and feet, 299–302, *299–303*
　myositis ossificans as, 294–295, *295–298*, 297, 299
　　vs. parosteal osteosarcoma, 211–212
　neurogenic, 294, 297
　pathogenesis of, 294
　radiologic-histologic correlations in, *12–13*
　total hip arthroplasty causing, 297–298
Histiocytoma, benign fibrous, 244, 248
　malignant fibrous, 250–252, *250–252*
　　chordoma with, 269
　　in dedifferentiated chondrosarcoma, 243
　　in dedifferentiated osteochondroma, 232
　　in Paget's disease, 171, 250, 252
　　malignant giant cell tumor with, 255
　　prosthesis associated with, 362
　　radiation causing, 150, 271
　　vs. fibrosarcoma, 249, 250
　　vs. metastatic carcinoma, 180
Histiocytosis, 119
　sinus, with massive lymphadenopathy, 123–124, *125–126*
Histochemistry. See *Immunohistochemical stains*.
Histologic-radiologic correlation, 8–9, *9–18*, 11, 15
Histology specimens. See *Pathology specimens*.
Histomorphometry of undecalcified bone, *23*, 23–24
　in aluminum bone disease, 88
　in osteomalacia, 82
　in osteoporosis, 92, 93, 94
　in primary hyperparathyroidism, 76, 77
　in renal osteodystrophy, 86, 87
HIV infection, bone and joint infections in, 159
Hodgkin's disease, of bone, 257–258, *258*
　vs. malignant fibrous histiocytoma, 251
Hoffa's disease. See *Synovial lipomatosis*.
Homogentisic acid, 57
Howship's lacunae, 30, *32*
Hunter syndrome, 55, 56
Hurler syndrome, 55, 56
Hyaline cartilage, *320*, 320–324, *322–324*
　calcification of, 9, 11, *11–12*
　lesions of, 220–221, *222*
Hyaluronic acid, 320, 322, *322*, 324
Hydroxyapatite, 25, 35, 44
1α-Hydroxylase, in oncogenic osteomalacia, 82
　in renal disease, 84
　in rickets, 78, 80
　parathyroid hormone and, 47
Hydroxyproline, 8, 33–34
　in Paget's disease, 169
Hypercalcemia, 43
　cancers causing, 47
　　metastatic carcinoma as, 178, 180
　　multiple myeloma as, 187
　in primary hyperparathyroidism, 76
　response to, 49
Hypercalciuria, disuse atrophy causing, 96
　in diabetes, 93
Hypercoagulability, osteonecrosis and, 137, 138
　in Legg-Calvé-Perthes disease, 145
Hyperlipidemia, osteonecrosis and, 137, 138
Hyperosteocytosis, in osteogenesis imperfecta, 61
Hyperosteoidosis, in renal osteodystrophy, 86, *following page 98*
Hyperostosis, diffuse idiopathic skeletal (DISH), 334–335, *336*, 343

Hyperostosis *(Continued)*
　infantile cortical, 302–303, *303*
Hyperparathyroidism, bed rest with, 96
　giant cell reparative granuloma of, 304, 305
　primary, 75–78, *77–78*
　secondary, histomorphometry in, 24
　　in calcipenic disorders, 78, 79, 82
　　in renal osteodystrophy, 83, 84, 86
Hyperphosphatemia, in familial tumoral calcinosis, 291
　in renal disease, 83–84, 87
Hypertrophic arthritis. See *Osteoarthritis*.
Hypertrophic nonunion, 112, *113*
Hypertrophic osteoarthropathy, 131–132, *131–132*, 132t
Hyperuricemia, 346
　in metastatic carcinoma, 178
　in multiple myeloma, 187
　treatment of, 348
Hypocalcemia, 43
　response to, 48, *48*
Hypochondroplasia, 66
Hypofibrinolysis, osteonecrosis and, 137, 138, 145
Hypogonadism, in men, osteoporosis caused by, 94
Hypophosphatemia, familial, 80–81
　in oncogenic osteomalacia, 83

Immune system. See also *Autoimmune disease(s)*.
　deficient, in osteopetrosis, 63
　vitamin D and, 46
Immunocompromised patient, infections in, 162
Immunoelectrophoresis, 185, 187
Immunoglobulins. See also *Light chains*.
　in plasma cell dyscrasia(s), 185
　　multiple myeloma and, 187
　　solitary myeloma and, 190
　in rheumatoid arthritis, 338
Immunohistochemical stains, 22
　in Ewing sarcoma/PNET, 260–261
　in metastatic carcinoma, 180
　specimens for, 366
Infarction. See *Osteonecrosis*.
Infection. See *Osteomyelitis*.
Inflammation phase, of fracture healing, 109, *109*
Inflammatory arthritis syndromes, 336–337. See also specific syndromes.
　histopathology of, 338
Inflammatory bowel disease, reactive arthritis of, 345–346
Insufficiency fractures, 113
Interferon-γ, for osteopetrosis, 64
Interleukin(s). See also *Cytokines*.
　in rheumatoid arthritis, 338
Interleukin–1, estrogen and, 91
　in cartilage metabolism, 327
　in metastatic carcinoma, 177
Interleukin–6, estrogen and, 91
　in Paget's disease, 166
Interstitial systems, 27
Intramembranous ossification, 37–38, *37–38*
Intraosseous ganglion, 277, 277t, 285, *286*
Intraosseous lipoma, 277, 277t, 286–287, *287–288*, 289
Intraosseous pressure, osteonecrosis and, 137
Intravascular bronchioalveolar tumor, 267
Involucrum, 154

Jaccoud's arthritis, 346
Jaffe-Campanacci syndrome, 244
Joint(s), laxity in, 326
　normal structure of, 319–324, *319–324*
　types of, 319
Joint capsule, 319
Joint diseases. See also *Bone diseases, diagnosis of*.
　categories of, 317, 318t
　history of, 317–318
　incidence of, 317

Joint replacement. See *Arthroplasty.*
Joint space, 319, *320*
Juxtacortical chondroma. See *Periosteal chondroma.*
Juxtacortical chondrosarcoma, 235, 240

Kappa light chains, in plasmacytosis, 185, 186
Keratan sulfate, 55, 322, *322*
    in osteoarthritis, 327
Ki-67 stain, in chondrosarcoma, 236, 240
    in enchondroma, 228
Kidney. See also *Renal* entries.
    parathyroid hormone and, 47, 48
Kienböck's disease, 147, *147*
Knee, spontaneous osteonecrosis of, 144–145, *145*
Köhler's disease, 147
Kyphoscoliosis, in mucopolysaccharidoses, 56
    in spondyloepiphyseal dysplasia, 68
Kyphosis, in primary osteoporosis, 91, *91–92*
    in Scheuermann's disease, 148, *148*
    in tuberculous spondylitis, 162

Laboratory studies, 8
Lactic dehydrogenase, in metastatic carcinoma, 178
Lacunae, 27, 29, *32*
    Howship's, 30, *32*
Lambda light chains, in amyloidoma, 191
    in osteosclerotic myeloma, 190
Lamellae, 27, *28,* 29
Lamellar bone, mineralization of, 35
    woven bone and, 38
Lamina splendens, 327
Langerhans' cell(s), 119, 121, *122*
Langerhans' cell granulomatosis, 119–122, *120–122,* 123t
Legg-Calvé-Perthes disease, 145–146, *146*
Leukemia(s), 127–128
    acute lymphoblastic, 127, 128
    fracturability and, 95
Ligaments, articular, 319
    laxity in, 326
Light chains, AL amyloid as, 190, 191
    Bence Jones proteins as, 185, 187, 190
    in chronic osteomyelitis, 186
Limb salvage surgery, 198
    in osteosarcoma, 219
Lining cells, 29
    osteoclasts and, 33, 36, *36,* 37
Link protein, 320, 322, *322,* 324
Lipoma, intraosseous, 277t, 286–287, *287–288,* 289
Lipoma arborescens. See *Lipomatosis, synovial.*
Lipomatosis, synovial, 307, 313–315, *314*
Lofgren's syndrome, 123
Long bones, zones of, 26, *27*
Looser lines, in rickets, 79–80
Looser zones, in osteomalacia, 82, *82–83,* 113
    in renal osteodystrophy, 86
Lubricin, 320
Lung. See also *Pulmonary* entries.
Lung carcinoma, metastatic, 175, 176, 178, *179, 181*
Lupus erythematosus, arthritis in, 346
    osteonecrosis in, 138
Lymphadenopathy, sinus histiocytosis with, 123–124, *125–126*
Lymphoma of bone, MRI of, *22*
    primary malignant, 256–257, *256–258*
        vs. Paget's disease, 172
        vs. small cell osteosarcoma, 216
    secondary malignant, 256
Lysosomal storage diseases, 53–57, *54–57*
Lysosomes, of osteoclasts, 30, 33
Lytic lesions, age of patient and, 7
    bone scan of, 17
    radiologic-histologic correlation with, 11, 15, *16–18*
    serum protein electrophoresis with, 8

M protein, 185
    in osteosclerotic myeloma, 190
Macrodactyly, in neurofibromatosis, 53
Macrophages, abnormal, in Gaucher disease, 54, 55
    in osteoclast differentiation, 36, 37, 63
Maffucci's syndrome, 230–231, *231*
Magnetic resonance imaging (MRI), 16, 19, *21–22*
Malignant tumors, 195, 197. See also specific tumors.
    fractures caused by, 117, *118*
    staging of, 198, 198t
    vs. disuse atrophy, 97
Marble bone disease. See *Osteopetrosis.*
Marble brain disease, 64
Marie-Strümpell disease, 343–344, *344–345*
Maroteaux-Lamy syndrome, 55, 57
Mastocytosis, 125–127, *126–127*
Matrix. See *Extracellular matrix; Osteoid.*
Matrix vesicles, 35, 38
McCune-Albright syndrome, 245–246, *247*
McKusick type metaphyseal chondrodysplasia, 70
Medullary canal, 26
Medullary infarcts, 140–141, *141*
Melorheostosis, 51, 70–71, *71*
    parosteal osteoma as, 200
Membranous bone, formation of, 37–38, *37–38*
Mendelian inheritance, 51–52
Menopause. See *Postmenopausal women.*
Mesenchymal chondrosarcoma, 235, 241–243, 244
Mesenchymoma, fibrocartilaginous, 247
Metabolic bone disease, 2–3, 75. See also specific diseases.
    pathologic fractures in, 95–96, 95t, 117–118
Metachronous multicentric osteosarcoma, 217
Metalloproteinases, in cartilage, 324, 327
Metaphyseal chondrodysplasia, 69–70, *70*
Metaphyseal flaring, in rickets, 79, *80*
Metaphysis, 26, *27*
    development of, 42, *43*
Metastatic disease in bone, 5, 175–180, 198, 198t
    clinical features of, 177–178
    clinical settings of, 175–176
    in pagetic bone, 171
    incidence of, 175
    osteoblastic, 178, *178–179*
    pathologic features of, 180, *181–182*
    pathologic fractures with, 4
    pathophysiology of, 176–177, *176–177*
    radiographic features of, 178, *178–179,* 180, *181*
    treatment of, 180, *182*
    vs. malignant lymphoma, 257
    vs. Paget's disease, 171–172
MGUS (monoclonal gammopathy of undetermined significance), 185
Milkman syndrome, 82
Mineralization. See also *Calcification.*
    disorders of, 78–83, 78t, *80, 82–84*
        aluminum bone disease as, 87–88
    of osteoid, 35, 37, *38*
Mineralization lag time, 23, 35
    in osteomalacia, 82, 87
Modeling of bone, 42
    calcitonin and, 48
    in Gaucher disease, 55
Monoclonal gammopathies. See *Plasma cell dyscrasias.*
Monoclonal gammopathy of undetermined significance (MGUS), 185
Morquio syndrome, 55, 56–57, *56–57*
MPS syndromes. See *Mucopolysaccharidoses.*
MRI (magnetic resonance imaging), 16, 19, *21–22*
Mucopolysaccharides. See *Proteoglycans.*
Mucopolysaccharidoses, 54, 55–57, *56–57*
Multicentric reticulohistiocytosis, 125
Multiple epiphyseal dysplasia, 68–69, *69*
Multiple exostosis, hereditary, 232, 234, *235,* 240
Multiple myeloma, 5–6, 186–189
    amyloidosis in, 191
    Bence Jones proteins in, 185, 191
    clinical features of, 186–187
    diagnosis of, 188–189, 189t

Multiple myeloma *(Continued)*
   epidemiology of, 186
   fracturability in, 95
   laboratory studies in, 187, 187t
   MGUS prior to, 185
   pathology of, 185–186
   pathophysiology of, 187, *187*
   physical examination in, 187
   radiographic features of, 188, *188–189*
   staging of, 189, 190t
   treatment of, 191–192
   types of, 186t
Münchmeyer's disease, 298
Mycobacteria, 162
Myelocele, in neurofibromatosis, 53
Myelofibrosis, 130–131, *130–131*. See also *Bone marrow, fibrosis of.*
Myeloma. See also *Multiple myeloma.*
   osteosclerotic, 190, 191
   solitary, of bone, 190, 191
Myeloma kidney, 187
Myocardial infarction, reflex sympathetic dystrophy following, 99
Myositis ossificans circumscripta, 294–295, *295–298,* 297, 299
   vs. parosteal osteosarcoma, 211–212

Necrosis. See *Osteonecrosis.*
Needle biopsy, 365
Neocortex, of prosthesis, 355
Neoplastic bone deposition, 11, *14.* See also *Tumor(s).*
Nephrolithiasis, in primary hyperparathyroidism, 76
Neuroectodermal tumor, peripheral (PNET), 258–261, *261*
   immunohistochemistry of, 260–261
   vs. small cell osteosarcoma, 216
Neurofibromatosis, 52–53, *53,* 53t
   osteomalacia caused by, 82–83
   segmental, 53
Neuron-specific enolase (NSE), 216, 260
Neuropathic joint, 335, *336–337*
Nonossifying fibroma, 244–245, *245*
Nonpenetrance, of genetic disease, 52
Nonunion, 3–4, 112, *112–113,* 112t
   strain intolerance causing, 111
Nora's lesion, 299
Normal stress, 105, *106*
NSE (neuron-specific enolase), 216, 260
Null allele effect, 60

O13 antibody, 22
   in Ewing sarcoma/PNET, 261
   in mesenchymal chondrosarcoma, 242–243
Ochronosis, 57–58, *58*
Ollier's disease, 228, 229–230, *230–231*
Open fractures, 108, 108t
Organic matrix. See *Osteoid.*
Osgood-Schlatter disease, 114, 147, *147*
Ossification, 37–38, *37–39*
   centers of, 38, 40–42, *40–43*
   radiodensity and, 11, *12*
Osteitis fibrosa, 86, *87*
Osteitis pubis, 160, *161*
Osteoarthritic cyst(s), 277, 277t, 284–285, *284–286*
   joint space narrowing and, 284, 285, *286,* 330, 331
   with rheumatoid arthritis, 341
Osteoarthritis, 324–335
   clinical presentation of, 329–332
   cyst(s) in. See *Osteoarthritic cyst(s).*
   DISH as, 334–335, *336*
   etiology of, 325–327, *326*
   general features of, 324, *325*
   generalized, 332
   history of, 318
   in alkaptonuria, 58
   in multiple epiphyseal dysplasia, 69

Osteoarthritis *(Continued)*
   in Paget's disease, 170
   incidence of, 324–325
   neuropathic joint as, 335, *336–337*
   of hip, 325, 331–332
   of spine, 332, 334, *335–336*
   pathology of, 327–329, *327–331*
   radiographic presentation of, 330–331, *332–334*
   secondary, 324, 325, 329–330
      to femoral head osteonecrosis, 4, 141t, 142
      to rheumatoid arthritis, 284, 341
   synovial chondromatosis secondary to, 310, *310*
   treatment of, 332
   vs. chronic pyrophosphate arthropathy, 349
Osteoarthropathy, hypertrophic, 131–132, *131–132,* 132t
Osteoarthrosis. See *Osteoarthritis.*
Osteoblastoma, 202–205, *204–207*
   vs. Paget's disease, 172
Osteoblasts, 29, *31*
   defective, in osteopetrosis, 63
      in progressive diaphyseal dysplasia, 64
      in X-linked hypophosphatemic rickets, 80
   glucocorticoid suppression of, 93
   in bone remodeling, 35, 36, *36,* 37
      senescence and, 90
   in bone resorption, 33, 46, 47
   in ossification, *37,* 37–38
   matrix proteins and, 34, 35
   measurements of, histomorphometry as, 23
      serum markers as, 8
   parathyroid hormone receptors on, 29, 33, 47
Osteocalcin, 8, 34
   in Paget's disease, 169
Osteochondral fragment, 135
Osteochondritis dissecans, 135, *136*
Osteochondroma, *222,* 231–232, *232–234*
   chondrosarcoma arising from, 240
   synovial chondromatosis with, *20,* 232, 307
   vs. parosteal osteosarcoma, 212
Osteochondromatosis. See *Exostosis(es), multiple hereditary.*
Osteochondromatous proliferation, bizarre parosteal, 299, *299–301*
Osteochondroses, 145–148, 145t, *146–148*
Osteoclastoma, 252
Osteoclasts, 30, *32,* 33. See also *Resorption of bone.*
   abnormal, in osteopetrosis, 62–63
   bisphosphonates and, 95
   calcitonin and, 33, 47, 48
   collagen breakdown by, 33–34
   in bone remodeling, 36, *36,* 37
   indices of bone turnover and, 8
   osteocalcin and, 34
   parathyroid hormone and, 33
   vitamin D and, 46
Osteocytes, 27, 29–30
   in membranous bone formation, 38, *38*
   parathyroid hormone and, 30, 47
Osteocytic membrane system, 29–30, *32*
   in calcium exchange, 44, 47
Osteocytic osteolysis, 30
   calcitonin and, 47
   parathyroid hormone and, 47, 48, 49
Osteodysplasia, radiation causing, 148–150, *149–150*
Osteodystrophy. See *Renal osteodystrophy.*
Osteofibrous dysplasia, 261–263, *262–263*
   vs. adamantinoma, 262–263, 264
   vs. differentiated adamantinoma, 264, *265*
   vs. fibrous dysplasia, 247
Osteogenesis imperfecta, 59–62, *60–62*
   fractures caused by, 59, 60, 95–96
   juvenile osteoporosis caused by, 94
   vs. osteoporosis, in men, 94
Osteoid, 29, *31*
   collagen in, 33–34, *34*
   in bone remodeling, 36
   in ossification, 37–38, *37–38*
   mineralization of, 35

Osteoid *(Continued)*
   noncollagenous proteins in, 34–35, 34t
Osteoid osteoma, 200–202, *201–204*
   vs. intracortical osteosarcoma, 217
   vs. parosteal osteoma, 200
Osteoid seam, *31,* 35
Osteolysis, osteocytic, 30
   calcitonin and, 47
   parathyroid hormone and, 47, 48, 49
Osteoma, 199–200, *200–201*
   osteoid, 200–202, *201–204*
      vs. intracortical osteosarcoma, 217
      vs. parosteal osteoma, 200
   parosteal, 199, 200, *200*
Osteomalacia, 78, 78t, 81–83, *82–84, following page 98*
   aluminum bone disease as, 24, 87–88
   diagnosis of, 24, 82
   fractures in, 82, 95t, 96, 113, 117–118
   in renal osteodystrophy, 83, 84, 86, 87
   oncogenic, 78, 82–83, *84,* 202
   osteoarthritis and, 332
   treatment of, 82
Osteomyelitis, 4–5, 153–163
   acute, 153, 154–155, *155, 157*
      pathology of, 156, *159*
   chronic, 153, 156, *157–158*
      appositional new bone in, *13–14*
      pathology of, 158, *160*
      recurrent multifocal, 163, *163*
      vs. Paget's disease, 172
      vs. plasmacytoma, 186
   fever in, 8
   fungal infections causing, 162
   general features of, 153
   hematogenous, 5, 153, 154–155, *155*
   history of, 153–154
   in AIDS patients, 159
   in drug abusers, 160
   in hemodialysis patients, 160
   in osteopetrosis, 63, 64
   in sickle cell anemia, 130, 138, 160
   pathology of, 156, 158, *159–160*
   secondary, 5, 153, 155
   subacute, 153, 155, *156–157*
      pathology of, 156, *159*
   syphilitic, 162, 163
   treatment of, 160–161
   vertebral, 158–159, *160,* 161
      vs. metastatic carcinoma, 180
   vs. acute leukemia, 127
   vs. Ewing sarcoma, 8
   vs. Hodgkin's disease, 258
   vs. malignant lymphoma, 257
   vs. neuropathic joint, 335
   vs. rheumatoid arthritis, 340, *341*
Osteonecrosis, 4
   calcification of infarct in, *9, 10*
   focal, 3, 4, 158
      in giant cell tumor, 254
   in Gaucher disease, 54–55
   in multiple epiphyseal dysplasia, 69
   in osteoarthritis, 328
   in osteochondroses, 145–147, 145t, *146–147*
   in radiation osteodysplasia, 148–150, *149–150*
   in sickle cell anemia, 129–130, *130*
      vs. osteomyelitis, 160
   infiltrative processes causing, 135
   intravascular occlusion causing, 135–145
      histopathology of, 138–140, *139–140*
      history of, 136
      in femoral head, 135, 137, 141–144, 141t, *142–144*
      in knee, 144–145, *145*
      medullary infarcts in, 140–141, *141*
      pathogenesis of, 136–137, 137t
      predisposing conditions with, 137–138, 137t
   malignant fibrous histiocytoma with, 251, 252

Osteonecrosis *(Continued)*
   of femoral head. See *Femoral head, osteonecrosis of.*
   of knee, 144–145, *145*
   radiation causing, 149, 150
   repair in, 139–140, *140*
   synovial chondromatosis with, 310
   transient osteoporosis and, 99
   trauma causing, 135
      in femoral head, 135
      in knee, 144
   vs. intraosseous lipoma, 289
Osteonectin, 34
Osteons, 27, *29–32*
Osteopenia, 2–3
   causes of, 95–96, 95t
   definitions of, 75
   histomorphometry in, 24
Osteopetrosis, 62–64, *63–64*
   fractures in, 63, 118
   malignant, 63–64
Osteophytes. See also *Bone spurs.*
   in CPPD, 349
   in DISH, *336*
   in neuropathic joint, 335
   in osteoarthritis, 328–329, 330–331, *330–333*
      Heberden's nodes and, 332
   in rheumatoid arthritis, 340, 341
   in spondylosis deformans, 334, *335–336*
Osteopoikilosis, 64–65, *66*
Osteopontin, 34
Osteoporosis, 3, 88–99
   definitions of, 75
   DEXA scan for, 19, 22, 88, 95
   fractures in, 117–118
      disuse atrophy and, 96
      healing of, 3
      in men, 94
      in primary osteoporosis, 89, 89t, 90, *90–91,* 91, 92
      in secondary osteoporosis, 92, 93
      prevention of, 95
      stress, 113
   high-turnover, 91, 92, 94
   idiopathic, 88, 94
      mastocytosis in, 126
   in disuse atrophy, 3, 96–97, *96–97*
      vs. multiple myeloma, 188, *188*
   in men, 93, 94
   in reflex sympathetic dystrophy, *99,* 99–100
   juvenile, 88, 94
   localized, 96–99, *96–99*
   low-turnover, 91, 92
   management of, 94–95
   osteoarthritis and, 326
   osteomalacia with, 81
   peak bone mass and, 88–89, 94–95
   postmenopausal, 88, 89, 91, *91*
   prevention of, 94–95
   primary, 88, 89–92, 89t, *90–92*
      histopathology of, 92, *following page 98*
      risk factors for, 91t
      type I, 88, 89, 91, *91*
      type II, 88, 90–91
   regional migratory, 98
   secondary, 88, 92–94, 92t
   senile, 3, 88, 90–91
   skeletal failure caused by, 88
   transient, 97–98, *98–99*
Osteoporosis circumscripta, 168
Osteosarcoma, 205–220
   conventional, 206, *207–211,* 208–210, *369*
   definition of, 205
   general features of, 205–206
   giant cell tumor with, 255
   high-grade surface, 217, 219
   in dedifferentiated chondrosarcoma, 243
   intracortical, 217

Osteosarcoma *(Continued)*
  low-grade central, 212
  multicentric, 217
  myositis ossificans with, 297
  osteoblastic, vs. osteoblastoma, 204–205
  Paget sarcoma as, 170–171, *172*
  prosthesis associated with, 362
  radiation causing, 150, 269, 271
  small cell, 216, *219*
  treatment of, 217, 219–220, *220–221*
  variants of, 206, 206t, *207*
    parosteal, *207,* 210–212, *212,* 217, 219
      vs. myositis ossificans, 297
      vs. parosteal osteoma, 200
    periosteal, *207,* 212, *213–214,* 219, *369*
    telangiectatic, *207,* 215–216, *216–218*
    well-differentiated intraosseus, *207,* 212–213, *214–215,* 215, 219
      vs. fibrous dysplasia, 247
  vs. distal femoral cortical irregularity syndrome, 116–117
  vs. malignant fibrous histiocytoma, 251
  vs. malignant lymphoma, 257
  vs. myositis ossificans, 297
  vs. reactive lesions, 299
Osteosclerosis, leukemia causing, 128
  myelofibrosis causing, 130–131, *130–131*
  renal osteodystrophy causing, 84, 86, *following page 98*
Osteosclerotic myeloma, 190, *191*
Otto pelvis, 331, *334*

Pachydermoperiostosis, 131, *131*
Paget sarcoma, 170–171, *172*
Paget's disease, 165–172
  bed rest in, hypercalcemia caused by, 96
  clinical features of, 165, *166*
  complication(s) of, 169–171, *171–172*
    fibrosarcoma as, 249
    giant cell reparative granuloma as, 304–305
    heterotopic ossification as, 298
  differential diagnosis of, 171–172
  epidemiology of, 165–166
  etiology of, 166
  histopathology of, 166–167, *166–167*
  history of, 165
  laboratory studies of, 168–169
  radiologic features of, 167–168, *168–171*
  treatment of, 172
  vs. malignant lymphoma, 256, *257*
Pain, as diagnostic clue, 7
Palsies, cranial nerve, in osteopetrosis, 63, *64*
  in Paget's disease, 170
Pamidronate, for Paget's disease, 172
Pancreatitis, osteonecrosis with, 137
Pannus, in ankylosing spondylitis, 343
  in rheumatoid arthritis, 339, *340,* 341
Parathyroid adenoma, 76, *77*
Parathyroid hormone, 46–47. See also *Hyperparathyroidism.*
  calcium balance and, *48,* 48–49
  in primary osteoporosis, 90
  osteoblast receptors for, 29, 33
  osteoclasts and, 33
  osteocytes and, 30
  vitamin D and, 46, 47, 84
Parathyroid hormone-related protein (PTHrP), 47, 178
Parosteal osteochondromatous proliferation, bizarre, 299, *299–301*
Parosteal osteoma, 199, 200, *200*
Parosteal osteosarcoma, *207,* 210–212, *212,* 217, 219
  vs. myositis ossificans, 297
  vs. parosteal osteoma, 200
Particle disease, 354, 356, 359, *360*
Pathology specimens, 365–371
  biopsy of, 365–366
    for histomorphometry, 24
  cutting of, through bone, 366–367, *366–367*
    through decalcified bone, 370–371

Pathology specimens *(Continued)*
  decalcification of, 366, 370, *370*
  from arthroplasty, 362, 367–368, *368*
  from skeletal dysplasias, 71–72
  from tumor resection, *369,* 369–370, 370t
  radiography of, 368–369, *368–369*
  staining of, 371
    immunohistochemical, 22, 366
Peak bone mass, 88–89, 94–95
Periosteal chondroma, *222,* 234–235, *235–237*
Periosteal chondrosarcoma, 235, 240
Periosteal desmoid, 116–117, *117*
Periosteal ganglion, 285
Periosteal osteosarcoma, *207,* 212, *213–214,* 219, *369*
Periosteum, 26, *28*
  joint capsule and, 319
  layers of, *109*
  stripping of, 4
Periostitis, florid reactive, 299, 300–301, *301–302*
  in acute leukemia, 127–128
  in hypertrophic osteoarthropathy, 132
  syphilitic, 162–163
Peripheral neuroectodermal tumor (PNET), 258–261, *261*
  immunohistochemistry of, 260–261
  vs. small cell osteosarcoma, 216
Permeative lesions, 15, *18*
Phenobarbital, mineralization and, 81
Phenytoin, mineralization and, 81
Phosphate diabetes, 80–81
Phosphatonin, 82
Phosphorus, 44–45
  deficiency of, 78–79
  parathyroid hormone and, 44–45, 47
  vitamin D and, 46
Physaliferous cells, of chordoma, 269, *271*
Physeal scar, 42
Physis. See *Epiphyseal plate.*
Piezoelectric currents, 3, 30, 96
Pigmented villonodular synovitis, 307, 310–312, *311–313*
  vs. synovial hemangioma, 313
Plasma cell dyscrasias, 5–6, 185–192, 186t
  amyloidoma of bone as, 191, *191*
  multiple myeloma as. See *Multiple myeloma.*
  osteosclerotic myeloma as, 190, *191*
  pathology of, 185–186, *186*
  solitary myeloma of bone as, 190, *191*
  treatment of, 191–192
  vs. chronic osteomyelitis, 186
Plasmacytoma, 186t
  solitary, of bone, 190, *191*
  vs. chronic osteomyelitis, 186
PNET (peripheral neuroectodermal tumor), 258–261, *261*
  immunohistochemistry of, 260–261
  vs. small cell osteosarcoma, 216
POEM syndrome, 190
Polygenic disorders, 51
Postmenopausal women, osteoarthritis in, 332
  osteoporosis in, 88, 89, 91, *91*
Post-traumatic cyst(s), 277, 277t, 285–286, *287*
Pott's disease, 162
Pregnancy, osteonecrosis in, 137
  transient osteoporosis in, 98–99
Preosteoblasts, 29
Primary spongiosa, 38, *39,* 40, 42, *43*
Procollagen, 33
Progressive diaphyseal dysplasia, 64, *65*
Prostate cancer, metastatic, 175
  immunohistochemical staining of, 180
  osteomalacia caused by, 83
  pathophysiology of, 176–177
  radiographic features of, 178, *178–179,* 181
Proteases, 30, 33. See also *Acid phosphatase.*
Proteoglycans, 55
  disorders of, mucopolysaccharidoses as, 55
    pseudoachondroplasia as, 68
  in bone, 34–35, 37

Proteoglycans *(Continued)*
   in hyaline cartilage, 320, 321, 322–323, *322–323,* 324
   in osteoarthritis, 326–327
Protocollagen, 33
Protrusio acetabuli, 331, *334*
Psammoma bodies, 9, 293
Pseudarthrosis, 4
   in failed arthroplasty, 360
   in neurofibromatosis, 53, *53*
   in osteofibrous dysplasia, 262
   synovial, 112
Pseudoabscess, prosthesis causing, 359
Pseudoachondroplasia, 68, *69*
Pseudogout, 349
   tophaceous, 293, *294,* 349
Pseudomalignant osseous tumor of soft tissue, 295
Pseudomonas aeruginosa, osteomyelitis caused by, 160
Pseudotumor, calcifying, of neural axis, 294
   granulomatous, prosthesis causing, 359, *360–361*
   hemophilic, 305–306
Psoriatic arthritis, 343, 346
PTHrP (parathyroid hormone–related protein), 47, 178
Pulmonary carcinoma, metastatic, 175, 176, 178, *179, 181*
Pulmonary hypertrophic osteoarthropathy, 131–132, 132t
Pulmonary metastasis, of chondroblastoma, 221
   of chordoma, 269
   of giant cell tumor, 255
   of osteosarcoma, 219
Pyarthrosis, 161
Pyridinoline cross-links, 8, 34
   in Paget's disease, 169
Pyrophosphate arthropathy, chronic, 349
   subchondral cysts in, 284

Rachitic rosary, 79
Radiation osteitis, fibrosarcoma with, 249
   malignant fibrous histiocytoma with, 250, 252
Radiation osteodysplasia, 148–150, *149–150*
Radiation therapy, for metastatic carcinoma, 180
   malignant giant cell tumor caused by, 255
   osteochondroma caused by, 231
   sarcomas caused by, 150, 269, 271
Radiodensity, patterns of, 9, *9–15,* 11
Radiofrequency ablation, of osteoid osteoma, 202
Radiography, ancillary techniques in, 16–22, *19–22*
   histologic correlations with, 8–9, *9–18,* 11, 15
   plain, 8–9, 16
Radiolysis, patterns of, 11, 15, *16–18*
Radionuclide bone scan, 16, *19*
Reactive arthritis, 343, 344–346, *345*
   genetic predisposition to, 51
   gonorrheal, 162
Reactive bone, appositional, 11, *13–14*
   in metastatic carcinoma, 180, *182*
   in osteoid osteoma, 201, *202–203*
   in osteomyelitis, 154, 156, 158, *158*
   radiologic-histologic correlations in, 11, *13–16,* 15
Reactive periostitis, florid, 299, 300–301, *301–302*
Reactive zone, of tumor, 198
Reconstructive surgery, with osteosarcoma, 219, *220*
Reflex sympathetic dystrophy, 99, *99–100*
Reiter's syndrome, 345
Remodeling lines, 27, *31,* 37
Remodeling of bone, 35–37, *36.* See also *Bone turnover; Resorption of bone.*
   calcitonin and, 48
   electrical activity in, 30, 37
Remodeling phase, of fracture healing, 109, *109,* 111, *111*
Renal. See also *Kidney.*
Renal cell carcinoma, metastatic, 178, 180, *181*
Renal dialysis, aluminum bone disease and, 87–88, *following page 98*
   amyloidosis and, 88
   osteomyelitis and, 160
   renal osteodystrophy and, 83, 86, 87

Renal dialysis *(Continued)*
   tumoral calcinosis and, 291
Renal osteodystrophy, 83–87, *85–87*
   adynamic, 86, 87
   high-turnover, 86, *87*
   histomorphometry in, 24, 86, 87
   hyperosteoidosis in, 86, *following page 98*
   low-turnover, 86, 87
   marrow fibrosis in, 86, *87, following page 98*
   osteosclerosis in, 84, 86, *following page 98*
   tunneling resorption in, 86, *following page 98*
   vs. osteomyelitis, 160
Renal pathology, in hyperparathyroidism, 76
   in multiple myeloma, 187, 189
   in oncogenic osteomalacia, 82
   in osteopetrosis, 64
   in X-linked hypophosphatemic rickets, 80
Renal rickets, 84
Reparative phase, of fracture healing, 109, *109–111,* 111
Resorption cavity, 37
Resorption of bone. See also *Bone turnover.*
   defective, in osteopetrosis, 62
   in remodeling of bone, 36, *36,* 37
   laboratory indices of, 8, 33–34
   of necrotic bone, 154
   osteoclasts in, 30, *32,* 33
   parathyroid hormone and, 47, 48, 49
   prosthesis causing, 359, *360*
   tunneling, 77, *78, following page 98*
   vitamin D and, 46
Resorption phase, of remodeling, 36, *36,* 37
Reticuloendothelial system, proliferative disorders of, 6, 119. See also specific disorders.
Reticulohistiocytoma, 125
Reticulohistiocytosis, multicentric, 125
Retinoblastoma, familial, osteosarcoma and, 206, 208
Rhabdomyosarcoma, in dedifferentiated chondrosarcoma, 243
Rheumatoid arthritis, 337–343
   clinical features of, 337–338
   genetic predisposition to, 337
   histopathology of, 338–340, *338–341*
   history of, 318
   incidence of, 337
   juvenile, 342–343, *343*
      vs. acute leukemia, 127
   pathogenesis of, 338
   radiologic features of, 340–341, *341–342*
   subchondral cysts in, 284, 341
   treatment of, 342
   vs. gout, 347
Rheumatoid factor, 338
   in juvenile rheumatoid arthritis, 342
Rice bodies, 339, *340*
Rickets, 78–81, *80*
   calcipenic, 79, 80
   causes of, 78–79, 78t
   nutritional, 79, 82
   renal, 84
   treatment of, 82
   Vitamin D–dependent, 78, 80
   vs. metaphyseal chondrodysplasia, 70
   X-linked hypophosphatemic, 78–79, *80,* 80–81, 82, *following page 98*
Rim sign, in subacute osteomyelitis, 155
Rosai-Dorfman disease, 124, *125–126*
Rothmund-Thomson syndrome, osteosarcoma and, 208

S-100 protein, 22
   in chondroblastoma, 221
   in chordoma, 269
   in Langerhans' cell granulomatosis, 121
   in sinus histiocytosis, 124
Saber shin, 163
Salmonella, osteomyelitis caused by, 130, 160
Sanfilippo syndrome, 55, 56

SAPHO syndrome, 163
Sarcoidosis of bone, 123, *124–125*
Sarcoma. See *Ewing sarcoma; Osteosarcoma.*
Scheie syndrome, 56
Scheuermann's disease, 148, *148*
Schmid type metaphyseal chondrodysplasia, 70
Schmorl's nodes, in Scheuermann's disease, 148, *148*
  in spondylosis deformans, 334, *336*
Scintigraphy, bone, 16–17, *19*
Sclerotic rim, 11, 15, *16*
Scoliosis, in neurofibromatosis, 53
  in osteogenesis imperfecta, 60
  osteoblastoma causing, 203
  osteoid osteoma causing, 201
Segmental fractures, 108
Septic arthritis, 153, 161–162
Sequestrum(a), 4, 5, 154, 156
Shear stress, 105, *106*
Shepherd's crook deformity, 246, *247*
Shoulder-hand syndrome, 99
Sialoproteins, of bone matrix, 34
Sickle cell anemia, 128–130, *130*
  osteomyelitis in, 130, 138, 160
  osteonecrosis in, 138, 140, 144
Silastic prosthesis(es), 353
  failure of, 358, *359*
Silicone synovitis, 358, *359*
Simple fractures, *107*
Sinus histiocytosis with massive lymphadenopathy, 123–124, *125–126*
Skeletal dysplasia(s), 1–2, 51, 58–59, 59t. See also specific dysplasias.
  osteochondromatosis as, 232, 234, *235*
  pathologist's role in, 71–72
Skeletal failure, 88
Sly syndrome, 55, 57
Small cell osteosarcoma, 216, *219*
Smoking, fracture healing and, 112
  osteoporosis and, 93–94
Solitary myeloma of bone, 6, 190, *191*
Spinal artery steal syndrome, 170
Spinal cord injury, heterotopic ossification with, 297
Spinal stenosis, in achondroplasia, 66
Spine, fractures of, in acute leukemia, 127
  osteoporosis causing, 89, *90*
  fungal infections of, 162
  osteoarthritis of, 332, 334, *335–336*
  osteomyelitis of, 158–159, *160*, 161
  vs. metastatic carcinoma, 180
Spiral fractures, *107–108*, 108
Spondylitis, 158–159, *160*, 161
  ankylosing, 343–344, *344–345*
    CT image of, 3-dimensional, *21*
    heterotopic ossification in, 298
  reactive arthritis causing, 345
  tuberculous, 162
Spondyloarthropathy, seronegative, 343
Spondyloepiphyseal dysplasia congenita, 67–68
Spondyloepiphyseal dysplasias, 67–68, *68*
  pseudoachondroplasia as, 68, *69*
Spondylosis deformans, 332, 334, *335–336*
Spongiosa, primary, 38, *39*, 40, 42, *43*
Spongy bone. See *Cancellous bone.*
Spotted bone disease. See *Osteopoikilosis.*
Squamous cell carcinoma, chronic osteomyelitis with, 156
  hypercalcemia in, 47
Staging, definition of, 198
Staphylococcus aureus, arthritis caused by, 161
  osteomyelitis caused by, 130, 154, 158, 159, 160
Stem cells, osteoblasts from, 29
  osteoclasts from, 62–63
Steroid therapy, osteonecrosis and, 137, 138, 140, 144
  osteoporosis caused by, 92–93
Stickler syndrome, 67
Still's disease, 342–343, *343*
Strain, definition of, 105
Strain intolerance, 111
Streaming potentials, 3, 30, 37, 96

Stress, mechanical, definition of, 105, *106*
  on bone, 36, 37, 96
  on cartilage, 324, 326
Stress fractures, 4, 112–114, *114–116*
  bone lesion(s) causing, 7
    enchondroma as, 239
  fatigue causing, 108
  in osteomalacia, 82, *82–84*, 113
  in Paget's disease, 169–170, *172*
  in renal osteodystrophy, 84, 86
  in rickets, 79–80
  locations of, 113, 113t
Stress-strain curve, 105, *106*
String sign, 210
Subchondral bone cyst(s), 277, 284, *284*
  amyloidosis causing, 88
  in CPPD, 349
  intraosseous ganglion as, 277, 277t, 285, *286*
  osteoarthritic, 277, 277t, 284–285, *284–286*, 328, *329–330*
  joint space narrowing and, 284, 285, *286*, 330, 331
    with rheumatoid arthritis, 341
  post-traumatic, 277, 277t, 285–286, *287*
Subungual exostosis, 299, 301–302, *302–303*
Sudeck's atrophy, *99*, 99–100
Superscan, in metastatic carcinoma, 178
Surgical margins, 198, 198t, 369
Surgical specimens. See *Pathology specimens.*
Swelling, as diagnostic clue, 7–8
Synchondroses, 319
Synchronous multicentric osteosarcoma, 217
Syndesmoses, 319
Synovial chondromatosis, 220, *222*
  primary, 307–310, *308–310*
  secondary, 307, 310, *310–311*
  vs. chondrosarcoma, 232, 236, 309
  with osteochondroma, *20*, 232, 307
Synovial chondrometaplasia. See *Synovial chondromatosis.*
Synovial chondrosarcoma, 309
Synovial fluid, 320, *321*
  cartilage metabolism and, 324
Synovial hemangioma, 307, 312–313, *314*
Synovial lipomatosis, 307, 313–315, *314*
Synovial membrane, 319–320, *321*
  in inflammatory arthritis syndromes, 337
  in osteoarthritis, 329, *331*
Synovial pseudarthrosis, 112
Synovitis. See also *Arthritis.*
  chronic, vs. synovial hemangioma, 313
  detritic, 329, *331*
  hemosiderotic, 312, *313*
  in alkaptonuria, 58
  pigmented villonodular, 307, 310–312, *311–313*
    vs. synovial hemangioma, 313
  rheumatoid, 338–339, *338–340*
  silicone, 358, *359*
  syphilitic, 162
Syphilitic bone infection, 162–163
Systemic disease, bone changes in, 6–7, 119. See also specific diseases.
Systemic lupus erythematosus, arthritis of, 346

Tartrate-resistant acid phosphatase, 8, 30, 33
Technetium bone scan, 16–17, *19*
Telangiectatic osteosarcoma, *207*, 215–216, *216–218*
Tendinitis, calcific, 291–292
Testosterone deficiency, osteoporosis caused by, 94
Tetracycline labeling, 23–24, 35
  in osteomalacia, 82
TGF-β, in giant cell tumors, 254
  osteoblasts and, 29, 35
Thalassemia, 128, *129*
Thanatophoric dysplasia, 2, 66–67
Thermocoagulation, of osteoid osteoma, 202
Thrombosis, osteonecrosis caused by, 136–137, 137t, 145
Thyroid carcinoma, metastatic, 178, 180

Thyroid gland. See *Calcitonin.*
Tide mark, 323, *323–324*
 duplication of, 326, *326*
Tissue sections. See *Pathology specimens.*
Tophaceous pseudogout, 293, *294,* 349
Tophus(i), in gout, 346–347, *347–348,* 348
Torus fractures, 108
Total joint arthroplasty. See *Arthroplasty.*
Total parenteral nutrition (TPN), aluminum bone disease and, 87
Trabeculae, 25–26, *25–27*
 in ossification, 37–38
 radiologic-histologic correlations with, 11, *12–15,* 15
Traction spurs, in DISH, 334–335, *336*
 in spinal osteoarthritis, 334
Transforming growth factor β, in giant cell tumors, 254
 osteoblasts and, 29, 35
Trauma. See also *Fracture(s).*
 cysts caused by, 277, 277t, 285–286, *287*
  aneurysmal bone cyst as, 280
  epidermal inclusion cyst as, *288,* 289
  subchondral cysts as, 284
 heterotopic ossification caused by, in hands and feet, 299, *300*
  in myositis ossificans, 294–295, *295–298,* 297, 299
  in neurologic trauma, 297
 osteoarthritis and, 325, 326, 328
 osteomas and, 200
 osteomyelitis and, 154
 osteonecrosis and, 135, 144, 145, 146, 147
Trevor's disease, 70, *71*
Tuberculosis, of bone, 162
Tumor(s). See also specific tumors.
 adenocarcinoma as, 176
  vs. chordoma, 269
 in cartilage, 220–221, *222*
 metastatic. See *Metastatic disease in bone.*
 pathology specimens from, *369,* 369–370, 370t
 primary, in bone, 5, 6, 195–271
  bone deposition in, 11, *14*
  classification of, 195
  clinical presentation of, 197
  evaluation of, 197
  general features of, 195
  history of, 196–197
  metastasis of, 198, 198t
  multiple myeloma as, 186
  staging of, 198, 198t
  treatment of, 197, 198, 198t
  vs. disuse atrophy, 97
 squamous cell carcinoma as, hypercalcemia in, 47, 178
  in chronic osteomyelitis, 156
 surgical margins for, 198, 198t, 369
Tumoral calcinosis, 9, *9,* 291–293, *292–293*
Tumoral calcium pyrophospate deposition disease, 293, *294,* 349
Tumor-like lesions, 291, 291t. See also specific lesions.
Tunneling resorption, 77, *78*
 in renal osteodystrophy, 86, *following page 98*
Turret exostoses, 299

Uncoupling, of osteoblasts, 3
 coupling and, 37
Undecalcified bone, 23, 23–24
Unicameral bone cyst, 117, 277–279, 277t, *278–281*
Urticaria pigmentosa, 125–126
Uveitis, in ankylosing spondylitis, 344
 in juvenile rheumatoid arthritis, 342

Vascular stasis, osteonecrosis and, 136–137
Vertebra plana, 120, *121*
Vitamin A toxicity, 334
Vitamin D, *45,* 45–46
 calcium balance and, 44, 45, 46, *48,* 48–49
 decreased synthesis of, in osteomalacia, 81, 82
  in osteoporosis, 90
  in renal disease, 84
  in vitamin D–dependent rickets, 78, 80
 deficiency of, in osteoarthritis, 332
  in osteomalacia, 78, 78t, 81, 82
  in osteoporosis, 90
  in rickets, 78, 78t, 79
 dietary requirement for, 45, 95
 elevated, in tumoral calcinosis, 291
 in osteoclast development, 33
 osteocalcin synthesis and, 34
 parathyroid hormone and, 46, 47, 84
 receptors for, genetic defects in, 78, 80, 90
  glucocorticoids and, 93
  on osteoblasts, 29, 46
Vitamin D–dependent rickets, 78, 80
Vitamin K, osteocalcin and, 34
Volkmann's canals, *25, 27, 30*

Wounds, gunshot, 106
Woven bone, definition of, 38
 in osteogenesis imperfecta, 61
 in osteosclerosis, 84, 86, *following page 98*
 lamellar bone formation from, 38
 mineralization of, 35
 parathyroid hormone and, 47

X-linked disorders, 51, 52
 hypophosphatemic rickets as, 78–79, *80,* 80–81, 82, *following page 98*

Yield point, 105, *106*

ISBN 0-7216-6336-2

90038